Maternal-Neonatal Nursing

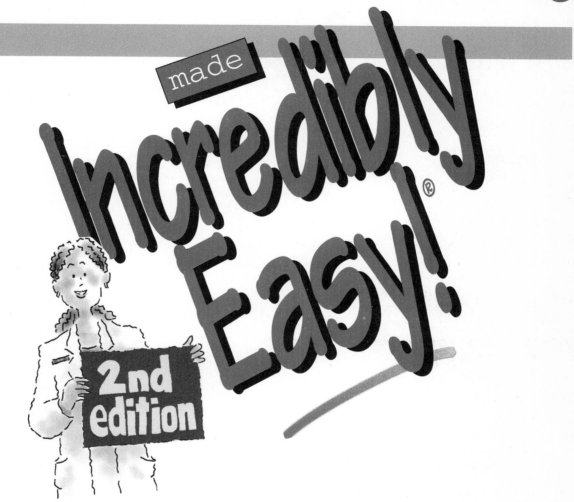

made

Incredibly Easy!®

2nd edition

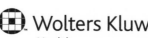

Wolters Kluwer | Lippincott Williams & Wilkins
Health

Philadelphia · Baltimore · New York · London
Buenos Aires · Hong Kong · Sydney · Tokyo

Staff

Executive Publisher
Judith A. Schilling McCann, RN, MSN

Editorial Director
David Moreau

Clinical Director
Joan M. Robinson, RN, MSN

Art Director
Mary Ludwicki

Electronic Producer
John Macalino

Senior Managing Editor
Tracy S. Diehl

Editorial Project Manager
Gabrielle Mosquera

Clinical Project Manager
Beverly Ann Tscheschlog, RN, BS

Editors
Laura Bruck, Karen C. Comerford

Copy Editors
Kimberly Bilotta (supervisor), Scotti Cohn, Jeannine Fielding, Shana Harrington, Pamela Wingrod

Designers
Lynn Foulk

Illustrator
Bot Roda

Digital Composition Services
Diane Paluba (manager), Joyce Rossi Biletz

Associate Manufacturing Manager
Beth J. Welsh

Editorial Assistants
Karen J. Kirk, Linda K. Ruhf, Jeri O'Shea

Indexer
Barbara Hodgson

MNIE2010907

Library of Congress Cataloging-in-Publication Data

Maternal-neonatal nursing made incredibly easy. — 2nd ed.
    p. ; cm.
    Includes bibliographical references and index.
    1. Maternity nursing. 2. Neonatology. I. Lippincott Williams & Wilkins.
    [DNLM: 1. Maternal-Child Nursing. WY 157.3 M42555 2008]
RG951.M3143 2008
618.2'0231—dc22
ISBN-13: 978-1-58255-651-2 (alk. paper)
ISBN-10: 1-58255-651-2 (alk. paper)   2007025528

Contents

Contributors and consultants iv

Foreword v

1   Introduction to maternal-neonatal nursing 1

2   Conception and fetal development 27

3   Family planning, contraception, and infertility 59

4   Physiologic and psychosocial adaptations to pregnancy 103

5   Prenatal care 147

6   High-risk pregnancy 209

7   Labor and birth 291

8   Complications of labor and birth 361

9   Postpartum care 417

10   Complications of the postpartum period 447

11   Neonatal assessment and care 475

12   High-risk neonatal conditions 517

Appendices and index

Laboratory values for pregnant and nonpregnant patients 561

Selected maternal daily dietary allowances 563

Normal neonatal laboratory values 565

NANDA-I taxonomy II 569

Glossary 573

Selected references 579

Index 581

Contributors and consultants

Christine C. Askham, RN, BSN
VN Faculty
Unitek College
Fremont, Calif.

Kimberly Attwood, RN, PhD(c)
Instructor
DeSales University
Center Valley, Pa.

Beatrice Beth Benda, RNC, MSN
Staff Nurse
Allina Hospitals & Clinics
University of Minnesota Fairview
    Riverside Maternal Fetal Medicine
    Clinic
Minneapolis

Anita Carroll, EdD, MSN
Nursing Instructor
West Texas A&M University
Canyon

Marsha L. Conroy, RN, MSN, APN
Nursing Instructor
Cuyahoga Community College
Cleveland

Kim Cooper, RN, MSN
Nursing Department Program Chair
Ivy Tech Community College of Indiana
Terre Haute

Patti F. Gardner, MSN, CNM, IBCLC
Clinical Nurse Specialist: Women's Health
    & Lactation
United Medical Center
Cheyenne, Wyo.

Valera A. Hascup, RNC, MSN, PhD (c), CCES, CTN
Assistant Professor of Nursing and
    Director of the Transcultural Nursing
    Institute
Kean University
Union, N.J.

Vivian Haughton, RN, MSN, CCE, IBCLC
Clinical Nurse Specialist–Maternal/Child
    Health
Good Samaritan Health System
Lebanon, Pa.

Dana M. L. Hinds, RN, MSN, FNP
Nursing Instructor, Family Nurse
    Practitioner
Central Maine Medical Center School of
    Nursing
Lewiston

Beverly Kass, RNC, MS
Faculty
William Paterson University
Wayne, N.J.

Randy S. Miller, RN-C, BS, MSN
Student Coordinator
Orlando (Fla.) Regional Healthcare

James F. Murphy, RNC, MS
Educator/Instructor
ViaHealth/Rochester General Hospital
Isabella Graham Hart School of Nursing
Rochester, N.Y.

Noel C. Piano, RN, MS
Instructor/Coordinator
Lafayette School of Practical Nursing
Adjunct Faculty
Thomas Nelson Community College
Williamsburg, Va.

Janet Somlyay, RN, MSN, CNS, CPNP
Clinical Nurse Specialist—Pediatrics and
    Nursery
United Medical Center
Cheyenne, Wyo.

Robin R. Wilkerson, RN, PHD
Associate Professor of Nursing
University of Mississippi
Jackson

Foreword

Nursing educators have long been tasked with making important nursing content stick in the minds of students and nurses. For this reason, we often find ourselves asking what it takes for nursing concepts, facts, and research findings to embed themselves in the brain, resulting in well-reasoned utilization of nursing processes and knowledgeable critical thinking. A couple of answers come to mind.

First, learning more readily occurs if there's a catalyst to assist it. Educators now realize that by encouraging students' active involvement in the learning process and using various adult learning methodologies, we can facilitate knowledge acquisition and application. Some of these methods include various forms of testing, case scenarios, and simulations.

Second, any way in which the educator can combine a fun experience with the learning process is a positive one. These experiences can come in the form of cartoons, funny poems, puzzles, contests, jokes, humorous or clever analogies, or even songs. There are no limits to the methods.

As a nursing educator, I'm drawn to resources that blend the elements of active learning and fun. This combination is what attracted me to the second edition of *Maternal-Neonatal Nursing Made Incredibly Easy.*

Those familiar with the first edition will be pleased to encounter the same well-loved features that helped make it an excellent resource. Comprehensive information is still conveyed succinctly in multiple forms that actively engage the reader. Original content has been updated and enhanced with tables, charts, diagrams, illustrations, quizzes, and delightful cartoons that help the reader focus on key facts. Additional content areas include information on grief and loss, bed rest, postpartum depression, alternative therapies, and substance abuse.

Some exciting additions include a CD with more than 300 NCLEX-style questions, including alternate-format questions. The CD also contains a list of nursing diagnoses by disorder, covering all of the disorders featured in the text. Concept maps for some nursing problems are also included.

In addition, icons draw your attention to important issues:

Advice from the experts—tips and tricks for maternal-neonatal nurses from the people who know best—other maternal-neonatal nurses.

Education edge—patient-teaching tips and checklists that help the nurse pass along information that can be vital to promoting a healthy pregnancy and preventing complications.

Bridging the gap—details on cultural differences that may affect care.

 Weighing the evidence—evidence-based practice pointers.

Enjoy this comprehensive resource that doesn't separate learning from fun. With the second edition of *Maternal-Neonatal Nursing Made Incredibly Easy,* it's a packaged deal!

Joan E. Edwards, RNC, MN, CNS
Assistant Clinical Professor
Texas Woman's University
Houston

Introduction to maternal-neonatal nursing

Just the facts

In this chapter, you'll learn:

♦ roles of maternal-neonatal nurses
♦ dynamics of family-centered nursing care
♦ structures and functions of families
♦ factors that influence a family's response to pregnancy
♦ legal and ethical issues associated with maternal-neonatal nursing.

A look at maternal-neonatal nursing

In North America, nurses care for more than four million pregnant patients each year. Providing this care can be challenging and rewarding. After all, you must use technology efficiently and effectively, offer thorough patient teaching, and remain sensitive to and supportive of patients' emotional needs.

Going down!

In recent decades, infant and maternal mortality rates have progressively declined, even among women older than age 35. Factors responsible for this decline include a reduction in such disorders as placenta previa and ectopic pregnancy, and prevention of related complications. Better control of complications associated with gestational hypertension and decreased use of anesthesia with childbirth also contribute to this decline.

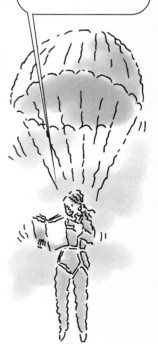

Infant and maternal mortality rates are going down—and so am I!

Room for improvement

Despite these advances, there's still room for improvement in maternal and neonatal health care. Infant and maternal mortality rates remain high for poor patients, minorities, and teenage mothers—largely because of a lack of good prenatal care.

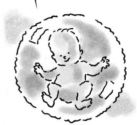

Your job is to take care of me and my mom and the rest of my family. I'll thank you when I arrive!

Maternal-neonatal nursing goals

The primary goal of maternal-neonatal nursing is to provide comprehensive family-centered care to the pregnant patient, the family, and the baby throughout pregnancy. (See *Three pregnancy periods.*)

Setting the standards

In 1980, the American Nurses Association's Maternal Child Health Nursing Practice division set standards for maternal-neonatal nursing. These standards provided guidelines for planning care and formulating desired patient outcomes. Later, the Association of Women's Health, Obstetric, and Neonatal Nurses built upon these standards to create the current practice standards to promote the health of women and newborns. Today, these standards form the principles to provide benchmarks for nurses who provide evidence-based nursing care to these patient populations.

Three pregnancy periods

Pregnancy can be broken down into three periods:

The *antepartum period* refers to the period from conception to the onset of labor.

The *intrapartum period* extends from the onset of contractions that cause cervical dilation to the first 1 to 4 hours after the birth of the neonate and delivery of the placenta.

The *postpartum period* refers to the 6 weeks after delivery of the neonate and the placenta. Also known as the *puerperium,* this stage ends when the reproductive organs return to the nonpregnant state.

Practice settings

Maternal-neonatal nurses practice in various settings. These include community-based health centers, doctors' offices, hospital clinics, acute care hospitals, maternity hospitals, birthing centers, and patients' homes.

There's no place like home...

Up until the year 2000, 98% of all births occurred in hospital labor and delivery suites or birthing units. Today, an increasing number of families are choosing to have their babies in alternative birth settings, such as birthing clinics or their homes. These alternative settings may give families more control over their birth experiences by allowing them to become more involved in the process.

...or a home away from home

In response to consumer demands for more relaxed, family-friendly birthing environments, hospitals have revamped their labor and delivery units to create more natural childbirth environments. Labor, delivery, and recovery rooms or labor, delivery, recovery, and postpartum suites are now found in most hospitals. In these homelike settings, partners, family members, and other support people may remain in the room throughout the birth experience. The patient then spends the postpartum-recovery period in the same room where she gave birth. These homelike environments allow for a more holistic and family-centered approach to maternal and neonatal health care.

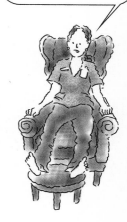

For some families, there's no place like home (or a homelike hospital setting) for having a baby!

Maternal-neonatal nursing roles and functions

Nurses involved in maternal-neonatal nursing assume many roles. These may include care provider, educator, advocate, and counselor. The functions involved for each of these roles depend on the nurse's level of education. Nurses involved in maternal-neonatal nursing may be registered nurses, certified nurse-midwives (CNMs), nurse practitioners (NPs), or clinical nurse specialists (CNSs).

Registered nurse

A registered nurse is a graduate of an accredited nursing program who has successfully passed the National Council Licensure Examination and is licensed by the state in which she works. To work in a maternal-neonatal department, a registered nurse goes through extensive on-site training, including competency checks and ongoing education. She plays a vital role in providing direct patient care, meeting the educational needs of the patient and her family, and functioning as an advocate and counselor.

Certified nurse-midwife

A CNM is a registered nurse who has achieved advanced education at a master's level or has obtained CNM certification. A CNM works independently and is able to care for a low-risk obstetric patient throughout her pregnancy. A CNM is also licensed to deliver a neonate.

Nurse practitioners

An NP is also a registered nurse who has received advanced education at a master's level or has obtained NP certification. An NP performs in an expanded advanced practice role. She obtains histories, performs physical examinations, and manages care (in consultation with a doctor) throughout the pregnancy and the postpartum period. She may practice as a women's health, family, neonatal, or pediatric NP.

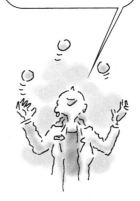

An NP is a master juggler of histories, physicals, and care management!

Women's health nurse practitioner

A women's health NP plays a vital role in educating women about their bodies and offering information on preventive health care. She cares for women with sexually transmitted diseases and counsels them about reproductive issues and contraceptive choices. A women's health NP helps women remain well so they can experience a healthy pregnancy and maintain good health throughout life.

Family nurse practitioner

A family nurse practitioner (FNP) provides care to all patients throughout the life cycle. She performs health physicals, prepares pregnancy histories, orders and performs diagnostic and obstetric examinations, plans care for the family throughout pregnancy and after birth, and can provide prenatal care in an uncomplicated pregnancy. An FNP cares for the entire family, focusing on health promotion, wellness, and optimal family functioning.

Neonatal nurse practitioner

A neonatal nurse practitioner (NNP) is highly skilled in the care of neonates and can work in practice settings with various care levels, from well-baby term nurseries to high-level intensive care and preterm nurseries. She can also work in neonatal intensive care units (NICUs) or neonatal follow-up clinics. An NNP's responsibilities include normal neonate assessment and physical examination as well as high-risk follow-up and discharge planning.

Pediatric nurse practitioner

A pediatric nurse practitioner (PNP) provides well-baby care and maternal counseling, performs physical assessments, and obtains detailed patient histories. The PNP serves as a primary health care provider. She can order diagnostic tests and prescribe appropriate drugs for therapy, although prescribing privileges depend on individual state regulations. If the PNP determines that a child has a major illness, such as heart disease, she may collaborate with a pediatrician or other specialists.

Clinical nurse specialist

A CNS is an RN who has received education at a master's level. The CNS focuses on health promotion, patient teaching, direct nursing care, and research activities. A CNS serves as a role model and teacher of quality nursing care. She may also serve as a consultant to registered nurses working in the maternal-neonatal field.

A special specialist

A CNS may be trained:
• to provide care in NICUs
• as a childbirth educator who develops and provides childbirth education programs, prepares the expectant patient and her family for labor and birth, and cares for the patient and her family in normal birth situations
• as a lactation consultant who teaches and assists the patient as she learns about breast-feeding.

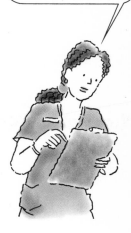

A CNS is an RN with a master's degree who teaches, does research, directs patient care, serves as a role mode ... and needs some sleep!

Family-centered care

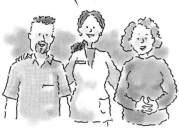

Maternal-neonatal nurses are responsible for providing comprehensive care to the pregnant woman, her fetus, and family members. This approach is known as *family-centered care*. Understanding the makeup and function of the family is essential to delivering family-centered care.

Family ties

A family is a group of two or more persons who possibly live together in the same household, perform certain interrelated social tasks, and share an emotional bond. Families can profoundly influence the individuals within them. Therefore, care that considers the family—not just the individual—has become a focus of modern nursing practice.

Changes such as the addition of a new family member alter the structure of the family. If one family member is ill or is going through a rough developmental period, other family members may feel a tremendous strain. Family roles must be flexible enough to adjust to the myriad changes that occur with pregnancy and birth.

Family structures

Several different family structures exist today. These structures may change over the life cycle of the family because of such factors as work, birth, death, and divorce. Family structures also may differ based on the family roles, generation issues, means of family support, and sociocultural issues.

Types of family structures include:
- nuclear family
- cohabitation family
- extended or multigenerational family
- single-parent family
- blended family
- communal family
- gay or lesbian family
- foster family
- adoptive family.

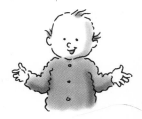

Nuclear family

A nuclear family is traditionally defined as a family consisting of a wife, a husband, and a child or children. A nuclear family can provide support to and feel affection for family members because of its relatively small size. However, small family size may also be a weakness for the nuclear family. For example, when a crisis arises, such as an illness, there are fewer family members to share the burden and provide support.

Cohabitation family

A cohabitation family is composed of a heterosexual couple who live together but aren't married. The living arrangement may be short- or long-term. A cohabitation family can offer psychological and financial support to its members in the same way as a traditional nuclear family.

Extended or multigenerational family

Extended or multigenerational families include members of the nuclear family and other family members, such as grandparents, aunts, uncles, cousins, and grandchildren. In this type of family, the main support person isn't necessarily a spouse or intimate partner. The primary caregiver may be a grandparent, an aunt, or an uncle. This type of family typically has more members to share burdens and provide support but may experience financial problems because income must be stretched to accommodate more people.

Single-parent family

Today, single-parent families account for 50% to 60% of families with school-age children. Although in many of these families the mother is the single parent present, an increasing number of fathers are also rearing children alone. Single-parent families exist for many reasons, including divorce, death of a spouse, and the decision to raise children outside of marriage.

Working hard for the money

Financial problems, such as low income, can be an issue for single parents. Even though an increasing number of single parents are fathers, most are mothers. Traditionally, women's salaries have been lower than men's salaries. This situation poses a problem when a mother's salary is the only source of income for the family.

Flying solo

Another difficulty for the single-parent family is the lack of family support for childcare, which can be problematic if the single parent becomes ill. A single parent may also have difficulty fulfilling the multitude of parental roles that are required of her, such as being a mother and a "father" in addition to being the sole income provider for the family.

Sometimes, being a single parent means flying solo.

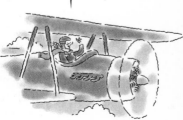

Blended family

In a blended family, two separate families have joined as one as a result of remarriage. Many times, conflicts and rivalries develop in these families when the children are exposed to new parenting methods. Jealousy and friction between family members may be an issue, especially when the new blended family has children of its own. On the other hand, children of blended families may also be more adaptable to new situations.

Communal family

A communal family is a group of people who have chosen to live together but aren't necessarily related by marriage or blood; instead, they may be related by social or religious values. People in communal families may not adhere to traditional health care practices, but they may proactively participate in their health care and be receptive to patient teaching.

Gay or lesbian family

Some gay and lesbian couples choose to include children in their families. These children may be adopted, or they may come from surrogate mothers, artificial insemination, or previous unions or marriages.

Foster family

Foster parents provide care for children whose biological parents can no longer care for them. Foster family situations are usually temporary arrangements until the biological parents can resume care or until a family can adopt the foster child. Foster parents may or may not have children of their own.

Adoptive family

Families of all types can become adoptive families. Families adopt children for various reasons, which may include the inability to have children biologically. In some cases, families choose to adopt foster children whose parents are unable to provide care and are willing to have their children adopted. Sometimes, adoptive parents are the child's biological siblings or a relative of the parent. This type of family can be very rewarding but also poses many challenges to the family unit, especially if biological children also live in the family. Adoptions can be arranged through an agency, an international adoption program, or private resources.

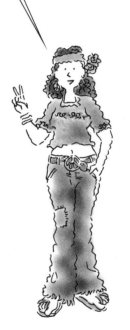

C'mon people now, smile on your brother. A communal family is a group of people who aren't related by blood or marriage but choose to live together. That's groovy!

Family tasks

A healthy family typically performs eight tasks to ensure its success as a working unit and the success of its members as individuals. These include:

- distribution of resources
- socialization of family members
- division of labor
- physical maintenance
- maintenance of order
- reproduction, release, and recruitment of family members
- placement of members into society
- safeguarding of motivation and morale.

Distribution of resources

Because each family has limited resources, the family needs to decide how those resources should be distributed. In some cases, certain family needs will be met and others won't. For example, one child may get new shoes whereas another gets hand-me-down shoes.

Money isn't everything

Money isn't the only resource. Such resources as affection and space must also be distributed. For example, the eldest child may get his own room, whereas younger children may have to share a room. Most families can make these decisions well. Dysfunctional families or those with financial problems may have problems completing these tasks.

Socialization of family members

Preparing children to live in society and to socialize with other individuals in their society is another important family task. If the culture of the family differs from the community in which it lives, this may be a difficult task.

Division of labor

Division of labor is the family task that involves assignment of responsibilities to each family member. For example, family members must decide who provides the family with monetary resources, who manages the home, and who cares for the children. The division of labor may change within a family when a new baby arrives, especially if both parents work full-time.

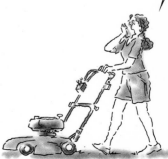

I sure could use some of that division of labor right about now!

Physical maintenance

The task of physical maintenance includes providing for basic needs, such as food, shelter, clothing, and health care. The family fulfills these needs by finding and maintaining employment and securing housing. It's important to have enough resources to complete these tasks or the family may find itself in crisis. Improper distribution of resources can also lead to problems related to providing for basic needs. Physical maintenance also includes providing emotional support and caring for family members who are ill.

Maintenance of order

The task of maintenance of order includes communication among family members. It also involves setting rules for family members and defining each individual's place within the family. For example, when a new baby arrives, a family with a healthy maintenance of order and well-defined rules and roles knows where that new member belongs. Family members welcome the new baby as a part of the family unit and understand the baby's role as a family member. An unhealthy family may find this task difficult. Members of a family without a healthy maintenance of order may feel threatened that the baby will change their roles or take their places in the family. They may see the new baby as an intruder.

Reproduction, release, and recruitment of family members

Reproduction, release, and recruitment of family members can occur in several ways. For example:
- a new child is born (reproduction)
- a child leaves home for college (release)
- a child is adopted (recruitment)
- elderly parents come to live with the nuclear family (recruitment).

Even though family members don't always control reproduction, release, and recruitment, accepting any of these life changes is a family task. A healthy family accepts the change and understands the effects that the change will have on family roles and functions.

Placement of members into society

Families also make decisions that define their place in society. In other words, when parents choose where to live and where to send their children to school, the family becomes part of a particular community within society. The activities they choose to par-

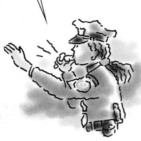

Hold it right there! Someone has to maintain order in the family, especially when a new member is on the way.

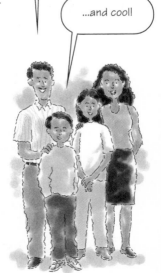

Change is a fact of life, and accepting and understanding that is part of what makes our family healthy...

...and cool!

ticipate in—such as church or synagogue, physical activities, and clubs—also define the family's place within the social community.

Safeguarding of motivation and morale

The task of safeguarding of motivation and morale is achieved though the development of family pride. Much of this is achieved through emotional encouragement and support. If family members are proud of their accomplishments, a sense of pride for each other and the family as a unit develops. This makes them more likely to care about one another and to defend the family and what the family does. They're also more likely to support one another during crises.

The nursing process

When providing care, maternal-neonatal nurses follow the nursing process steps, which are:
- assessment
- nursing diagnosis
- planning
- implementation
- outcome evaluation.
    These steps help to ensure quality and consistent care.

Assessment

A maternal-neonatal nursing assessment should include an assessment of the patient and her family. Assessment involves continually collecting data to identify a patient's actual and potential health needs. According to the American Nurses Association guidelines, data should accurately reflect the patient's life experiences and patterns of living. To accomplish this, adopt an objective and nonjudgmental approach when gathering data. Data can be obtained through a nursing history, physical examination, and review of pertinent laboratory and medical information.

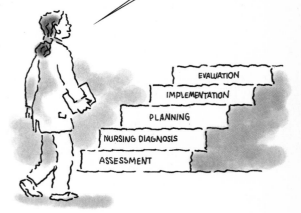

The nursing process steps help to ensure high-quality, consistent care. They're also great for exercising my glutes!

EVALUATION
IMPLEMENTATION
PLANNING
NURSING DIAGNOSIS
ASSESSMENT

Mommy factors

During pregnancy, assess such maternal factors as:
- patient's age
- past medical, pregnancy, and birth history
- reaction to fetal movement
- nutritional status.

Remember that the mother's health directly affects the well-being of the fetus.

Baby factors

After birth, assess such neonatal factors as:
- Apgar score
- gestational age
- weight in relation to gestational age
- vital signs
- feeding patterns
- muscle tone
- condition of the fontanels
- characteristics of the neonate's cry.

Here you go, ma'am. It's our healthy mother–healthy fetus special, and it's just what the doctor ordered!

Family factors

Assessment should always reflect a family-centered approach. Be sure to assess family status, and note how it's affected by the pregnancy and birth. Be aware of how the family is coping with the new arrival and how parents, siblings, and other family members are affected. Also, assess how the mother, father, siblings, and other family members bond with the neonate.

Nursing diagnosis

In 1990, NANDA-International defined a nursing diagnosis as "a clinical judgment about individual, family, or community responses to actual or potential health problems or life processes." It went on to say that nursing diagnoses provide the basis for the selection of nursing interventions to achieve outcomes for which the nurse is accountable.

Fussy factor

In maternal-neonatal nursing, you'll develop nursing diagnoses for the patient, family, and neonate that are appropriate for the prenatal, intrapartum, and postpartum periods. The information gathered during your nursing assessment can be used to help you formulate appropriate nursing diagnoses. For example, a new mother might experience frustration because her neonate is fussing and crying within the first hour after breast-feeding. Based on this assessment data, the patient would be assigned a nursing diagnosis of *Ineffective breast-feeding*.

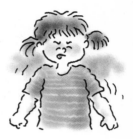

I'm supposed to express my feelings about the new baby? Well, get ready! You asked for it!

Planning

After establishing a nursing diagnosis, you'll develop a care plan. A care plan serves as a communication tool among health care team members and helps ensure continuity of care. The plan consists of expected outcomes that describe behaviors or results to be achieved within a specified time, as well as the nursing interventions needed to achieve these outcomes.

Keep it in the family

Be sure to include the patient and her family when planning and implementing the care plan. For example, when you're developing a care plan for a patient who has a nursing diagnosis of *Interrupted family process*, you should make sure that the care plan encourages family members to express their feelings about the pregnancy. Be aware of the family's changing needs, and be aware of the new mother's sensitivity and emotional concerns. (See *Ensuring a successful care plan*.)

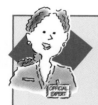

Advice from the experts

Ensuring a successful care plan

Your care plan must rest on a solid foundation of carefully chosen nursing diagnoses. It also must fit your patient's needs, age, developmental level, culture, strengths, weaknesses, and willingness and ability to take part in her care. Your plan should help the patient attain the highest functional level possible while posing minimal risk and not creating new problems. If complete recovery isn't possible, your plan should help the patient cope physically and emotionally with her impaired or declining health.

Use the following guidelines to help ensure that your care plan is effective.

Be realistic

Avoid setting a goal that's too difficult for the patient to achieve. The patient may become discouraged, depressed, and apathetic if she can't achieve expected outcomes.

Tailor your approach to each patient's problem

Individualize your outcome statements and nursing interventions. Keep in mind that each patient is different; no two patient problems are exactly alike.

Avoid vague terms

It's best to use precise, quantitative terms rather than vague ones. For example, if your patient seems ambivalent toward her neonate, describe this behavior: "doesn't respond when the baby cries," "watches television when changing the baby's diaper," or "frequently asks to take the baby back to the nursery so she can talk on the phone." To indicate that the patient's vital signs are stable, document specific measurements, such as "heart rate less than 100 beats/minute" or "systolic blood pressure greater than 100 mm Hg."

Implementation

During the implementation phase of the nursing process, you put your care plan into action. Implementation encompasses all nursing interventions directed at solving the patient's problems and meeting her health care needs. When you're coordinating implementation, seek help from the patient as well as the patient's family and other caregivers.

Review, revise, regroup

After implementing the care plan, continue to monitor the patient to gauge the effectiveness of interventions and to adjust them as her condition changes. Expect to review, revise, and update the entire care plan regularly, according to facility policy.

Outcome evaluation

The outcome evaluation step of the nursing process evaluates how well the patient met her care plan goals, or outcomes. It also evaluates the effectiveness of the care plan. To evaluate the plan effectively, you must establish criteria for measuring the goals and the outcomes of the plan. Then you must assess the patient's responses to these interventions. These responses help determine whether the care plan should be continued, discontinued, or changed. Inevitably, this evaluation brings about new assessment information, which necessitates the creation of new nursing diagnoses and a modification of the plan.

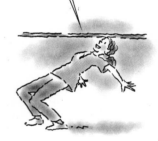

When it comes to care plans, remaining flexible is key. Be ready to monitor, review, revise, and update.

Frequent follow-up plan

Evaluate the care plan frequently. This allows for changes and revisions as the needs of the patient and her family change, ensuring that the care plan accurately reflects the family's current needs.

Family response to pregnancy

Several factors can influence a family's response to pregnancy. These factors include:
- maternal age
- cultural beliefs
- whether the pregnancy was planned
- family dynamics
- social and economic resources
- age and health status of other family members
- mother's medical and obstetric history.

Maternal age

The mother's age can affect how family members respond to a pregnancy. Whether the mother is nearing menopause or just a teenager, family members may respond negatively to the pregnancy.

Waiting it out

Today, more families are waiting to have children until later in life. The number of women age 40 and older having children has risen dramatically in the past 10 years. The number of women who have their first child after age 40 has also increased. If an older woman becomes pregnant, especially one who's already a mother, the family may react unfavorably. For example, older children may be disgusted by the idea that their parents are having sex, or by the pregnancy itself. Also, some family members may perceive pregnancy as the role of a young mother—not one nearing menopause.

A lion-taming career and motherhood—not the best mix! No wonder so many women today are waiting to have children until later in life.

Aren't you a little young?

Teenage pregnancy rates have also changed dramatically. According to the Centers for Disease Control and Prevention, the birth rate for teenagers in the United States declined steadily throughout the 1990s, falling from 62.1 births per 1,000 teenagers ages 15 to 19 in 1991 to 48.5 births in 2000—a reduction of 22%.

If the mother is a young teenager who isn't married, the family may view the pregnancy unfavorably for several reasons. For example, family members may fear that the single mother won't be able to provide for her baby or that she won't finish her schooling. Family members may also be concerned about how their own roles will change as a result of the pregnancy. They may fear that they'll become full-time caregivers for the child. In addition, the family's religious beliefs may lead them to view the pregnancy as unacceptable or even sinful; they may reject the pregnant teenager as well as the child she carries.

Cultural beliefs

Cultural values can influence how a family plans for or reacts to childbearing. Some cultures view childbearing as something to be shared with others as soon as the pregnancy is known. Families in other cultures, such as the Jewish culture, shy away from being public about the pregnancy until it has reached a certain gestational stage.

Woman's work

Cultural norms affect family roles, behaviors, and expectations. For example, culture may influence how a man participates in the pregnancy and childbirth. Members of some cultures, such as Mexican-Americans and Arab-Americans, allow only women in the birthing room during childbirth. In some cases, the birthing room is considered a woman's place—not a man's.

Cultural cues

Cultural values can also influence nursing care. Acknowledging the cultural characteristics and beliefs of a patient and her family is an important part of family-centered care. To provide culturally competent care for women during pregnancy, a nurse needs to familiarize herself with the practices and customs of various cultures. (See *Childbearing practices of selected cultures.*)

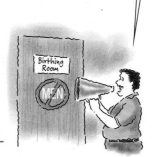

In some cultures, the birthing room is considered women-only territory. Push, honey, push!

Planned versus unplanned pregnancy

Some women view pregnancy as a natural and desired outcome of marriage. To them, having children is a natural progression after marriage. They may plan to have children, or they may not plan the pregnancy but are accepting when it happens. Women who are prepared to accept a pregnancy tend to seek medical validation when the first signs of pregnancy appear.

For other women, pregnancy may be unplanned; the woman may react with ambivalence, or she may deny her symptoms and postpone seeking medical validation. If the father doesn't want a child or the parents are having other difficulties in their relationship, family upheaval can result. In some cases, especially in some adolescents, pregnancy may be an unwanted result of sexual experimentation without contraception.

Expecting to be expecting

Just because a pregnancy is planned, however, doesn't mean that no family member will have trouble accepting it—possibly, even the mother or father. The mother may initially want the pregnancy but may be ambivalent, about how the pregnancy is changing her body. The parents as a unit may feel they aren't prepared to be parents or that they don't have enough experience around children. In addition, one family member may feel that the family's resources can't provide for a new addition. This too can lead to turmoil over the pregnancy.

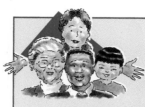

Bridging the gap

Childbearing practices of selected cultures

A patient's cultural beliefs can affect her attitudes toward illness, traditional medicine, pregnancy, and childbirth. By trying to accommodate these beliefs and practices in your care plan, you can increase the patient's willingness to learn and comply with treatment regimens. Because cultural beliefs may vary within particular groups, individual practices may differ from those described here.

Culture	Childbearing practices
Asian-American	• View pregnancy as a natural process • Believe mother has "happiness in her body" • Omit milk from diet because it causes stomach distress • Believe inactivity and sleeping late can result in difficult birth • Believe childbirth causes a sudden loss of "yang forces," resulting in an imbalance in the body • Believe hot foods, hot water, and warm air restore the yang forces • Are attended to during labor by other women (usually the patient's mother)—not the father of the baby • Have stoic response to labor pain • May prefer herbal medicine • Restrict activity for 40 to 60 days postpartum • Believe that colostrum is harmful (old, stale, dirty, poisonous, or contaminated) to baby so may delay breast-feeding until milk comes in
Native-American	• View pregnancy as a normal, natural process • May start prenatal care late • Prefer a female birth attendant or a midwife • May be assisted in birth by mother, father, or husband • View birth as a family affair and may want entire family present • May use herbs to promote uterine contractions, stop bleeding, or increase flow of breast milk • Use cradle boards to carry baby and don't handle baby much • May delay breast-feeding because colostrum is considered harmful and dirty • May plan on taking the placenta home for burial
Hispanic-American	• View pregnancy as normal, healthy state • May delay prenatal care • Prefer a "patera," or midwife • Are strongly influenced by the mother-in-law and mother during labor and may listen to them rather than the baby's father during birth • View crying or shouting out during labor as acceptable • Bring together mother's legs after childbirth to prevent air from entering uterus • May wear a religious necklace that's placed around the neonate's neck after birth • Believe in maintaining good health by keeping a balance of hot and cold foods • Restricted to boiled milk and toasted tortillas for first 2 days after birth • Must remain on bed rest for 3 days after birth • Delay bathing for 14 days after childbirth

(continued)

Childbearing practices of selected cultures (continued)

Culture	Childbearing practices
Hispanic-American *(continued)*	• Delay breast-feeding because colostrum is considered dirty and spoiled • Don't circumcise male infants • May place a bellyband on the neonate to prevent umbilical hernia
Arab-American	• May not seek prenatal care • Seek medical assistance when medical resources at home fail • Fast during pregnancy to produce a son • May labor in silence to be in control • Limit male involvement during childbirth
African-American	• View pregnancy as a state of well-being • May delay prenatal care • Believe that taking pictures during pregnancy may cause stillbirth • Believe that reaching up during pregnancy may cause the umbilical cord to strangle the baby • May use self-treatment for discomfort • May cry out during labor or may be stoic • May receive emotional support during birth from mother or another woman • May view vaginal bleeding during postpartum period as sickness • May prohibit tub baths and shampooing hair in the postpartum period • May view breast-feeding as embarrassing and, therefore, bottle-feed • Consider infant who eats well "good" • May introduce solid food early • May oil the baby's skin • May place a bellyband on the neonate to prevent umbilical hernia

Family dynamics

Family dynamics—including a family's structure and how it functions—also affect how a new pregnancy is perceived. Family members are influenced by their changing roles as well as by the physical and emotional changes the pregnant woman experiences. Some family members accept the pregnancy as a part of the family's growth. Other family members may view the pregnancy as a stressor and consider the new member an intruder.

For many families, pregnancy causes career and lifestyle changes that must be made to accommodate the new addition. The parents' ability to meet the physical and emotional needs of existing children in the family also changes.

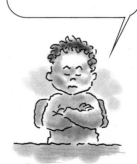

Some family members might be less than thrilled about a new baby. Not me! I'm ecstatic!

Coping or moping?

The family support system may be affected as it attempts to cope with the pregnancy. Effective coping methods are demonstrated by the family's participation in parenting classes, childbirth education classes, and prenatal care. Ineffective coping mechanisms are evidenced by delaying confirmation of the pregnancy, hiding the pregnancy, or delaying prenatal care.

Social and economic resources

Economic status can also affect how a family responds to pregnancy. A pregnant woman living in a family whose financial responsibilities are stretched may delay prenatal care or choose not to take prenatal vitamins because of their cost. Many families are barely able survive on two incomes; a pregnancy may reduce that income, which places emotional and financial strain on the family.

Age and health status of other family members

The health of other family members is another factor that can affect how a family views a pregnancy. If one family member is sick or has a long-term illness that requires a lot of family time and support, the addition of another family member may not be viewed favorably. It also affects the time family members have available to spend with the sick family member. As a result, family roles may have to change.

He ain't heavy—he's my brother

Siblings may also be influenced by the arrival of a new family member. Some siblings may perceive the new addition as a threat to their position in the family and become jealous. Such threats can be real or perceived, especially when the sibling experiences separation from the mother when she's hospitalized.

What a difference a year makes

Sibling reaction depends on the child's age. For instance, toddlers are aware of the mother's changing appearance and may have difficulty with separation when the mother leaves. A toddler exhibits this stress by showing signs of regression. Preschoolers and school-age children are likely to be interested in the pregnancy and may ask a lot of questions. They may also express a willingness to participate in childcare. Adolescents, on the other hand, are more likely to be embarrassed by the mother's pregnancy be-

Because you're all participating in parenting and childbirth education classes, I can tell that you're coping well with pregnancy.

cause it represents sexual activity between their parents. However, they may also be very attentive to the needs of the mother.

Medical and obstetric history of the mother

Ideally, a woman should be in good health when she begins her pregnancy. Sometimes, however, a woman with an ongoing illness (such as cardiac disease) becomes pregnant. Such an illness can complicate the pregnancy and cause problems for the woman, affecting how the mother and other members of the family respond to the news. Family members may be concerned that a pregnancy could jeopardize the mother's health. Likewise, if a woman has an obstetric history that includes some difficult labors or births, the family may react unfavorably out of concern for the mother's health.

Ethical and legal issues

Some of the most difficult decisions made in the health care setting are those that involve children and their families. Because maternal-neonatal nursing is so family-centered, conflicts commonly arise because family members don't agree on how a situation should be handled. In addition, the values of the health care provider may conflict with those of the family. Legal and ethical issues that may arise in maternal-neonatal care include abortion, prenatal screening, conception issues, fetal tissue research, eugenics and gene manipulation, and treatment of preterm and high-risk neonates. (See *Dealing with ethical and legal issues*.)

Abortion

Abortion can pose a complex ethical dilemma for a nurse and her patients. A nurse who's ethically or morally opposed to abortion can't be forced to participate in the procedure. However, the nurse's employer can insist that she provide nursing care to all patients.

Practice, don't preach

No matter what your opinions are regarding abortion, don't allow personal feelings to interfere with your care for a postabortion patient and don't try to impose your values on the patient. A nurse's role is to provide the best possible care, not to judge or make comments about a patient's personal decision.

Regardless of our own views, it isn't a nurse's job to pass judgment on patients.

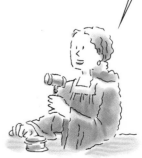

Dealing with ethical and legal issues

When you're faced with an ethical or a legal issue in your practice, such as abortion or in vitro fertilization, be sure to follow these guidelines to ensure that you're providing the best care to your patient and fulfilling your nursing duties.

Inform and be informed

Nurses can help their patients make informed decisions by providing factual information, by practicing supportive listening, and by helping the family clarify its values.

Be self-aware

To reach your own resolutions about legal and ethical issues, you'll need to examine your views honestly and carefully. You'll want to periodically reevaluate your position in light of new medical information and your own experi-

ence. If you feel strongly about a particular issue, you should consider working for a facility that matches your views.

Remember your role

Every nurse has an ethical obligation to provide competent, compassionate care. Even if your views on a particular issue differ greatly from those of your patient, don't allow your personal feelings to interfere with the quality of care you provide.

Prenatal screening

Thanks to such diagnostic procedures as amniocentesis, ultrasound, alpha-fetoprotein screening, and chorionic villi sampling, it's now possible to detect inherited and congenital abnormalities long before birth. In a few cases, the diagnosis has paved the way for repair of a defect in utero. However, because it's easier to detect genetic disorders than to treat them, prenatal screening commonly forces a patient to choose between having an abortion and taking on the emotional and financial burden of raising a severely disabled child.

Benefits vs. risks

Prenatal diagnostic procedures involve some risk to the fetus. Amniocentesis, for example, causes serious complications or death in about 0.5% of patients. Some people feel that this risk creates a conflict between the rights of the fetus and the parents' right to know his health status.

Knowing is half the battle

If testing is to be considered ethical by patients and their families, the nurse must take steps to help the patients fully understand the procedure, comprehend what the test can and can't tell them, and be informed about other available options. Thus, effective pretest and posttest counseling sessions are essential parts of an ethical prenatal screening program.

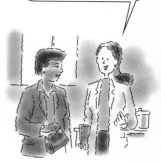

Effective pretest and posttest counseling sessions are essential parts of an ethical prenatal screening program.

Conception issues

Infertility can have devastating effects on the emotional well-being of a couple who yearns for children. As a result, many couples spend time and money to conceive or adopt a child. When medical procedures (such as fertility medications, hysterosalpingostomy, and artificial insemination) fail and adoption isn't an option, infertile couples may turn to in vitro fertilization (IVF), or surrogate motherhood.

In vitro fertilization

In IVF, ova are removed from a woman's ovaries, placed in a petri dish filled with a sterilized growth medium, and covered with healthy motile spermatozoa for fertilization. Three to five embryos are then implanted in the woman's uterus 10 to 14 days after fertilization, and the remaining fertilized ova are frozen for future use or discarded. IVF can be performed using the partner's sperm (homologous) or a donor's sperm (heterologous).

What about the leftovers?

Some people hail the scientific manipulation of ova and sperm as a medical miracle. Others are concerned that IVF circumvents the natural process of procreation. Another IVF issue involves leftover embryos. About 15 to 20 embryos may result from a single fertilization effort, but only 3 to 5 of them are implanted in the woman's uterus. Some individuals question whether it's ethical to discard these leftover embryos, destroy them, or use them for scientific study.

No matter what your values are concerning IVF, keep in mind that your goal is to provide the best nursing care possible to your patients.

Surrogate motherhood

A surrogate mother is a woman who gives birth after carrying the fertilized ovum of another woman or, more commonly, after being artificially inseminated with sperm from the biological father. In the latter case, the biological father then legally adopts the infant.

Offering hope

Surrogate motherhood offers hope for infertile couples in which the woman is the infertile partner. It's also an option for a woman whose age or health makes pregnancy risky. A surrogate birth poses no greater risk to the fetus (or surrogate mother) than any average birth.

> When it comes to modern treatments for infertility, one person's medical miracle is another person's controversy.

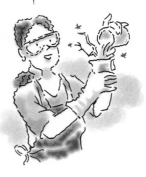

Whose rights are right?

One ethical concern about surrogate motherhood involves the potential conflicts concerning the rights of the surrogate mother, the infertile couple, the fetus, and society. The basic dispute involves who has the strongest claim to the child. Does the surrogate mother have rights by virtue of her biological connection? Does the surrogate contract guarantee the infertile couple the right to the child? Courts of law usually rule in favor of the infertile couple.

Support systems

In a surrogate mother situation, the nurse's role is to support her patient. If the patient is the surrogate mother, collaboration with a social worker or a psychologist may be necessary.

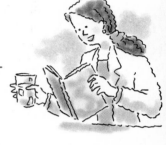

Staying in the research loop will help you provide the most up-to-date information to your patients.

Fetal tissue research

Transplants using stem cells from aborted fetuses offer hope for treating Parkinson's disease, Alzheimer's disease, diabetes, and other degenerative disorders. Stem cells have the ability to become any body cell, but only for a short period of time before they become differentiated into specific cells. Stem cells also carry a reduced risk of rejection because of their immaturity. Currently, bone marrow stem cells are the only stem cells commonly used to treat disease.

Stay in the loop

Such treatment is controversial and may conflict with your values or those of your patient. As a nurse, you'll need to stay informed about developing research so that you can provide your patients with the most current information.

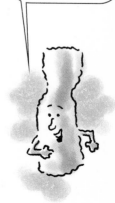

More and more, scientists are using genes like me to screen for disease.

Eugenics and gene manipulation

Eugenics is the science of improving a species through control of hereditary factors—in other words, by manipulating the gene pool. In the past, medical research has been limited to efforts to repair or halt the damage caused by disease and injury. Today, however, genetic manipulation and engineering have tremendous potential for altering the course of human development.

It's all in the genes

Using current techniques, researchers can learn many things about a fetus before it's born, including its sex or whether it suffers from certain serious medical conditions. Deoxyribonucleic acid (DNA) can even tell parents what color hair their child will have or how tall he'll be.

Mr. Screen Genes

The identification of the genes responsible for inherited diseases and congenital malformations has spurred the development of new screening tests. Genetic testing is now a fairly common component of prenatal care, facilitating the identification of fetuses with such disorders as Down syndrome and Tay-Sachs disease. The screening of neonates for phenylketonuria is legally required in most states.

Harnessing the power of heredity

Many medical conditions don't have safe and effective treatments. In some cases, gene therapy can change that. Gene therapy using DNA can be used to:
- increase the activity of a gene in the body
- decrease the activity of a gene in the body
- introduce a new gene into the body.

Genetic engineering can even give science the ability to re-create the human body. Scientists frequently discover new ways to identify and manipulate the genetic material of everything from single-cell organisms to human beings.

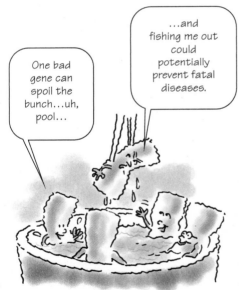

Designer genes

There's little controversy about the ethics of gene therapy as it's currently practiced. However, some groups express concerns about the future. Genetic engineering can potentially allow parents to choose what traits they want their child to have. These "designer babies" may pose ethical dilemmas for some health care practitioners. Although enormous advances in technology are still needed before selecting such complicated traits as hair color, intelligence, and height becomes a reality, it's possible that these choices will be available to parents in the near future.

Keep informed

Genetic manipulation and gene therapy are still experimental in some cases. As a result, few nurses are directly involved in these aspects of genetic research. Nonetheless, you have an ethical obligation to stay informed and to support efforts to establish legal and technological safeguards.

Preterm and high-risk neonates

Twenty years ago, an infant born at 26 weeks' gestation had almost no chance of survival. This is no longer the case. Advances in neonatology, such as intrauterine surgery, synthetic lung surfactant, and new antibiotics, help save increasingly smaller and sicker infants.

Matters of life and death

When you care for an extremely premature or a critically ill infant and his mother, family members look to you to assist them with life-and-death decisions. To help the parents of an extremely premature or critically ill neonate reach ethically sound decisions, you'll need to present all available options in a compassionate, unbiased manner using simple terms. By carefully helping family members consider the pros and cons of both initiating and withholding treatment, you can help them come to terms with the neonate's condition and reach a decision with which they'll be able to live.

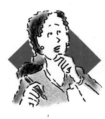

Quick quiz

1. The intrapartum period starts:
   A.   after delivery of the neonate and placenta.
   B.   at the onset of contractions.
   C.   at conception.
   D.   during the second trimester.

Answer: B. The intrapartum period starts at the onset of contractions that cause cervical dilation and lasts through the first 1 to 4 hours after the birth of the neonate and delivery of the placenta.

2. A registered nurse who has achieved advanced education at a master's level or through certification, cares for low-risk obstetric patients, and is licensed to deliver a neonate is called a:
   A.   nurse practitioner.
   B.   clinical nurse specialist.
   C.   pediatric nurse practitioner.
   D.   certified nurse-midwife.

Answer: D. A certified nurse-midwife is a registered nurse with advanced education who cares for low-risk obstetric patients and is licensed to deliver a neonate.

3. A family that consists of parents, grandparents, and grand-children is known as:
- A. a cohabitation family.
- B. an extended family.
- C. a blended family.
- D. a communal family.

Answer: B. An extended or multigenerational family consists of the nuclear family as well as other family members, such as grandparents, aunts, uncles, cousins, and grandchildren.

4. When a woman gives birth after carrying the fertilized ovum of another woman, it's called:
- A. in vitro fertilization.
- B. cesarean birth.
- C. surrogate motherhood.
- D. gamete fertilization.

Answer: C. Surrogate motherhood involves one woman giving birth after carrying the fertilized ovum of another woman or after being inseminated with sperm from the biological father.

5. The science of improving a species through control of heredi-tary factors by manipulation of the gene pool is called:
- A. eugenics.
- B. in vitro fertilization.
- C. fetal tissue research.
- D. genealogy.

Answer: A. Eugenics is the science of improving a species through control of hereditary factors by manipulation of the gene pool.

Scoring

☆☆☆ If you answered all five questions correctly, fantastic! Your labor is paying off!

☆☆ If you answered four questions correctly, good work! You're sure to reproduce these results in later chapters!

☆ If you answered fewer than four questions correctly, don't worry! Just breathe, relax, and push (through a review of the chapter, that is).

2

Conception and fetal development

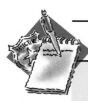

Just the facts

In this chapter, you'll learn:

♦ anatomic structures and functions of the male and female reproductive systems

♦ effects of hormone production on sexual development

♦ the process of fertilization

♦ stages of fetal development

♦ structural changes that result from pregnancy.

A look at conception and fetal development

Development of a functioning human being from a fertilized ovum involves a complex process of cell division, differentiation, and organization. Development begins with the union of spermatozoon and ovum (conception) to form a composite cell containing chromosomes from both parents. This composite cell (called a *zygote*) divides repeatedly. Finally, groups of differentiated cells organize into complex structures, such as the brain, spinal cord, liver, kidneys, and other organs that function as integrated units.

To fully understand the dramatic physical changes that occur during pregnancy, you must be familiar with reproductive anatomy and physiology and the stages of fetal development. Let's start with the male reproductive system.

Here's looking at you, kid.

Can you even conceive of it!? When we get together, we form a new cell called a zygote.

Male reproductive system

Anatomically, the main distinction between a male and a female is the presence of conspicuous external genitalia in the male. In contrast, the major reproductive organs of the female lie within the pelvic cavity.

Making introductions

The male reproductive system consists of the organs that produce, transfer, and introduce mature sperm into the female reproductive tract, where fertilization occurs. (See *Structures of the male reproductive system*.)

Multitasking

In addition to supplying male sex cells (spermatogenesis), the male reproductive system plays a part in the secretion of male sex hormones.

Penis

The organ of copulation, the penis deposits sperm in the female reproductive tract and acts as the terminal duct for the urinary tract. The penis also serves as the means for urine elimination. It consists of an attached root, a free shaft, and an enlarged tip.

What's inside

Internally, the cylinder-shaped penile shaft consists of three columns of erectile tissue bound together by heavy fibrous tissue. Two corpora cavernosa form the major part of the penis. On the underside, the corpus spongiosum encases the urethra. Its enlarged proximal end forms the bulb of the penis.

The glans penis, at the distal end of the shaft, is a cone-shaped structure formed from the corpus spongiosum. Its lateral margin forms a ridge of tissue known as the *corona*. The glans penis is highly sensitive to sexual stimulation.

What's outside

Thin, loose skin covers the penile shaft. The urethral meatus opens through the glans to allow urination and ejaculation.

In a different vein

The penis receives blood through the internal pudendal artery. Blood then flows into the corpora cavernosa through the penile artery. Venous blood returns through the internal iliac vein to the vena cava.

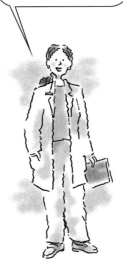

Here's the main difference—males have external genitalia, whereas most female reproductive organs are inside the pelvic cavity.

Structures of the male reproductive system

The male reproductive system consists of the penis, the scrotum and its contents, the prostate gland, and the inguinal structures.

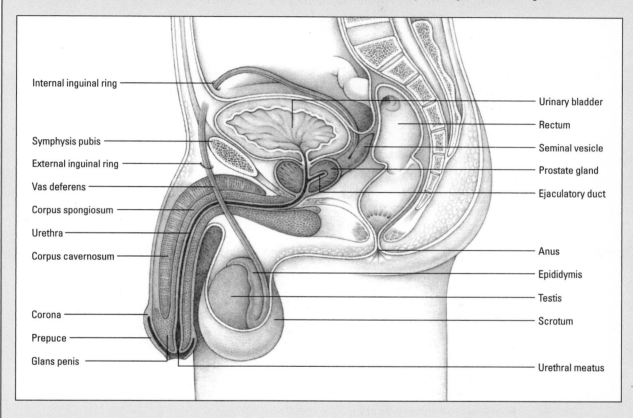

Internal inguinal ring

Symphysis pubis

External inguinal ring

Vas deferens

Corpus spongiosum

Urethra

Corpus cavernosum

Corona

Prepuce

Glans penis

Urinary bladder

Rectum

Seminal vesicle

Prostate gland

Ejaculatory duct

Anus

Epididymis

Testis

Scrotum

Urethral meatus

Scrotum

The penis meets the scrotum, or scrotal sac, at the penoscrotal junction. Located posterior to the penis and anterior to the anus, the scrotum is an extra-abdominal pouch that consists of a thin layer of skin overlying a tighter, musclelike layer. This musclelike layer, in turn, overlies the tunica vaginalis, a serous membrane that covers the internal scrotal cavity.

Canals and rings

Internally, a septum divides the scrotum into two sacs, which each contain a testis, an epididymis, and a spermatic cord. The spermatic cord is a connective tissue sheath that encases autonomic nerve fibers, blood vessels, lymph vessels, and the vas deferens (also called the *ductus deferens*).

The spermatic cord travels from the testis through the inguinal canal, exiting the scrotum through the external inguinal ring and entering the abdominal cavity through the internal inguinal ring. The inguinal canal lies between the two rings.

Loads of nodes

Lymph nodes from the penis, scrotal surface, and anus drain into the inguinal lymph nodes. Lymph nodes from the testes drain into the lateral aortic and pre-aortic lymph nodes in the abdomen.

Testes

The testes are enveloped in two layers of connective tissue called the *tunica vaginalis* (outer layer) and the *tunica albuginea* (inner layer). Extensions of the tunica albuginea separate the testes into lobules. Each lobule contains one to four seminiferous tubules, small tubes where spermatogenesis takes place.

Climate control

Spermatozoa development requires a temperature lower than that of the rest of the body. The dartos muscle, a smooth muscle in the superficial fasciae, causes scrotal skin to wrinkle, which helps regulate temperature. The cremaster muscle, rising from the internal oblique muscle, helps to govern temperature by elevating the testes.

Duct system

The male reproductive duct system, consisting of the epididymis, vas deferens, and urethra, conveys sperm from the testes to the ejaculatory ducts near the bladder.

Swimmers, take your mark!

The epididymis is a coiled tube that's located superior to and along the posterior border of the testis. During ejaculation, smooth muscle in the epididymis contracts, ejecting spermatozoa into the vas deferens.

Descending tunnel

The vas deferens leads from the testes to the abdominal cavity, extends upward through the inguinal canal, arches over the urethra, and descends behind the bladder. Its enlarged portion, called the *ampulla*, merges with the duct of the semi-

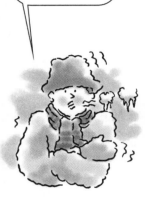

Brrrr! One of the jobs of the scrotum is to keep the testes cooler than the rest of the body.

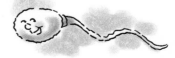

During ejaculation, smooth muscle in the epididymis contracts, sending spermatozoa into the vas deferens.

nal vesicle to form the short ejaculatory duct. After passing through the prostate gland, the vas deferens joins with the urethra.

Tube to the outside

A small tube leading from the floor of the bladder to the exterior, the urethra consists of three parts:

- prostatic urethra, which is surrounded by the prostate gland and drains the bladder

- membranous urethra, which passes through the urogenital diaphragm

- spongy urethra, which makes up about 75% of the entire urethra.

Accessory reproductive glands

The accessory reproductive glands, which produce most of the semen, include the seminal vesicles, bulbourethral glands (Cowper's glands), and prostate gland.

A pair of pairs

The seminal vesicles are paired sacs at the base of the bladder. The bulbourethral glands, also paired, are located inferior to the prostate.

Improving the odds

The walnut-size prostate gland lies under the bladder and surrounds the urethra. It consists of three lobes: the left and right lateral lobes and the median lobe.

The prostate gland continuously secretes prostatic fluid, a thin, milky, alkaline fluid. During sexual activity, prostatic fluid adds volume to semen. It also enhances sperm motility and improves the odds of conception by neutralizing the acidity of the man's urethra and the woman's vagina.

Basically basic

Semen is a viscous, white secretion with a slightly alkaline pH (7.8 to 8) that consists of spermatozoa and accessory gland secretions. The seminal vesicles produce roughly 60% of the fluid portion of semen, whereas the prostate gland produces about 30%. A viscid fluid secreted by the bulbourethral glands also becomes part of semen.

Spermatogenesis

Sperm formation (also called *spermatogenesis*) begins when a male reaches puberty and usually continues throughout life.

Divide and conquer

Spermatogenesis occurs in four stages:

In the first stage, the primary germinal epithelial cells, called *spermatogonia*, grow and develop into primary spermatocytes. Both spermatogonia and primary spermatocytes contain 46 chromosomes, consisting of 44 autosomes and the two sex chromosomes, X and Y.

Next, primary spermatocytes divide to form secondary spermatocytes. No new chromosomes are formed in this stage; the pairs only divide. Each secondary spermatocyte contains one-half of the number of autosomes, 22; one secondary spermatocyte contains an X chromosome; the other, a Y chromosome.

In the third stage, each secondary spermatocyte divides again to form spermatids (also called *spermatoblasts*).

Finally, the spermatids undergo a series of structural changes that transform them into mature spermatozoa, or sperm. Each spermatozoa has a head, neck, body, and tail. The head contains the nucleus; the tail, a large amount of adenosine triphosphate, which provides energy for sperm motility.

Queuing up

Newly mature sperm pass from the seminiferous tubules through the vasa recta into the epididymis. Only a small number of sperm can be stored in the epididymis. Most of them move into the vas deferens, where they're stored until sexual stimulation triggers emission.

Check the expiration date?

After ejaculation, sperm can survive for 24 to 72 hours at body temperature. Sperm cells retain their potency and can survive for up to 4 days in the female reproductive tract.

Hormonal control and sexual development

Androgens (male sex hormones) are produced in the testes and adrenal glands. Androgens are responsible for the development of male sex organs and secondary sex characteristics. One major androgen is testosterone.

Memory jogger

To remember the meaning of spermatogenesis, keep in mind that genesis means "beginning" or "new." Therefore, spermatogenesis means beginning of new sperm.

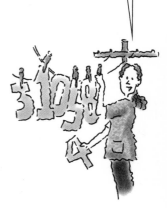

The number of sperm and their motility affect fertility. A low sperm count (less than 20 million per milliliter of semen) may be a cause of infertility.

Team captain

Leydig cells, located in the testes between the seminiferous tubules, secrete testosterone, the most significant male sex hormone. Testosterone is responsible for the development and maintenance of male sex organs and secondary sex characteristics, such as facial hair and vocal cord thickness. Testosterone is also required for spermatogenesis.

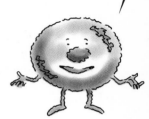

Just call me the captain of team testosterone!

Calling the plays

Testosterone secretion begins approximately 2 months after conception, when the release of chorionic gonadotropins from the placenta stimulates Leydig cells in the male fetus. The presence of testosterone directly affects sexual differentiation in the fetus. With testosterone, fetal genitalia develop into a penis, scrotum, and testes; without testosterone, genitalia develop into a clitoris, vagina, and other female organs.

During the last 2 months of gestation, testosterone usually causes the testes to descend into the scrotum. If the testes don't descend after birth, exogenous testosterone may correct the problem.

Other key players

Other hormones also affect male sexuality. Two of these, luteinizing hormone (LH)—also called *interstitial cell-stimulating hormone*—and follicle-stimulating hormone (FSH), directly affect secretion of testosterone.

Waiting on the bench

During early childhood, a boy doesn't secrete gonadotropins and thus has little circulating testosterone. Secretion of gonadotropins from the pituitary gland, which usually occurs between ages 11 and 14, marks the onset of puberty. These pituitary gonadotropins stimulate testis functioning as well as testosterone secretion.

Put me in, coach!

During puberty, the penis and testes enlarge and the male reaches full adult sexual and reproductive capability. Puberty also marks the development of male secondary sexual characteristics, including:
• distinct body hair distribution
• skin changes (such as increased secretion by sweat and sebaceous glands)
• deepening of the voice (from laryngeal enlargement)
• increased musculoskeletal development
• other intracellular and extracellular changes.

Star player

After a male achieves full physical maturity, usually by age 20, sexual and reproductive function remain fairly consistent throughout life.

Subtle changes

With aging, a man may experience subtle changes in sexual function but he doesn't lose the ability to reproduce. For example, an elderly man may require more time to achieve an erection, experience less firm erections, and have reduced ejaculatory volume. After ejaculation, he may take longer to regain an erection.

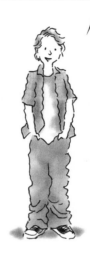

Hey, I've almost reached full physical maturity. Now can I borrow the car?

Female reproductive system

Unlike the male reproductive system, the female system is largely internal, housed within the pelvic cavity.

External genitalia

The external female genitalia, or vulva, include the mons pubis, labia majora, labia minora, clitoris, and adjacent structures. These structures are visible on inspection. (See *Structures of the female reproductive system*, pages 36 and 37.)

Mons pubis

The mons pubis is a rounded cushion of fatty and connective tissue covered by skin and coarse, curly hair in a triangular pattern over the symphysis pubis (the joint formed by the union of the pubic bones anteriorly).

Labia majora

The labia majora are two raised folds of adipose and connective tissue that border the vulva on either side, extending from the mons pubis to the perineum. After onset of the first menses (called *menarche*), the outer surface of the labia is covered with pubic hair. The inner surface is pink and moist.

Labia minora

The labia minora are two moist folds of mucosal tissue, dark pink to red in color, that lie within and alongside the labia majora. Each upper section divides into an upper and lower lamella. The two upper lamellae join to form the prepuce, a hoodlike covering over

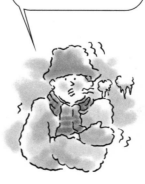

The labia are highly vascular and have many nerve endings— making them sensitive to pain, pressure, touch, sexual stimulation, and temperature extremes.

the clitoris. The two lower lamellae form the frenulum, the posterior portion of the clitoris.

The lower labial sections taper down and back from the clitoris to the perineum, where they join to form the fourchette, a thin tissue fold along the anterior edge of the perineum.

Minor in name only

The labia minora contain sebaceous glands, which secrete a lubricant that also acts as a bactericide. Like the labia majora, they're rich in blood vessels and nerve endings, making them highly responsive to stimulation. They swell in response to sexual stimulation, a reaction that triggers other changes that prepare the genitalia for coitus.

Clitoris

The clitoris is the small, protuberant organ just beneath the arch of the mons pubis. It contains erectile tissue, venous cavernous spaces, and specialized sensory corpuscles, which are stimulated during sexual activity.

Adjacent structures

The vestibule is an oval area bounded anteriorly by the clitoris, laterally by the labia minora, and posteriorly by the fourchette.

Featuring glands

The mucus-producing Skene's glands are found on both sides of the urethral opening. Openings of the two mucus-producing Bartholin's glands are located laterally and posteriorly on either side of the inner vaginal orifice.

The urethral meatus is the slitlike opening below the clitoris through which urine leaves the body. In the center of the vestibule is the vaginal orifice. It may be completely or partially covered by the hymen, a tissue membrane.

Not too simple

Located between the lower vagina and the anal canal, the perineum is a complex structure of muscles, blood vessels, fasciae, nerves, and lymphatics.

Internal genitalia

The female internal genitalia include the vagina, cervix, uterus, fallopian tubes, ovaries, and mammary glands. The main function of these specialized organs is reproduction.

(Text continues on page 38.)

Structures of the female reproductive system

The female reproductive system consists of external and internal genitalia. These structures include the vagina, cervix, uterus, fallopian tubes, ovaries, and other structures. Reproductive, urinary, and GI structures are housed in the female pelvis. These include the bladder, anus, and rectum.

View of external genitalia in lithotomy position

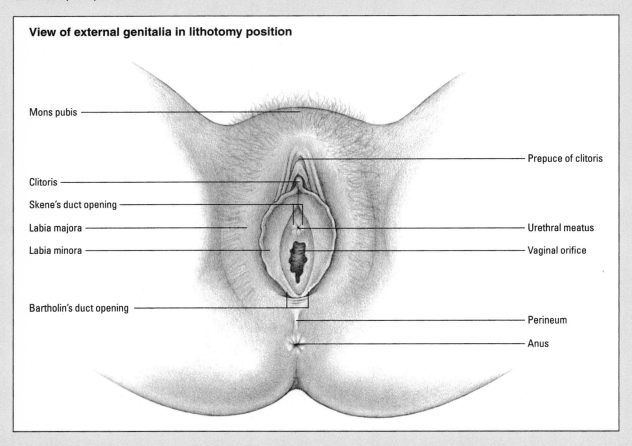

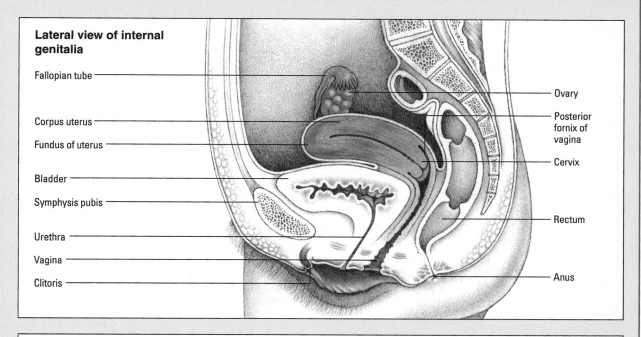

Lateral view of internal genitalia

Fallopian tube

Corpus uterus

Fundus of uterus

Bladder

Symphysis pubis

Urethra

Vagina

Clitoris

Ovary

Posterior fornix of vagina

Cervix

Rectum

Anus

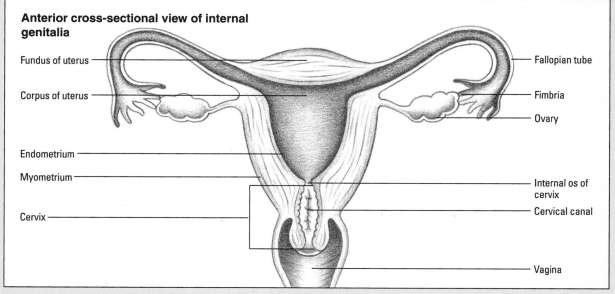

Anterior cross-sectional view of internal genitalia

Fundus of uterus

Corpus of uterus

Endometrium

Myometrium

Cervix

Fallopian tube

Fimbria

Ovary

Internal os of cervix

Cervical canal

Vagina

Vagina

The vagina, a highly elastic muscular tube, is located between the urethra and the rectum.

Three layers...

The vaginal wall has three tissue layers: epithelial tissue, loose connective tissue, and muscle tissue. The uterine cervix connects the uterus to the vaginal vault. Four fornices, recesses in the vaginal wall, surround the cervix.

...three functions

The vagina has three main functions:

to accommodate the penis during coitus

to channel blood discharged from the uterus during menstruation

to serve as the birth canal during childbirth.

Separate but equal

The upper, middle, and lower vaginal sections have separate blood supplies. Branches of the uterine arteries supply blood to the upper vagina, the inferior vesical arteries supply blood to the middle vagina, and the hemorrhoidal and internal pudendal arteries feed into the lower vagina.

Blood returns through a vast venous plexus to the hemorrhoidal, pudendal, and uterine veins, and then to the hypogastric veins. This plexus merges with the vertebral venous plexus.

Cervix

The cervix is the lowest portion of the uterus. It projects into the upper portion of the vagina. The end that opens into the vagina is called the *external os;* the end that opens into the uterus, the *internal os.* The cervix is sealed with thick mucus. This prevents sperm from entering except for a few days around ovulation when the plug becomes thinner.

Kids change everything!

Childbirth permanently alters the cervix. In a female who hasn't delivered a child, the external os is a round opening about 3 mm in diameter; after the first childbirth, it becomes a small transverse slit with irregular edges.

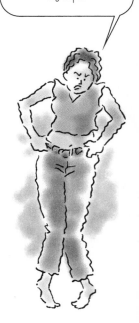

Over time, everything changes— the size and shape of the cervix, and the size and shape of my hips!

Uterus

The uterus is a small, firm, pear-shaped, muscular organ situated between the bladder and rectum. It typically lies at almost a 90-degree angle to the vagina. The mucous membrane lining of the uterus is called the *endometrium*, and the muscular layer of the uterus is called the *myometrium*.

Fundamental fundus

During pregnancy, the elastic, upper portion of the uterus, called the *fundus*, accommodates most of the growing fetus until term. The uterine neck joins the fundus to the cervix, the uterine part extending into the vagina. The fundus and neck make up the main uterine body, called the *corpus*.

Fallopian tubes

Two fallopian tubes attach to the uterus at the upper angles of the fundus. These narrow cylinders of muscle fibers are where fertilization occurs.

Riding the wave

The curved portion of the fallopian tube, called the *ampulla*, ends in the funnel-shaped infundibulum. Fingerlike projections in the infundibulum, called *fimbriae*, move in waves that sweep the mature ovum (female gamete, or sex cell) from the ovary into the fallopian tube.

Ovaries

The ovaries are located on either side of the uterus. The size, shape, and position of the ovaries vary with age. Round, smooth, and pink at birth, they grow larger, flatten, and turn grayish by puberty. During the childbearing years, they take on an almond shape and a rough, pitted surface; after menopause, they shrink and turn white.

Swept away

The ovaries' main function is to produce mature ova. At birth, each ovary contains approximately 400,000 graafian follicles. During the childbearing years, one graafian follicle produces a mature ovum during the first half of each menstrual cycle. As the ovum matures, the follicle ruptures and the ovum is swept into the fallopian tube.

The ovaries also produce estrogen and progesterone as well as a small amount of androgens.

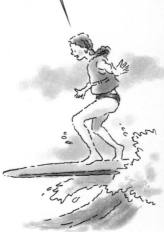

Fingerlike projections called *fimbriae* move in waves, sweeping the ovum from the ovary to the fallopian tube.

Mammary glands

The mammary glands, located in the breast, are specialized accessory glands that secrete milk. Although present in both sexes, they typically function only in the female.

Thanks for the mammaries

Each mammary gland contains 15 to 20 lobes that are separated by fibrous connective tissue and fat. Within the lobes are clustered acini—tiny, saclike duct terminals that secrete milk during lactation.

The ducts draining the lobules converge to form excretory (*lactiferous*) ducts and sinuses (*ampullae*), which store milk during lactation. These ducts drain onto the nipple surface through 15 to 20 openings. (See *The female breast.*)

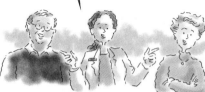

Both males and females have mammary glands—but they typically function only in the female.

The female breast

The breasts are located on either side of the anterior chest wall over the greater pectoral and the anterior serratus muscles. Within the areola, the pigmented area in the center of the breast, lies the nipple. Erectile tissue in the nipple responds to cold, friction, and sexual stimulation.

Support and separate

Each breast is composed of glandular, fibrous, and adipose tissue. Glandular tissue contains 15 to 20 lobes made up of clustered acini, tiny saclike duct terminals that secrete milk. Fibrous Cooper's ligaments support the breasts; adipose tissue separates the two breasts.

Produce and drain

Milk glands in each breast produce milk by acini cells and then deliver it to the nipple by a lactiferous duct.

Sebaceous glands on the areolar surface, called Montgomery's tubercles, produce sebum, which lubricates the areola and nipple during breast-feeding.

Lateral cross section

Clavicle

Adipose tissue

Acini of lobule

Glandular lobe

Collecting and main ducts

Areola

Montgomery's tubercle

Nipple

Lactiferous duct orifice

Lactiferous duct

Lactiferous sinus

Fibrous septa

Hormonal function and the menstrual cycle

Like the male body, the female body changes as it ages in response to hormonal control. When a female reaches the age of menstruation, the hypothalamus, ovaries, and pituitary gland secrete hormones—estrogen, progesterone, FSH, and LH—that affect the buildup and shedding of the endometrium during the menstrual cycle. (See *Events in the female reproductive cycle*, pages 42 and 43.)

A spurt of growth

During adolescence, the release of hormones causes a rapid increase in physical growth and spurs the development of secondary sex characteristics. This growth spurt begins at approximately age 11 and continues until early adolescence, or about 3 years later.

Irregularity of the menstrual cycle is common during this time because of failure of the female to ovulate. With menarche, the uterine body flexes on the cervix and the ovaries are situated in the pelvic cavity.

A monthly thing

The menstrual cycle is a complex process that involves both the reproductive and endocrine systems. The cycle averages 28 days.

Supply exhausted

In contrast to the slowly declining hormones of the aging male, the aging female's hormones decline rapidly in a process called *menopause*. Although the pituitary gland still releases FSH and LH, the body has exhausted its supply of ovarian follicles that respond to these hormones and menstruation no longer occurs.

Cessation of menses usually occurs between ages 45 and 55. Some women experience menopause early, possibly as a result of genetics, ovarian damage, autoimmune disorders, or surgical interventions such as hysterectomy. When menopause occurs before age 45, it's known as *premature menopause*.

Menopause can be broken down into three stages: perimenopause, menopause, and postmenopause.

Climactic climacteric

Perimenopause consists of the 8 to 10 years (called the *climacteric years*) of declining ovarian function that occur before menopause. During this time, the ovaries gradually begin to produce less estrogen and the woman may experience irregular menses that become further apart and produce a lighter flow. As menopause progresses, the ovaries stop producing progesterone and estrogen altogether.

(Text continues on page 44.)

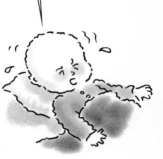

Are you telling me I have to wait until I'm 11 before I'll have my growth spurt? That is so unfair!

Events in the female reproductive cycle

The female reproductive cycle usually lasts 28 days. During this cycle, three major types of changes occur simultaneously: ovulatory, hormonal, and endometrial (involving the lining [endometrium] of the uterus).

Ovulatory

• Ovulatory changes, which usually last 5 days, begin on day 1 of the menstrual cycle.
• As the cycle begins, low estrogen and progesterone levels in the bloodstream stimulate the hypothalamus to secrete gonadotropin-releasing hormone (Gn-RH). In turn, Gn-RH stimulates the anterior pituitary gland to secrete follicle-stimulating hormone (FSH) and luteinizing hormone (LH).
• Follicle development within the ovary (in the follicular phase) is spurred by increased levels of FSH and, to a lesser extent, LH.
• When the follicle matures, a spike in the LH level occurs, causing the follicle to rupture and release the ovum, thus initiating ovulation.
• After ovulation (in the luteal phase), the collapsed follicle forms the corpus luteum, which degenerates if fertilization doesn't occur.

Hormonal

• During the follicular phase of the ovarian cycle, the increasing FSH and LH levels that stimulate follicle growth also stimulate increased secretion of the hormone estrogen.
• Estrogen secretion peaks just before ovulation. This peak sets in motion the spike in LH levels, which causes ovulation.
• After ovulation (about day 14), estrogen levels decline rapidly. In the luteal phase of the ovarian cycle, the corpus luteum is formed and begins to release progesterone and estrogen.
• As the corpus luteum degenerates, levels of both of these ovarian hormones decline.

Endometrial

• The endometrium is receptive to implantation of an embryo for only a short time in the reproductive cycle. Thus, it's no accident that its most receptive phase occurs about 7 days after the ovarian cycle's release of an ovum—just in time to receive a fertilized ovum.
• In the first 5 days of the reproductive cycle, the endometrium sheds its functional layer, leaving the basal layer (the deepest layer) intact. Menstrual flow consists of this detached layer and accompanying blood from the detachment process.
• The endometrium begins regenerating its functional layer at about day 6 (the proliferative phase), spurred by rising estrogen levels.
• After ovulation, increased progesterone secretion stimulates conversion of the functional layer into a secretory mucosa (secretory phase), which is more receptive to implantation of the fertilized ovum.
• If implantation doesn't occur, the corpus luteum degenerates, progesterone levels drop, and the endometrium again sheds its functional layer.

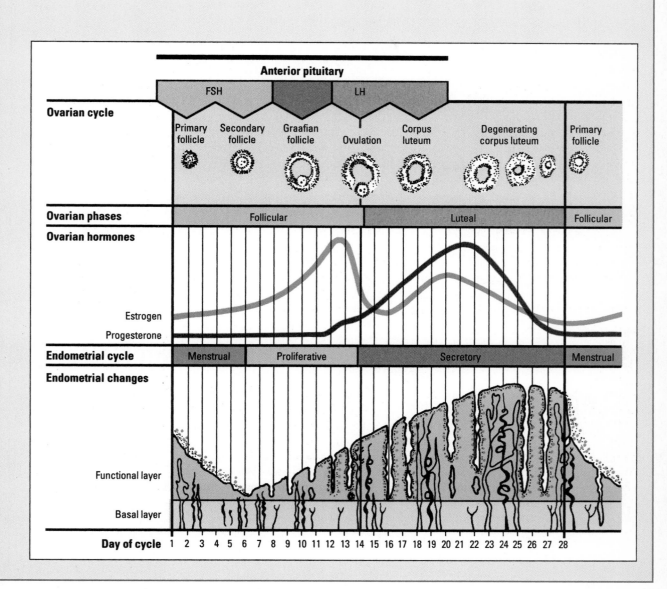

Out of eggs

A woman is considered to have reached the menopause stage after menses are absent for 1 year. At this stage, the ovaries have stopped producing eggs and have almost completely stopped producing estrogen.

Signs and symptoms of menopause include:
- hot flashes (sudden feelings of warmth that spread throughout the upper body and may be accompanied by blushing or sweating)
- irregular or skipped menses
- mood swings and irritability
- fatigue
- insomnia
- headaches
- changes in sex drive
- vaginal dryness.

Menopause can be confirmed through analysis of FSH levels or a Pap-like test that assesses for vaginal atrophy.

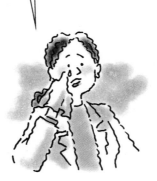

Mood swings—just one of the possible signs and symptoms of menopause (sniff).

One thing leads to another

Postmenopause refers to the years after menopause. During this stage, the symptoms of menopause cease for most women. However, the risk of other health problems increases as a result of declining estrogen levels. These problems include:
- osteoporosis
- heart disease
- decreased skin elasticity
- vision deterioration.

Fertilization

Production of a new human being begins with *fertilization*, the union of a spermatozoon and an ovum to form a single new cell. After fertilization occurs, dramatic changes begin inside a woman's body. The cells of the fertilized ovum begin dividing as the ovum travels to the uterine cavity, where it implants itself in the uterine lining. (See *How fertilization occurs*.)

Survivial of the fittest

For fertilization to take place, however, the spermatozoon must first reach the ovum. Although a single ejaculation deposits several hundred million spermatozoa, many are destroyed by acidic vaginal secretions. The only spermatozoa that survive are those that enter the cervical canal, where cervical mucus protects them.

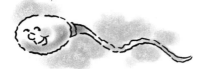

It's a lot of work for one sperm! After I make my way through the cervical mucus, uterine contractions help me to penetrate the fallopian tubes.

How fertilization occurs

Fertilization begins when the spermatozoon is activated upon contact with the ovum. Here's what happens.

The spermatozoon, which has a covering called the *acrosome,* approaches the ovum.

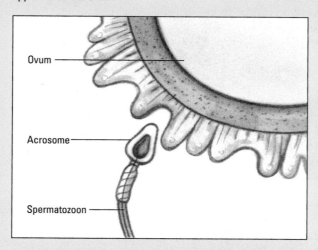

The acrosome develops small perforations through which it releases enzymes necessary for the sperm to penetrate the protective layers of the ovum before fertilization.

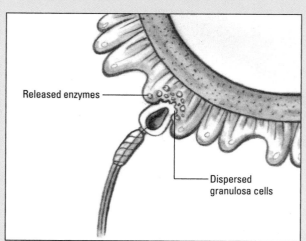

The spermatozoon then penetrates the zona pellucida (the inner membrane of the ovum). This triggers the ovum's second meiotic division (following meiosis), making the zona pellucida impenetrable to other spermatozoa.

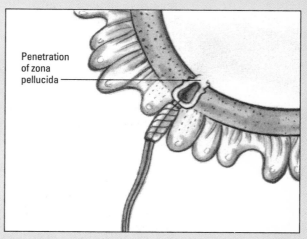

After the spermatozoon penetrates the ovum, its nucleus is released into the ovum, its tail degenerates, and its head enlarges and fuses with the ovum's nucleus. This fusion provides the fertilized ovum, called a *zygote,* with 46 chromosomes.

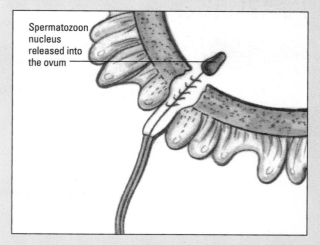

Timing is everything

The ability of spermatozoa to penetrate the cervical mucus depends on the phase of the menstrual cycle at the time of transit:
- Early in the cycle, estrogen and progesterone levels cause the mucus to thicken, making it more difficult for spermatozoa to pass through the cervix.
- During midcycle, however, when the mucus is relatively thin, spermatozoa can pass readily through the cervix.
- Later in the cycle, the cervical mucus thickens again, hindering spermatozoa passage.

Help along the way

Spermatozoa travel through the female reproductive tract by means of flagellar movements (whiplike movements of the tail). After spermatozoa pass through the cervical mucus, however, the female reproductive system assists them on their journey with rhythmic contractions of the uterus that help the spermatozoa to penetrate the fallopian tubes. Spermatozoa are typically viable (able to fertilize the ovum) for up to 2 days after ejaculation; however, they can survive in the reproductive tract for up to 4 days.

Disperse and penetrate

Before a spermatozoon can penetrate the ovum, it must disperse the granulosa cells and penetrate the zona pellucida, the thick, transparent layer surrounding the incompletely developed ovum. Enzymes in the acrosome (head cap) of the spermatozoon permit this penetration. After penetration, the ovum completes its second meiotic division and the zona pellucida prevents penetration by other spermatozoa.

The spermatozoon's head then fuses with the ovum nucleus, creating a cell nucleus with 46 chromosomes. The fertilized ovum is called a *zygote*.

Pregnancy

Pregnancy starts with fertilization and ends with childbirth; on average, its duration is 38 weeks. During this period (called *gestation*), the zygote divides as it passes through the fallopian tube and attaches to the uterine lining by implantation. A complex sequence of pre-embryonic, embryonic, and fetal developments transforms the zygote into a full-term fetus.

Making predictions

Because the uterus grows throughout pregnancy, uterine size serves as a rough estimate of gestation. The fertilization date is rarely known, so the woman's expected delivery date is typically calculated from the beginning of her last menses. The tool used for calculating delivery dates is known as *Nägele's rule*.

Here's how it works: If you know the 1st day of the last menstrual cycle, simply count back 3 months from that date and then add 7 days. For example, let's say that the 1st day of the last menses was April 29. Count back 3 months, which gets you to January 29, and then add 7 days for an approximate due date of February 5.

> Nägele's rule can't predict the future, but it can provide a good estimation of when a baby will be born.

Stages of fetal development

During pregnancy, the fetus undergoes three major stages of development:

- pre-embryonic period (fertilization to week 3)
- embryonic period (weeks 4 through 7)
- fetal period (week 8 through birth).

It all starts here

The pre-embryonic phase starts with ovum fertilization and lasts 3 weeks. As the zygote passes through the fallopian tube, it undergoes a series of mitotic divisions, or cleavage. (See *Pre-embryonic development*, page 48.)

Zygote to embryo

During the embryonic period (the 4th through the 7th week of gestation), the developing zygote starts to take on a human shape and is now called an *embryo*. Each germ layer—the ectoderm, mesoderm, and endoderm—eventually forms specific tissues in the embryo. (See *Embryonic development*, page 49.)

Organ systems form during the embryonic period. During this time, the embryo is particularly vulnerable to injury by maternal drug use, certain maternal infections, and other factors.

Baby on the way!

During the fetal stage of development, which extends from the 8th week until birth, the maturing fetus enlarges and grows heavier. (See *From embryo to fetus*, page 50.)

(Text continues on page 51.)

Pre-embryonic development

The pre-embryonic phase lasts from conception until approximately the end of week 3 of development.

Zygote...

As the fertilized ovum advances through the fallopian tube toward the uterus, it undergoes mitotic division, forming daughter cells, initially called *blastomeres,* that each contain the same number of chromosomes as the parent cell. The first cell division ends about 30 hours after fertilization; subsequent divisions occur rapidly.

The *zygote,* as it's now called, develops into a small mass of cells called a *morula,* which reaches the uterus at about day 3 after fertilization. Fluid that amasses in the center of the morula forms a central cavity.

...into blastocyst

The structure is now called a *blastocyst.* The blastocyst consists of a thin trophoblast layer, which includes the blastocyst cavity, and the inner cell mass. The trophoblast develops into

fetal membranes and the placenta. The inner cell mass later forms the embryo (late blastocyst).

Getting attached: Blastocyst and endometrium

During the next phase, the blastocyst stays within the zona pellucida, unattached to the uterus. The zona pellucida degenerates and, by the end of week 1 after fertilization, the blastocyst attaches to the endometrium. The part of the blastocyst adjacent to the inner cell mass is the first part to become attached.

The trophoblast, in contact with the endometrial lining, proliferates and invades the underlying endometrium by separating and dissolving endometrial cells.

Letting it all sink in

During the next week, the invading blastocyst sinks below the endometrium's surface. The penetration site seals, restoring the continuity of the endometrial surface.

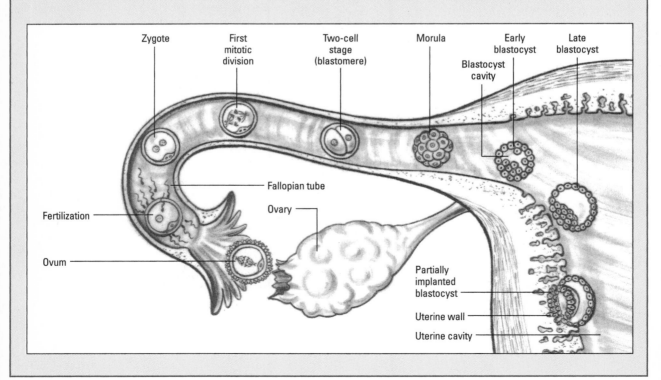

Embryonic development

Each of the three germ layers—ectoderm, mesoderm, and endoderm—forms specific tissues and organs in the developing embryo.

Ectoderm

The ectoderm, the outermost layer, develops into the:
- epidermis
- nervous system
- pituitary gland
- tooth enamel
- salivary glands
- optic lens
- lining of lower portion of anal canal
- hair.

Mesoderm

The mesoderm, the middle layer, develops into:
- connective and supporting tissue
- the blood and vascular system
- musculature
- teeth (except enamel)
- the mesothelial lining of pericardial, pleural, and peritoneal cavities
- the kidneys and ureters.

Endoderm

The endoderm, the innermost layer, becomes the epithelial lining of the:
- pharynx and trachea
- auditory canal
- alimentary canal
- liver
- pancreas
- bladder and urethra
- prostate.

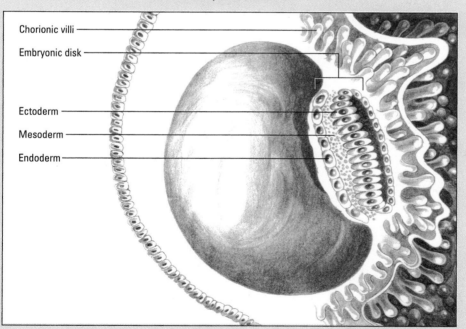

Chorionic villi
Embryonic disk
Ectoderm
Mesoderm
Endoderm

From embryo to fetus

Significant growth and development take place within the first 3 months following conception, as the embryo develops into a fetus that nearly resembles a full-term neonate.

Month 1

At the end of the first month, the embryo has a definite form. The head, the trunk, and the tiny buds that will become the arms and legs are discernible. The cardiovascular system has begun to function, and the umbilical cord is visible in its most primitive form.

Month 2

During the second month, the embryo—called a *fetus* from week 8—grows to 1" (2.5 cm) and weighs 1 g (⅓₀ oz). The head and facial features develop as the eyes, ears, nose, lips, tongue, and tooth buds form. The arms and legs also take shape. Although the gender of the fetus isn't yet discernible, all external genitalia are present. Cardiovascular function is complete, and the umbilical cord has a definite form. At the end of the second month, the fetus resembles a full-term neonate except for size.

Month 3

During the third month, the fetus grows to 7.6 cm (3") and weighs 28.3 g (1 oz). Teeth and bones begin to appear, and the kidneys start to function. The fetus opens its mouth to swallow, grasps with its fully developed hands, and prepares for breathing by inhaling and exhaling (although its lungs aren't functioning). At the end of the first *trimester* (the 3-month periods into which pregnancy is divided), its gender is distinguishable.

Months 3 to 9

Over the remaining 6 months, fetal growth continues as internal and external structures develop at a rapid rate. In the third trimester, the fetus stores the fats and minerals it will need to live outside the womb. At birth, the average full-term fetus measures 50.1 cm (20") and weighs 3 to 3.5 kg (7 to 7½ lb).

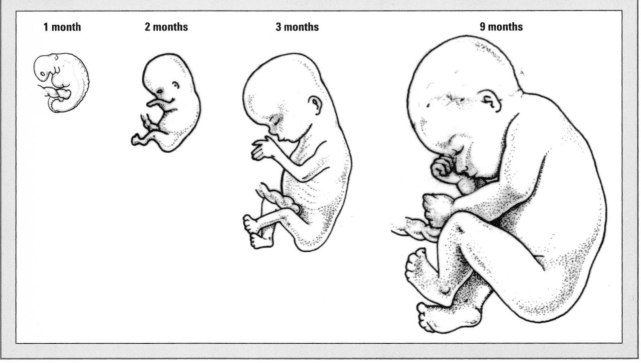

| 1 month | 2 months | 3 months | 9 months |

Two unusual features appear during this stage:

☝ The fetus's head is disproportionately large compared to its body. (This feature changes after birth as the infant grows.)

✌ The fetus lacks subcutaneous fat. (Fat starts to accumulate shortly after birth.)

Structural changes in the ovaries and uterus

During pregnancy, the reproductive system undergoes a number of changes.

Corpus luteum

Pregnancy changes the usual development of the corpus luteum and results in the development of the following structures:
• decidua
• amniotic sac and fluid
• yolk sac
• placenta.

Normal functioning of the corpus luteum requires continuous stimulation by LH. Progesterone produced by the corpus luteum suppresses LH release by the pituitary gland. If pregnancy occurs, the corpus luteum continues to produce progesterone until the placenta takes over. Otherwise, the corpus luteum atrophies 3 days before menstrual flow begins.

Hormone soup

With age, the corpus luteum grows less responsive to LH. Therefore, the mature corpus luteum degenerates unless stimulated by progressively increasing amounts of LH.

Pregnancy stimulates the placental tissue to secrete large amounts of human chorionic gonadotropin (HCG), which resembles LH and FSH. HCG prevents corpus luteum degeneration, stimulating the corpus luteum to produce large amounts of estrogen and progesterone.

Ups and downs of HCG

The corpus luteum, stimulated by the hormone HCG, produces the estrogen and progesterone needed to maintain the pregnancy during the first 3 months. HCG can be detected as early as 9 days after fertilization and can provide confirmation of pregnancy even before the woman has missed her first menses.

The HCG level gradually increases during this time, peaks at about 10 weeks' gestation, and then gradually declines.

> The fetus isn't the only thing changing during pregnancy—the mother's reproductive system undergoes changes as well.

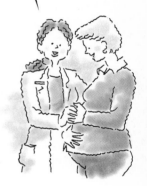

Decidua

The decidua is the endometrial lining of the uterus that undergoes hormone-induced changes during pregnancy. Decidual cells secrete the following three substances:

• the hormone *prolactin*, which promotes lactation
• a peptide hormone, *relaxin*, which induces relaxation of the connective tissue of the symphysis pubis and pelvic ligaments and promotes cervical dilation
• a potent hormonelike fatty acid, *prostaglandin*, which mediates several physiologic functions. (See *Development of the decidua and fetal membranes*.)

Amniotic sac and fluid

The amniotic sac, enclosed within the chorion, gradually grows and surrounds the embryo. As it enlarges, the amniotic sac expands into the chorionic cavity, eventually filling the cavity and fusing with the chorion by the 8th week of gestation.

A warm, protective sea

The amniotic sac and amniotic fluid serve the fetus in two important ways, one during gestation and the other during delivery. During gestation, the fluid gives the fetus a buoyant, temperature-controlled environment. Later, amniotic fluid serves as a fluid wedge that helps to open the cervix during birth.

Some from mom, some from baby

Early in pregnancy, amniotic fluid comes chiefly from three sources:

☝ fluid filtering into the amniotic sac from maternal blood as it passes through the uterus

✌ fluid filtering into the sac from fetal blood passing through the placenta

🖖 fluid diffusing into the amniotic sac from the fetal skin and respiratory tract.

Later in pregnancy, when the fetal kidneys begin to function, the fetus urinates into the amniotic fluid. Fetal urine then becomes the major source of amniotic fluid.

Every sea has its tides

Production of amniotic fluid from maternal and fetal sources balances amniotic fluid that's lost through the fetal GI tract. Typically, the fetus swallows up to several hundred milliliters of amniotic fluid each day. The fluid is absorbed into the fetal circulation from

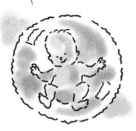

Amniotic fluid protects me during pregnancy—and later helps open the cervix for delivery.

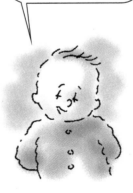

I've always had a good appetite—even as a fetus, when I slurped down lots of amniotic fluid each day! (Frankly, I prefer milk.)

Development of the decidua and fetal membranes

Specialized tissues support, protect, and nurture the embryo and fetus throughout its development. Among these tissues, the decidua and fetal membranes begin to develop shortly after conception.

Decidua

During pregnancy, the endometrial lining is called the *decidua*. It provides a nesting place for the developing ovum and has some endocrine functions.

Based primarily on its position relative to the embryo, the decidua may be known as the *decidua basalis,* which lies beneath the chorionic vesicle; the *decidua capsularis,* which stretches over the vesicle; or the *decidua parietalis,* which lines the remainder of the endometrial cavity.

Fetal membranes

The *chorion* is a membrane that forms the outer wall of the blastocyst. Vascular projections, called *chorionic villi,* arise from its periphery. As the chorionic vesicle enlarges, villi arising from the superficial portion of the chorion, called the *chorion laeve,* atrophy, leaving this surface smooth. Villi arising from the deeper part of the chorion, called the *chorion frondosum,* proliferate, projecting into the large blood vessels within the decidua basalis through which the maternal blood flows.

Blood vessels that form within the growing villi become connected with blood vessels that form in the chorion, in the body stalk, and within the body of the embryo. Blood begins to flow through this developing network of vessels as soon as the embryo's heart starts to beat.

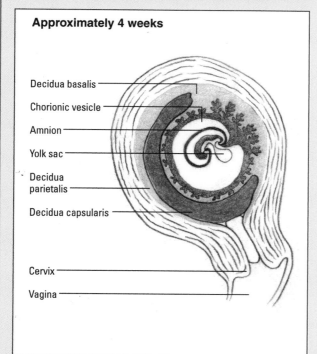

Approximately 4 weeks

- Decidua basalis
- Chorionic vesicle
- Amnion
- Yolk sac
- Decidua parietalis
- Decidua capsularis
- Cervix
- Vagina

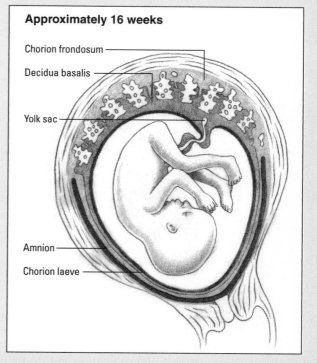

Approximately 16 weeks

- Chorion frondosum
- Decidua basalis
- Yolk sac
- Amnion
- Chorion laeve

the fetal GI tract; some is transferred from the fetal circulation to the maternal circulation and excreted in maternal urine.

Yolk sac

The yolk sac forms next to the endoderm of the germ disk; a portion of it is incorporated in the developing embryo and forms the GI tract. Another portion of the sac develops into primitive germ cells, which travel to the developing gonads and eventually form *oocytes* (the precursor of the ovum) or *spermatocytes* (the precursor of the spermatozoon) after gender has been determined.

Here today, gone tomorrow

During early embryonic development, the yolk sac also forms blood cells. Eventually, it undergoes atrophy and disintegrates.

Placenta

Using the umbilical cord as its conduit, the flattened, disk-shaped placenta provides nutrients to and removes wastes from the fetus from the 3rd month of pregnancy until birth. The placenta is formed from the chorion, its chorionic villi, and the adjacent decidua basalis.

A fetal lifeline

The umbilical cord contains two arteries and one vein and links the fetus to the placenta. The umbilical arteries, which transport blood from the fetus to the placenta, take a spiral course on the cord, divide on the placental surface, and branch off to the chorionic villi. (See *Picturing the placenta.*)

In a helpful vein

The placenta is a highly vascular organ. Large veins on its surface gather blood returning from the villi and join to form the single umbilical vein, which enters the cord, returning blood to the fetus.

Specialists on the job

The placenta contains two highly specialized circulatory systems:
• The *uteroplacental* circulation carries oxygenated arterial blood from the maternal circulation to the intervillous spaces—large spaces separating chorionic villi in the placenta. Blood enters the intervillous spaces from uterine arteries that penetrate the basal part of the placenta; it leaves the intervillous spaces and flows back into the maternal circulation through veins in the basal part of the placenta near the arteries.

> The placenta has two circulation systems—one involving maternal blood and another transporting fetal blood.

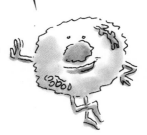

Picturing the placenta

At term, the placenta (the spongy structure within the uterus from which the fetus derives nourishment) is flat, cakelike, and round or oval. It measures 15 to 19.5 cm (6″ to 7¾″) in diameter and 2 to 3 cm (¾″ to 1¼″) in breadth at its thickest part. The maternal side is lobulated; the fetal side is shiny.

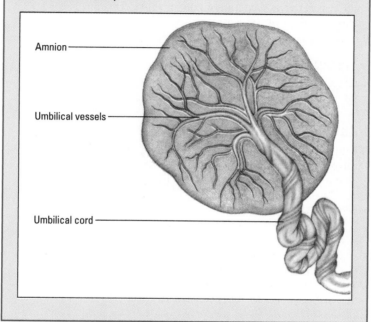

Amnion

Umbilical vessels

Umbilical cord

• The *fetoplacental* circulation transports oxygen-depleted blood from the fetus to the chorionic villi by the umbilical arteries and returns oxygenated blood to the fetus through the umbilical vein.

Placenta takes charge

For the first 3 months of pregnancy, the corpus luteum is the main source of estrogen and progesterone—hormones required during pregnancy. By the end of the third month, however, the placenta produces most of the hormones; the corpus luteum persists but is no longer needed to maintain the pregnancy.

Hormones on the rise

The levels of estrogen and progesterone, two steroid hormones, increase progressively throughout pregnancy. Estrogen stimulates uterine development to provide a suitable environment for the fetus.

Progesterone, synthesized by the placenta from maternal cholesterol, reduces uterine muscle irritability and prevents spontaneous abortion of the fetus.

Keep those acids coming

The placenta also produces human placental lactogen (HPL), which resembles growth hormone. HPL stimulates maternal protein and fat metabolism to ensure a sufficient supply of amino acids and fatty acids for the mother and fetus. HPL also stimulates breast growth in preparation for lactation. Throughout pregnancy, HPL levels rise progressively.

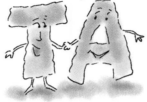

That placenta thinks of everything!

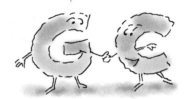

It produces HPL to make sure mom and fetus get enough of us—amino acids!

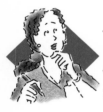

Quick quiz

1. Spermatogenesis is:
   A. the growth and development of sperm into primary spermatocytes.
   B. the division of spermatocytes to form secondary spermatocytes.
   C. the structural changing of spermatids.
   D. the entire process of sperm formation.

   Answer: D. Spermatogenesis refers to the entire process of sperm formation—from the development of primary spermatocytes to the formation of fully functional spermatozoa.

2. The primary function of the scrotum is to:
   A. provide storage for newly developed sperm.
   B. maintain a cool temperature for the testes.
   C. deposit sperm in the female reproductive tract.
   D. provide a place for spermatogenesis to take place.

   Answer: B. The function of the scrotum is to maintain a cool temperature for the testes, which is necessary for spermatozoa formation.

3. The main function of the ovaries is to:
   A.   secrete hormones that affect the buildup and shedding of the endometrium during the menstrual cycle.
   B.   accommodate a growing fetus during pregnancy.
   C.   produce mature ova.
   D.   channel blood discharged from the uterus during menstruation.

Answer: C. The main function of the ovaries is to produce mature ova.

4. The corpus luteum degenerates in which phase of the female reproductive cycle?
   A.   Luteal
   B.   Follicular
   C.   Proliferative
   D.   Ovarian

Answer: A. The corpus luteum degenerates in the luteal phase of the ovarian cycle of reproduction.

5. The four hormones involved in the menstrual cycle are:
   A.   LH, progesterone, estrogen, and testosterone.
   B.   estrogen, FSH, LH, and androgens.
   C.   estrogen, progesterone, LH, and FSH.
   D.   LH, estrogen, testosterone, and androgens.

Answer: C. The four hormones involved in the menstrual cycle are estrogen, progesterone, LH, and FSH.

6. Each of the three germ layers forms specific tissues and organs in the developing:
   A.   zygote.
   B.   ovum.
   C.   embryo.
   D.   fetus.

Answer: C. Each of the three germ layers (ectoderm, mesoderm, and endoderm) forms specific tissues and organs in the developing embryo.

7. The structure that guards the fetus is the:
   A.   decidua.
   B.   amniotic sac.
   C.   corpus luteum.
   D.   yolk sac.

Answer: B. The structure that guards the fetus by producing a buoyant, temperature-controlled environment is the amniotic sac.

Scoring

☆☆☆   If you answered all seven questions correctly, fantastic! You're
         fertilization-friendly!

 ☆☆   If you answered five or six questions correctly, excellent! Now re-
         produce that success in the chapters ahead!

  ☆   If you answered fewer than five questions correctly, don't fear!
         Your concept of conception will improve after a little review.

3

Family planning, contraception, and infertility

Just the facts

In this chapter, you'll learn:

♦ goals of family planning

♦ various methods of contraception, including the advantages and disadvantages of each

♦ surgical methods of family planning

♦ issues related to elective termination of pregnancy

♦ causes of infertility

♦ treatments and procedures used to correct infertility.

A look at family planning

Family planning involves the decisions couples or individuals make regarding when (and if) they should have children, how many children to have, and how long to wait between pregnancies. Family planning also consists of choices to prevent or achieve pregnancy and to control the timing and number of pregnancies. Family planning is a personal topic that has many ethical, physical, emotional, religious, and legal implications. Effectiveness, cost, contraindications, and adverse effects for all contraceptives should be presented to the patient and her partner so that they can make an informed decision.

> Information is power. Keep couples informed so they can make the family planning decisions that are best for them.

A look at contraception

Contraception is the deliberate prevention of conception, using a method or device to avert fertilization of an ovum.

Choosing a contraceptive

When discussing with a patient the contraceptive methods that are most appropriate for her and her partner, remember that a contraceptive should be safe, easily obtained, free from adverse effects, affordable, acceptable to the user and her partner, and free from effects on future pregnancies. In addition, couples should use a contraceptive that's as close as possible to being 100% effective.

History lesson

Information from the patient's menstrual and obstetric history should be used to determine which contraceptive method is best for her. The patient's history is also used to plan appropriate patient teaching.

An assessment for family planning involves collecting a reproductive history, including:
- interval between menses
- duration and amount of flow
- problems that occur during menses
- number of previous pregnancies
- number of previous births (and date of each)
- duration of each pregnancy
- type of each delivery
- gender and weight of children when delivered
- problems during previous pregnancies
- problems after delivery.

Scope out potential complications

The patient's health history may also identify potential risks of complications and help to determine whether hormonal contraceptives are safe for the patient to use. For example, a breast-feeding patient may be prescribed progesterone alone or a low-dose combination of hormonal contraceptives, which may cause her milk supply to decrease.

Factor in the partner

In some cases, the health of the patient's sexual partner influences which contraception method is used. For example, if the patient's

> It's elementary, my dear Watson! A patient's health history will provide clues about which contraceptive method is best for her.

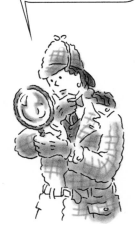

sexual partner is infected with human immunodeficiency virus (HIV), ideally, she should practice abstinence. If this isn't an option for your patient, encourage her to use a condom to prevent conception as well as infection transmission.

Implementing the chosen contraceptive

The effectiveness and safety of any contraceptive depends greatly on the patient's knowledge of and compliance with the chosen method. The patient's inability to understand proper use of the contraceptive device or an unwillingness to use it correctly or consistently may result in pregnancy. That's why patient teaching is such an important component of family planning. (See *Teaching tips on contraception*.)

With proper instruction and information, the patient should be able to:
• describe the use of the selected contraceptive correctly
• describe adverse reactions to the selected contraceptive and state her responsibility to report any that occur
• state that she'll make an appointment for her next visit (if indicated)
• express that the current method of birth control is an acceptable method for her.

> Where are those instructions? Having the right information and instructions is key to the proper use of contraceptives—and to fixing this bike!

Education edge

Teaching tips on contraception

Here are some points you should cover when teaching a patient about contraception:
• Teach proper use of the selected contraceptive, and describe the procedure for the chosen method accurately.
• Discuss possible adverse reactions. Direct the patient to report adverse reactions to her health care provider.
• Stress the importance of keeping follow-up appointments. During follow-up visits, contraceptive use and adverse reactions are evaluated and a repeat Papanicolaou test is performed. Follow-up visits also provide an opportunity to address any questions the patient may have.
• Answer all questions in a manner that's easily understood by the patient.

Methods of contraception

Contraceptive methods include abstinence, natural family planning methods, oral contraceptives, the morning-after pill (MAP), the intravaginal method, transdermal contraceptive patches, I.M. injections, intrauterine devices, and mechanical and chemical barrier methods.

Abstinence

Abstinence, or refraining from having sexual intercourse, has a 0% failure rate. It's also the most effective way to prevent the transmission of sexually transmitted diseases (STDs). However, most individuals—especially adolescents—don't consider it an option or a form of contraception. Abstinence should always be presented as an option to the patient in addition to information about other forms of contraception.

The plus side

Here are the advantages of abstinence:
• It's the only method that's 100% effective against pregnancy and STDs.
• It's free.
• There are no contraindications.

The minus side

Here are the disadvantages of abstinence:
• Partners and peers may have negative reactions to it.
• It requires commitment and self-control from both partners.

Natural family planning methods

Natural family planning methods are contraceptive methods that don't use chemicals or foreign material or devices to prevent pregnancy. Religious beliefs may prevent some individuals from using hormonal or internal contraceptive devices. Others just prefer a more natural method of planning or preventing pregnancy. Natural family planning methods include the rhythm (calendar) method, basal body temperature method, cervical mucus (Billings) method, symptothermal method, ovulation awareness, and coitus interruptus.

Keeping count

For most natural family planning methods, the woman's fertile days must be calculated so that she can abstain from intercourse on those days. Various methods are used to determine the woman's fertile period. The effectiveness of these methods depends on the patient's and partner's willingness to refrain from sex on the female partner's fertile days. Failure rates vary from 10% to 20%.

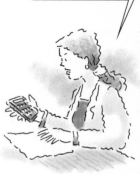

> Calculate the woman's fertile days? Nobody told me there would be a math test!

Rhythm method

The rhythm, or calendar, method requires that the couple refrain from intercourse on the days that the woman is most likely to conceive based on her menstrual cycle. This fertile period usually lasts from 3 or 4 days before until 3 or 4 days after ovulation.

Dear diary

Teach the woman to keep a diary of her menstrual cycle to determine when ovulation is most likely to occur. She should do this for 6 consecutive cycles. To calculate her safe periods, tell her to subtract 18 from the shortest cycle and 11 from the longest cycle that she has documented. For instance, if she had 6 menstrual cycles that lasted 26 to 30 days, her fertile period would be from the 8th day (26 minus 18) to the 19th day (30 minus 11). To ensure that pregnancy doesn't occur, she and her partner should abstain from intercourse during days 8 to 19 of her menstrual cycle. During those fertile days, she and her partner may also choose to use contraceptive foam. (See *Using the calendar method*, page 64.)

> I've got rhythm, I've got music…but that won't necessarily keep me from getting pregnant. The rhythm method requires meticulous record-keeping and the ability to monitor body changes.

The plus side

Here are the advantages of the rhythm method:
• No drugs or devices are needed.
• It's free.
• It may be acceptable to members of religious groups that oppose birth control.
• It encourages couples to learn more about how the female body functions.
• It encourages communication between partners.
• It can also be used to plan a pregnancy.

The minus side

Here are the disadvantages of the rhythm method:
• It requires meticulous record-keeping as well as an ability and willingness for the woman to monitor her body changes.
• It restricts sexual spontaneity during the woman's fertile period.

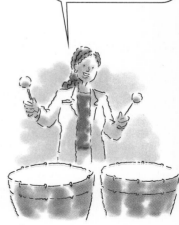

Using the calendar method

This illustration demonstrates how the calendar method would be used to determine the woman's fertile period (ovulation) and when she should abstain from coitus.

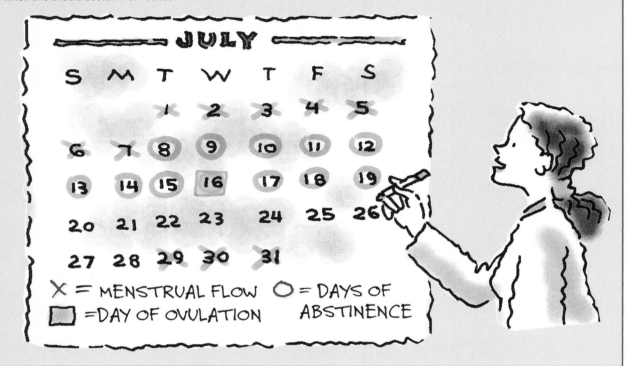

- It requires extended periods of abstinence from intercourse.
- It's only reliable for women with regular menstrual cycles.
- It may be unreliable during periods of illness, infection, or stress.

Basal body temperature

Just before the day of ovulation, a woman's basal body temperature (BBT) falls about one-half of a degree. At the time of ovulation, her BBT rises a full degree because of progesterone influence.

Ups and downs, highs and lows

To use the BBT method of contraception, a woman must take her temperature every morning before sitting up, getting out of bed, or beginning her morning activity. (See *Teaching a patient how to take BBT*, pages 66 and 67.) By recording this daily temperature, she can see a slight dip and then an increase in body temperature. The increase in temperature indicates that she has ovulated. She should refrain from intercourse for the next 3 days. Three days is significant because this is the lifespan of a discharged ovum. Because sperm can survive in the female reproductive tract for 4 days, the BBT method of contraception is typically combined with the calendar method so that the couple can abstain from intercourse a few days before ovulation as well.

Various variables

One problem with this method is that many things can affect BBT. The woman may forget and take her temperature after rising out of bed or she may have a slight illness. These situations cause a rise in temperature. If the woman changes her daily routine, the change in activity could also affect her body temperature, which may lead her to mistakenly interpret a fertile day as a safe day and vice versa.

The plus side

Here are the advantages of the BBT method:
• It's inexpensive. The only expense involved is the cost of a BBT thermometer, which is calibrated in tenths of a degree.
• No drugs are needed.
• It may be acceptable to members of religious groups that oppose birth control.
• It encourages couples to learn more about how the female body functions.
• It encourages communication between partners.
• It can also be used to plan a pregnancy.

The minus side

Here are the disadvantages of the BBT method:
• It requires meticulous record-keeping and an ability and willingness to monitor the woman's body changes.
• It restricts sexual spontaneity during the woman's fertile period.
• It requires extended periods of abstinence from intercourse.
• It's reliable only for women with regular menstrual cycles.
• It may be unreliable during periods of illness, infection, or stress.
• It's contraindicated in women who have irregular menses.

Cervical mucus

The cervical mucus method (also known as the *Billings method*) predicts changes in the cervical mucus during ovulation. Each month, before a woman's menses, the cervical mucus becomes thick and stretches when pulled between the thumb and forefin-

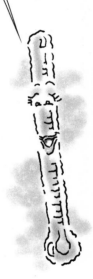

To get an accurate reading, a patient should take her basal body temperature before rising from bed.

Education edge

Teaching a patient how to take BBT

Here are tips to help you teach your patient about recording basal body temperature (BBT). Remind the patient that BBT is lower during the first 2 weeks of the menstrual cycle, before ovulation. Immediately after ovulation, the temperature begins to rise. It continues to rise until it's time for the next menses. This rise in temperature indicates that progesterone has been released into the system, which, in turn, means that the woman has ovulated.

Charting BBT doesn't predict the exact day of ovulation; it just indicates that ovulation has occurred. However, this can be used to help the patient to monitor her ovulatory pattern and give her a timeframe during which ovulation occurs.

Getting started

Tell your patient to follow these instructions for taking BBT:
• Advise the patient to chart the days of menstrual flow by darkening the squares above the 98° F (36.7° C) mark. She should start with the first day of her menses (day 1) and then take her temperature each day after her menses ends.
• Tell the patient to use a thermometer that measures tenths of a degree.
• Instruct the patient to take her temperature as soon as she wakes up. Tell her that it's important to do this at the same time each morning.

• The patient should then place a dot on the graph's line that matches the temperature reading. (Tell her not to be surprised if her waking temperature before ovulation is 96° or 97° F [35.6° or 36.1° C].) If she forgets to take her temperature on one day, instruct her to leave that day blank on the graph and not to connect the dots.
• Instruct her to make notes on the graph if she misses taking her temperature, feels sick, can't sleep, or wakes up at a different time. Advise her also that if she's taking any medicine—even aspirin—it may affect her temperature. Remind her to mark the dates when she has sexual intercourse.

Sample chart

Look over the sample temperature chart, recorded by "Susan Jones." Ms. Jones used an S to record sexual intercourse and made notes showing she had insomnia on September 27. She forgot to take her temperature on September 19. Notice that she didn't connect the dots on this day. Her temperature dipped on September 24 (day 15 of the cycle) and began rising afterward.

Of course, your patient's chart will be larger and will probably include temperatures over 99.3° F (37.4° C) and under 97° F.

ger. The normal stretchable amount of cervical mucus (also known as *spinnbarkeit*) is 8 to 10 cm (3″ to 4″). Just before ovulation, the cervical mucus becomes thin, watery, transparent, and copious.

Slippery peaks

During the peak of ovulation, the cervical mucus becomes slippery and stretches at least 2.5 cm (1″) before the strand breaks. Breast tenderness and anterior tilt of the cervix also occur with ovulation. The fertile period consists of all the days that the cervical mucus is copious and the 3 days after the peak date. During these days, the woman and her partner should abstain from intercourse to avoid conception.

Sample temperature chart

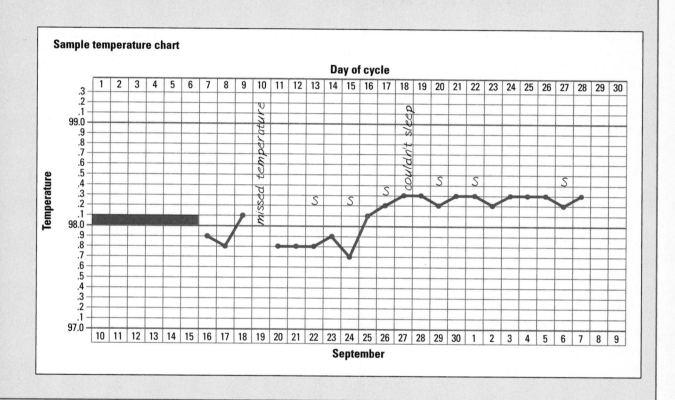

Consistently checking consistency

Cervical mucus must be assessed every day for changes in consistency and amounts to be sure that those changes signify ovulation. Assessing cervical mucus after intercourse is unreliable because seminal fluid has a watery, postovulatory consistency, which can be confused with ovulatory mucus.

The plus side

Here are the advantages of the cervical mucus method:
• No drugs or devices are needed.
• It's free.
• It may be acceptable to members of religious groups that oppose birth control.

• It encourages couples to learn more about how the female body functions.
• It encourages communication between partners.
• It can also be used to plan a pregnancy.
• There are no contraindications.

The minus side

Here are the disadvantages of the cervical mucus method:
• It requires meticulous record-keeping and an ability and willingness to monitor the woman's body changes.
• It restricts sexual spontaneity during the woman's fertile period.
• It requires extended periods of abstinence from intercourse.
• It's reliable only for women with regular menstrual cycles.
• It may be unreliable during periods of illness, infection, or stress.

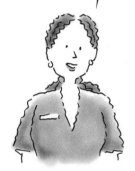

Combining the BBT and cervical mucus methods is more effective than using just one method.

Symptothermal method

The symptothermal method combines the BBT method with the cervical mucus method. The woman takes her daily temperature and watches for the rise in temperature that signals the onset of ovulation. She also assesses her cervical mucus every day. The couple abstains from intercourse until 3 days after the rise in basal temperature or the fourth day after the peak day (indicating ovulation) of cervical mucus because these signs signify the woman's fertile period. Combining these two methods is more effective than using either method alone.

The plus side

Here are the advantages of the symptothermal method:
• It's inexpensive. The only expense involved is the cost of a BBT thermometer, which is calibrated in tenths of a degree.
• No drugs are needed.
• It may be acceptable to members of religious groups that oppose birth control.
• It encourages patients and their partners to learn more about how the female body functions.
• It encourages communication between partners.
• It can also be used to plan a pregnancy.

The minus side

Here are the disadvantages of the symptothermal method:
• It requires meticulous record-keeping and ability and willingness of a woman to monitor body changes.
• It restricts sexual spontaneity during the woman's fertile period.
• It requires extended periods of abstinence from intercourse.
• It's reliable only for women with regular menstrual cycles.

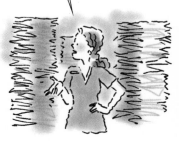

Phew! The symptothermal method certainly requires meticulous record-keeping!

• It may be unreliable during periods of illness, infection, or stress.

Ovulation awareness

Over-the-counter ovulation detection kits determine when ovulation occurs by measuring luteinizing hormone (LH) in the urine. Usually, during each menstrual cycle, LH levels rise suddenly (called an *LH surge*), causing an ovum to be released from the ovary 24 to 36 hours later (ovulation). This test determines the midcycle surge of LH, which can be detected in the urine as early as 12 to 24 hours after ovulation. These kits are about 98% to 100% accurate, but they're fairly expensive to use as a primary means of birth control. (See *Performing a home ovulation test*, page 70.)

The plus side

Here are the advantages of the ovulation awareness method:
• It's an easier way to determine ovulation than the BBT or cervical mucus methods.
• It may be less offensive to a woman than the cervical mucus method.
• It has a high rate of accuracy.
• There are no contraindications.

The minus side

Here are the disadvantages of the ovulation awareness method:
• It's expensive.
• It requires extended periods of abstinence from intercourse.
• It's reliable only for women with regular menstrual cycles.

Coitus interruptus

Coitus interruptus, one of the oldest known methods of contraception, involves withdrawal of the penis from the vagina during intercourse before ejaculation. However, because pre-ejaculation fluid that's deposited outside the vagina may contain spermatozoa, fertilization can occur.

The plus side

Here are the advantages of the coitus interruptus method:
• It's free.
• It doesn't involve record-keeping.
• There are no contraindications.

The minus side

Here are the disadvantages of the coitus interruptus method:
• It isn't reliable.
• It restricts sexual spontaneity.

Education edge

Performing a home ovulation test

A home ovulation test helps the patient determine the best time to try to become pregnant or to prevent pregnancy by monitoring the amount of luteinizing hormone (LH) that's found in her urine. These test kits can be purchased over-the-counter.

Normally, during each menstrual cycle, levels of LH rise suddenly, causing an egg to be released from the ovary 24 to 36 hours later.

Getting ready
Tell your patient to follow these instructions before performing a home ovulation test:
• Read the kit's directions thoroughly before performing the test.
• Before testing, calculate the length of the menstrual cycle. Count from the beginning of one menses to the beginning of the next menses. (The patient should count her first day of bleeding as day 1. She can use a chart such as the one shown at right to determine when to begin testing.)
• This test can be performed any time of the day or night, but it should be performed at the same time every day.
• Don't urinate for at least 4 hours before taking the test, and don't drink a lot of fluids for several hours before the test.

Taking the test
Tell your patient to follow these instructions for performing a home ovulation test:
• Remove the test stick from the packet.
• Sit on the toilet and direct the absorbent tip of the test stick downward and directly into the urine stream for at least 5 seconds or until it's thoroughly wet.
• Be careful not to urinate on the window of the stick.
• Alternatively, urinate in a clean, dry cup or container and then dip the test stick (absorbent tip only) into the urine for at least 5 seconds.
• Place the stick on a clean, flat, dry surface.

Reading the results
Explain to your patient the following instructions for reading home ovulation test results:
• Wait at least 5 minutes before reading the results. When the test is finished, a line appears in the small window (control window).
• If there's no line in the large rectangular window (test window) or if the line is lighter than the line in the small rectangular window (control window), the patient hasn't begun an LH surge. She should continue testing daily.
• If she sees one line in the large rectangular window that's similar to or darker than the line in the small window, she's experiencing an LH surge.

This means that ovulation should occur within the next 24 to 36 hours.
• Once the patient has determined that she's about to ovulate, she'll know she's at the start of the most fertile time of her cycle and should use this information to plan accordingly.

Length of cycle	Start test this many days after last menses begins	Length of cycle	Start test this many days after last menses begins
21	5	31	14
22	5	32	15
23	6	33	16
24	7	34	17
25	8	34	18
26	9	36	19
27	10	37	20
28	11	38	21
29	12	39	22
30	13	40	23

Oral contraceptives

Oral contraceptives (birth control pills) are hormonal contraceptives that consist of synthetic estrogen and progesterone. The estrogen suppresses production of follicle-stimulating hormone (FSH) and LH, which, in turn, suppresses ovulation. The progesterone complements the estrogen's action by causing a decrease in cervical mucus permeability, which limits sperm's access to the ova. Progesterone also decreases the possibility of implantation by interfering with endometrial proliferation.

Dosage duo

There are two types of oral contraceptives:

☞ Monophasic oral contraceptives provide fixed doses of estrogen and progesterone throughout a 21-day cycle. These preparations provide a steady dose of estrogen but an increased amount of progestin during the last 11 days of the menstrual cycle.

✌ Triphasic oral contraceptives maintain a cycle more like a woman's natural menstrual cycle because they vary the amount of estrogen and progestin throughout the cycle. Triphasic oral contraceptives have a lower incidence of breakthrough bleeding than monophasic oral contraceptives.

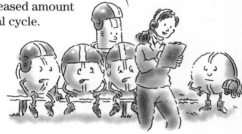

What a team! The estrogen in oral contraceptives suppresses ovulation and the progesterone decreases the permeability of cervical mucus.

Small but powerful

A mini pill is available for women who can't take estrogen-based pills because of a history of thrombophlebitis. This type of pill is taken every day—even when the woman has her menses. Progestins in the pill inhibit the development of the endometrium, thus preventing implantation.

21- or 28-day package deals

Monophasic and triphasic oral contraceptives are dispensed in either 21- or 28-day packs. The first pill is usually taken on the first Sunday following the start of a woman's menses, but it's possible to start oral contraceptives on any day. For a woman who has recently given birth, oral contraceptives can be started on the first Sunday 2 weeks after delivery. Patients should be advised to use an additional form of contraception for the first week after starting an oral contraceptive because the drug doesn't take effect for 7 days. (See *Teaching tips on oral contraceptives*, page 72.)

Birth control pills that are prescribed in a 21-day dispenser allow the woman to take a pill every day for 3 weeks. She should expect to start her menstrual flow about 4 days after she takes a cycle of pills. The 28-day pills are packaged with 21 days of birth

Education edge

Teaching tips on oral contraceptives

Be sure to include these tips when teaching patients about oral contraceptives:
• Inform the patient about possible adverse reactions, such as fluid retention, weight gain, breast tenderness, headache, breakthrough bleeding, chloasma, acne, yeast infection, nausea, and fatigue. It may be necessary to change the type or dosage of the contraceptive to relieve these adverse reactions.
• Instruct the patient on the dietary needs of a woman who's taking an oral contraceptive. Tell her to increase her intake of foods high in vitamin B_6 (wheat, corn, liver, meat) and folic acid

(liver; green, leafy vegetables). About 20% to 30% of oral contraceptive users have dietary deficiencies of vitamin B_6 and folic acid. Moreover, health care professionals speculate that oral contraceptive users should also increase their intake of vitamins A, B_2, B_{12}, C, and niacin.
• Advise the patient to use an additional form of contraception for the first 7 days after starting the drug because it doesn't take effect for 7 days.
• Advise the patient to use an additional form of contraception when taking antibiotics.

control pills and 7 days of placebos. The woman starts the new pack of pills when she finishes the last pack, eliminating the risk of forgetting to start a new pack.

It's seasonal

The newest type of oral contraceptive on the market is a combination of levonorgestrel and ethinyl estradiole called Seasonale. This once-daily pill extends the time between periods, allowing a woman to have a period four times a year as opposed to monthly.

The plus side

Here are the advantages of oral contraceptives:
• Monophasic and triphasic oral contraceptives are 99.5% effective. The failure rate is about 3%; failure usually occurs because the woman forgets to take the pill or because of other individual differences in the woman's physiology.
• They don't inhibit sexual spontaneity.
• They may reduce the risk of endometrial and ovarian cancer, ectopic pregnancy, ovarian cysts, and noncancerous breast tumors.
• They decrease the risk of pelvic inflammatory disease (PID) and dysmenorrhea.
• They regulate the menstrual cycle and may diminish or eliminate premenstrual tension.

The minus side

Here are the disadvantages of oral contraceptives:
• They don't protect the woman or her partner from STDs.
• They must be taken daily.

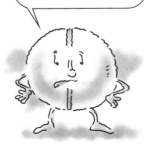

Oral contraceptives can help to regulate the menstrual cycle and decrease premenstrual symptoms. However, they need to be taken daily and they don't protect against STDs.

- They can be expensive (from $25 to $45 monthly).
- Illnesses that cause vomiting may reduce their effectiveness.
- Some antibiotics reduce their effectiveness.
- They're contraindicated in women who are breast-feeding or pregnant; those who have a family history of stroke, coronary artery disease, thrombohemolytic disease, or liver disease; and those who have undiagnosed vaginal bleeding, malignancy of the reproductive system, malignant cell growth, or hypertension.
- Women who are older than age 40, and those who have a history of or have been diagnosed with diabetes mellitus, elevated triglyceride or cholesterol level, breast or reproductive tract malignancy, high blood pressure, obesity, seizure disorder, sickle cell disease, mental depression, and migraines or other vascular-type headaches, should be strongly cautioned about taking oral contraceptives for birth control. The possible side effects of oral contraceptives may be more severe in women who fall under these categories.
- A patient older than age 35 is at increased risk for a fatal heart attack if she smokes more than 15 cigarettes per day and takes oral contraceptives.
- Adverse effects include nausea, headache, weight gain, depression, mild hypertension, breast tenderness, breakthrough bleeding, and monilial vaginal infections.
- When a woman wants to conceive, she may not be able to for up to 8 months after stopping oral contraceptives. The pituitary gland requires a recovery period to begin the stimulation of cyclic gonadotropins, such as FSH and LH, which help regulate ovulation. In addition, many practitioners recommend that women not become pregnant within 2 months of stopping oral contraceptives.

Morning-after pill

Also called *emergency contraception*, the MAP prevents pregnancy in the event of unprotected sexual intercourse or failure of a birth control method (such as a broken condom). It may be obtained from various doctors' offices and family planning clinics. The MAP is a pregnancy prevention measure, not an abortion pill.

The MAP is given as two doses of hormones: progesterone alone, estrogen alone, or a combination of both. The first dose must be taken within 72 hours of sexual intercourse; a second dose is taken 12 hours later. A woman may be prescribed a certain number of oral hormonal contraceptive pills from a birth control pack (estrogen and progesterone combination) or she may be prescribed a "plan B" pack, which contains 0.75 mg of levonorgestrel.

Medications for nausea may also be prescribed, and the woman is instructed to return to the office or clinic in 3 weeks.

She must also be instructed to use a birth control method consistently until her menstrual period begins.

The plus side

Here are the advantages of the MAP:
- It's 75% to 95% effective, depending on which product is used, when in the cycle intercourse occurred, how soon the woman uses the method, and whether she has had unprotected intercourse within the past 72 hours.
- It doesn't inhibit sexual spontaneity.
- It's readily available when unforeseen circumstances occur.

The minus side

Here are the disadvantages of the MAP:
- It doesn't offer protection from STDs.
- It must be taken within a 72-hour period after intercourse, and again 12 hours later.
- The hormone dosage is larger than that of oral hormonal contraceptives and commonly causes nausea, vomiting, and malaise.
- It can be expensive.
- Contraindications and precautions are similar to those for other oral hormonal contraceptives.

Intravaginal method

Another method of introducing hormones into the woman's circulation is the intravaginal route by a cervical ring that slowly releases contraceptive hormones. Called the NuvaRing, the woman inserts it into her vagina, where it stays held in by the vaginal walls, for 3 weeks. She then removes it, allowing her menstruation to occur, and then reinserts it after 1 week.

The plus side

Here are the advantages of the intravaginal method:
- It's inserted only every 3 weeks.
- The woman doesn't have to remember to take a pill every day.
- The woman has fewer hormonal peaks and decreases because of the slow but steady release.
- It's 99% effective.
- It allows sexual spontaneity.
- It's discreet.
- It's easy to insert.

The minus side

Here are the disadvantages of the intravaginal method:
- It doesn't protect the woman or her partner from STDs.
- It's contraindicated in women who are pregnant or may become pregnant; those who are breast-feeding; those who have a family history of stroke, coronary artery disease, thrombohemolytic disease, or liver disease; those who have undiagnosed vaginal bleeding; and those who are sensitive to the material in the ring.
- Women who are over age 40; women who have a history of or have been diagnosed with diabetes mellitus, elevated triglycerides or cholesterol level, breast or reproductive tact malignancy, high blood pressure, obesity, seizure disorder, sickle cell disease, mental depression, and migraines or other vascular-type headaches; and women who smoke should be strongly cautioned about using a hormonal contraceptive ring. The possible side effects of hormonal contraceptives may be greater in women with a history of these disorders.

Transdermal contraceptive patches

The transdermal contraceptive patch is a highly effective, weekly hormonal birth control patch that's worn on the skin. A combination of estrogen and progestin is integrated into the patch. The hormones are absorbed into the skin and then transferred into the bloodstream.

Patchwork

The patch is very thin, beige, and smooth, and measures 1¾″ (4.4 cm) square. It can be worn on the upper outer arm, buttocks, abdomen, or upper torso. The patch is worn for 1 week and replaced on the same day of the week for 3 consecutive weeks. No patch is worn during the fourth week. Studies have shown that the patch remains attached and effective when the patient bathes, swims, exercises, or wears it in humid weather.

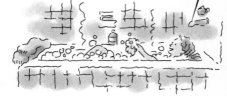

What a trooper! The transdermal contraceptive patch remains attached to the skin, even when the patient bathes, swims, or exercises.

The plus side

Here are the advantages of the transdermal contraceptive patch:
- It's 99% effective in preventing pregnancy if used exactly as directed.
- It's convenient. No preparation is needed before intercourse.
- It's a good alternative for patients who commonly forget to take oral contraceptives.

The minus side

Here are the disadvantages of the transdermal patch:
• It doesn't protect the woman or her partner from STDs.
• It's contraindicated in women who are breast-feeding; those who have a family history of stroke, coronary artery disease, thrombohemolytic disease, or liver disease; those who have undiagnosed vaginal bleeding; and those who are sensitive to the adhesive used on the patch.
• Women who are over age 40; women who have a history of or have been diagnosed with diabetes mellitus, elevated triglycerides or cholesterol level, breast or reproductive tract malignancy, high blood pressure, obesity, seizure disorder, sickle cell disease, mental depression, and migraines or other vascular-type headaches; and women who smoke should be strongly cautioned about using a transdermal contraceptive patch for birth control. The possible side effects of hormonal contraceptives may be more severe in women who fall under these categories.
• It has been found to be slightly less effective in women who weigh more than 198 lbs (89.8 kg). These women may need to consider another form of contraception.
• Some antibiotics reduce its effectiveness.

I.M. injections

I.M. injections of medroxyprogesterone (Depo-Provera) are administered every 12 weeks. Depo-Provera stops ovulation from occurring by suppressing the release of gonadotropic hormones. It also changes the cervical mucosa to prevent sperm from entering the uterus.

The plus side

Here are the advantages of I.M. Depo-Provera:
• It doesn't inhibit sexual response.
• Except for abstinence, it's more effective than other birth control methods.
• It helps prevent endometrial cancer.

The minus side

Here are the disadvantages of I.M. Depo-Provera:
• It requires an injection every 12 weeks.
• It can be expensive. Each injection costs about $35, including injection fees.
• If the patient wants to become pregnant, it may take 9 to 24 months after the last injection to conceive.
• It doesn't protect against STDs.

- Its effects can't be reversed after it's injected.
- It may cause changes in the menstrual cycle.
- It may cause weight gain because of an increase in appetite.
- It may cause headache, fatigue, and nervousness.
- It's contraindicated if the patient is pregnant or has liver disease, undiagnosed vaginal bleeding, breast cancer, blood clotting disorders, or cardiovascular disease.

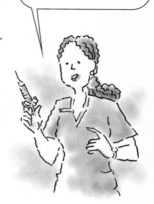

Depo-Provera is highly effective, but it does require a bit of an "Ouch!" every 12 weeks.

Intrauterine device

The intrauterine device (IUD) is a plastic contraceptive device that's inserted into the uterus through the cervical canal. (See *IUD insertion*, page 78.) The IUD is inserted into and removed from the uterus most easily during the woman's menses, when the cervical canal is slightly dilated. Inserting the device during menses also reduces the likelihood of inserting an IUD into a woman who's pregnant.

Copper interference

One type of IUD, the ParaGard-T, is a T-shaped, polyethylene device with copper wrapped around its vertical stem. The copper interferes with sperm mobility, decreasing the possibility of sperm crossing the uterine space. A knotted monofilament retrieval string is attached through a hole in the stem.

Progesterone reserve

Another type of IUD, the Progestasert IUD system, is a T-shaped device made of an ethylene vinyl acetate copolymer with a knotted monofilament retrieval string attached through a hole in the vertical stem. Progesterone is stored in the hollow vertical stem, suspended in an oil base. The drug gradually diffuses into the uterus and prevents endometrium proliferation. This IUD must be replaced annually to replenish the progesterone. The Progestasert system may relieve excessive menstrual blood loss and dysmenorrhea.

If a woman becomes pregnant with an IUD in place, the device can be left; however, it's usually removed to prevent spontaneous abortion and infection.

The plus side

Here are the advantages of an IUD:
- It doesn't inhibit sexual spontaneity.
- Neither partner feels the device during intercourse.

IUD insertion

An intrauterine device (IUD) is a plastic contraceptive device that's inserted into a woman's uterus through the cervical canal. This is performed most easily during menses. A bimanual examination is performed to determine uterine position, shape, and size.

Before IUD insertion, make sure that the procedure has been explained to the patient and that her questions have been addressed. Also, be sure to obtain informed consent.

How it's done
Here's how the device is inserted.

The movable flange on the inserter barrel of the IUD is set to the depth of the uterus (measured in centimeters). The loaded inserter tube is introduced through the cervical canal and into the uterus.

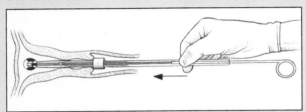

The IUD is inserted by retracting the inserter slowly about ½" (1.3 cm) over the plunger while the plunger is held still. This allows the arms to open.

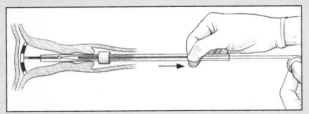

The plunger is gently advanced until resistance is felt. This action ensures high fundal placement of the IUD and may reduce the potential for expulsion.

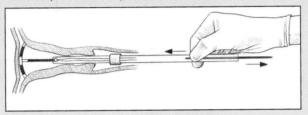

The solid rod is withdrawn while the inserting barrel is held stationary. The insertion barrel is then withdrawn from the cervix. The strings are clipped about 1" to 3" (2.5 to 7.5 cm) from the cervical os. This action leaves sufficient string for checking the placement of and removing the IUD.

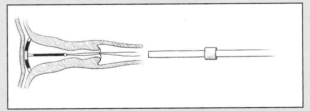

The minus side

Here are the disadvantages of an IUD:
- It's expensive.
- It may cause uterine cramping on insertion.
- It may cause infection, especially in the initial weeks after insertion.
- It can be spontaneously expelled in the first year by 5% to 20% of women.

- It doesn't protect against STDs.
- The incidence of PID increases with IUD use. Most cases of PID occur during the first 3 months after insertion. After 3 months, the risk of PID is lower unless preinsertion screening failed to identify a person at risk for STDs. The patient should be instructed to watch for signs of PID. (See *Signs of PID*.)
- It increases the risk of ectopic pregnancy.
- It's contraindicated in women who have Wilson's disease (because of the inability to metabolize copper properly).
- It's contraindicated in women who have active, recent, or recurrent PID; infection or inflammation of the genital tract; STDs; diseases that suppress immune function, including HIV; unexplained cervical or vaginal bleeding; previous problems with IUDs; cancer of the reproductive organs; or a history of ectopic pregnancy. Insertion is also contraindicated in patients who have severe vasovagal reactivity, difficulty obtaining emergency care, valvular heart disease, anatomic uterine deformities, anemia, or nulliparity.

Barrier methods

In the barrier methods of contraception, a chemical or mechanical barrier is inserted between the cervix and the sperm to prevent the sperm from entering the uterus, traveling to the fallopian tubes, and fertilizing the ovum. Because barrier methods don't use hormones, they're sometimes favored over hormonal contraceptives, which can cause many adverse effects. However, failure rates for barrier methods are higher than for hormonal contraceptives.

Barrier methods include spermicidal products, diaphragms, cervical caps, vaginal rings, and male and female condoms.

Spermicidal products

Before intercourse, spermicidal products are inserted into the vagina. Their goal is to kill sperm before the sperm enter the cervix. Spermicides also change the pH of the vaginal fluid to a strong acid, which isn't conducive to sperm survival. Vaginally inserted spermicides are available in gels, creams, films, foams, and suppositories.

The gels, foams, and creams are inserted using an applicator and should be inserted at least 1 hour before intercourse. The woman should be instructed not to douche for 6 hours after intercourse to ensure that the agent has completed its spermicidal action in the vagina and cervix.

Spermicidal films are made of glycerin that's impregnated with nonoxynol 9. The film is folded and then inserted into the

Education edge

Signs of PID

If your patient has an intrauterine device, tell her that untreated vaginal infections can progress to pelvic inflammatory disease (PID). Instruct the patient to watch for signs and symptoms of PID, such as:
- fever of 101° F (38.3° C)
- purulent vaginal discharge
- painful intercourse
- abdominal or pelvic pain
- suprapubic tenderness or guarding
- tenderness on bimanual examination.

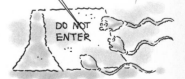

Barrier methods block us from entering the uterus and fertilizing the ovum.

That doesn't seem fair!

DO NOT ENTER

vagina. When the film makes contact with vaginal secretions or precoital penile emissions, it dissolves and carbon dioxide foam forms to protect the cervix against invading spermatozoa.

Spermicidal suppositories consist of cocoa butter and glycerin and are filled with nonoxynol 9. The suppositories are inserted into the vagina, where they dissolve to release the spermicide. The suppository takes 15 minutes to dissolve, so patients should be instructed to insert it 15 minutes before intercourse.

The plus side

Here are the advantages of spermicidal products:
- They're inexpensive.
- They may be purchased over-the-counter, which makes them easily accessible.
- They don't require a visit to a health care provider.
- Spermicidal films wash away with natural body fluids.
- Nonoxynol 9, one of the most preferred spermicides, may also help prevent the spread of STDs.
- Vaginally inserted spermicides may be used in combination with other birth control methods to increase their effectiveness.
- They're useful in emergency situations such as when a condom breaks.

The minus side

Here are the disadvantages of spermicidal products:
- They need to be inserted from 15 minutes to 1 hour before intercourse, so they may interfere with sexual spontaneity.
- Some spermicides may be irritating to the vagina and penile tissue.
- Some women are bothered by the vaginal leakage that can occur, especially after using cocoa- and glycerin-based suppositories.
- The film foam's effectiveness depends on vaginal secretions; therefore, it isn't recommended for women who are nearing menopause because decreased vaginal secretions make the film less effective.
- Spermicidal products may be contraindicated in women who have acute cervicitis because of the risk of further irritation.

Diaphragm

The diaphragm is another barrier-type contraceptive that mechanically blocks sperm from entering the cervix. It's composed of a soft, latex dome that's supported by a round, metal spring on the outside. A diaphragm can be inserted up to 2 hours before intercourse. Optimum effectiveness is achieved by using it in combination with spermicidal jelly that's applied to the rim of the diaphragm before it's inserted. Diaphragms are available in various sizes and must be fitted to the individual. (See *Inserting a diaphragm*, page 82.)

The plus side

Here are the advantages of the diaphragm:
• It's a good choice for women who choose not to use hormonal contraceptives or don't feel that they can use natural family planning methods effectively.
• When combined with spermicidal jelly, its effectiveness ranges from 80% to 93% for new users and increases to 97% for long-term users.
• It causes few adverse reactions.
• It helps protect against STDs when used with spermicide.
• It doesn't alter the body's metabolic or physiologic processes.
• It can be inserted up to 2 hours before intercourse.
• Providing it's correctly fitted and inserted, neither partner can feel it during intercourse.

The minus side

Here are the disadvantages of the diaphragm:
• It must be inserted before intercourse and may interfere with spontaneity.
• Although it can be left in place for up to 24 hours, if intercourse is repeated before 6 hours (which is how long the diaphragm *must* be left in place after intercourse) more spermicidal gel must be inserted. The diaphragm can't be removed and replaced because this could cause sperm to bypass the spermicidal gel and fertilization could occur.
• The pressure it creates on the urethra may cause a higher incidence of upper urinary tract infections (UTIs).
• It must be refitted after birth, cervical surgery, miscarriage, dilatation and curettage (D&C), therapeutic abortion, or weight gain or loss of more than 15 lb (6.8 kg) because of cervical shape changes.
• It's contraindicated in women who have a history of cystocele, rectocele, uterine retroversion, prolapse, retroflexion, or anteflexion because the cervix position may be displaced, making insertion and proper fit questionable.
• It's contraindicated in patients with a history of toxic shock syndrome or repeated UTIs, vaginal stenosis, pelvic abnormalities, or allergy to spermicidal jellies or rubber. It's also contraindicated in patients who show an unwillingness to learn proper techniques for diaphragm care and insertion.
• It can't be used in the first 6 weeks postpartum.

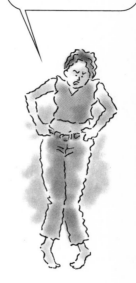

Size really does matter when it comes to diaphragms—not to mention jeans!

Education edge

Inserting a diaphragm

As you insert a diaphragm, instruct the patient to prepare her for inserting the diaphragm herself. Identify structures and the feelings associated with proper insertion. Follow these steps for insertion.

After putting on gloves, lubricate the rim or dome of the fitting ring or diaphragm to lessen the discomfort of insertion.

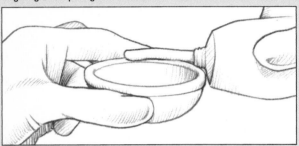

Fold the diaphragm in half with one hand by pressing the opposite sides together. Hold the vulva open with your other hand.

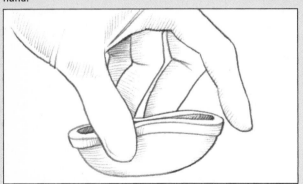

Slide the folded diaphragm into the vagina and toward the posterior cervicovaginal fornix.

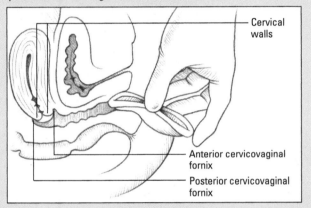

Cervical walls

Anterior cervicovaginal fornix

Posterior cervicovaginal fornix

The diaphragm should fit below the symphysis and cover the cervix. The proximal ring should fit behind the pubic arch with minimal pressure. Note that the cervix is palpable behind the diaphragm. The cervix feels like a "nose."

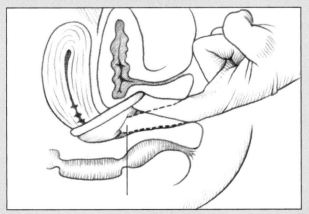

Cervical cap

The cervical cap is another barrier-type method of contraception. It's similar to the diaphragm but smaller. It's a thimble-shaped, soft rubber cup that the patient places over the cervix. The cap is held in place by suction. The addition of a spermicide creates a chemical barrier as well. Women who aren't suited for diaphragms may use cervical caps. Failure of the cervical cap is commonly due to failure to use the device or inappropriate use of the device. (See *Recognizing a correct fit.*)

Along with a spermicide, a cervical cap creates a mechanical and chemical barrier.

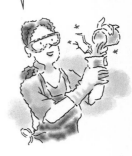

The plus side

Here are the advantages of the cervical cap:
• It requires less spermicide, is less likely to become dislodged during intercourse, and doesn't require refitting with a change in weight.
• It's 85% effective for nulliparous women and 70% effective for parous women when used correctly and consistently.

Advice from the experts

Recognizing a correct fit

With the proper fit, the gap or space between the base of the cervix and the inside of the cervical cap ring should be 1 to 2 mm (to reduce the possibility of dislodgment), and the rim should fill the cervicovaginal fornix.

To verify a good fit, leave the cervical cap in place for 1 to 2 minutes. Then, with the cap in place, pinch the dome until there's a dimple. A dimple that takes about 30 seconds to resume a domed appearance indicates good suction and a good fit. If the cap is too small, the rim leaves a gap where the cervix remains exposed. If the cap is too large, it isn't snug against the cervix and is more easily dislodged.

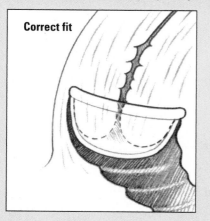

Correct fit

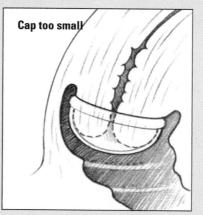

Cap too small

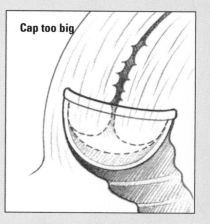

Cap too big

• It doesn't alter hormones.
• It can be inserted up to 8 hours before intercourse.
• It doesn't require reapplication of spermicide before repeated intercourse.
• It can remain in place longer than a diaphragm because it doesn't exert pressure on the vaginal walls or urethra.

The minus side

Here are the disadvantages of the cervical cap:
• It requires possible refitting after weight gain or loss of 15 lb (6.8 kg) or more, recent pregnancy, recent pelvic surgery, or cap slippage.
• It may be difficult to insert or remove.
• It may cause an allergic reaction or vaginal lacerations and thickening of the vaginal mucosa.
• It may cause a foul odor if left in place for more than 36 hours.
• It can't be used during menstruation or during the first 6 postpartum weeks.
• It shouldn't be left in place longer than 24 hours.
• It's contraindicated in patients with a history of toxic shock syndrome, a previously abnormal Pap test, allergy to latex or spermicide, an abnormally short or long cervix, history of PID, cervicitis, papillomavirus infection, cervical cancer, or undiagnosed vaginal bleeding.

Male condom

A male condom is a latex or synthetic sheath that's placed over the erect penis before intercourse. It prevents pregnancy by collecting spermatozoa in the tip of the condom, preventing them from entering the vagina.

Position is important

The condom should be positioned so that it's loose enough at the penis tip to collect ejaculate but not so loose that it comes off the penis. The penis must be withdrawn before it becomes flaccid after ejaculation or sperm can escape from the condom into the vagina.

The plus side

Here are the advantages of the male condom:
• Many women favor male condoms because they put the responsibility of birth control on the male.
• No health care visit is needed.
• It's available over-the-counter in pharmacies and grocery stores.

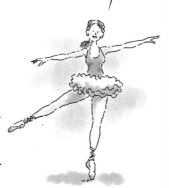

In ballet as well as condom usage, exact position is critical.

- It's easy to carry.
- It prevents the spread of STDs.

The minus side

Here are the disadvantages of the male condom:
- It must be applied before any vulvar penile contact takes place because pre-ejaculation fluid may contain sperm.
- It may cause an allergic reaction if the product contains latex and either partner is allergic.
- It may break during use if it's used incorrectly or is of poor quality.
- It can't be reused.
- Sexual pleasure may be affected.
- It may interfere with spontaneity.

Female condom

A female condom is made of latex and lubricated with nonoxynol 9. The inner ring (closed end) covers the cervix. The outer ring (open end) rests against the vaginal opening. Female condoms are intended for one-time use and shouldn't be used in combination with male condoms. (See *Inserting a female condom*, page 86.)

The plus side

Here are the advantages of the female condom:
- It's 95% effective.
- It helps prevent the spread of STDs.
- It can be purchased over-the-counter.

The minus side

Here are the disadvantages of the female condom:
- It's more expensive than the male condom.
- It's difficult to use and hasn't gained as much acceptance as a male condom.
- Pregnancy can occur as a result of failure to use or incorrect use.
- It may break or become dislodged.
- It's contraindicated in patients or partners with latex allergies.
- It may interfere with spontaneity.

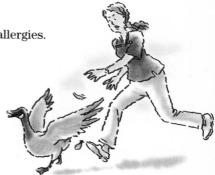

A female condom? What's good for the goose is 95% effective for the gander!

Education edge

Inserting a female condom

A female condom is made of latex and lubricated with nonoxynol 9. It has an inner ring that covers the cervix and an outer ring that rests against the vaginal opening, as shown below.

Inserting the condom
Inform your patient to take these steps when inserting the condom.

Fold the inner ring in half with one hand by pressing the opposite sides together, as shown below. When inserted, the inner ring covers the cervix.

After the condom is inserted, the outer ring (open end) rests against the vaginal opening.

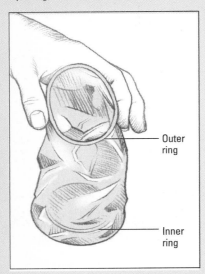

Outer ring

Inner ring

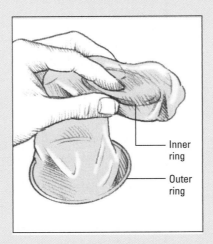

Inner ring

Outer ring

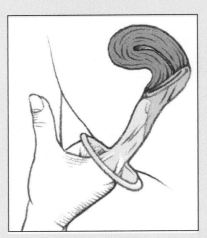

Surgical methods of family planning

Surgical methods of family planning include vasectomy (for men) and tubal ligation (for women). These procedures are the most commonly chosen contraceptive methods for couples over age 30.

Reversal reality

It's possible to reverse these procedures, but it's expensive and isn't always effective. Therefore, surgical sterilization should be chosen only when the patient and her partner, if applicable, have thoroughly discussed the options and know that these procedures are for permanent contraception.

Vasectomy

Vasectomy is a procedure in which the pathway for spermatozoa is surgically severed. Incisions are made on each side of the scrotum, and the vas deferens is cut and tied, then plugged or cauterized. This blocks the passage of sperm. The testes continue to produce sperm as usual, but the sperm can't pass the severed vas deferens. (See *A closer look at vasectomy*.)

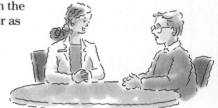

Vasectomy is 99.6% effective, and it can be done as an outpatient procedure with little or no pain.

Lying in wait

The patient should be cautioned that sperm remaining in the vas deferens at the time of surgery may remain viable for as long as 6 months. An additional form of contraception should be used until two negative sperm reports have been obtained. These reports confirm that all of the remaining sperm in the vas deferens has been ejaculated.

To prevent your patients from making a rash decision regarding vasectomy, explain that this procedure

A closer look at vasectomy

In a vasectomy, the vas deferens is surgically altered to prohibit the passage of sperm. Here's how.

✌ The surgeon makes two small incisions, one on each side of the scrotum.

✌ He then cuts the vas deferens with scissors.

✌ The vas deferens is then cauterized or plugged to block the passage of sperm.

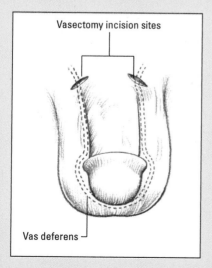

Vasectomy incision sites

Vas deferens

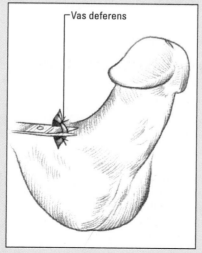

Vas deferens

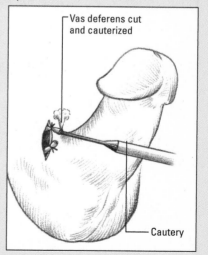

Vas deferens cut and cauterized

Cautery

should be viewed as irreversible, although reversal is possible in 95% of cases.

The plus side

Here are the advantages of vasectomy:
• It can be done as an outpatient procedure, with little anesthesia and minimal pain.
• It's 99.6% effective.
• It doesn't interfere with male erection, and the male still produces seminal fluid—it just doesn't contain sperm.

The minus side

Here are the disadvantages of vasectomy:
• Misconceptions about the procedure may lead some men to resist it.
• Some reports indicate that vasectomy may be associated with the development of kidney stones.
• It's contraindicated in individuals who aren't entirely certain of their decision to choose permanent sterilization, and in those with specific surgical risks such as an anesthesia allergy.

Tubal sterilization

In tubal sterilization, a laparoscope is used to cauterize, crush, clamp, or block the fallopian tubes, thus preventing pregnancy by blocking the passage of ova and sperm. The procedure is performed after menses and before ovulation. It can also be performed 4 to 6 hours (although it's usually performed within 12 to 24 hours) after the birth of a baby or after an abortion.

Here's how it works:

A small incision is made in the abdomen.

Carbon dioxide is pumped into the abdominal cavity to lift the abdominal wall, providing an easier view of the surgical area.

A lighted laparoscope is inserted, and the fallopian tubes are located.

An electric current is then used to cauterize the tubes, or the tubes are clamped and cut.

After surgery, patients may notice some abdominal bloating from the carbon dioxide, but this subsides. (See *A closer look at tubal sterilization.*)

A closer look at tubal sterilization

In a laparoscopic tubal sterilization, the surgeon inserts a laparoscope and occludes the fallopian tube by cauterizing, crushing, clamping, or blocking. This prevents the passage of ova and sperm.

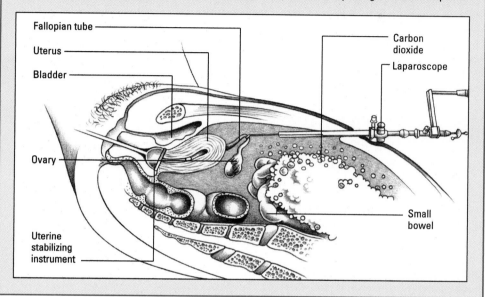

Fallopian tube

Uterus

Bladder

Carbon dioxide

Laparoscope

Ovary

Uterine stabilizing instrument

Small bowel

Sneak attack

Women should be cautioned to not have unprotected intercourse before the procedure because sperm that can become trapped in the tube could fertilize an ovum, resulting in an ectopic pregnancy.

This procedure should be viewed as irreversible. Although reversal is successful in 40% to 75% of patients, this process is difficult and could cause an ectopic pregnancy.

The plus side

Here are the advantages of tubal sterilization:
• It can be performed on an outpatient basis, and the patient is usually discharged within a few hours after the procedure.
• It's 99.6% effective.
• It's been associated with a decreased incidence of ovarian cancer.
• A woman can resume intercourse 2 to 3 days after having the procedure.

The minus side

Here are the disadvantages of tubal sterilization:

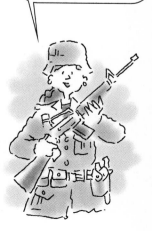

Women should protect themselves from unwanted pregnancy before undergoing tubal sterilization. Trapped sperm could launch a sneak attack, resulting in an ectopic pregnancy.

- Some woman may be reluctant to choose it because it requires a small surgical incision and general anesthesia.
- Complications include a risk of bowel perforation and hemorrhage and the typical risks of general anesthesia (allergy, arrhythmia) during the procedure.
- Contraindications include umbilical hernia and obesity.
- Posttubal ligation syndrome may occur. This includes vaginal spotting and intermittent vaginal bleeding as well as severe lower abdominal cramping.
- It isn't recommended for individuals who aren't certain of their decision to choose permanent sterilization.

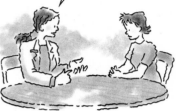

Tubal sterilization is 99.6% effective and can be performed on an outpatient basis.

Elective termination of pregnancy

A procedure that's performed to deliberately end a pregnancy is known as an *elective termination of pregnancy*. Also known as an *induced abortion*, elective termination of pregnancy can be performed for many reasons, some of which involve:
- pregnancy that threatens a woman's life
- pregnancy in which amniocentesis identifies a chromosomal defect in the fetus
- pregnancy that results from rape or incest
- pregnancy in which the woman chooses not to have a child.

Elective terminations of pregnancy can be medically or surgically induced.

Medically induced abortion

In the medically induced method of abortion, a progesterone antagonist called *mifepristone* (Mifeprex [RU-486]) is taken to block the effect of progesterone and prevent implantation of the fertilized ovum. The drug is taken as a single dose at any time within 28 days' gestation. If a spontaneous abortion doesn't occur, misoprostol ([Cytotec], a prostaglandin E1 analog) is administered 3 days later.

Uterine contractions occur with mild cramping, and the products of conception are expelled. One advantage to using this method is that it decreases the risk of damage to the uterus that can occur from instruments used in surgically induced abortions.

Consider this

Disadvantages of medically induced elective termination include the possibility of incomplete abortion as well as prolonged bleeding. Medically induced abortion is contraindicated in patients with suspected or confirmed ectopic pregnancy (unless the patient is

(Text continues on page 91.)

Female pelvic organs

The female pelvis includes reproductive, urinary, and GI structures. Reproductive structures include the internal and external genitalia. Hormonal influences determine the development and function of these structures and affect fertility and childbearing.

Most of the structures of the female reproductive system are internal, housed within the pelvic cavity.

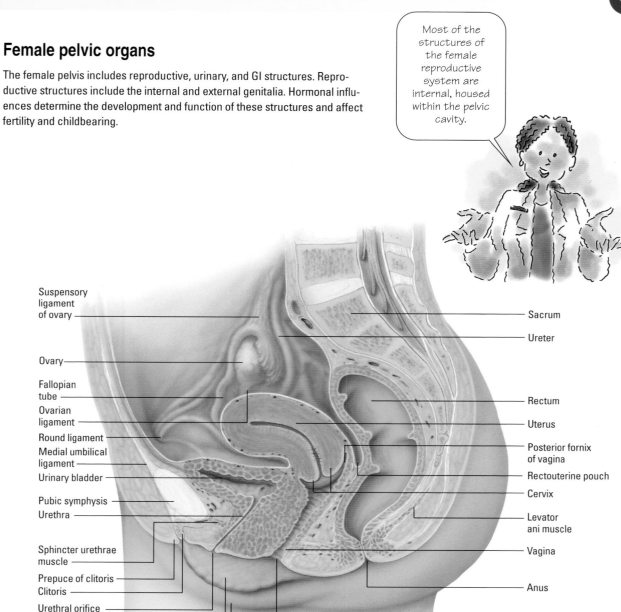

Suspensory ligament of ovary

Ovary

Fallopian tube

Ovarian ligament

Round ligament

Medial umbilical ligament

Urinary bladder

Pubic symphysis

Urethra

Sphincter urethrae muscle

Prepuce of clitoris

Clitoris

Urethral orifice

Labium minus

Labium majus

Vaginal orifice

Sacrum

Ureter

Rectum

Uterus

Posterior fornix of vagina

Rectouterine pouch

Cervix

Levator ani muscle

Vagina

Anus

Ovarian and uterine changes during the menstrual cycle

The hypothalamus, ovaries, and pituitary gland secrete hormones that effect the buildup and shedding of the endometrium during the menstrual cycle. The menstrual cycle normally occurs over 28 days, although it may range from 22 to 34 days. The cycle is regulated by fluctuating hormone levels that, in turn, are regulated by negative and positive feedback mechanisms involving the hypothalamus, pituitary glands, and ovaries.

The hormonal changes of the menstrual cycle trigger a series of changes in the uterine endometrium as follows:
• menstrual (preovulatory) phase—endometrium exfoliates and sheds
• proliferative (follicular) phase and ovulation—endometrium proliferates
• luteal (secretory) phase—endometrium becomes thick and secretory to prepare for the implantation of a fertilized ovum
• premenstrual phase—in absence of fertilization, estrogen and progesterone levels drop and the endometrium sheds.

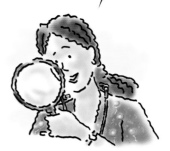

These illustrations show the relationship between ovarian changes and uterine changes during the menstrual cycle.

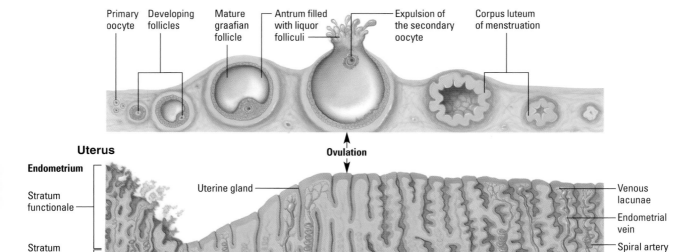

Ovary

Primary oocyte — Developing follicles — Mature graafian follicle — Antrum filled with liquor folliculi — Expulsion of the secondary oocyte — Corpus luteum of menstruation

Ovulation

Uterus

Endometrium

Stratum functionale

Uterine gland

Venous lacunae

Endometrial vein

Stratum basale

Spiral artery

Basal artery

Myometrium

Arcuate artery

Day 0 — 4 — 14 — 26 — 28

Menstrual phase — Proliferative phase — Luteal phase — Premenstrual phase

Fertilization and implantation

During monthly ovulation, an ovum is released from the ovary into the fallopian tube, where it travels toward the uterus. If present, sperm from the male move through the fallopian tube, where they meet the ovum.

If a sperm penetrates the ovum, fertilization occurs and the ovum is called a *zygote.* The zygote continues to travel toward the uterus, dividing many times until it becomes a blastocyst. When the blastocyst reaches the uterus, it implants in the uterine wall and continues to develop over the next 9 months.

Ovum (Egg)   **Spermatozoon (Sperm)**

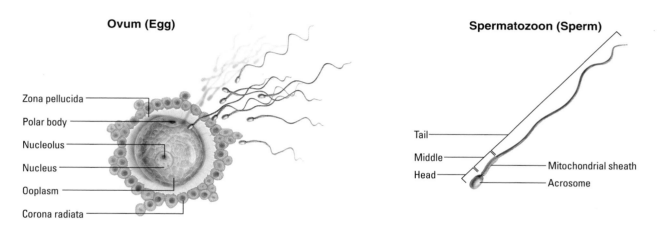

Fertilization and implantation

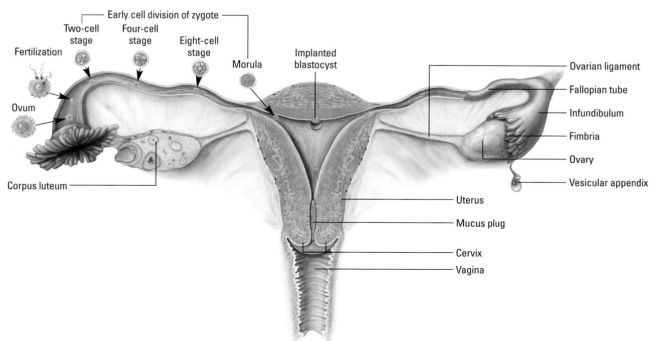

Male pelvic structures

In the male, pelvic structures include GI, reproductive, and urinary organs. These structures are illustrated below.

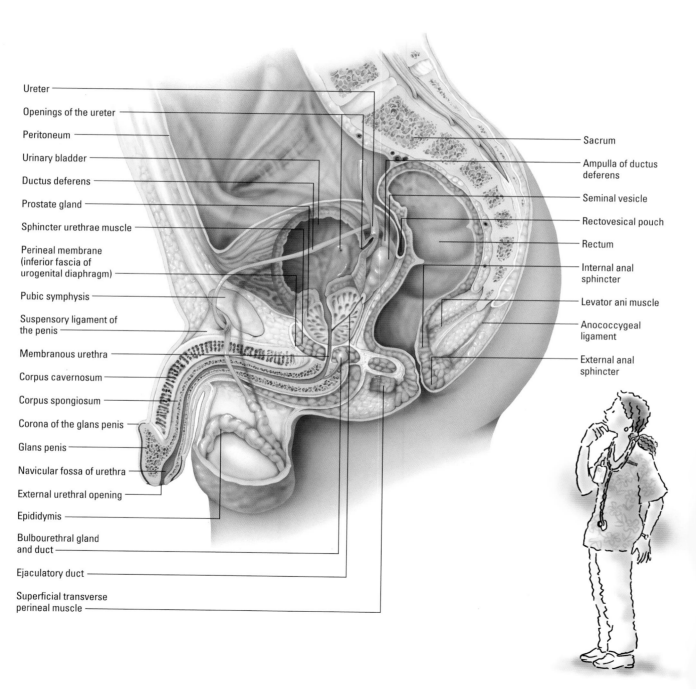

Ureter

Openings of the ureter

Peritoneum

Urinary bladder

Ductus deferens

Prostate gland

Sphincter urethrae muscle

Perineal membrane
(inferior fascia of
urogenital diaphragm)

Pubic symphysis

Suspensory ligament of
the penis

Membranous urethra

Corpus cavernosum

Corpus spongiosum

Corona of the glans penis

Glans penis

Navicular fossa of urethra

External urethral opening

Epididymis

Bulbourethral gland
and duct

Ejaculatory duct

Superficial transverse
perineal muscle

Sacrum

Ampulla of ductus
deferens

Seminal vesicle

Rectovesical pouch

Rectum

Internal anal
sphincter

Levator ani muscle

Anococcygeal
ligament

External anal
sphincter

closely monitored and the pregnancy is at fewer than 6 weeks' gestation); hemorrhage disorders; current long-term systemic corticosteroid therapy; history of allergy to mifepristone, misoprostol, or other prostaglandins; an IUD; or chronic adrenal failure.

Surgically induced abortions

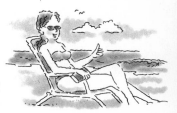

Got seaweed? It's actually used to help maintain the integrity of the cervix during D&E.

Depending on the gestation at the time of the abortion, surgical abortion can be performed several ways. These include D&C, dilatation and vacuum extraction (D&E), saline induction, and hysterotomy.

Dilatation and vacuum extraction

D&E uses the same technique as D&C except that the products of conception are removed by vacuum extraction. Some facilities admit the patient the day before the procedure to begin cervical dilation. This is achieved by inserting into the cervix a laminaria tent made of seaweed that has been dried and sterilized. This helps maintain the integrity of the cervix so that future pregnancies aren't threatened. As the seaweed from the laminaria tent absorbs the moisture from the cervix and vagina, it begins to swell and dilate the cervix. Then a small catheter is inserted, and the products of conception are extracted by the vacuum over a 5-minute period.

This procedure can be performed between 12 and 16 weeks' gestation as either an outpatient or inpatient procedure. Complications such as uterine puncture and infections can occur.

Saline induction

Saline induction can be performed to terminate pregnancy if gestation is between 16 and 24 weeks. In saline induction, hypertonic saline solution is inserted through the uterine cavity into the amniotic fluid, which forces fluid to shift, causing the placenta and endometrium to slough.

Hysterotomy

A hysterotomy is the removal of the products of conception through a surgical incision in the uterus. This procedure, which is similar to a cesarean birth, can be performed for a pregnancy that's more than 18 weeks' gestation. Hysterotomy is usually performed because the cervix has become resistant to the effect of oxytocin and may not respond to saline induction. When it's determined that an abortion must be performed, gestation is more than 18 weeks, and other methods have failed, this procedure is still possible.

Infertility

Infertility is defined as the inability to conceive after 1 year of consistent attempts without using contraception. As many as 10% to 15% of couples who desire children experience infertility. (See *What's behind rising infertility rates?*)

Infertility can be considered primary or secondary:

• *Primary infertility* refers to infertility that occurs in couples who have not previously conceived.

• *Secondary infertility* refers to infertility that occurs in couples who have previously conceived.

Skillful and sensitive

Talking to a couple about infertility and its treatment requires many skills. For instance, you need to guide them sensitively through rigorous tests and treatments—some of which may be painful and embarrassing. At the same time, you need to help them deal with their own emotions.

Bittersweet emotions

A diagnosis of infertility may stir up many feelings and conflicts, such as anger, guilt, and blame, which may disrupt relationships and alter self-esteem. What's more, although treatment heightens the hope of conception, it can also lead to deep disappointment if fertility measures fail. (See *Infertility teaching topics.*)

Infertile couples need open communication to help build their trust and confidence in the health care team. Understandably, many couples feel uncomfortable discussing their sex life, let alone having intercourse assigned on a rigid schedule that's designed to take advantage of peak fertile days.

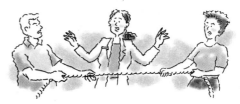

Infertility can be an emotional tug-of-war for many couples. You'll need to guide them sensitively through many tests and treatments.

What's behind rising infertility rates?

Childless couples need to feel that they aren't alone. Let them know that the number of couples dealing with infertility has doubled in recent years. Factors that may contribute to rising infertility rates include:

• aging—more and more couples postpone childbearing until age 30 or older, allowing age and concomitant disease processes to affect fertility

• sexually transmitted diseases, which may be responsible for up to 20% of infertility cases

• intrauterine devices, which can cause pelvic inflammatory disease and consequent infertility

• environmental factors such as toxins

• complications of abortion or childbirth.

There's also a higher incidence of infertility in females who:

• have irregular or absent periods

• experience pain during sexual intercourse

• have had ruptured appendices or other abdominal surgeries.

Conditions for conception

Many couples think that conception occurs easily when, in fact, certain conditions must be present for conception to occur. These include:
- sufficient and motile sperm
- mucus secretions that promote sperm movement in the reproductive tract
- unobstructed uterus and open fallopian tubes that allow sperm free passage
- regular ovulation and healthy ova
- hormonal sufficiency and balance that support implantation of the embryo in the uterus
- sexual intercourse timed so that sperm fertilize the ovum within 24 hours of the ovum's release.

Sex-specific causes of infertility

Many conditions can cause infertility in men and women.

Just for him

Some causes of male infertility remain unknown, but factors that have been identified include:
- structural abnormalities, such as varicoceles (enlarged, varicose veins in the scrotum that can affect sperm number and motility) and hypospadias
- infection, possibly from an STD
- hormonal imbalances that reduce the amount of spermatozoa produced or disrupt their ability to travel effectively in the female reproductive tract
- heat (produced by wearing tight-fitting underwear or jeans, sitting in a hot tub or hot bath water, or driving long distances) that adversely affects sperm number and motility
- fever-producing illnesses that adversely affect sperm number and motility
- penile or testicular injury or congenital anomalies that diminish sperm
- certain prescription drugs known to affect sperm quality
- use of substances such as alcohol, marijuana, cocaine, and tobacco, that are suspected of affecting sperm quality
- coital frequency—either too often or too seldom—which may decrease sperm number and motility
- environmental agents, such as exposure to radiation or other industrial and environmental toxins
- psychological and emotional stress.

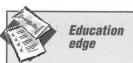

Education edge

Infertility teaching topics

When teaching patients about infertility, be sure to cover these topics.
- Definition of infertility
- Possible causes, such as ovulatory dysfunction and structural abnormalities
- Fertility drugs, including menotropins (Pergonal) and clomiphene (Clomid)
- Explanation of in vitro fertilization–embryo transfer and gamete intrafallopian transfer, if appropriate
- Artificial insemination
- Surgery to promote fertility, including varicocelectomy, hysteroscopy, laparoscopy, and laparotomy
- Psychological counseling

Just for her

Female infertility usually stems from anovulation (ovulatory dysfunction), fallopian tube obstruction, uterine conditions, or pelvic abnormalities caused by one or more of the following factors:
• hormonal imbalances that prevent the ovary from releasing ova regularly (or at all) or from producing enough progesterone to support growth and maintain the uterine lining needed for implantation of the embryo
• infection or inflammation (past, chronic, or current) that damages the ovaries and fallopian tubes, such as from PID, STDs, appendicitis, childhood disease, or surgical trauma
• structural abnormalities, such as a uterus scarred by infection or one that's abnormally shaped or positioned since birth, deformed by fibroid tumors, exposed to diethylstilbestrol, or injured by conization
• mucosal abnormalities caused by infection, inadequate hormone levels, or antibodies to sperm, which may create a hostile environment that prevents sperm from entering the uterus and continuing to the fallopian tubes
• endometriosis (in some women), in which the endometrial tissue—usually confined to the inner lining of the uterine cavity—is deposited outside the uterus on such structures as the ovaries or fallopian tubes, causing inflammation and scarring
• endocrine abnormalities, such as elevated prolactin levels and pituitary, thyroid, or adrenal dysfunction
• recreational drug use (including tobacco, marijuana, and cocaine) and environmental and occupational factors (exposure to heat and chemicals).

Normogonadotrophic anovulation

Normogonadotrophic anovulation is usually seen in women with polycystic ovary syndrome and in those who are overweight. Patients with normogonadotrophic anovulation have normal FSH levels but elevated LH levels. They may also bleed in response to a progesterone withdrawal test.

Hyperprolactinemic anovulation

In hyperprolactinemic anovulation, excessive prolactin secretion impairs ovarian function. Elevated levels of prolactin in the blood are normal during lactation but are otherwise pathologic. Hyperprolactinemic anovulation may also be caused by physical or emotional stress, rapid weight loss, or a pituitary adenoma.

Hypogonadotrophic anovulation

Hypogonadotrophic anovulation may be caused by stress, weight loss, or excessive exercise. In many cases, this type of anovulation is functional and transient. An organic cause should be excluded, however, particularly if the patient displays neurologic symptoms. Patients with hypogonadotrophic anovulation typically have low levels of FSH, LH, and estrogen and an absence of withdrawal bleeding after a progesterone challenge test.

Hypergonadotrophic anovulation

Hypergonadotrophic anovulation results from ovarian resistance or failure. It's commonly diagnosed when repeated measurements show plasma levels of FSH are higher than 20 mIU/ml.

Treatment options

Infertility can be treated with drugs, special procedures, or various types of surgery.

Medications

Drugs can be used in several ways to help treat infertility. They may be prescribed to treat certain conditions that inhibit fertility. For example, antibiotics may be prescribed for infections or danazol (Danocrine) may be ordered for a patient with endometriosis. (See *Explaining how danazol affects fertility*.) Drugs designed to initiate ovulation, improve cervical mucus, or stimulate sperm production may also be prescribed.

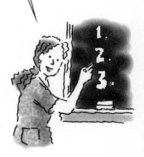

> Infertility can be treated with drugs, special procedures, or surgery.

Education edge

Explaining how danazol affects fertility

If the patient's primary health care practitioner finds that endometriosis interferes with your patient's ability to conceive, he may recommend treatment with danazol (Danocrine).

Effects of hormonal suppression
Inform the patient that danazol suppresses her hormonal cycle, so she won't menstruate while she's taking it. This gives endometrial tissue, which usually swells and bleeds during menses, a rest. The endometrial implants deposited on her ovaries or fallopian tubes should also recede and refrain from bleeding, helping inflammation subside as well.

The patient can then stop taking the drug and try to become pregnant. Alternatively, the primary health care practitioner may suggest surgery to remove the implants while they're small.

Adverse reactions
Warn the patient to promptly report adverse reactions, such as voice changes and other signs of virilization. Some androgenic effects, such as deepening of the voice, may not be reversible after stopping the drug.

Just for him

For men whose infertility is caused by hypogonadism secondary to pituitary or hypothalamic failure, treatment may include human menopausal gonadotropins (hMGs), human chorionic gonadotropin (HCG), or pulsatile gonadotropin-releasing hormone (Gn-RH). These medications are highly effective in achieving sperm quality that's sufficient to induce pregnancy.

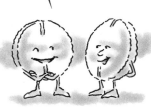

hMGs, HCG, and Gn-RH all help to achieve sperm quality that's sufficient to induce pregnancy.

Just for her

For women, the type of fertility drug prescribed depends on the type of anovulation.

Normogonadotrophic anovulation

Recommended treatments for normogonadotrophic anovulation include clomiphene (Clomid) or tamoxifen (Nolvadex) combined with weight reduction.

Invigorating the ovaries

Clomiphene (Clomid) is an estrogen agonist used to stimulate the ovaries. The drug binds to estrogen receptors, decreasing the number available, and falsely signals the hypothalamus to increase FSH and LH, resulting in the release of more ova.

The drug is taken on cycle days 5 through 10 and may produce ovulation 6 to 11 days after the last dose. The patient needs to have intercourse every other day for 1 week beginning 5 days after she takes her last dose. The initial dose may not cause ovulation, and the dosage may be adjusted later. The patient should document the ovulatory process by keeping a BBT chart or by using an ovulation prediction kit (or both).

Additional effects

The drug may trigger multiple ova development and release, but the incidence of multiple births (mostly twins) stays near 5%. The drug may also make the patient feel moody from fluctuating hormone levels. If the patient fails to have a normal menses, she should contact her primary health care practitioner, who may withhold the drug and order a pregnancy test.

The patient may experience slight bloating and hot flashes (caused by a release of LH, which indicates that the drug is working). She may also experience dysmenorrhea as a result of the drug triggering the ovulatory cycle (the first cycle the patient has had in a while).

Instruct the patient to report blurred vision; other visual changes, such as spots or flashing lights; and severe headaches that are unrelieved by acetaminophen (Tylenol). Additionally, instruct the patient to tell her primary health care practitioner if ab-

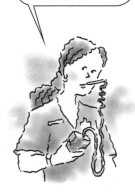

Is it hot in here? Clomiphene may cause hot flashes in some patients.

dominal distention, bloating, pain, or weight gain occurs. These effects may signal ovarian enlargement or ovarian cysts, and treatment may need to be discontinued.

And another thing

Another therapy for normogonadotrophic anovulation is the administration of pulsatile Gn-RH or FSH to induce multiple follicular growth, followed by HCG and timed intercourse or assisted reproductive techniques.

Hyperprolactinemic anovulation

Treatment for hyperprolactinemic anovulation includes bromocriptine (Parlodel) or chemically related dopamine agonists, such as pergolide (Permax) or cabergoline (Dostinex). If pituitary function is normal, these drugs can be combined with clomiphene or tamoxifen to induce ovulation.

Hypogonadotrophic anovulation

Treatment of hypogonadotrophic anovulation varies depending on the cause. In the presence of primary pituitary failure, ovulation can be induced with pulsatile Gn-RH. In women with suspected luteal phase defects, progesterone may be administered during the luteal phase for three to six cycles.

Hypergonadotrophic anovulation

No current drug therapy has restored ovulation in patients with hypergonadotrophic anovulation. Adoption or ova donation may be recommended.

Infertility procedures

Such procedures as in vitro fertilization–embryo transfer (IVF-ET), gamete intrafallopian transfer (GIFT), zygote intrafallopian transfer (ZIFT), intracytoplasmic sperm injection (ICSI), embryo donation, and intrauterine insemination (sometimes called *artificial insemination*) may be recommended to help treat infertility.

In vitro fertilization–embryo transfer

IVF-ET refers to the removal of one or more mature oocytes from a woman's ovary by laparoscopy. After removal, these oocytes are fertilized by exposing them to sperm under laboratory conditions outside the woman's body. Embryo transfer (ET) is the insertion of these laboratory-grown fertilized ova (zygotes) into the woman's uterus. This is performed approximately 40 hours after fertilization. Ideally, one or more of the zygotes implant. IVF-ET circumvents the need for a fallopian tube to pick up an ovum or to propel a fertilized ovum to the uterus.

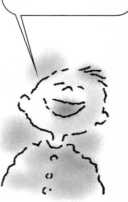

Can you believe it? I started life as a laboratory-grown zygote, transferred into my mom's uterus. What a hoot!

The perfect candidates

IVF-ET is performed for couples who haven't been able to conceive as a result of damaged or blocked fallopian tubes. It can also be used if the man has oligospermia (low sperm count) or if the woman lacks the cervical mucus that enables sperm to travel from the vagina into the cervix.

Agents of ovulation

The woman is given an ovulation drug, such as clomiphene or menotropins (Pergonal). On about the tenth day of her menstrual cycle, the ovaries are examined; when the size of the follicles appears to be mature, the woman is given an injection of HCG hormone. This causes ovulation to occur within 38 to 42 hours. Then the IVF-ET procedure is performed. (See *How IVF works.*)

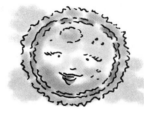

Although it can be expensive, ova donation may be a good alternative for a woman who doesn't ovulate.

Ova donation

Donor ovum may be used in IVF-ET instead of the woman's ovum if the woman doesn't ovulate or if she carries a sex-linked disease that she doesn't want to pass on to her offspring.

Alternate eggs

In ova donation, ova that are retrieved from a well-screened and hormonally stimulated donor are fertilized in a petri dish by sperm from the recipient's partner or a sperm donor. After an incubation period, the best embryos are transferred into the recipient's uterus. The rest may be frozen for possible use in a second transfer if necessary or if the recipient desires a second child genetically related to the first. Ova donation is an emotional, expensive, and time-intensive experience. However, it offers a realistic, successful option for patients who otherwise have no way to have a child. Experienced programs report clinical pregnancy rates of 50 percent per ova donation cycle. These success rates are better than pregnancy rates with IVF cycles using a woman's own ova.

Meet the candidates

Good recipient candidates for ova donation include women who:
• have never had a spontaneous menses
• stopped menstruating at an early age
• produced few or no eggs, or an elevated FSH level, in a previous in vitro fertilization (IVF) cycle
• have stopped menstruating (usually in their 40s) or don't respond well to fertility drugs
• have an FSH level of 15 or more on day 3 of a Clomiphene Challenge Test. (Research suggests these women won't be successful with IVF using their own eggs.)
• have had multiple IVF cycles and failed to achieve a pregnancy.

How IVF works

For patients who meet the necessary criteria, in vitro fertilization–embryo transfer (IVF-ET) bypasses the barriers to in vivo fertilization.

In IVF-ET, after the ovaries receive hormonal stimulation, laparoscopy may be used to visualize and aspirate fluid (containing eggs) from the ovarian follicles. (To avoid using laparoscopy and a general anesthetic, an ultrasound technique may be used, first to visualize the ovarian follicles and then to guide a needle through the back of the vagina to retrieve fluid and eggs from the ovarian follicles.) The eggs are then placed in a test tube or a laboratory dish containing a culture medium for 3 to 6 hours.

Next, sperm from the patient's partner (or a donor) is added to the dish. Two days after insemination, the now-fertilized egg or embryo is transferred into the patient's uterus, where it may implant and establish a pregnancy.

IVF-ET

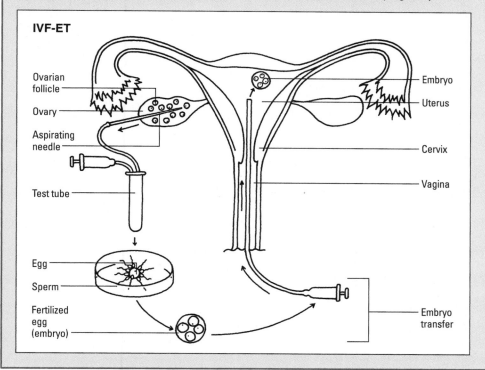

Second surprise

In addition to the usual risks of IVF, approximately 15% to 20% of ova donation pregnancies result in miscarriage and 20% to 25% result in multiple births (such as twins, triplets, or more).

Gamete intrafallopian transfer

In GIFT, the ovaries are stimulated with fertility drugs and the results are monitored. Next, ova are collected from the ovaries transvaginally by needle aspiration. They're placed in a catheter with sperm and then transferred into the fallopian tube, allowing fertilization and implantation to occur naturally from that point.

Embryo donation or surrogate embryo transfer

Embryo donation or surrogate embryo transfer can be used when the woman doesn't ovulate or if the woman has ovarian failure but a functioning uterus. The partner or donor sperm can be used to fertilize a donated ovum so that the embryo contains one-half of the pair's gene pool. The fertilized oocyte is then placed in the woman's uterus by ET or GIFT. Some patients see this option as an advantage over adoption because it allows them to experience pregnancy and they may have a shorter wait for a child.

Surgery

Surgeries for infertility include varicocelectomy, laparoscopy, and laparotomy. If surgery is required to enhance fertility, be sure to explain the procedure to the patient.

Varicocelectomy

A varicocele is a varicosity (abnormality) of the spermatic vein. It allows blood to pool in the scrotum and raises the temperature around the sperm. This, in turn, may reduce sperm production and motility.

A surgery called varicocelectomy can be performed to repair or remove a varicocele. A small incision is made in the scrotum, and the enlarged, varicose-like vein that causes this condition is tied off.

Laparoscopy

A female patient may need surgery to treat tubal disease, endometriosis, or such pelvic conditions as adhesions. A laparoscopy is used to visualize the pelvic and upper abdominal organs and peritoneal surfaces. It can also be used to visualize the distance between the fallopian tubes and the ovaries. If this distance is too large, the discharged ovum can't enter the tube. Dye can be injected into the uterus to assess tubal patency. The laparoscope can also be used to examine the fimbria (the fingerlike projections in the fallopian tubes that accept the ovum as it's released from the ovary and heads toward the fallopian tubes). If PID has damaged them, normal conception is unlikely.

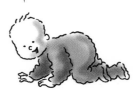

Ova donation pregnancies can result in twins, triplets, or even more! Stock up on those diapers!

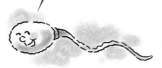

I don't function well when the heat is turned up.

Complications of laparoscopy include excessive bleeding, abdominal cramps, and shoulder pain resulting from the abdomen being inflated with carbon dioxide.

Hysteroscopy

A hysteroscopy is the visualization of the uterus through insertion of a hysteroscope. A hysteroscope is a thin, hollow, fiber-optic tube that's inserted through the vagina and cervix into the uterus. This procedure is done to remove uterine polyps and small fibroid tumors.

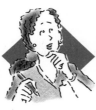

Quick quiz

1. Which family planning method requires assessment of the quality of cervical mucus throughout the menstrual cycle?
   A. Rhythm method
   B. Coitus interruptus
   C. Billings method
   D. Basal body temperature

Answer: C. The Billings method requires assessment of cervical mucus, which is minimal and not stretchy until ovulation occurs. At the time of ovulation, the cervical mucus is present in greater quantity, is stretchy, and is more favorable to penetration by sperm.

2. A vasectomy is considered 100% effective after:
   A. approximately 2 weeks.
   B. approximately 4 weeks.
   C. two consecutive sperm counts show zero sperm.
   D. six consecutive sperm counts show zero sperm.

Answer: C. A vasectomy is considered 100% effective after two consecutive sperm counts show zero sperm. Some sperm remain in the proximal vas deferens after vasectomy. It may take up to several months to clear the proximal ducts of sperm.

3. Which woman is the best candidate for using an IUD?
   A. A woman with Wilson's disease
   B. A mother of two with no history of PID
   C. A mother of one who has a history of severe dysmenorrhea
   D. A 35-year-old woman with recent PID

Answer: B. An IUD is an optimal contraceptive for a woman who has no history of PID, dysmenorrhea, or previous IUD failures.

4. A 20-year-old woman arrives at a family planning clinic seeking emergency contraception 48 hours after she had unprotected sexual intercourse. The nurse correctly responds by saying:

    A.   "Come right in so we can get you started."
    B.   "You must wait 72 hours before the pill will work."
    C.   "You need to wait until you have missed your period."
    D.   "The pills must be started the morning after intercourse."

Answer: A. The first dose of hormones must be taken within 72 hours of sexual intercourse.

5. A 38-year-old woman asks about IVF-ET. Which statement about IVF-ET is correct ?

    A.   Oocytes are retrieved from the ovary, placed in a catheter with washed motile sperm, and transferred into the fallopian tube.
    B.   An indication for this procedure would be unexplained infertility with normal tubal anatomy and patency and absence of previous tubal disease.
    C.   The woman's ova are collected from the ovaries, fertilized in the laboratory with sperm, and transferred to her uterus after normal embryo development has occurred.
    D.   Blastocytes are retrieved from the ovary and transferred into the fallopian tube.

Answer: C. IVF-ET refers to fertilization of the ovum in a laboratory. The woman's ova are collected from the ovaries, fertilized in the laboratory with sperm, and transferred to her uterus after normal embryo development has occurred.

Scoring

☆☆☆ If you answered all five questions correctly, super! Your conception of the material is right on target!

☆☆ If you answered three or four questions correctly, smile! Your planning method seems to work!

☆ If you answered fewer than three questions correctly, don't worry. Just make plans to do some extra family planning review.

4

Physiologic and psychosocial adaptations to pregnancy

Just the facts

In this chapter, you'll learn:

♦ presumptive, probable, and positive signs of pregnancy

♦ ways in which the major body systems are affected by pregnancy

♦ methods of promoting acceptance of pregnancy

♦ psychosocial changes that occur during each trimester.

A look at pregnancy changes

During pregnancy, a woman undergoes many physiologic and psychosocial changes. Her body adapts in response to the demands of the growing fetus while her mind prepares for the responsibilities that come with becoming a parent. Physiologic changes initially indicate pregnancy; these changes continue to affect the body throughout pregnancy as the fetus grows and develops. Psychosocial changes occur in both the mother and father and may vary from trimester to trimester.

Physiologic signs of pregnancy

Pregnancy produces several types of physiologic changes that must be evaluated before a definitive diagnosis of pregnancy is made. The changes can be:
• presumptive (subjective)
• probable (objective)
• positive.

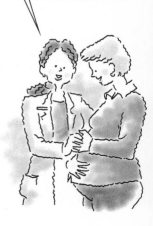

Women can expect a wide range of changes during pregnancy—good practice for all those diaper changes once the baby is born!

Neither presumptive nor probable signs confirm pregnancy because both can be caused by other medical conditions; they simply suggest pregnancy, especially when several are present at the same time. (See *Making sense out of pregnancy signs.*)

Presumptive signs of pregnancy

Presumptive signs of pregnancy are those that can be assumed to indicate pregnancy until more concrete signs develop. These signs include breast changes, nausea and vomiting, amenorrhea, urinary frequency, fatigue, uterine enlargement, quickening, and skin changes. A pregnant patient typically reports some presumptive signs.

Breast changes

Tingling, tender, or swollen breasts can occur as early as a few days after conception. The areola may darken and tiny glands around the nipple, called *Montgomery's tubercles,* may become elevated.

Nausea and vomiting

At least 50% of pregnant women experience nausea and vomiting early in pregnancy (commonly called *morning sickness*). These symptoms are typically the first sensations experienced during pregnancy. Nausea and vomiting usually begin at 4 to 6 weeks' gestation. These symptoms usually stop at the end of the first trimester, but they may last slightly longer in some patients.

Amenorrhea

Amenorrhea is the cessation of menses. For a woman who has regular menses, this may be the first indication that she's pregnant.

Urinary frequency

A pregnant woman may notice an increase in urinary frequency during the first 3 months of pregnancy. This symptom continues until the uterus rises out of the pelvis and relieves pressure on the bladder.

When lightening strikes

Urinary frequency may return at the end of pregnancy as lightening occurs (the fetal head exerts renewed pressure on the bladder).

Memory jogger

To remember the three categories of pregnancy signs, think of the three **Ps**:

Presumptive—Think of a presumptive sign as one that suggests, "If I had to guess, I'd say yes!"

Probable—Think of a probable sign as one that means, this lady is most likely going to give birth!

Positive—Think of a positive sign as one that confirms, in about 9 months, this woman is going to have a baby!

When it rains, it pours! Urinary frequency may increase during the first 3 months of pregnancy—and again at the end of pregnancy.

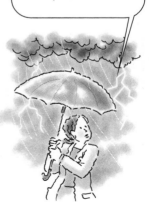

Making sense out of pregnancy signs

This chart classifies the signs of pregnancy into three categories: presumptive, probable, and positive.

Sign	Weeks from implantation	Other possible causes
Presumptive		
Breast changes, including feelings of tenderness, fullness, or tingling, and enlargement or darkening of areola	2	• Hormonal contraceptives • Hyperprolactinemia induced by tranquilizers • Infection • Prolactin-secreting pituitary tumor • Pseudocyesis • Premenstrual syndrome
Feeling of nausea or vomiting upon arising	2	• Gastric disorders • Infections • Psychological disorders, such as pseudocyesis and anorexia nervosa
Amenorrhea	2	• Anovulation • Blocked endometrial cavity • Endocrine changes • Illness • Medications (phenothiazines, Depo-Provera) • Metabolic changes • Stress
Frequent urination	3	• Emotional stress • Pelvic tumor • Renal disease • Urinary tract infection
Fatigue	12	• Anemia • Chronic illness • Depression • Stress
Uterine enlargement in which the uterus can be palpated over the symphysis pubis	12	• Ascites • Obesity • Uterine or pelvic tumor
Quickening (fetal movement felt by the woman)	18	• Excessive flatus • Increased peristalsis

(continued)

Making sense out of pregnancy signs *(continued)*

Sign	Weeks from implantation	Other possible causes
Presumptive (continued)		
Linea nigra (line of dark pigment on the abdomen)	24	• Cardiopulmonary disorders • Estrogen-progestin hormonal contraceptives • Obesity • Pelvic tumor
Melasma (dark pigment on the face)	24	• Cardiopulmonary disorders • Estrogen-progestin hormonal contraceptives • Obesity • Pelvic tumor
Striae gravidarum (red streaks on the abdomen)	24	• Cardiopulmonary disorders • Estrogen-progestin hormonal contraceptives • Obesity • Pelvic tumor
Probable		
Serum laboratory tests revealing the presence of human chorionic gonadotropin (hCG) hormone	1	• Cross-reaction of luteinizing hormone (similar to hCG) • Hydatidiform mole
Chadwick's sign (vagina changes color from pink to violet)	6	• Hyperemia of cervix, vagina, or vulva
Goodell's sign (cervix softens)	6	• Estrogen-progestin hormonal contraceptives
Hegar's sign (lower uterine segment softens)	6	• Excessively soft uterine walls
Sonographic evidence of gestational sac in which characteristic ring is evident	6	None
Ballottement (fetus can be felt to rise against abdominal wall when lower uterine segment is tapped on during bimanual examination)	16	• Ascites • Uterine tumor or polyps
Braxton Hicks contractions (periodic uterine tightening)	20	• GI distress • Hematometra • Uterine tumor
Palpation of fetal outline through abdomen	20	• Subserous uterine myoma

Making sense out of pregnancy signs *(continued)*

Sign	Weeks from implantation	Other possible causes
Positive		
Sonographic evidence of fetal outline	8	None
Fetal heart audible by Doppler ultrasound	10 to 12	None
Palpation of fetal movement through abdomen	20	None

Fatigue

A pregnant woman may report that she's often fatigued. During the first trimester, the woman's body works hard to manufacture the placenta and to adjust to the many other physical demands of pregnancy, while she mentally and emotionally prepares for motherhood. Around 16 weeks' gestation, the body has adjusted to the pregnancy, the placenta's development is complete, and the patient should start to have more energy.

Uterine enlargement

Softening of the uterus and fetal growth cause the uterus to enlarge and stretch the abdominal wall.

Quickening

Quickening is recognizable movements of the fetus. It can occur anywhere between the 14th and 26th weeks of pregnancy but typically is noticed between weeks 18 and 22.

Fluttering flutterflies

To the patient, quickening may feel like fluttering movements in her lower abdomen.

Skin changes

Numerous skin changes occur during pregnancy, including those listed here:
• *Linea nigra* refers to a dark line that extends from the umbilicus or above to the mons pubis. In the primigravid patient, this line develops at approximately the third month

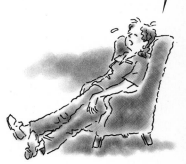

Pregnancy can be tiring—especially during the first 16 weeks.

of pregnancy. In the multigravid patient, linea nigra typically appears before the third month. (See *Skin changes during pregnancy*.)

• *Melasma*, also known as *chloasma* or the "mask of pregnancy," are darkened areas that may appear on the face, especially on the cheeks and across the nose. Melasma appears after the 16th week of pregnancy and gradually becomes more pronounced. After childbirth, it typically fades.

• *Striae gravidarum* are red or pinkish streaks that appear on the sides of the abdominal wall and sometimes on the thighs.

Skin changes during pregnancy

Linea nigra and striae gravidarum are two skin changes that occur during pregnancy. Both fade after pregnancy, with striae gravidarum fading to glistening silvery lines.

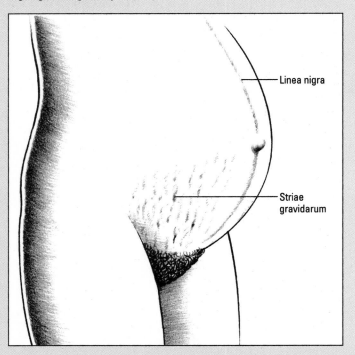

Probable signs of pregnancy

Probable signs of pregnancy strongly suggest pregnancy. They're more reliable indicators of pregnancy than presumptive signs, but they can also be explained by other medical conditions. Probable signs include positive laboratory tests, such as serum and urine tests; positive results on a home pregnancy test; Chadwick's sign; Goodell's sign; Hegar's sign; sonographic evidence of a gestational sac; ballottement; and Braxton Hicks contractions.

Laboratory tests

Laboratory tests for pregnancy are used to detect the presence of human chorionic gonadotropin (hCG)—a hormone created by the chorionic villi of the placenta—in the urine or blood serum of the woman. Because hCG is produced by trophoblast cells—preplacental cells that wouldn't be present in a nonpregnant woman—detection of hCG is considered a sign of pregnancy. Because laboratory tests for diagnosing pregnancy are accurate only 95% to 98% of the time, positive hCG results are considered probable rather than positive.

Looking for hCG in all the right places

Tests for hCG include radioimmunoassay, enzyme-linked immunosorbent assay, and radioreceptor assay. For these tests, hCG is measured in milli-international units (mIU). In pregnant women, trace amounts of hCG appear in the serum as early as 24 to 48 hours after implantation of the fertilized ovum. They reach a measurable level of about 50 mIU/mL between 7 and 9 days after conception. Levels peak at about 100 mIU/mL between the 60th and 80th days of gestation. After this point, the level declines. At term, hCG is barely detectable in serum or urine.

Home pregnancy tests

Home pregnancy tests, which are available over-the-counter, are 97% accurate when performed correctly. They're convenient and easy to use, taking only 3 to 5 minutes to perform.

Dip stick

Here's how the home pregnancy test works:
- A reagent strip is dipped into the urine stream.
- A color change on the strip denotes pregnancy.

Most manufacturers suggest that a woman wait until the day of the missed menstrual period to test for pregnancy.

Chadwick's sign

Chadwick's sign is a bluish coloration of the mucous membranes of the cervix, vagina, and vulva. It can be observed at 6 to 8 weeks' gestation by bimanual examination.

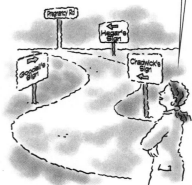

Goodell's sign

Goodell's sign is a softening of the cervix that occurs at 6 to 8 weeks' gestation. The cervix of a nonpregnant woman typically has the same consistency as a nose; the cervix of a pregnant woman feels more like an earlobe.

Hegar's sign

Hegar's sign is a softening of the uterine isthmus that can be felt on bimanual examination at 6 to 8 weeks' gestation. As pregnancy advances, the isthmus becomes part of the lower uterine segment. During labor, it expands further.

Ultrasonography

Ultrasonography, or sonographic evaluation, can detect probable and positive signs of pregnancy. At 4 to 6 weeks' gestation, a characteristic ring indicating the gestational sac is visible on sonographic evaluation.

Ballottement

Ballottement is passive movement of the fetus. It can be identified at 16 to 18 weeks' gestation.

Braxton Hicks contractions

Braxton Hicks contractions are uterine contractions that begin early in pregnancy and become more frequent after 28 weeks' gestation. Typically, they result from normal uterine enlargement that occurs to accommodate the growing fetus. Sometimes, however, they may be caused by a uterine tumor.

Positive signs of pregnancy

Positive signs of pregnancy include sonographic evidence of the fetal outline, an audible fetal heart rate, and fetal movement that's felt by the examiner. These signs confirm pregnancy because they can't be attributed to other conditions.

Ultrasonography

Ultrasonography can confirm pregnancy by providing an image of the fetal outline, which can typically be seen by the 8th week. The fetal outline on the ultrasound is so clear that a crown to rump measurement can be made to establish gestational age. Fetal heart movement may be visualized as early as 7 weeks' gestation.

Audible fetal heart rate

Fetal heart rate can be confirmed by auscultation or visualization during an ultrasound. Fetal heart sounds may be heard as early as the 10th to 12th week by Doppler ultrasonography.

Fetal movement

Even though the pregnant woman can feel fetal movement at a much earlier date (usually around 16 to 20 weeks), other people aren't able to feel fetal movement until the 20th to 24th week. Obese patients may not feel fetal movement until later in pregnancy because of excess adipose tissue.

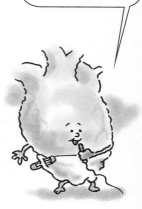

Testing...testing... one, two, three. Can anybody hear me out there?

Physiologic changes in body systems

As the fetus grows and hormones shift during pregnancy, physiologic adaptations occur in every body system to accommodate the fetus. These changes help a pregnant woman to maintain health throughout the pregnancy and to physically prepare for childbirth. Physiologic changes also create a safe and nurturing environment for the fetus. Some of these changes take place even before the woman knows that she's pregnant.

Reproductive system

In addition to the physical changes that initially indicate pregnancy, such as Hegar's sign and Goodell's sign, the reproductive system undergoes significant changes throughout pregnancy.

Out and about

External reproductive structures affected by pregnancy include the labia majora, labia minora, clitoris, and vaginal introitus. These structures enlarge because of increased vascularity. Fat deposits also contribute to the enlargement of the labia majora and labia minora. These structures reduce in size after childbirth, but may not return to their prepregnant state because of loss of mus-

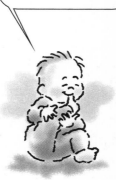

Sometimes, an external or internal structure that changes during pregnancy may not return to its prepregnant state. But that's a small price to pay for all this cuteness!

cle tone or perineal injury (such as from an episiotomy or a vaginal tear). For example, in many patients, the labia majora remain separated and gape after childbirth. In addition, varices may be caused by pressure on vessels in the perineal and perianal areas.

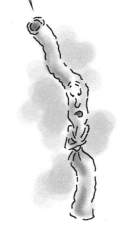

Look out! Pressure on vessels in the perineal area can cause varices.

The inside story

Internal reproductive structures, including the ovaries, uterus, and other structures, change dramatically to accommodate the developing fetus. These internal structures may not regain their pre-pregnant states after childbirth.

Ovaries

When fertilization occurs, ovarian follicles cease to mature and ovulation stops. The chorionic villi, which develop from the fertilized ovum, begin to produce hCG to maintain the ovarian corpus luteum. The corpus luteum produces estrogen and progesterone until the placenta is formed and functioning. At 8 to 10 weeks' gestation, the placenta assumes production of these hormones. The corpus luteum, which is no longer needed, then involutes (becomes smaller due to a reduction in cell size).

Uterus

In a nonpregnant woman, the uterus is smaller than the size of a fist, measuring approximately 7.5 cm × 5 cm × 2.5 cm (3″ × 2″ × 1″). It can weigh 60 to 70 g (2 to 2½ oz) in a nulliparous patient (a patient who has never been pregnant) and 100 g (3½ oz) in a parous patient (a patient who has given birth). In a nonpregnant state, a woman's uterus can hold up to 10 ml of fluid. Its walls are composed of several overlapping layers of muscle fibers that adapt to the developing fetus and help in expulsion of the fetus and placenta during labor and childbirth.

More strength, more stretch

After conception, the uterus retains the developing fetus for approximately 280 days, or 9 calendar months. During this time, the uterus undergoes progressive changes in size, shape, and position in the abdominal cavity. In the first trimester, the pear-shaped uterus lengthens and enlarges in response to elevated levels of estrogen and progesterone. This hormonal stimulation primarily increases the size of myometrial cells (hypertrophy), although a small increase in cell number (hyperplasia) also occurs. These changes increase the amount of fibrous and elastic tissue to more than 20 times that of the nonpregnant uterus. Uterine walls become stronger and more elastic.

During the first few weeks of pregnancy, the uterine walls remain thick and the fundus rests low in the abdomen. The uterus can't be palpated through the abdominal wall. After 12 weeks of pregnancy, however, the uterus typically reaches the level of the symphysis pubis (the joint at the pubic bone) and then may be palpated through the abdominal wall.

Shape shifters

In the second trimester, the corpus and fundus become globe-shaped. As pregnancy progresses, the uterus lengthens and becomes oval in shape. The uterine walls thin as the muscles stretch; the uterus rises out of the pelvis, shifts to the right, and rests against the anterior abdominal wall. At 20 weeks' gestation, the uterus is palpable just below the umbilicus and reaches the umbilicus at 22 weeks' gestation. As uterine muscles stretch, Braxton Hicks contractions may occur, helping to move blood more quickly through the intervillous spaces of the placenta.

Reach and descend

In the third trimester, the fundus reaches nearly to the xiphoid process (the lower tip of the breast bone). Between weeks 38 and 40, the fetus begins to descend into the pelvis (lightening), which causes fundal height to gradually drop. The uterus remains oval in shape. Its muscular walls become progressively thinner as it enlarges, finally reaching a muscle wall thickness of 5 mm (¼″) or less. At term (40 weeks), the uterus typically weighs approximately 1,100 g (2 lb), holds 5 to 10 L of fluid, and has stretched to approximately 28 cm × 24 cm × 21 cm (11″ × 9½″ × 8¼″). (See *Fundal height throughout pregnancy*, page 114.)

Endometrial development

During the menstrual cycle, progesterone stimulates increased thickening and vascularity of the endometrium, preparing the uterine lining for implantation and nourishment of a fertilized ovum. After implantation, menstruation stops.

The endometrium then becomes the decidua, which is divided into three layers:

decidua capsularis, which covers the blastocyst (fertilized ovum)

decidua basalis, which lies directly under the blastocyst and forms part of the placenta

decidua vera, which lines the rest of the uterus.

Fundal height throughout pregnancy

This illustration shows approximate fundal heights at various times during pregnancy. The times indicated are in weeks. Note that between weeks 38 and 40, the fetus begins to descend into the pelvis.

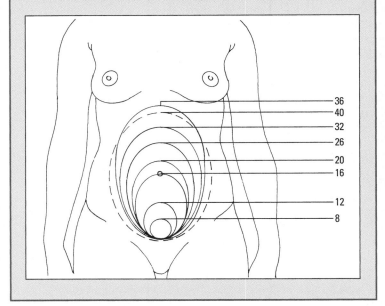

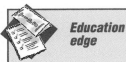

Education edge

Uterine bleeding

Uterine bleeding in a pregnant patient is always potentially serious because it can result in major blood loss. A pregnant woman should be warned that such blood loss poses a major health risk. Advise the pregnant patient to contact her practitioner if uterine bleeding occurs.

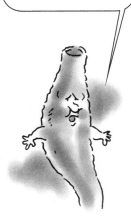

During pregnancy, it's okay for my waistline to expand a bit, too. I have to be ready to handle increased blood flow to the uterus and placenta.

Vascular growth

As the fetus grows and the placenta develops, uterine blood vessels and lymphatics increase in number and size. Vessels must enlarge to accommodate the increased blood flow to the uterus and placenta. By the end of pregnancy, an average of 500 ml of blood may flow through the maternal side of the placenta each minute. Maternal arterial pressure, uterine contractions, and maternal position affect uterine blood flow throughout pregnancy.

Because one-sixth of the body's blood supply is circulating through the uterus at any given time, uterine bleeding during pregnancy is always potentially serious and can result in major blood loss. (See *Uterine bleeding*.)

Cervical changes

The cervix consists of connective tissue, elastic fibers, and endocervical folds. This composition allows it to stretch during childbirth. During pregnancy, the cervix softens. It also takes on a bluish color during the second month due to increased vasculature. It becomes edematous and may bleed easily on examination or sexual activity.

Bacteria blocker

During pregnancy, hormonal stimulation causes the glandular cervical tissue to increase in cell number and become hyperactive, secreting thick, tenacious mucus. This mucus thickens into a mucoid weblike structure, eventually forming a mucus plug that blocks the cervical canal. This creates a protective barrier against bacteria and other substances attempting to enter the uterus.

Vagina

During pregnancy, estrogen stimulates vascularity, tissue growth, and hypertrophy in the vaginal epithelial tissue. White, thick, odorless, and acidic vaginal secretions increase. The acidity of these secretions helps prevent bacterial infections but, unfortunately, also fosters yeast infections, a common occurrence during pregnancy. (See *Fighting* Candida *infection*.)

Other vaginal changes include:
- development of a bluish color due to increased vascularity
- hypertrophy of the smooth muscles and relaxation of connective tissues, which allow the vagina to stretch during childbirth
- lengthening of the vaginal vault
- possible heightened sexual sensitivity.

Breasts

In addition to the presumptive signs that occur in the breasts during pregnancy (such as tenderness, tingling, darkening of the areola, and appearance of Montgomery's tubercles), the nipples enlarge, become more erectile, and darken in color. The areolae widen from a diameter of less than 3 cm (1½″) to 5 or 6 cm (2″ or 3″) in the primigravid patient.

Rarely, patches of brownish discoloration appear on the skin adjacent to the areolae. These patches, known as *secondary areolae*, may indicate pregnancy if the patient has never breast-fed an infant.

Lactation preparation

The breasts also undergo several changes in preparation for lactation. As blood vessels enlarge, veins beneath the skin of the breasts become more visible and may appear as intertwining patterns over the anterior chest wall. Breasts become fuller and heavier as lactation approaches. They may throb uncomfortably.

Increasing hormone levels cause the secretion of colostrum (a yellowish, viscous fluid) from the nipples. High in protein, antibodies, and minerals—but low in fat and sugar relative to mature human milk—colostrum may be secreted as early as week 16 of pregnancy,

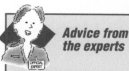

Advice from the experts

Fighting *Candida* infection

Changes in the pH of vaginal secretions during pregnancy favor the growth of *Candida albicans,* a species of yeast-like fungi. This infection can be transmitted to the neonate as he passes through the birth canal during delivery, at which point it's called *thrush* or *oral monila.*

Medication is prescribed to treat and prevent transmission of *Candida* infection if it's properly diagnosed beforehand. Keep on top of possible infections by asking the patient if she has experienced signs and symptoms, such as itching, burning, and a cream cheese–like discharge.

but it's most common during the last trimester. It continues secreting until 2 to 4 days after delivery and is followed by mature milk production.

More change for first-timers

Breast changes are more pronounced in a primigravida patient than in a multigravida patient. In a multigravida patient, changes are even less significant if the patient has breast-fed an infant within the past year because her areola are still dark and her breasts enlarged. (See *Comparing the nonpregnant and pregnant breast*.)

Comparing the nonpregnant and pregnant breast

Subtle changes appear in the breasts of a pregnant patient because of increased estrogen and progestin production.

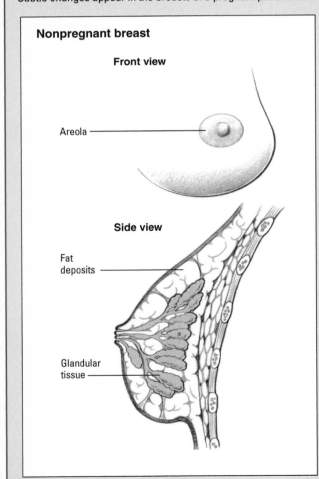

Nonpregnant breast

Front view

Areola

Side view

Fat deposits

Glandular tissue

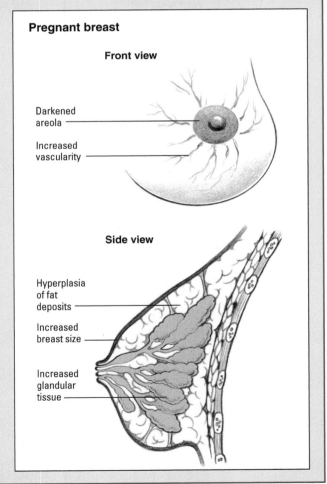

Pregnant breast

Front view

Darkened areola

Increased vascularity

Side view

Hyperplasia of fat deposits

Increased breast size

Increased glandular tissue

Endocrine system

The endocrine system undergoes many fluctuations during pregnancy. Changes in hormone levels and protein production help support fetal growth and maintain body functions.

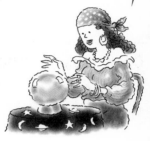

I predict palmar erythema caused by the estrogen produced by the placenta.

Placenta

The most striking change in the endocrine system during pregnancy is the addition of the placenta. The placenta is an endocrine organ that produces large amounts of estrogen, progesterone, hCG, human placental lactogen (hPL), relaxin, and prostaglandins.

The estrogen produced by the placenta causes breast and uterine enlargement as well as palmar erythema (redness in the palm of the hand). Progesterone helps maintain the endometrium by inhibiting uterine contractility. It also prepares the breasts for lactation by stimulating breast tissue development.

Maxin' and relaxin

Relaxin is secreted primarily by the corpus luteum. It helps inhibit uterine activity. It also helps to soften the cervix, which allows for dilation at delivery, and soften the collagen in body joints, which allows for laxness in the lower spine and helps enlarge the birth canal.

How stimulating!

Secreted by the trophoblast cells of the placenta in early pregnancy, hCG stimulates progesterone and estrogen synthesis until the placenta assumes this role.

Alternate energy source

Also called *human chorionic somatomammotropin*, the hormone hPL is secreted by the placenta. It promotes fat breakdown (lipolysis), providing the patient with an alternate source of energy so that glucose is available for fetal growth. This hormone, however, has a complicating effect. Along with estrogen, progesterone, and cortisol, hPL inhibits the action of insulin, resulting in an increased insulin need throughout pregnancy.

Prostaglandins

Prostaglandins are found in high concentration in the female reproductive tract and the decidua during pregnancy. They affect smooth muscle contractility to such an extent that they may trigger labor at the pregnancy's term.

Pituitary gland

The pituitary gland undergoes various changes during pregnancy. High estrogen and progesterone levels in the placenta stop the pituitary gland from producing follicle-stimulating hormone and luteinizing hormone. Increased production of growth hormone and melanocyte-stimulating hormone causes skin pigment changes.

Late-breaking developments

Late in pregnancy, the posterior pituitary gland begins to produce oxytocin, which stimulates uterine contractions during labor. Prolactin production also starts late in pregnancy as the breasts prepare for lactation after birth.

Thyroid gland

As early as the second month of pregnancy, the thyroid gland's production of thyroxine-binding protein increases, causing total thyroxine (T_4) levels to rise. Because the amount of unbound T_4 doesn't increase, these thyroid changes don't cause hyperthyroidism; however, they increase basal metabolic rate (BMR), cardiac output, pulse rate, vasodilation, and heat intolerance. BMR increases by about 20% during the second and third trimesters as the growing fetus places additional demands for energy on the woman's system. By term, the woman's BMR may increase by 25%. It returns to the prepregnant level within 1 week after childbirth.

In addition to T_4 level changes, increased estrogen levels augment the circulating amounts of triiodothyronine (T_3). Like the elevation of T_4, the elevation of T_3 levels doesn't lead to a hyperthyroid condition during pregnancy because much of this hormone is bound to proteins and, therefore, nonfunctional.

Parathyroid gland

As pregnancy progresses, fetal demands for calcium and phosphorus increase. The parathyroid gland responds by increasing hormone production during the third trimester to as much as twice the prepregnancy level.

Adrenal gland

Adrenal gland activity increases during pregnancy as production of corticosteroids and aldosterone escalates.

Corticosteroids deployed

Some researchers believe that increased corticosteroid levels suppress inflammatory reactions and help to reduce the possibility of

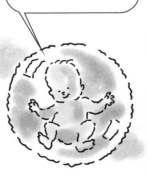

I want calcium! I want phosphorus! Hey, if you think I'm demanding now, just wait until I'm born!

the woman's body rejecting the foreign protein of the fetus. Corticosteroids also help to regulate glucose metabolism in the woman.

Aldosterone zone

Increased aldosterone levels help to promote sodium reabsorption and maintain the osmolarity of retained fluid. This indirectly helps to safeguard the blood volume and provide adequate perfusion pressure across the placenta.

Pancreas

Although the pancreas itself doesn't change during pregnancy, maternal insulin, glucose, and glucagon production do. In response to the additional glucocorticoids produced by the adrenal glands, the pancreas increases insulin production. Insulin is less effective than normal, however, because estrogen, progesterone, and hPL all act as antagonists to it. Despite insulin's diminished action and increased fetal demands for glucose, maternal glucose levels remain fairly stable because the mother's fat stores are used for energy.

Respiratory system

Throughout pregnancy, changes occur in the respiratory system in response to hormonal changes. These changes can be anatomic (biochemical) or functional (mechanical). As pregnancy advances, these respiratory system changes promote gas exchange, providing the woman with more oxygen.

Anatomic changes

The diaphragm rises by approximately 1⅝″ (4 cm) during pregnancy, which prevents the lungs from expanding as much as they normally do on inspiration. The diaphragm compensates for this by increasing its excursion (outward expansion) ability, allowing more normal lung expansion. In addition, the anteroposterior and transverse diameters of the rib cage increase by approximately ¾″ (2 cm), and the circumference increases by 2″ to 2 ¾″ (5 to 7 cm). This expansion is possible because increased progesterone relaxes the ligaments that join the rib cage. As the uterus enlarges, thoracic breathing replaces abdominal breathing.

All that vascularization

Increased estrogen production leads to increased vascularization of the upper respiratory tract. As a result, the patient may develop respiratory congestion, voice changes, and epistaxis as capillaries become engorged in the nose, pharynx, larynx, trachea, bronchi, and vocal cords. Increased vascularization may also cause the eustachian tubes to swell, leading to such problems as impaired hearing, earaches, and a sense of fullness in the ears. This increased stuffiness in the nose, pharynx, and larynx—combined with the pressure the enlarged uterus places on the patient's diaphragm—may make the patient feel as if she's short of breath.

Functional changes

Changes in pulmonary function improve gas exchange in the alveoli and facilitate oxygenation of blood flowing through the lungs. Respiratory rate typically remains unaffected in early pregnancy. By the third trimester, however, increased progesterone may increase the rate by approximately two breaths per minute. (See *Helping patients breathe easier*.)

Rising tide

Tidal volume (the amount of air inhaled and exhaled) rises throughout pregnancy as a result of increased progesterone and increased diaphragmatic excursion. In fact, a pregnant patient breathes 30% to 40% more air during pregnancy than she does when she isn't pregnant. Minute volume (the amount of air expired per minute) increases by approximately 50% by term.

The difference between changes in tidal volume and minute volume creates a slight hyperventilation, which decreases carbon dioxide in the alveoli. The resulting lowered partial pressure of arterial carbon dioxide in maternal blood leads to a greater partial pressure difference of carbon dioxide between fetal and maternal blood, which facilitates diffusion of carbon dioxide from the fetus.

Hyperprotective

An elevated diaphragm decreases functional residual capacity (the volume of air remaining in the lungs after exhalation), which contributes to hyperventilation. Maternal hyperventilation is considered a protective measure that prevents the fetus from being exposed to excessive levels of carbon dioxide. Vital capacity (the largest volume of air that can be expelled voluntarily after maximum inspiration) increases slightly during pregnancy. These changes, along with increased cardiac output and blood volume, provide adequate blood flow to the placenta.

Assorted aberrations

During the third month of pregnancy, increased progesterone sensitizes respiratory receptors and increases ventilation, leading to a drop in carbon dioxide levels. This increases pH, which might cause mild respiratory alkalosis; however, the decreased level of bicarbonate present in a pregnant woman partially or completely compensates for this tendency.

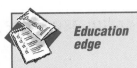

Education edge

Helping patients breathe easier

Pregnant women commonly experience chronic dyspnea (shortness of breath). Advise the patient that, although her breathing rate is more rapid than usual (18 to 20 breaths per minute), this rate is normal during pregnancy.

To help your patient cope with dyspnea, tell her to try holding her arms above her head. This raises the rib cage and temporarily gives the patient more room to breath. She can also try sleeping on her side with her head elevated by pillows. Show her how to practice slow, deep breathing and tell her to take her time when climbing stairs.

Cardiovascular system

Pregnancy alters the cardiovascular system so profoundly that its changes would be considered pathologic, and even life-threatening, outside of this situation. During pregnancy, however, these changes are vital.

Anatomic changes

The heart enlarges slightly during pregnancy, probably because of increased blood volume and cardiac output. This enlargement isn't marked and reverses after childbirth. As pregnancy advances, the uterus moves up and presses on the diaphragm, displacing the heart upward and rotating it on its long axis. The amount of displacement varies depending on the position and size of the uterus, the firmness of the abdominal muscles, the shape of the abdomen, and other factors.

Auscultatory changes

Changes in blood volume, cardiac output, and the size and position of the heart alter heart sounds during pregnancy. These altered heart sounds would be considered abnormal in a patient who isn't pregnant.

During pregnancy, S_1 tends to exhibit a pronounced splitting, and each component tends to be louder. An occasional S_3 sound may occur after 20 weeks' gestation. Many pregnant patients exhibit a systolic ejection murmur over the pulmonic area.

Break in rhythm

Cardiac rhythm disturbances, such as sinus arrhythmia, premature atrial contractions, and premature ventricular contractions, may occur. In the pregnant patient with no underlying heart disease, these arrhythmias don't require therapy and don't indicate the development of myocardial disease.

Hemodynamic changes

Hemodynamically, pregnancy affects heart rate and cardiac output, venous and arterial blood pressures, circulation and coagulation, and blood volume.

Heart rate and cardiac output

During the second trimester, heart rate gradually increases. It may reach 10 to 15 beats/minute above the patient's prepregnancy rate. During the third trimester, heart rate may increase by 15 to 20 beats/minute above the patient's prepregnancy rate. The patient may

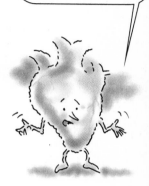

The vital changes that occur in the cardiovascular system during pregnancy would be considered life-threatening if they occurred at another time.

feel palpitations occasionally throughout pregnancy. In the early months, these palpitations result from sympathetic nervous stimulation.

All about output

Increased tissue demands for oxygen and increased stroke volume raise cardiac output by up to 50% by the 32nd week of pregnancy. The increase is highest when the patient is lying on her side and lowest when she's lying on her back. The side-lying position reduces pressure on the great vessels, which increases venous return to the heart. Cardiac output peaks during labor, when tissue demands are greatest.

Venous and arterial blood pressure

When the patient lies on her back, femoral venous pressure increases threefold from early pregnancy to term. This occurs because the uterus exerts pressure on the inferior vena cava and pelvic veins, slowing venous return from the legs and feet. The patient may feel light-headed if she rises abruptly after lying on her back. Edema in the legs and varicosities in the legs, rectum, and vulva may occur.

Progesterone to smooth muscles: Relax!

Early in pregnancy, increased progesterone levels relax smooth muscles and dilate arterioles, resulting in vasodilation. Despite the hypervolemia that occurs during pregnancy, the woman's blood pressure doesn't normally rise because the increased action of the heart enables the body to handle the increased amount of circulating blood. In most women, blood pressure actually decreases slightly during the second trimester because of the lowered peripheral resistance to circulation that occurs as the placenta rapidly expands. Systolic and diastolic pressures may decrease by 5 to 10 mm Hg. The pregnant patient's blood pressure is at its lowest during the second half of the second trimester; it gradually returns to first trimester levels during the third trimester. By term, arterial blood pressure approaches prepregnancy levels.

Position, position, position

Brachial artery pressure is lowest when the pregnant patient lies on her left side because this relieves uterine pressure on the vena cava. Brachial artery pressure is highest when the patient lies on her back (supine). The weight of the growing uterus presses the vena cava against the vertebrae, obstructing blood flow from the lower extremities. This results in a decrease in blood return to the heart and, consequently, immediate decreased cardiac output and hypotension. (See *A look at supine hypotension.*)

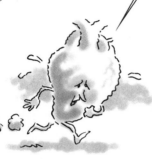

A pregnant woman's heart rate increases during the second trimester, and again during the third!

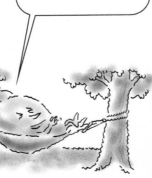

A pregnant patient should avoid lying in a supine position. The weight of the uterus on the vena cava could lead to supine hypotension.

A look at supine hypotension

When a pregnant woman lies on her back, the weight of the uterus presses on the vena cava and aorta, as shown below left. This obstructs blood flow to and from the legs, resulting in supine hypotension. In a side-lying position, shown below right, pressure on the vessels is relieved, allowing blood to flow freely.

Back-lying position

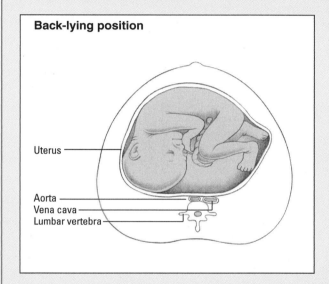

Uterus

Aorta
Vena cava
Lumbar vertebra

Side-lying position

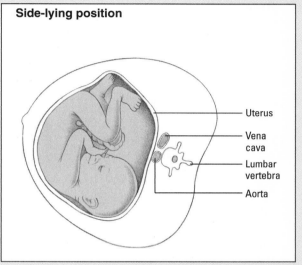

Uterus

Vena cava

Lumbar vertebra

Aorta

Circulation and coagulation

Venous return decreases slightly during the eighth month of pregnancy and, at term, increases to normal levels. Blood is able to clot more easily during pregnancy and the postpartum period because of increased levels of clotting factors VII, IX, and X.

Blood volume

Total intravascular volume increases beginning between 10 and 12 weeks' gestation and peaks with an increase of approximately 40% between weeks 32 and 34. This increase can total 5,250 ml in a pregnant patient compared with 4,000 ml in a nonpregnant patient. Volume decreases slightly in the 40th week and returns to normal several weeks after delivery.

The ABCs of RBCs

Increased blood volume, which consists of two-thirds plasma and one-third red blood cells (RBCs), performs several functions.

• It supplies the hypertrophied vascular system of the enlarging uterus.
• It provides nutrition for fetal and maternal tissues.
• It serves as a reserve for blood loss during childbirth and puerperium.

As the plasma volume first increases, the concentration of hemoglobin and erythrocytes may decline, giving the woman physiologic anemia or pseudoanemia. The woman's body compensates for this change by producing more RBCs. The body can create nearly normal levels of RBCs by the second trimester.

Hematologic changes

Hematologic changes also occur during pregnancy. Pregnancy affects iron demands and absorption as well as RBC, white blood cell (WBC), and fibrinogen levels. In addition, bone marrow becomes more active during pregnancy, producing an excess of RBCs of up to 30%.

Ironing out deficiencies

During pregnancy, the body's demand for iron increases. Not only does the developing fetus require approximately 350 to 400 mg of iron per day for healthy growth, but the mother's iron requirement increases as well—by 400 mg per day. This iron increase is necessary to promote RBC production and accommodate the increased blood volume that occurs during pregnancy. The total daily iron requirements of a woman and her fetus amount to roughly 800 mg. Because the average woman's store of iron is only about 500 mg, a pregnant woman should take iron supplements.

Iron supplements may also be necessary to accommodate for impaired iron absorption. Absorption of iron may be hindered during pregnancy as a result of decreased gastric acidity (iron is absorbed best from an acid medium). In addition, increased plasma volume (from 2,600 ml in a nonpregnant woman to 3,600 ml in a pregnant woman) is disproportionately greater than the increase in RBCs, which lowers the patient's hematocrit (the percentage of RBCs in whole blood) and may cause anemia. Hemoglobin level also decreases. Hematocrit below 35% and hemoglobin level below 11.5 g/dl indicate pregnancy-related anemia. Iron supplements are commonly prescribed during pregnancy to reduce the risk of this complication.

WBC mystery

The WBC count rises from 7,000 ml before pregnancy to 20,500 ml during pregnancy. The reason for this is unknown. The count may increase to 25,000 ml or more during labor, childbirth, and the early postpartum period.

Fibrin factor

Fibrinogen (a protein in blood plasma) is converted to fibrin by thrombin and is known as *coagulation factor I*. In a nonpregnant patient, levels average 250 mg/dl. In a pregnant patient, levels average 450 mg/dl, increasing as much as 50% by term. This increase in the coagulation factor plays an important role in preventing maternal hemorrhage during childbirth.

Urinary system

The kidneys, ureters, and bladder undergo profound changes in structure and function during pregnancy.

Anatomic changes

Significant dilation of the renal pelves, calyces, and ureters begins as early as 10 weeks' gestation, probably due to increased estrogen and progesterone levels. As pregnancy advances and the uterus undergoes dextroversion (movement toward the right), the ureters and renal pelves become more dilated above the pelvic brim, particularly on the right side. In addition, the smooth muscle of the ureters undergoes hypertrophy and hyperplasia and muscle tone decreases, primarily because of the muscle-relaxing effects of progesterone. These changes slow the flow of urine through the ureters and result in hydronephrosis and hydroureter (distention of the renal pelves and ureters with urine), predisposing the pregnant patient to urinary tract infections (UTIs). In addition, because of the delay between urine's formation in the kidneys and its arrival in the bladder, inaccuracies may occur during clearance tests.

Maximal capacity, minimal comfort

Hormonal changes cause the bladder to relax during pregnancy, permitting it to distend to hold approximately 1,500 ml of urine. However, hormonal changes and pressure from the growing uterus cause bladder irritation, manifested as urinary frequency and urgency, even if the bladder contains little urine. Bladder vascularity increases and the mucosa bleeds easily.

When the uterus rises out of the pelvis, urinary symptoms reduce. As term approaches, however, the presenting part of the fetus engages in the pelvis, which exerts pressure on the bladder again, causing symptoms to return.

Functional changes

Pregnancy affects fluid retention; renal, ureter, and bladder function; renal tubular resorption; and nutrient and glucose excretion.

Fluid retention

Water is retained during pregnancy to help handle the increase in blood volume and to serve as a ready source of nutrients for the fetus. Because nutrients can only pass to the fetus when dissolved in or carried by fluid, this ready fluid supply is a fetal safeguard. This excess fluid also replenishes the mother's blood volume in case of hemorrhage.

A running theme

To provide sufficient fluid volume for effective placental exchange, a pregnant woman's total body water increases about 7.5 L from prepregnancy levels of 30 to 40 L. To maintain osmolarity, the body has to increase sodium reabsorption in the tubules. To accomplish this, the body's increased progesterone levels stimulate the angiotensin-renin system in the kidneys to increase aldosterone production. Aldosterone helps with sodium reabsorption. Potassium levels, however, remain adequate despite the increased urine output during pregnancy because progesterone is potassium-sparing and doesn't allow excess potassium to be excreted in the urine.

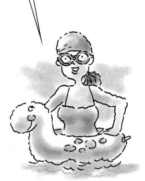

A pregnant woman's body retains water to ensure there's a medium in which nutrients can travel to get to the fetus.

Renal function

During pregnancy, the kidneys must excrete the waste products of the mother's body as well as those of the growing fetus. Also, the kidneys must be able to break down and excrete additional protein and manage the demands of increased renal blood flow. The kidneys may increase in size, which changes their structure and ultimately affects their function.

During pregnancy, urine output gradually increases to 60% to 80% more than prepregnancy output (1,500 ml/day). In addition, urine specific gravity decreases. The glomerular filtration rate (GFR) and renal plasma flow (RPF) begin to increase in early pregnancy to meet the increased needs of the circulatory system. By the second trimester, the GFR and RPF have increased by 30% to 50% and remain at this level for the duration of the pregnancy. This rise is consistent with that of the circulatory system increase, peaking at about 24 weeks' gestation. This efficient GFR level leads to lowered blood urea nitrogen and lowered creatinine levels in maternal plasma.

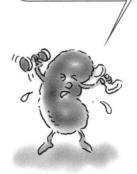

During pregnancy, I put in a double workout of excreting maternal AND fetal waste.

Glucose spill

An increased GFR leads to increased filtration of glucose into the renal tubules. Because reabsorption of glucose by the tubule cells occurs at a fixed rate, glucose sometimes is excreted, or spills, into urine during pregnancy. (See *When glucose enters urine.*) Lactose, which is being produced by the mammary glands during pregnancy but isn't being used, also spills into the urine.

Ureter and bladder function

During pregnancy, the uterus is pushed slightly toward the right side of the abdomen by the increased bulk of the sigmoid colon. The pressure on the right ureter caused by this movement may lead to urinary stasis and pyelonephritis (inflammation of the kidney cased by bacterial infection). Pressure on the urethra may lead to poor bladder emptying and possible bladder infection, which can become more dangerous if it results in kidney infection. Infection in the kidneys, which serve as the filtering system for toxins in the blood, can be extremely dangerous to the mother. UTIs are also potentially dangerous to the fetus because they're associated with preterm labor.

Renal tubular resorption

To maintain sodium and fluid balance, renal tubular resorption increases by as much as 50% during pregnancy. The patient's sodium requirement increases because she needs more intravascular and extracellular fluid. She may accumulate 6.2 to 8.5 L of water to meet her needs and those of the fetus and placenta. Up to 75% of maternal weight gain is due to increased body water in the extracellular spaces. Amniotic fluid and the placenta account for about one-half of this amount; increased maternal blood volume and enlargement of the breasts and uterus account for the rest.

Posture of elimination

Late in pregnancy, changes in the patient's posture affect sodium and water excretion. For example, the patient excretes less when lying on her back because the enlarged uterus compresses the vena cava and aorta, causing decreased cardiac output. This decreased cardiac output reduces renal blood flow, which in turn decreases kidney function. The patient excretes more when lying on her left side because, in this position, the uterus doesn't compress the great vessels and cardiac output and kidney function remain unchanged.

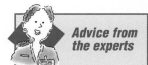

Advice from the experts

When glucose enters urine

During each prenatal visit, the patient's urine should be checked for glucose. A finding of more than a trace of glucose in a routine sample of urine from a pregnant patient is considered abnormal until proven otherwise.

Glycosuria on two consecutive occasions that isn't related to carbohydrate intake warrants further investigation. It may indicate gestational diabetes. Such a finding should be reported to the practitioner. In many cases, an oral glucose screening test is ordered. A small percentage of women have glycosuria of pregnancy that isn't diabetes-related but is due to a decreased kidney threshold for glucose.

Nutrient and glucose excretion

A pregnant patient loses increased amounts of some nutrients, such as amino acids, water-soluble vitamins, folic acid, and iodine. Proteinuria (protein in the urine) can occur during pregnancy because the filtered load of amino acids may exceed the tubular reabsorptive capacity. When the renal tubules can't reabsorb the amino acids, protein may be excreted in small amounts in the patient's urine. Values of +1 protein on a urine dipstick aren't considered abnormal until the levels exceed 300 mg/24 hours. Glycosuria (glucose in the urine) may also occur as GFR increases without a corresponding increase in tubular resorptive capacity.

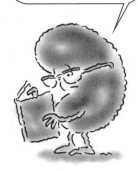

Use it or lose it! My tubules can't reasborb amino acids, so I have to excrete protein in the urine.

GI system

Changes during pregnancy affect anatomic elements in the GI system and alter certain GI functions. These changes are associated with many of the most commonly discussed discomforts of pregnancy.

Anatomic changes

The mouth, stomach, intestines, gallbladder, and liver are affected during pregnancy. (See *Crowding of abdominal contents*.)

Mouth

The salivary glands become more active in the pregnant patient, especially in the latter half of pregnancy. The gums become edematous and bleed easily because of increased vascularity.

Stomach and intestines

As progesterone increases during pregnancy, gastric tone and motility decrease, thus slowing the stomach's emptying time and possibly causing regurgitation and reflux of stomach contents. This may cause the patient to complain of heartburn. Progesterone also makes smooth muscle—including that which appears in the intestine—less active.

Make room for the uterus

As the uterus enlarges, it tends to displace the stomach and intestines toward the back and sides of the abdomen. About halfway through the pregnancy, the pressure may be sufficient enough to slow intestinal peristalsis and the emptying time of the stomach, leading to heartburn, constipation, and flatulence. Relaxin may contribute to decreased gastric motility, which may cause a de-

Crowding of abdominal contents

As the uterus enlarges as a result of the growing fetus, the intestinal contents are pushed upward and to the side. The uterus usually remains midline, although it may shift slightly to the right because of the increased bulk of the sigmoid colon on the left.

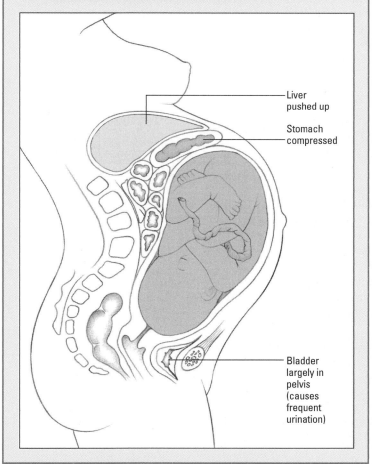

Liver pushed up

Stomach compressed

Bladder largely in pelvis (causes frequent urination)

I can tell them not to push, but I know it's no use. Crowding of abdominal contents occurs late in pregnancy as a result of uterine enlargement.

crease in blood supply to the GI tract as blood is drawn to the uterus.

The enlarged uterus also displaces the large intestine and puts increased pressure on veins below the uterus. This may predispose the patient to hemorrhoids.

Gallbladder and liver

As smooth muscles relax, the gallbladder empties sluggishly. This can lead to reabsorption of bilirubin into the maternal bloodstream, causing subclinical jaundice (generalized itching). A woman who has had previous gallstone formation may have an increased tendency for stone formation during pregnancy as a result of the increased plasma cholesterol level and additional cholesterol incorporated in bile. A patient with a peptic ulcer generally finds her condition improved during pregnancy because the acidity of the stomach decreases.

Biliary overtime

The liver doesn't enlarge or undergo major changes during pregnancy. However, hepatic blood flow may increase slightly, causing the liver's workload to increase as BMR increases. Factors within the liver as well as increased estrogen and progesterone decrease bile flow.

Some liver function studies show drastic changes during pregnancy, possibly caused by increased estrogen levels. Test results may show:
- doubled alkaline phosphatase levels, caused in part by increased alkaline phosphatase isoenzymes from the placenta
- decreased serum albumin
- increased plasma globulin levels, causing decreases in albumin globulin ratios
- decreased plasma cholinesterase levels.

These changes would suggest hepatic disease in a nonpregnant patient but are considered normal in the pregnant patient.

Functional changes

Nausea and vomiting during pregnancy may affect appetite and food consumption, even when the patient's energy demand increases.

Appetite and food consumption

A pregnant patient's appetite and food consumption fluctuate. This may be due to several things. For example, the patient may experience nausea and vomiting that decrease her appetite and, therefore, food consumption. These symptoms are more noticeable in the morning when the patient first arises, hence the term *morning sickness*. Nausea and vomiting can also occur when the woman experiences fatigue, and may be more frequent if the patient smokes. Nausea and vomiting tend to be noticeable when hCG and progesterone levels begin to rise. These conditions may also be a reaction to decreased glucose levels (because glucose is

Nausea and vomiting may decrease a pregnant patient's appetite and food consumption.

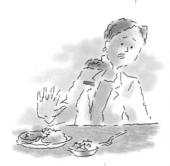

being used in great quantities by the growing fetus) or increased estrogen levels.

In addition to the reduced appetite caused by nausea and vomiting, increased hCG levels and changes in carbohydrate metabolism may reduce the patient's appetite. When nausea and vomiting stop, the patient's appetite and metabolic needs increase.

Carbohydrate, lipid, and protein metabolism

The patient's carbohydrate needs rise to meet increasing energy demands. The patient needs more glucose, especially during the second half of pregnancy. Plasma lipid levels increase starting in the first trimester, rising at term to 40% to 50% above prepregnancy levels. Cholesterol, triglyceride, and lipoprotein levels increase as well. The total concentration of serum proteins decreases, especially serum albumin and, perhaps, gamma globulin. The primary immunoglobulin transferred to the fetus is lowered in the patient's serum.

Musculoskeletal system

The patient's musculoskeletal system changes in response to hormones, weight gain, and the growing fetus. These changes may affect the patient's gait, posture, and comfort. In addition, increased maternal metabolism creates the need for greater calcium intake. If the patient ingests insufficient calcium, hypocalcemia and muscle cramps may occur. Musculoskeletal changes during pregnancy include changes to the skeleton, muscles, and nerves.

Skeleton

The enlarging uterus tilts the pelvis forward, shifting the patient's center of gravity. The lumbosacral curve increases, accompanied by a compensatory curvature in the cervicodorsal region. The lumbar and dorsal curves become even more pronounced as breasts enlarge and their weight pulls the shoulders forward, producing a stoop-shouldered stance. Increasing sex hormones (and possibly the hormone relaxin) relax the sacroiliac, sacrococcygeal, and pelvic joints. These changes cause marked alterations in posture and gait. Relaxation of the pelvic joints may also cause the patient's gait to change. Shoe and ring sizes tend to increase because of weight gain, hormonal changes, and dependent edema. Although these changes may persist after childbirth, in most cases they return to prepregnancy states.

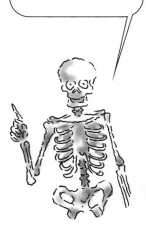

Pregnancy can make my joints relax.

Muscles

In the third trimester, the prominent rectus abdominis muscles (rectus muscles of the abdomen) separate, allowing the abdominal contents to protrude at the midline. Occasionally, the abdominal wall may not be able to stretch enough and the rectus muscles may actually separate, a condition known as *diastasis*. If this happens, a bluish groove appears at the site of separation after pregnancy.

Inny to outty

The umbilicus is stretched by pregnancy to such an extent that, by the week 28 of gestation, its depression becomes obliterated and smooth because it has been pushed so far outward. In most women, it may appear as if it has turned inside out, protruding as a round bump at the center of the abdominal wall.

Nerves

In the third trimester, carpal tunnel syndrome may occur when the median nerve of the carpal tunnel of the wrist is compressed by edematous surrounding tissue. The patient may notice tingling and burning in the dominant hand, possibly radiating to the elbow and upper arm. Numbness or tingling in the hands also may result from pregnancy-related postural changes such as slumped shoulders that pull on the brachial plexus.

Integumentary system

Skin changes vary greatly among pregnant patients. Of those patients who experience skin changes, Blacks and Whites with brown hair typically show more marked changes.

Because some skin changes may remain after childbirth, they aren't considered important signs of pregnancy in a patient who has given birth before. The patient may need the nurse's help to integrate these skin changes into her self-concept. Skin changes associated with pregnancy include striae gravidarum, pigment changes, vascular markings, and other changes.

Striae gravidarum

The patient's weight gain and enlarging uterus, combined with the action of adrenocorticosteroids, lead to stretching of the underlying connective tissue of the skin, creating striae gravidarum in the second and third trimesters. Better known as *stretch marks*, striae on light-skinned patients appear as pink or slightly reddish streaks with slight depressions; on dark-skinned patients, they appear

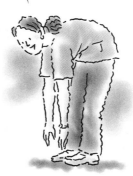

Stretch marks are most common on the skin covering the breasts, abdomen, buttocks, and thighs.

lighter than the surrounding skin tone. They develop most commonly on the skin covering the breasts, abdomen, buttocks, and thighs. After labor, they typically grow lighter until they appear silvery white on light-skinned patients and light brown on dark-skinned patients.

Pigment changes

Pigmentation begins to change at approximately 8 weeks' gestation, partly because of melanocyte-stimulating and adrenocorticotropic hormones and partly because of estrogen and progesterone. These changes are more pronounced in hyperpigmented areas, such as the face, breasts (especially nipples), axillae, abdomen, anal region, inner thighs, and vulva. Specific changes may include linea nigra and melasma.

Vascular markings

Tiny, bright-red angiomas may appear during pregnancy as a result of estrogen release, which increases subcutaneous blood flow. They're called *vascular spiders* because of the branching pattern that extends from each spot. Occurring mostly on the chest, neck, arms, face, and legs, they disappear after childbirth.

Pink-handed

Palmar erythemas, commonly seen along with vascular spiders, are well-delineated, pinkish areas over the palmar surface of the hands. When pregnancy ends and estrogen levels decrease, this condition reverses.

Bubbled gums

Epulides, also known as *gingival granuloma gravidarum*, are raised, red, fleshy areas that appear on the gums as a result of increased estrogen. They may enlarge, cause severe pain, and bleed profusely. An epulis that grows rapidly may require excision.

Other integumentary changes

Nevi (circumscribed, benign proliferations of pigment-producing cells in the skin) may develop on the face, neck, upper chest, or arms during pregnancy. Oily skin and acne from increased estrogen may also occur. Hirsutism (excessive hair growth) may occur, but this reverses when pregnancy ends. By the sixth week of pregnancy, fingernails may soften and break easily—a problem that may be exacerbated by nail polish removers.

Immune system

Immunologic competency naturally decreases during pregnancy, most likely to prevent the woman's body from rejecting the fetus. To the immune system, the fetus is a foreign object. In most cases, the immune system responds to foreign objects by sending defense cells that gang up on the foreign objects and try to destroy them. For certain types of foreign objects, such as a cold virus, this immune response is necessary to protect the body. In a situation such as organ transplantation, however, the patient must be given medications to reduce the immune system response so that the body doesn't attack the transplant.

Make yourself at home

A similar process occurs naturally in a pregnant woman, whereby her immune system response decreases, allowing the fetus to remain. In particular, immunoglobulin G (IgG) production is decreased, which increases the risk of infection during pregnancy. A simultaneous increase in the WBC count may help to counteract the decrease in IgG response.

Neurologic system

Changes in the neurologic system during pregnancy are poorly defined and aren't completely understood. For most patients, neurologic changes are temporary and revert back to normal after pregnancy is over.

Nervous reactions

Functional disturbances called *entrapment neuropathies* occur in the peripheral nervous system as a result of mechanical pressure. In other words, nerves become trapped and pinched by the enlarging uterus and enlarged edematous vessels, making them less functional. For example, the patient may experience meralgia paresthetica, a tingling and numbness in the anterolateral portion of the thigh that results when the lateral femoral cutaneous nerve becomes entrapped in the area of the inguinal ligaments. This feeling is more pronounced in late pregnancy, as the gravid uterus presses on the nerves and as vascular stasis occurs.

Psychosocial changes

Pregnancy and childbirth are events that deeply affect the lives of parents, partners, and family members. A nurse faces many responsibilities and challenges regarding the expectant family's psychosocial care. Psychological, social, economic, and cultural factors as well as family and individual influences toward sex-specific and family roles affect the parents' response to pregnancy and childbirth. All of these aspects of childbearing affect the health of the parents and their children.

Phases of acceptance

A patient's acceptance of the pregnancy can progress through different phases:

- During the first stage, called *full embodiment*, a patient may become dependent on her partner or significant others and may be introspective and calm. The patient, especially if she's a new mother, may initially feel some ambivalence about finding out that she's pregnant. She may spend the first few weeks imagining how the pregnancy will change her life. As the pregnancy progresses, however, the mother incorporates the fetus into her body image.
- Next comes the developmental stage of *fetal distinction*. In this stage, the patient starts to view her fetus as a separate individual. She begins to accept her new body image and may even characterize it as being "full of life." She may become closer or more dependent on her mother at this stage.
- The next stage is *role transition*. During this stage, the patient prepares to separate from and give up her attachment to the fetus. She may become anxious about labor and delivery. Discomfort and frustration over the awkwardness of her body may lead the patient to become impatient about the impending delivery. During this stage, the patient also begins to get ready for the baby and to mentally prepare for her role as mother.

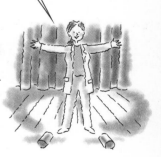

A woman's acceptance of her pregnancy can be viewed in three stages: full embodiment, fetal distinction, and role transition.

Influences affecting acceptance

Such factors as cultural background, family influences, and individual temperaments can affect a patient's acceptance of her pregnancy.

Cultural background

A woman's cultural background may strongly influence how she progresses through the stages of acceptance. They may also guide how actively the woman participates in her pregnancy. Certain beliefs and taboos may place restrictions on her behavior and activities. For example, Native Americans may not seek prenatal care as soon as other pregnant women because they view pregnancy as a normal condition.

Family influences

The home in which a woman was raised can also influence her beliefs about and her acceptance of pregnancy. If a woman was raised in a home in which children were loved and viewed as pleasant additions to a happy family, she'll probably have a more positive attitude toward pregnancy. If she was raised in a home in which children were considered intruders or were blamed for the breakup of a marriage, the woman's view of pregnancy may not be a positive one.

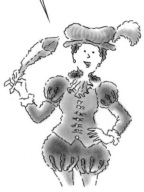

During the role transition stage, the patient begins to prepare for her new role as mother.

Like mother, like daughter

More specifically, the views of the patient's mother commonly influence the patient's attitudes about pregnancy. If her mother hated being pregnant and always reminded her that she was a burden and that children weren't always wanted, she may view her own pregnancy in the same way.

Individual temperament

A woman's temperament and ability to cope with or adapt to stress plays a role in how she resolves conflict and adapts to her new life after childbirth. How she accepts her pregnancy depends on her self-image and the support that's given to her. For example, a woman may view pregnancy as a situation that robs her of her career, looks, and freedom.

Make room for daddy?

A woman's relationship with the child's father also influences her acceptance of the pregnancy. If the father is there to provide emotional support, acceptance of the pregnancy is likely to be easier for the woman than if he isn't a part of the pregnancy. Whether the father of the child is able to accept the pregnancy depends on the same factors that affect the mother: cultural background, past experiences, relationship with family members, and individual temperament.

Promoting acceptance of pregnancy

Pregnancy is a time of profound psychological, social, and biological changes that affect the parents' responsibilities, freedoms, values, priorities, social status, relationships, and self-images. The events of the childbearing year (9 antenatal and 3 postpartum months) also may be unpredictable. Although expectant parents can control some events (for example, obtaining early prenatal care) and adopt positive attitudes, they can't control all that happens during that year.

Cheerleader for change

The nurse must promote family adaptation to the new family member. To achieve these goals, the nurse should take these steps, as expertise allows:
• Promote each family member's self-esteem.
• Elicit questions and concerns from the family and listen to them attentively.
• Discuss the roles and tasks for each family member, affirm their efforts, and inquire about and show concern for each family member's health care needs. Make referrals as needed.
• Involve all family members in prenatal visits, as appropriate.
• Facilitate communication among family members and offer anticipatory guidance about family changes during pregnancy and the postpartum period.
• Help to mobilize the family's resources.
• Offer sexual counseling to the patient and her partner.
• Help the patient maximize her family's positive contributions and minimize negative ones.

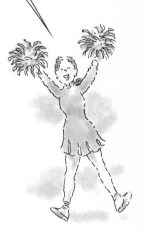

Give me an A! Give me a D! Give me an APT! What does it spell? Adapt!

Good job!

• Praise the family's efforts.
• Offer books and other materials that address all family members.
• Promote the family's prenatal bonding (sometimes called *attachment*) with the fetus by sharing information about fetal development and helping the family identify fetal heart tones, position, and movements. Reinforce bonding behaviors, such as patting the abdomen or talking to the fetus, by asking the patient or her partner to note and report fetal movements.

Conquering conflicts

• Facilitate conflict resolution related to pregnancy and childbirth. Help identify underlying conflicts through reflective communication, validation of feelings, and exploration of dreams and fantasies. Promote conflict resolution by teaching such techniques as personal affirmation and dream interpretation and by suggest-

ing literature that helps identify and resolve conflicts. Refer any patient who can't resolve conflicts to counseling.
• Support adaptive coping patterns through realistic patient and family education about pregnancy, childbirth, and the postpartum period. Discuss childbirth and human responses accurately and realistically. Frankly discuss the challenges of parenting.

Proceed with care

• Deliver culturally sensitive nursing care. Gather information about the family's customs and beliefs to add to assessment data and to individualize care.
• Identify personal attitudes and feelings about childbearing. Avoid imposing personal values, feelings, and emotional reactions on others. Also avoid making assumptions about the patient and her preferences. Allow her to share her feelings freely.

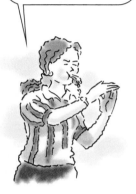

Time out! A nurse can promote adaptation during pregnancy by helping family members to identify underlying conflicts and teaching them techniques for conflict resolution.

First trimester

During the first trimester, the family's key psychosocial challenge is to resolve any ambivalence. The mother copes with the common discomforts and changes of the first trimester; the father begins to accept the reality of the pregnancy.

Other psychosocial challenges that the parents face include maternal acceptance of physical changes and paternal acceptance of and preparation for fatherhood.

Ambivalence

The first trimester is known as the *trimester of ambivalence* because parents experience mixed feelings. Many women have unrealistic ideas about maternal instincts, expecting to feel only loving, happy thoughts about the fetus and motherhood. In fact, most women feel some ambivalence about pregnancy and motherhood. Pregnancy involves stressful changes that force women to think and behave differently than they have in the past.

Sharing the joy (and the doubt)

Feelings of ambivalence are inevitable and normal. Encourage the parents to communicate these feelings to each other. Partners who discuss these feelings usually can resolve their concerns and fears and enjoy the gratifications of expecting a child. When partners share feelings, they may find they're experiencing similar conflicts.

Dream a little dream

During this time, both partners may experience vivid dreams about the impending birth. The woman may recall her dreams with greater intensity, however, because she typically is awakened more often at night by heartburn, fetal activity, and a need to urinate. Dreams tend to follow a predictable pattern during pregnancy. By exploring them, expectant parents can better understand themselves and any subconscious conflicts they may have. Dream analysis may be used to help resolve these psychosocial conflicts.

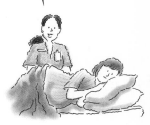

During the first trimester, it's perfectly normal for the woman to have especially vivid dreams about what's to come.

Psychological responses to physical changes

In the early weeks of the first trimester, the woman watches for body changes that confirm her pregnancy. Her body image (her mental image of how her body looks, feels, and moves, and how others see her) changes as her breasts enlarge, her menses cease, and she begins to experience nausea, fatigue, waist thickening, and general weight gain. Depending on her acceptance of the pregnancy, the woman may enjoy or dread these changes.

In the mood...or not!

A woman's response to the physical changes her body incurs during pregnancy, as well as other factors, can affect the sexual relationship between her and her partner. Women's sexual responses during pregnancy vary widely. Some women are too uncomfortable during the first trimester to enjoy sexual intercourse. Others, especially those who have had a past spontaneous abortion, may fear fetal injury. Those who believe sex is only for procreation may feel guilty about sexual activity during pregnancy. Conversely, some patients may feel sexually stimulated by the freedom from contraception, the joy of conception, or the lack of pressure to avoid pregnancy or to have sex on a regular schedule to achieve pregnancy.

A man's sexual response also may change during his partner's pregnancy. Typically, the man worries about how the pregnancy will change his relationship with his partner. He may feel personally rejected when his partner's fatigue, nausea, and other first trimester discomforts diminish her sexual interest. He may also fear causing spontaneous abortion or fetal injury during intercourse. These concerns may increase as the pregnancy advances.

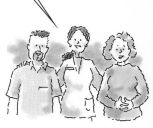

A healthy dose of affection and communication will go a long way toward helping an expectant couple to deal with their fears and concerns.

Affection prescription

Because of these fears and concerns, both partners may need extra affection from each other, especially during the first trimester. The nurse should encourage them to communicate and share their feelings and preferences about sexual activities.

Acceptance of and preparation for fatherhood

During the first trimester, the father typically finds the pregnancy unreal and intangible. The idea of the fetus may be abstract to him because he can't observe physical changes in his partner. Accepting the reality of pregnancy is the father's main psychological task in the first trimester.

You've got style

Because he isn't physically pregnant, the father can choose his degree and type of involvement in the pregnancy. There are three fathering styles:

The *observer* style describes a father who's happy about the pregnancy and provides much support to his partner. However, due to personal shyness or cultural values, he doesn't participate in such activities as attending parenting education classes or helping to choose the mode of infant feeding.

The *expressive* style describes a man who shows a strong emotional response to the pregnancy and wishes to be fully involved in it. He demonstrates the same emotional lability and ambivalence as the pregnant woman and may even experience common pregnancy symptoms, such as nausea, vomiting, and fatigue.

In the *instrumental* style of fathering, the man takes on the role of "manager" of the pregnancy. He asks questions and takes pictures throughout the pregnancy, carefully plans for the birthing event, prepares to serve as labor coach, and plans for the infant's arrival home. He's protective and supportive of his wife and feels responsible for the pregnancy outcome.

None of these styles is more competent or mature than another. Although each father becomes more involved as the pregnancy advances, fathering style usually remains consistent. Regardless of fathering style, the man may experience two psychosocial phenomena during the pregnancy: obsession with his role as provider and couvade symptoms.

Show baby the money

Because society values a man's provider role, the expectant father usually ponders the increased financial responsibilities a child brings. Finances remain a major focus throughout pregnancy, and the man may exert tremendous effort to attain financial security. A disproportionate emphasis on finances may reflect deep doubts about his competence as a father. The more secure he feels about his family's economic status, the more open and nurturing he can be with his partner.

Sympathy pains

Couvade syndrome describes physical symptoms—such as backache, nausea, and vomiting—experienced by the man that mimic the symptoms experienced by the pregnant woman. These symptoms commonly result from stress, anxiety, and empathy for the woman. Couvade symptoms aren't associated with the father's attachment to the fetus and aren't limited to first-time fathers. However, they occur most frequently in fathers who are greatly involved in the pregnancy.

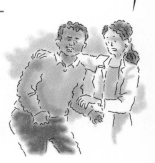

Congratulations! You're experiencing backaches and nausea and your wife is pregnant. You're the proud father of couvade symptoms.

Second trimester

During the second trimester, psychosocial tasks include mother-image development, father-image development, coping with body image and sexuality changes, and development of prenatal attachment. Parents may experience various fears. Feeling dependent and vulnerable, the woman may fear for her partner's safety. In touch with mortality, the man may consider how his death would affect his family. He may recall risks he has taken, such as driving recklessly; as a result, he may commit to being more careful to avoid the risk of abandoning his partner and fetus.

Dreams with meaning

During the second trimester, the parents' dreams may reflect concerns about the normalcy of the fetus, parental abilities, divided loyalties, and related subjects. To accomplish these tasks, the couple may examine their dreams and fears.

Mother-image development

As the second trimester begins, expectant parents have completed much of the first trimester's conflicts or ambivalence. The woman has abandoned old roles and has started to determine what kind of mother she wants to be. Her mother image is a composite of mothering characteristics she has gleaned from role models, readings, and her imagination.

Four aspects of the mother-daughter relationship influence the woman's mother image:

Introspection is common during the second trimester. The pregnant woman takes a good look at herself and begins to see a mother!

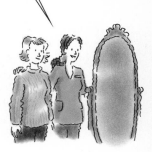

- her mother's availability in the past and during the pregnancy

- her mother's reaction to the pregnancy, her acceptance of the grandchild, and her acknowledgment of her daughter as a mother

- her mother's respect for the daughter's autonomy and acceptance of her as a mature adult her mother's willingness to reminisce about her own child-bearing and child-rearing experiences.

Expect introspection

The new mother's preoccupation with forming a mother image causes a period of introspection. As a result, she may show less affection, become more passive, or withdraw from her other children, who react by becoming more demanding. Her partner also may feel neglected during this period.

Father-image development

While the woman develops her mother image, the man begins to form his father image, which is based on his relationship with his father, previous fathering experiences, the fathering styles of friends and family members, and his partner's view of his role in the pregnancy.

Reach out and touch someone

As he starts to develop his father image, the man remembers his relationship with his father and sometimes increases contact with his parents. He may have difficulty viewing his father as a grandfather and coming to terms with his position as a father.

Generally, the woman's expectations about her partner's involvement and the quality of their relationship predict the man's role in delivery and child-rearing. Some women desire privacy and modesty during childbirth and don't expect or desire to involve their partners. Others expect their partner's full involvement in tracking fetal movements, attending prenatal visits, and acting as coach, advocate, and primary emotional support during labor. When the patient's expectations about her partner's role don't match those of her partner, the couple may need to be referred for counseling.

Prenatal bonding

A new phase begins at approximately 17 to 20 weeks' gestation, when the woman feels fetal movements for the first time. Because fetal movements are a sign of good health and may dispel the fear of spontaneous abortion, the woman almost always experiences the first flutter of movement positively, even when the pregnancy is unwanted. As a result, she becomes attentive to the type and timing of movements and to fetal responses to environmental factors, such as music, abdominal strokes, and meals.

Yes, sir, that's my baby

The woman may demonstrate bonding behaviors, such as stroking and patting her abdomen, talking to the fetus about eating while she eats, reprimanding the fetus for moving too much, engaging her partner in conversations with the fetus, eating a balanced diet, and engaging in other health-promoting behaviors. Bonding is influenced by the woman's health, developmental stage, and culture—not by obstetric complications, general anxiety, or demographic variables such as socioeconomic level.

This prenatal bonding requires positive self-esteem, positive role models, and acceptance of the pregnancy. Social support improves this attachment, which in turn increases the woman's feelings of maternal competence and effectiveness. In general, a woman who displays more bonding behaviors during pregnancy has more positive feelings about the neonate after delivery.

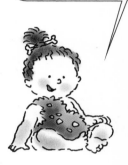

When parents bond with me in utero, they develop positive feelings about their roles as parents.

Third trimester

As the third trimester begins, the woman feels a sense of accomplishment because her fetus has reached the age of viability. She may feel sentimental about the approaching end of her pregnancy, when the mother-child relationship replaces the mother-fetus relationship. At the same time, however, she may look forward to giving birth because the last months of pregnancy involve bulkiness, insomnia, childbirth anxieties, and concern about the neonate's normalcy.

Time to address the special delivery

During the third trimester, the woman and her partner must adapt to activity changes, prepare for parenting, provide partner support, accept body image and sexuality changes, develop birth plans, and prepare for labor. At this time, the woman needs to overcome any fears she may have about the unknown, labor pain, loss of self-esteem, loss of control, and death. The technique of dream and fear examination may help the couple accomplish these tasks.

Adaptation to activity changes

The growing fetus makes daily activities more difficult for the woman and forces her to slow down. This change can affect her emotional state and her family relationships. Decreased social support for the woman on maternity leave can add to anxiety.

Preparation for parenting

Because the pregnant woman is more aware of what's going on in her body, she may begin to prepare for parenting before her partner. As the woman's body grows, however, typically so does the partner's acceptance of the pregnancy and anticipation of fatherhood. To prepare for parenting, the couple may now focus on concrete tasks, such as preparing the nursery, making decisions about childcare, and planning postpartum events.

Partner support and nurture

The couple's ability to support each other through the childbearing cycle is paramount. In many families, men and women get their support from each other.

Easy does it

In relationships in which neither partner is dominant, there may be greater satisfaction and greater closeness during the pregnancy. Relationships that allow flexibility, growth, and risk-taking ease the transition into parenthood.

Acceptance of body image and sexuality changes

A woman's body image can change as the pregnancy progresses and she gains weight. She may begin to feel less attractive. Her body image and her partner's feelings affect her sexual drive. Poor body image may cause the woman's interest in sex to drop off. Some men also experience diminished sexual interest as pregnancy advances. Couples that desire sexual intimacy in the third trimester must be creative, using new positions and techniques.

Preparation for labor

Childbirth education classes can prepare the woman and her partner for labor and delivery. The partner's attendance at prenatal classes and his participation in all aspects of pregnancy correlate with his degree of relationship satisfaction. Women who feel supported during the pregnancy and delivery may make the transition to motherhood more easily.

Development of birth plans

A highly dependent woman may allow the practitioner to make decisions about the birth plans, assuming that the practitioner's decisions are the wisest. A more independent woman may seek health care that's comfortable to her and that fits with her beliefs and knowledge, thus ensuring that her wishes are honored during

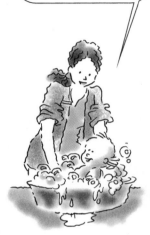

During the third trimester, it's time to prepare for the concrete realities of parenting.

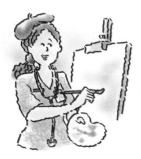

Creativity is key for the couple that wants to stay sexually intimate during the third trimester.

labor. A woman who shapes her childbirth experience and who develops realistic expectations of the event has dealt with her fears.

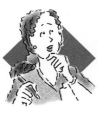

Quick quiz

1. Nausea and vomiting are common during pregnancy because of:

    A.   increased progesterone levels.
    B.   decreased progesterone levels.
    C.   increased estrogen levels.
    D.   decreased estrogen levels.

Answer: C. Nausea and vomiting may occur as a systemic reaction to increased estrogen levels.

2. Which change in respiratory function during pregnancy is considered normal?

    A.   Increased tidal volume
    B.   Increased expiratory volume
    C.   Decreased inspiratory capacity
    D.   Decreased oxygen consumption

Answer: A. A pregnant woman breathes more deeply, which increases the tidal volume of gas moving in and out of the respiratory tract with each breath.

3. Decreased gastric motility may occur around midpregnancy because of:

    A.   estrogen.
    B.   progesterone.
    C.   relaxin.
    D.   folic acid.

Answer: C. Relaxin (a hormone produced by the ovaries) can contribute to decreased gastric motility, which may cause a decrease in blood supply to the GI tract as blood is drawn into the uterus.

4. Which condition is common in the second trimester of pregnancy?

    A.   Mastitis
    B.   Metabolic acidosis
    C.   Physiologic anemia
    D.   Respiratory acidosis

Answer: C. Hemogoloin and hematocrit values decrease during pregnancy and the increase in plasma volume exceeds the increase in red blood cell production.

5. Which cardiac condition is normal during pregnancy?

    A.   Cardiac tamponade
    B.   Heart failure
    C.   Endocarditis
    D.   Systolic murmur

Answer: D. Systolic murmurs are heard in up to 90% of pregnant patients, and the murmur disappears soon after birth.

Scoring

☆☆☆ If you answered all five questions correctly, bravo! You're a pregnancy adaptations star!

☆☆ If you answered three or four questions correctly, take a bow! Your brain has adapted to all of your new knowledge!

☆ If you answered fewer than three questions correctly, the show must go on! Do a quick review, then get ready for the next act!

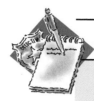

5

Prenatal care

Just the facts

In this chapter, you'll learn:

♦ components of a prenatal patient history and physical assessment

♦ different types of prenatal testing

♦ nutritional needs of the pregnant patient

♦ common discomforts of pregnancy and ways to minimize them.

A look at prenatal care

Prenatal care is essential to the overall health of the neonate and the mother. Traditional elements of prenatal care include assessing the patient, performing prenatal testing, providing nutritional care, and minimizing the discomforts of pregnancy. However, that isn't where prenatal care ends—or, should we say, where it begins.

Pre-pregnancy prenatal

Believe it or not, prenatal care begins long before pregnancy, when the expectant mother herself is still a child! Ideally, to reduce the risk of complications during pregnancy, a woman needs to maintain good health and nutrition throughout her life. For example, adequate calcium and vitamin D intake during the woman's infancy and childhood helps to prevent rickets, which can distort pelvic size, resulting in difficulties during birth. Maintaining immunizations protects her from viral diseases such as rubella. In addition, such healthy lifestyle practices as eating a nutritious diet, having positive attitudes about sexuality, practicing safer sex, having regular pelvic examinations, and receiving prompt treatment for sexually transmitted diseases (STDs) also contribute to the patient's health status throughout pregnancy.

Clean your room! Do your homework! Prevent rickets? A kid's work is never done!

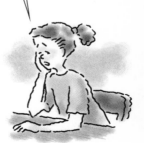

After the fact

Prenatal care after the patient has conceived consists of a thorough assessment, including a health history and physical examination, prenatal testing, nutritional care, and reduction of discomfort. Each of these factors should be addressed at the first prenatal visit.

Occasion for education

The first prenatal visit is also the time when the pregnant woman and her family can receive information on and counseling about what to expect during pregnancy, including necessary care. This promotes the development of healthy behaviors and helps to prevent complications. Keep in mind that the patient education you provide during pregnancy should vary depending on the age and parity of the woman as well as her cultural background. Warn the patient ahead of time that her first visit may be a long one.

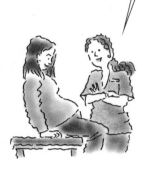

Developing and maintaining healthy behaviors during pregnancy helps prevent complications.

Assessment

The first prenatal visit is the best time to establish baseline data for the pregnant patient. A thorough assessment of the reproductive system should be included. As with other body systems, this assessment depends on an accurate history (see *Tips for a successful interview*) and a thorough physical examination.

Share and share alike

Remember to keep the patient informed about assessment findings. Sharing this information with her may help her to comply with health care recommendations and encourage her to seek additional information about any problems or questions that she has later in the pregnancy.

Health history

Information obtained from the patient's health history helps establish baseline data, which can be used to plan health-promotion strategies for every subsequent visit and identify potential complications. (See *Formidable findings*, page 150.)

The health history you conduct should be extensive. Be sure to include biographic data, information on the patient's nutritional status, a medical history, a family history, a gynecologic history, and an obstetric history.

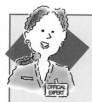

Advice from the experts

Tips for a successful interview

Here are some tips that can help you obtain an accurate and thorough patient history.

Location

Pregnancy is too private to be discussed in public areas. Make every effort to interview your patient in a private, quiet setting. Trying to talk to a pregnant woman in a crowded area, such as a busy waiting room in a clinic, is rarely effective. Remember patient confidentiality and respect the patient's privacy, especially when discussing intimate topics.

Checklist

To ensure that your history is complete, be sure to ask about:
• the patient's overall patterns of health and illness
• the patient's medical and surgical history
• the patient's history of pregnancy or abortion
• the date of the patient's last menses and whether her menses are regular or irregular
• the patient's sexual history, including number of partners, frequency, current method of birth control, and satisfaction with chosen method of birth control
• the patient's family history
• any allergies the patient has
• health-related habits, such as smoking and alcohol use.

Biographic data

When obtaining biographic data, assure the patient that the information will remain confidential. Topics to discuss include age; cultural considerations, such as race and religion; marital status; occupation; and education.

Age

The patient's age is an important factor because reproductive risks increase among adolescents younger than age 15 and women older than age 35. For example, pregnant adolescents are more likely to have preeclampsia, also known as *gestational hypertension*. Expectant mothers older than age 35 are at risk for other problematic conditions, including placenta previa; hydatidiform mole; and vascular, neoplastic, and degenerative diseases. (See chapter 6, High-risk pregnancy.)

Formidable findings

When performing your health history and assessment, look for the following findings to determine if a pregnant patient is at risk for complications.

Obstetric history

- History of infertility
- Grandmultiparity
- Incompetent cervix
- Uterine or cervical anomaly
- Previous preterm labor or preterm birth
- Previous cesarean birth
- Previous infant with macrosomia
- Two or more spontaneous or elective abortions
- Previous hydatidiform mole or chorio-carcinoma
- Previous ectopic pregnancy
- Previous stillborn neonate or neonatal death
- Previous multiple gestation
- Previous prolonged labor
- Previous low-birth-weight infant
- Previous midforceps delivery
- Diethylstilbestrol exposure in utero
- Previous infant with neurologic deficit, birth injury, or congenital anomaly
- Less than 1 year since last pregnancy

Medical history

- Cardiac disease
- Metabolic disease
- Renal disease
- Recent urinary tract infection or bacteriuria
- GI disorders
- Seizure disorders
- Family history of severe inherited disorders
- Surgery during current pregnancy
- Emotional disorders or mental retardation

- Previous surgeries, particularly those involving the reproductive organs
- Pulmonary disease
- Endocrine disorders
- Hemoglobinopathies
- Sexually transmitted disease (STD)
- Chronic hypertension
- History of abnormal Papanicolaou smear
- Malignancy
- Reproductive tract anomalies

Current obstetric status

- Inadequate prenatal care
- Intrauterine growth-restricted fetus
- Large-for-gestational-age fetus
- Gestational hypertension (preeclampsia)
- Abnormal fetal surveillance tests
- Polyhydramnios
- Placenta previa
- Abnormal presentation
- Maternal anemia
- Weight gain of less than 10 lb (4.5 kg)
- Weight loss of more than 5 lb (2.3 kg)
- Overweight or underweight status
- Fetal or placenta malformation
- Rh sensitization
- Preterm labor
- Multiple gestation
- Premature rupture of membranes
- Abruptio placentae
- Postdate pregnancy
- Fibroid tumors
- Fetal manipulation
- Cervical cerclage (purse string suture placed around incompetent cervix to

prevent premature opening and subsequent spontaneous abortion)
- STD
- Maternal infection
- Poor immunization status

Psychosocial factors

- Inadequate finances
- Social problems
- Adolescent
- Poor nutrition
- More than two children at home with no additional support
- Lack of acceptance of pregnancy
- Attempt at or ideation of suicide
- Poor housing
- Lack of involvement of father of baby
- Minority status
- Parental occupation
- Inadequate support systems
- Dysfunctional grieving
- Psychiatric history

Demographic factors

- Maternal age younger than 16 or older than 35
- Fewer than 11 years of education

Lifestyle

- Smoking (more than ten cigarettes per day)
- Substance abuse
- Long commute to work
- Refusal to use seatbelts
- Alcohol consumption
- Heavy lifting or long periods of standing
- Unusual stress
- Lack of smoke detectors in the home

Race and religion

The patient's race and religion, as well as other cultural considerations, may also impact a pregnancy. Obtaining information from your patient about these topics can help you plan patient care. (See *Cultural considerations for assessment.*) It also gives you greater insight into the patient's behavior, potential problems in health promotion and maintenance, and ways of coping with illness.

It's important to learn about the cultural communities in which you work, and become familiar with the cultural practices of those communities. (See *Southeast Asian views of pregnancy.*)

A race to detect disease

Because some diseases are more common among certain cultural groups, asking the patient about her race can be an important part of your assessment. It may help guide your prenatal testing. For example, a pregnant black woman should be screened for sickle cell trait because this trait primarily occurs in people of African or Mediterranean descent. A Jewish woman of Eastern European ancestry should be screened for Tay-Sachs disease.

Believe it or not

Religious beliefs and practices can also affect the patient's health during pregnancy and can predispose her to complications. For example, Amish women may not be immunized against rubella, putting them at risk. In addition, Seventh-Day Adventists traditionally exclude dairy products from their diets, and Jehovah's Witnesses refuse blood transfusions. Because these practices could impact prenatal care and the patient's risk of complications and, thus, you should ask about them when you take the patient's health history.

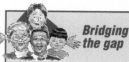

Bridging the gap

Cultural considerations for assessment

Encourage the patient to discuss her cultural beliefs regarding health, illness, and health care. Be considerate of the patient's cultural background. Also, be aware that members of many cultures are reluctant to talk about sexual matters and, in some cultures, sexual matters aren't discussed freely with members of the opposite sex.

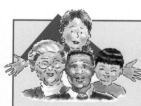

Bridging the gap

Southeast Asian views of pregnancy

Many women from Southeast Asia (Cambodia, Laos, and Vietnam) don't seek care during pregnancy because they don't see it as a time when medical intervention is necessary. In many cases, they're extremely modest and may find pelvic examinations embarrassing. They may rely on herbs and folk remedies to manage common discomforts of pregnancy. In addition, they may hold the belief that blood isn't replaceable, which may prevent them from agreeing to laboratory blood studies. Planning care for these patients may require interpreters, classes in prenatal health, and explanations of how health promotion regimens can fit within their cultural belief systems.

Marital status

Knowing the patient's marital status may help you determine whether family support systems are available. Marital status can also provide information on the size of the patient's home, her sexual practices, and possible stress factors.

Occupation

Ask about the patient's occupation and work environment to assess possible risk factors. If the patient works in a high-risk environment that exposes her to such hazards as chemicals, inhalants, or radiation, inform her of the dangers of these substances as well as the possible effects on her pregnancy. Knowing the patient's occupation can also help you to identify such risks as working long hours, lifting heavy objects, and standing for prolonged periods.

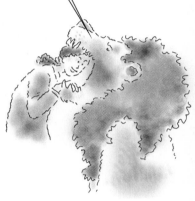

Asking about a patient's occupation will help to identify potential risks during pregnancy.

Education

The patient's formal education and her life experiences may influence several aspects of the pregnancy, including:
- her attitude toward the pregnancy
- her willingness to seek prenatal care
- the adequacy of her at-home prenatal care and nutritional status
- her knowledge of infant care
- her emotional response to childbirth and the responsibilities of parenting.

Obtaining information about the patient's education can help you to plan appropriate patient teaching.

Nutritional status

Adequate nutrition is especially vital during pregnancy. During the prenatal assessment, take a 24-hour diet history (recall). For more information, see the section on nutritional care later in this chapter.

Medical history

When taking a medical history, find out whether the patient is taking any prescription or over-the-counter (OTC) drugs, including vitamins and herbal remedies. Also ask about her smoking practices, alcohol use, and use of illegal drugs. Many drugs—except those with very large molecules, such as insulin and heparin—are able to cross the placenta and affect the fetus. All of the medications the patient is currently taking (including vitamins and herbal remedies) should be carefully evaluated, and the benefits of each medication should be weighed against the risk to the fetus.

Brushing up on current events

Ask the patient about previous and current medical problems that may jeopardize the pregnancy. For example:
• Diabetes can worsen during pregnancy and harm the mother and fetus. Even a woman who has been successfully managing her diabetes may find it challenging during pregnancy because the glucose-insulin regulatory system changes during pregnancy. Every woman appears to develop insulin resistance during pregnancy. In addition, the fetus uses maternal glucose, which may lead to hypoglycemia in the mother. When glucose regulation is poor, the mother is at risk for gestational hypertension and infection, especially monilial infection. The fetus is at risk for asphyxia and stillbirth. Macrosomia (an abnormally large body) may also occur, resulting in an increased risk of birth complications.
• Maternal hypertension, which is more common in women with essential hypertension, renal disease, or diabetes, increases the risk of abruptio placentae.
• Rubella infection during the first trimester can cause malformation in the developing fetus.
• Genital herpes can be transmitted to the neonate during birth. A woman with a history of this disease should have cultures done throughout her pregnancy and may need to deliver by cesarean birth to reduce the risk of transmission.

Obstacle course

Specific problems that you should ask the pregnant patient about include cardiac disorders, respiratory disorders such as tuberculosis; reproductive disorders, such as STDs and endometriosis; phlebitis; epilepsy; and gallbladder disorders. Also, ask the patient if she has a history of urinary tract infections (UTIs), cancer, alcoholism, smoking, drug addiction, or psychiatric problems.

Consider the patient's education level when using medicinal or scientific terms. For example, she may answer "No" when asked if she has hypertension, but "Yes" when asked if she has high blood pressure.

Family history

Knowing the medical histories of the patient's family members can help you plan care and guide your assessment by identifying complications for which the patient may be at greater risk. For example, if the patient has a family history of varicose veins, she may inherit a weakness in blood vessel walls that becomes evident when she develops varicosities during pregnancy. Gestational hypertension has also been shown to have a familial tendency, so a family history of gestational hypertension means that the patient is at greater risk for this complication. Be sure to ask whether there's a family history of multiple births, congenital diseases or deformities, or mental disability.

Don't dis Dad!

When possible, obtain a medical history from the child's father as well. Note that some fetal congenital anomalies may be traced to the father's exposure to environmental hazards.

Gynecologic history

The gynecologic portion of your assessment should include a menstrual history and contraceptive history.

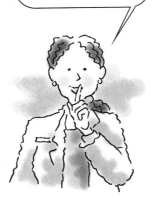

No need to whisper; menstrual and contraceptive information are important parts of a pregnant woman's gynecologic history.

Menstrual history

When obtaining a menstrual history, be sure to ask the patient:
• When did your last menstrual period begin?
• How many days are there between the start of one of your periods and the start of the next?
• Was your last period normal? Was the one before that normal?
• How many days does your flow usually last, and is it light, moderate, or heavy?
• Have you had bleeding or spotting since your last normal menstrual period?

Menarche plays a part

Age at menarche is important when determining pregnancy risks in adolescents. When pregnancy occurs within 3 years of menarche, there's an increased risk of maternal and fetal mortality. Such a pregnancy also increases the risk of delivering a neonate who's small for gestational age. Keep in mind that pregnancy can also occur before regular menses are established.

Cramping her style

Ask the patient to describe the intensity of her menstrual cramps. If she indicates that her cramps are very painful, anticipate the need for counseling to help her prepare for labor.

Contraceptive history

To obtain a contraceptive history, ask the patient:
• What form of contraception did you use before your pregnancy?
• How long did you use it?
• Were you satisfied with the method?
• Did you experience any complications while on this type of birth control?

Patients who took hormonal contraceptives before becoming pregnant should be asked how long it took to become pregnant once the contraceptives were stopped.

Contraceptive catastrophes

A woman whose pregnancy results from contraceptive failure needs special attention to ensure her medical and emotional well-being. Because the pregnancy wasn't planned, the woman may have emotional and financial issues. Offering support and referring her to counselors may help her work through these issues and resolve any ambivalence.

If the patient has an intrauterine device (IUD) in place when she becomes pregnant, it will ned to be removed immediately because of the risk of spontaneous abortion or preterm labor and delivery.

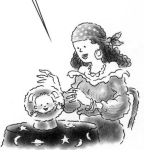

A crystal ball is fun, but Nägele's rule is much more reliable for calculating a patient's estimated date of delivery.

Calculating estimated date of delivery

Based on information obtained in the patient's menstrual history, you can calculate the patient's estimated date of delivery (EDD) using Nägele's rule: first day of last normal menses, minus 3 months, plus 7 days. Because Nägele's rule is based on a 28-day cycle, you may need to vary the calculation for a woman whose menstrual cycle is irregular, prolonged, or shortened.

Obstetric history

Obtaining an obstetric history is another important part of your assessment. The obstetric history provides important information about the patient's past pregnancies. No matter what age the patient is, don't assume that this is her first pregnancy. (See *Pregnancy classification system*, page 156.)

Getting the details

The obstetric history should include specific details about past pregnancies, including whether the patient had difficult or long labors and whether she experienced complications. Be sure to document each child's sex and the location and date of birth.

Do it in order

Always record the patient's obstetric history chronologically. For a list of the types of information you should include in a complete obstetric history, see *Taking an obstetric history*, page 157.

What's your type?

In addition to asking about pregnancy history, ask the woman if she knows her blood type. If the woman's blood type is Rh-negative, ask if she received $Rh_o(D)$ immune globulin (RhoGAM) after miscarriages, abortions, or previous births so that you'll know whether Rh sensitization occurred. If she didn't receive RhoGAM after any of these situations, her present pregnancy may be at risk for Rh sensitization. Also ask if she's ever had a blood transfusion to establish possible risk of hepatitis B and human immunodeficiency virus (HIV) exposure.

Gravida and para

Two important components of a patient's obstetric history are her gravida and para status. *Gravida* represents the number of times the patient has been pregnant. *Para* refers to the number of children above the age of viability the patient has delivered. The age of viability is the earliest time at which a fetus can survive outside the womb, generally at age 24 weeks or at a weight of more than 400 g (14.1 oz). These two pieces of information are important but provide only the most rudimentary information about the patient's obstetric history.

The gravida-para code

A slightly more informative system reflects the gravida and para numbers and includes the number of abortions in the patient's history. For example, G-3, P-2, Ab-1 describes a patient who has been pregnant three times, has had two deliveries after 20 weeks' gestation, and has had one abortion.

TPAL, GTPAL, and GTPALM

In an attempt to provide more detailed information about the patient's obstetric history, many facilities now use one of the following classification systems: TPAL, GTPAL, or GTPALM. These systems involve the assignment of numbers to various aspects of a patient's obstetric past. They offer health care practitioners a way to quickly obtain fairly comprehensive information about a patient's obstetric history. In particular, these systems offer more detailed information about the patient's para history.

How often, how many, how viable

In TPAL, the most basic of the three systems, the patient is assigned a four-digit number as follows:
• T is the number of pregnancies that ended at term (38 weeks' gestation or later).
• P is the number of pregnancies that ended after 20 weeks' gestation and before the end of 37 weeks' gestation.
• A is the number of pregnancies that ended in spontaneous or induced abortions.

Pregnancy classification system

When referring to the obstetric and pregnancy history of a patient, keep these terms in mind:
• A *primigravida* is a woman who's pregnant for the first time.
• A *primipara* is a woman who has delivered one child past the age of viability.
• A *multigravida* is a woman who has been pregnant before but may not necessarily have carried to term.
• A *multipara* is a woman who has carried two or more pregnancies to viability.
• A *nulligravida* is a woman who has never been and isn't currently pregnant.

Taking an obstetric history

When taking the pregnant patient's obstetric history, be sure to ask her about:
• genital tract anomalies
• medications used during this pregnancy
• history of hepatitis, pelvic inflammatory disease, acquired immunodeficiency syndrome, blood transfusions, and herpes or other sexually transmitted diseases (STDs)
• partner's history of STDs
• previous abortions
• history of infertility.

Pregnancy particulars

Also ask the patient about past pregnancies. Be sure to note the number of past full-term and preterm pregnancies and obtain the following information about each of the patient's past pregnancies, if applicable:
• Was the pregnancy planned?

• Did any complications—such as spotting, swelling of the hands and feet, surgery, or falls—occur?
• Did the patient receive prenatal care? If so, when did she start?
• Did she take any medications? If so, what were they? How long did she take them? Why?
• What was the duration of the pregnancy?
• How was the pregnancy overall for the patient?

Birth and baby specifics

Also obtain the following information about the birth and postpartum condition of all previous pregnancies:
• What was the duration of labor?
• What type of birth was it?
• What type of anesthesia, if any, did the patient have?
• Did the patient experience any

complications during pregnancy or labor?
• What were the birthplace, condition, sex, weight, and Rh factor of the neonate?
• Was the labor as she had expected it? Better? Worse?
• Did she have stitches after birth?
• What was the condition of the infant after birth?
• What was the infant's Apgar score?
• Was special care needed for the infant? If so, what?
• Did the neonate experience any problems during the first several days after birth?
• What's the child's present state of health?
• Was the infant discharged from the heath care facility with the mother?
• Did the patient experience any postpartum problems?

• L is the number of children who are alive at the time the history is obtained.

Note that the patient's gravida number remains the same, but the TPAL systems allow subclassification of her para status. In most cases, a practitioner includes the patient's gravida status in addition to her TPAL number. Here are some examples:
• A woman who has had two previous pregnancies, has delivered two term children, and is pregnant again is a gravida 3 and is assigned a TPAL of 2-0-0-2.
• A woman who has had two abortions at 12 weeks (under the age of viability) and is pregnant again is a gravida 3 and is assigned a TPAL of 0-0-2-0.
• A woman who is pregnant for the sixth time, has delivered four term children and one preterm child, and has had one spontaneous abortion and one elective abortion is a gravida 6 and is assigned a TPAL of 4-1-2-5.

> The TPAL, GTPAL, and GTPALM systems are easy ways to share information about the patient's obstetric history with other members of the health care team.

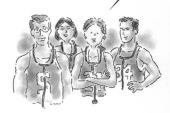

Details, details

More comprehensive systems for classifying pregnancy status include the GTPAL and GTPALM systems. These classification tools provide greater detail about the patient's pregnancy history. In the GTPAL system, the patient's gravida status is incorporated into her TPAL number. In GTPALM, a number is added to the GTPAL to represent the number of multiple pregnancies the patient has experienced (M). Note that a patient who hasn't given birth to multiple pregnancies doesn't receive a number to represent M.

Here are some examples:
• If a woman has had two previous pregnancies, has delivered two term children, and is currently pregnant, she's assigned a GTPAL of 3-2-0-0-2.
• If a woman who's pregnant with twins delivers at 35 weeks' gestation and the neonates survive, she's classified as a gravida 1, para 2 and is assigned a GTPAL of 1-0-2-0-2. Using the GTPALM system, the same woman would be identified as 1-0-2-0-2-1.

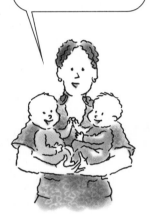

The mom of these two cuties delivered at 35 weeks. When she was pregnant, she was classified as a gravida 1, para 2 and assigned a GTPAL of 1-0-2-0-2.

Preventing history from repeating itself

If the patient is a multigravida, you'll want to know about any complications that affected her previous pregnancies. A woman who has delivered one or more large neonates (more than 4.1 kg [9 lb]) or who has a history of recurrent *Candida* infections or unexplained unsuccessful pregnancies should be screened for obesity and a family history of diabetes. A history of recurrent second-trimester abortions may indicate an incompetent cervix.

Physical assessment

Physical assessment should occur throughout pregnancy, starting with the mother's first prenatal visit and continuing throughout labor, delivery, and the postpartum period. Physical assessment includes evaluation of maternal and fetal well-being. At each assessment stage, keep in mind the interdependence of the mother and fetus. Changes in the mother's health may affect fetal health, and changes in fetal health may affect the mother's physical and emotional health.

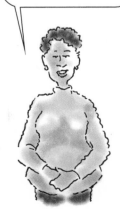

We're in this together! Changes in my health affect my baby and changes in my baby's health affect me.

Rounding the baselines

At the first prenatal visit, measurements of height and weight establish baselines for the patient and allow comparison with expected values throughout the pregnancy. Vital signs, including blood pressure, respiratory rate, and pulse rate, are also measured for baseline assessment. (See *Monitoring vital signs.*)

Scheduled surveillance

Prenatal care visits are usually scheduled every 4 weeks for the first 28 weeks of pregnancy, every 2 weeks until the 36th week, and then weekly until delivery, which usually occurs between weeks 38 and 42. Women who have known risk factors for complications and those who develop complications during the pregnancy require more frequent visits.

And now back to our regularly scheduled visit

Regular prenatal visits usually consist of weight measurements, vital sign checks, palpation of the abdomen, and fundal height checks. You should also assess the patient for preterm labor symptoms, fetal heart tones, and edema. Also, be sure to ask her if she has felt her baby move. (See *Assessing pregnancy by weeks*, page 160.)

Getting started

At the start of a prenatal visit, the woman should undress, put on a gown, and empty her bladder. Emptying the bladder makes the pelvic examination more comfortable for her, allows for easier identification of pelvic organs, and provides a urine specimen for laboratory testing.

Head-to-toe assessment

A thorough physical assessment should include inspection of the patient's general appearance, head and scalp, eyes, nose, ears, mouth, neck, breasts, heart, lungs, back, rectum, extremities, and skin.

> A prenatal visit should include a thorough physical assessment that's toe-to-head... oops... head-to-toe.

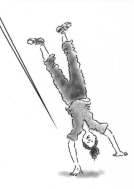

General appearance

Inspect the patient's general appearance. This helps form an impression of the woman's overall health and well-being. The manner in which a patient dresses and speaks, in addition to her body posture, can reveal how she feels about herself. Also inspect for signs of intimate partner violence. Be sure to document your findings.

Head and scalp

Examine the head and scalp for symmetry, normal contour, and tenderness. Check the hair for distribution, thickness, dryness or oiliness, and use of hair dye. Look for chloasma, an extra pigment on the face that may accompany pregnancy. Dryness or sparseness of hair suggests poor nutrition. Lack of cleanliness may suggest fatigue.

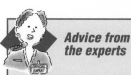

Advice from the experts

Monitoring vital signs

Monitoring the patient's vital signs, especially blood pressure, during each prenatal visit is an important part of ongoing assessment. A sudden increase in blood pressure is a danger sign of gestational hypertension. Likewise, a sudden increase in pulse or respiratory rate may suggest bleeding, such as in an early placenta previa or an abruption.

Be sure to report any of these signs or alterations in the patient's vital signs to the health care practitioner for further assessment and evaluation.

Assessing pregnancy by weeks

Here are some assessment findings you can expect as pregnancy progresses.

Weeks 1 to 4
- Amenorrhea occurs.
- Breasts begin to change.
- Immunologic pregnancy tests become positive: Radioimmunoassay test results are positive a few days after implantation; urine human chorionic gonadotropin test results are positive 10 to 14 days after amenorrhea occurs.
- Nausea and vomiting may begin between the 4th and 6th weeks.

Weeks 5 to 8
- Goodell's sign occurs (softening of cervix and vagina).
- Ladin's sign occurs (softening of uterine isthmus).
- Hegar's sign occurs (softening of lower uterine segment).
- Chadwick's sign appears (purple-blue coloration of the vagina, cervix, and vulva).
- McDonald's sign appears (easy flexion of the fundus toward the cervix).
- Braun von Fernwald's sign occurs (irregular softening and enlargement of the uterine fundus at the site of implantation).
- Piskacek's sign may occur (asymmetrical softening and enlargement of the uterus).
- The cervical mucus plug forms.
- Uterus changes from pear shape to globular.
- Urinary frequency and urgency occur.

Weeks 9 to 12
- Fetal heartbeat is detected using an ultrasonic stethoscope.
- Nausea, vomiting, and urinary frequency and urgency lessen.
- By the 12th week, the uterus is palpable just above the symphysis pubis.

Weeks 13 to 17
- Mother gains 10 to 12 lb (4.5 to 5.5 kg) during the second trimester.
- Uterine soufflé (sound made by the blood within the arteries of a gravid uterus) is heard on auscultation.
- Mother's heartbeat increases by about 10 beats/minute between 14 and 30 weeks' gestation. The rate is maintained until 40 weeks' gestation.
- By the 16th week, the mother's thyroid gland enlarges by about 25%, and the uterine fundus is palpable halfway between the symphysis pubis and the umbilicus.
- Maternal recognition of fetal movements, or quickening, occurs between 16 and 20 weeks' gestation.

Weeks 18 to 22
- The uterine fundus is palpable just below the umbilicus.
- Fetal heartbeats are heard with a fetoscope at 20 weeks' gestation.
- Fetal rebound or ballottement is possible.

Weeks 23 to 27
- The umbilicus appears to be level with abdominal skin.

- Striae gravidarum are usually apparent.
- The uterine fundus is palpable at the umbilicus.
- The shape of the uterus changes from globular to ovoid.
- Braxton Hicks contractions start.

Weeks 28 to 31
- The patient gains 8 to 10 lb (3.5 to 4.5 kg) in the third trimester.
- The uterine wall feels soft and yielding.
- The uterine fundus is halfway between the umbilicus and xiphoid process.
- Fetal outline is palpable.
- The fetus is mobile and may be found in any position.

Weeks 32 to 35
- The mother may experience heartburn.
- Striae gravidarum become more evident.
- The uterine fundus is palpable just below the xiphoid process.
- Braxton Hicks contractions increase in frequency and intensity.
- The mother may experience shortness of breath.

Weeks 36 to 40
- The umbilicus protrudes.
- Varicosities, if present, become very pronounced.
- Ankle edema is evident.
- Urinary frequency recurs.
- Engagement, or lightening, occurs.
- The mucus plug is expelled.
- Cervical effacement and dilation begin.

Eyes

Be sure to perform a careful inspection of the eyes. Look for edema in the eyelids. Ask the patient if she ever sees spots before her eyes or has diplopia (double vision) or other vision problems. (See *Watching for vision changes*.) These assessment findings may indicate gestational hypertension. In addition, an ophthalmoscopic examination may reveal that the optic disk appears swollen from edema associated with gestational hypertension.

Nose

Inspect the nose for nasal congestion and nasal membrane swelling, which may result from increased estrogen levels. If these conditions occur, advise the patient to avoid using topical medicines and nose sprays for relief without her health care practitioner's consent. These medications can be absorbed into the bloodstream and may harm the fetus.

Ears

During early pregnancy, nasal stuffiness may lead to blocked eustachian tubes, which can cause a feeling of "fullness" and dampening of sound. This disappears as the body adjusts to the new estrogen level.

Mouth

Examine the inside and outside of the mouth. Cracked corners may reveal a vitamin A deficiency. Pinpoint lesions with an erythematous base on the lips suggest herpes infection. Gingival (gum) hypertrophy may result from estrogen stimulation during pregnancy; the gums may be slightly swollen and tender to the touch. (See *Taking care of the teeth*, page 162.)

> The patient's hearing may be affected early in pregnancy because of blocked eustachian tubes.

Neck

Slight thyroid hypertrophy may occur during pregnancy because overall metabolic rate is increased. Lymph nodes normally aren't palpable and, if enlarged, may indicate an infection.

Breasts

During pregnancy, the areola may darken, breast size increases, and breasts become firmer. Blue streaking of veins may occur on the breasts. Colostrum may be expressed as early as 16 weeks' gestation. Montgomery's tubercles may become more prominent.

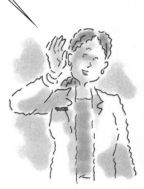

BSE basics

Instruct the patient on how to perform a breast self-examination (BSE), and tell her to perform a BSE monthly. Also educate her on the ongoing changes she'll experience during pregnancy, as appropriate.

Heart

Assess the patient's heart. Heart rate should range from 70 to 80 beats/minute. Occasionally, a benign functional heart murmur that's caused by increased vascular volume may be auscultated. If this occurs, the patient needs further evaluation to ensure that the condition is only a physiologic change related to the pregnancy and not a previously undetected heart condition.

Lungs

Assess respiratory rate and rhythm. Vital capacity (the amount of air that can be exhaled after maximum inspiration) shouldn't be reduced despite the fact that lung tissue assumes a more horizontal appearance as the growing uterus pushes up on the diaphragm. Late in pregnancy, diaphragmatic excursion (diaphragm movement) is reduced because the diaphragm can't descend as fully as usual because of the distended uterus.

Back

When examining the patient's back, be sure to assess for scoliosis. If she has scoliosis, refer her to an orthopedic surgeon to make sure the condition doesn't worsen during pregnancy. Typically, the lumbar curve is accentuated when standing so the patient can maintain body posture in the face of increasing abdominal size. If she has scoliosis, however, the added pressure of the growing fetus on the back may be more bothersome and painful.

Rectum

Assess the rectum for hemorrhoidal tissue, which commonly results from pelvic pressure that prevents venous return.

Extremities and skin

Assess for palmar erythema, an itchy redness in the palms that occurs early in pregnancy as a result of high estrogen levels. Assess for varicose veins and check the filling time of nailbeds. Observe for edema, and assess the patient's gait. The patient should be taught proper posture and walking to prevent musculoskeletal and gait problems later in pregnancy.

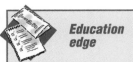

Education edge

Taking care of the teeth

Advise the patient that dental hygiene and taking care of dental caries are important during pregnancy. Dental X-rays can be taken during pregnancy as long as the woman reminds her dentist that she's pregnant and needs a lead apron. Extensive dental work requiring anesthesia shouldn't be done during pregnancy without approval from the woman's practitioner.

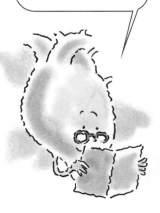

A pregnant patient's heart rate should range from 70 to 80 beats per minute. I can handle that!

Pelvic examination

A pelvic examination provides information on the health of internal and external reproductive organs and is valuable in assessment.

Patient prep

Take the following steps to prepare the patient for the pelvic examination:
• Ask the patient if she has douched within the past 24 hours. Explain that douching can wash away cells and organisms that the examination is designed to evaluate.
• For the patient's comfort, instruct her to empty her bladder before the examination. Provide a urine specimen container, if needed.
• To help the patient relax, which is essential for a thorough pelvic examination, explain what the examination entails and why it's necessary. The patient may desire to have a person in the room with her for support. It may also be beneficial to review some relaxation techniques with the patient such as deep breathing.
• If the patient is scheduled for a Papanicolaou (Pap) test, inform her that she may have to return later for another test if the findings of the first test aren't conclusive. Reassure her that this is done to confirm the results of the first test. If she has never had a Pap test, tell her that the test shouldn't hurt.
• Explain to the patient that a bimanual examination is performed to assess the size and location of the ovaries and uterus.

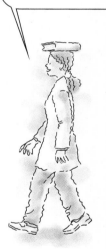

Even a charm-school dropout should be taught that proper posture and walking prevent musculoskeletal and gait problems later in pregnancy.

Shall I compare thee?

During the examination, record the patient's uterine fundal height and fetal heart sounds. Compare the new fundal height findings with the information obtained in the patient's history. In other words, make sure that the information you obtained about the patient's last menstrual period and her estimated date of delivery correlate with the current fundal height.

On the move

At about 12 to 14 weeks' gestation, the uterus is palpable over the symphysis pubis as a firm globular sphere. It reaches the umbilicus at 20 to 22 weeks, the xiphoid at 36 weeks, and then, in many cases, returns to about 4 cm below the xiphoid due to lightening at 40 weeks. (See *Measuring fundal height*, page 164.)

If the woman is past 12 weeks of pregnancy, palpate fundus location, measure fundal height (from the notch above the symphysis pubis to the superior aspect of the uterine fundus), and plot the height on a graph. This information helps detect variations in

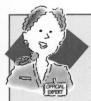

Advice from the experts

Measuring fundal height

Measuring the height of the uterus above the symphysis pubis reflects the progress of fetal growth, provides a gross estimate of the duration of pregnancy, and may indicate intrauterine growth retardation. Excessive increase in fundal height could mean multiple pregnancy or hydramnios (an excess of amniotic fluid).

To measure fundal height, use a pliable (not stretchable) tape measure or pelvimeter to measure from the notch of the symphysis pubis to the top of the fundus, without tipping back the corpus. During the second and third trimesters, make the measurement more precise by using the following calculation, known as McDonald's rule:

height of fundus (in centimeters) $\times$ $\frac{8}{7}$ = duration of pregnancy in weeks.

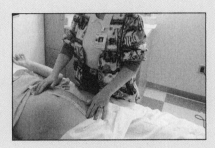

fetal growth. If an abnormality is detected, it can be further investigated with ultrasound to determine the cause.

After the examination, offer the patient premoistened tissues to clean the vulva.

Estimation of pelvic size

The size and shape of woman's pelvis can affect her ability to deliver her neonate vaginally. It's impossible to predict from a woman's outward appearance if her pelvis is adequate for the passage of a fetus. For example, a woman may look as if she has a wide pelvis, but she may only have a wide iliac crest and a normal, or smaller than normal, internal ring. (See *Pelvic shape and potential problems*.)

Clearly clearance counts

Internal pelvic measurements give actual diameters of the inlet and outlet through which the fetus passes. The internal pelvis must be large enough to allow a patient to give birth vaginally without difficulty. Differences in pelvic contour develop mainly because of heredity factors. However, such diseases as rickets may cause contraction of the pelvis, and pelvic injury may also be responsible for pelvic distortion.

Now or later?

Pelvic measurements can be taken at the initial visit or at a visit later in pregnancy, when the woman's pelvic muscles are more re-

There's no need to take pelvic measurements again if a woman has previously given birth vaginally. She has already passed the test! (My test, however, is a different story!)

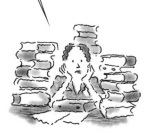

Pelvic shape and potential problems

The shape of a woman's pelvis can affect the delivery of her fetus. Her pelvis may be one of four types.

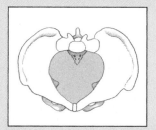 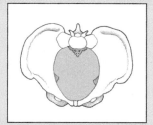 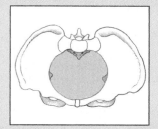 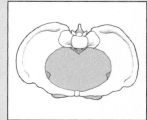

Android pelvis

In an *android* pelvis, the pelvic arch forms an acute triangle, making the lower dimensions of the pelvis extremely narrow. A pelvis of this shape is typically associated with males, but can also occur in women. A pregnant woman with this pelvic shape may experience difficulty delivering the fetus because the narrow shape makes it difficult for the fetus to exit.

Anthropoid pelvis

In an *anthropoid* pelvis, also known as an *apelike pelvis,* the transverse diameter is narrow and the anteroposterior diameter of the inlet is larger than normal. This pelvic shape doesn't accommodate a fetal head as well as a gynecoid pelvis because the transverse diameter is narrow.

Gynecoid pelvis

In a *gynecoid* pelvis, the inlets are well-rounded in both the forward and backward diameters and the pubic arch is wide. This type of pelvis is ideal for childbirth.

Platypelloid pelvis

In a *platypelloid,* or flattened, pelvis, the inlet is oval and smoothly curved but the anteroposterior diameter is shallow. Problems may occur during childbirth for a patient with this pelvic shape if the fetal head is unable to rotate to match the curves of the spine because the anteroposterior diameter is shallow and the pelvis is flat.

laxed. If a routine ultrasound is scheduled, estimations of pelvic size may be made through a combination of pelvimetry and fetal ultrasound.

Estimation of pelvic adequacy should be done by the 24th week of pregnancy because, by this time, the fetal head may grow large enough to interfere with safe passage and birth if the pelvic measurements are small. In this case, the woman should be advised that she may not be able to deliver her fetus vaginally and may require a cesarean birth. If a woman has already given birth vaginally, her pelvis has proven to be adequate. You don't need to remeasure her pelvis unless it has sustained trauma since her last vaginal birth.

Diagonal conjugate

The diagonal conjugate is the distance between the anterior surface of the sacral prominence and the anterior surface of the inferior margin of the symphysis pubis. It's the most useful gauge of pelvic size because it indicates the anteroposterior diameter of the pelvic inlet (the narrower diameter). (See *Diagonal conjugate measurement.*)

Ample room

If the measurement obtained is more than 5″ (12.5 cm), the pelvic inlet is considered adequate for childbirth (the diameter of the fetal head that must pass that point averages 3½″ [9 cm]).

True conjugate

The true conjugate, also known as the *conjugate vera*, is the measurement between the anterior surface of the sacral prominence and the posterior surface of the inferior margin of the symphysis pubis. This measurement can't be made directly but is estimated from the measurement of the diagonal conjugate.

Diagonal conjugate measurement

The diagonal conjugate is measured while the woman is in the lithotomy position. Two fingers of the examining hand are placed in the vagina and pressed inward and upward until the middle finger touches the sacral prominence. (The woman may feel the pressure of the examining finger.) The location where the examining hand touches the symphysis pubis is marked by the other hand. After withdrawing the examining hand, the distance between the tip of the middle finger and the marked point is measured with a ruler or a pelvimeter.

If the examining hand is small with short fingers, the fingers may not reach the sacral prominence, making manual pelvic measurements impossible.

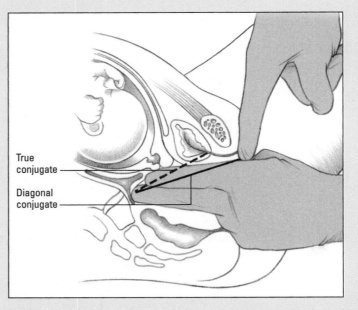

True conjugate

Diagonal conjugate

Tried and true

Here's how it's done:

The usual depth of the symphysis pubis (½″ to ¾″ [1 to 2 cm]) is subtracted from the diagonal conjugate measurement.

The distance remaining is the true conjugate, or the actual diameter of the pelvic inlet through which the fetal head must pass. The average true conjugate diameter is 4″ to 4¼″ (10 to 11 cm).

Ischial tuberosity

The ischial tuberosity is the transverse diameter of the pelvic outlet. This measurement is made at the medial and lowermost aspect of the ischial tuberosities, at the level of the anus. A pelvimeter is generally used to measure the diameter, although it can be measured using a ruler or by comparing it with a known handspan or clenched fist measurement. A diameter of 10.5 cm (4¼″) is considered adequate for passage of the fetal head through the outlet.

Prenatal testing

The fetus is assessed by using direct and indirect monitoring techniques. Common tests include fetal heart rate (FHR) monitoring, ultrasonography, fetal activity determination, maternal urinalysis and serum assays, amniocentesis, chorionic villi sampling (CVS), percutaneous umbilical blood sampling (PUBS), fetoscopy, blood studies, prepartum nonstress test (NST), prepartum contraction stress test (CST), and nipple stimulation CST.

Fetal heart rate

You can obtain an FHR by placing a fetoscope or Doppler ultrasound stethoscope on the mother's abdomen and counting fetal heartbeats. Simultaneously palpating the mother's pulse helps you to avoid confusion between maternal and fetal heartbeats.

Heart to heart

A fetoscope can detect fetal heartbeats as early as 20 weeks' gestation. The Doppler ultrasound stethoscope, a more sensitive instrument, can detect fetal heartbeats as early as 10 weeks' gestation and remains a useful tool throughout labor.

To determine the FHR at fewer than 20 weeks' gestation, place the head of the Doppler stethoscope at the midline of the patient's abdomen above the pubic hairline. After 20 weeks' gestation,

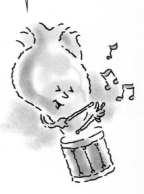

Whose beat is whose? Mom's may be louder, so avoid confusion by palpating her pulse while you listen for my FHR.

when fetal position can be determined, palpate for the back of the fetal thorax and position the instrument directly over it. Locate the loudest heartbeats and palpate the maternal pulse. Count fetal heartbeats for at least 15 seconds while monitoring maternal pulse. Leopold's maneuvers can be used to determine fetal position, presentation, and attitude. However, because the presentation and position of the fetus may change, most practitioners don't perform Leopold's maneuvers until 32 to 34 weeks' gestation. (See *Performing Leopold's maneuvers.*)

Advice from the experts

Performing Leopold's maneuvers

You can determine fetal position, presentation, and attitude by performing Leopold's maneuvers. Ask the patient to empty her bladder, assist her to a supine position, and expose her abdomen. Then perform the following four maneuvers in order.

First maneuver
Face the patient and warm your hands. Place your hands on the patient's abdomen to determine fetal position in the uterine fundus. Curl your fingers around the fundus. When the fetus is in the vertex position (head first), the buttocks should feel irregularly shaped and firm. When the fetus is in breech position, the head should feel hard, round, and movable.

Second maneuver
Move your hands down the side of the abdomen, applying gentle pressure. If the fetus is in the vertex position, you'll feel a smooth, hard surface on one side—the fetal back. On the opposite side, you'll feel lumps and knobs—the knees, hands, feet, and elbows. If the fetus is in the breech position, you may not feel the back at all.

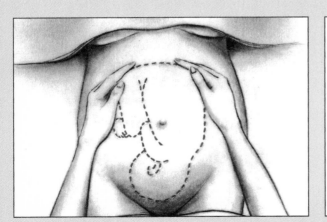

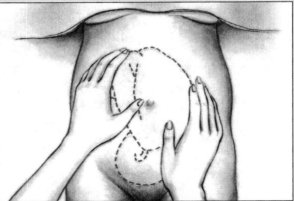

Because FHR usually ranges from 120 to 160 beats/minute, auscultation yields only an average rate at best. It can detect gross (but commonly late) signs of fetal distress, such as tachycardia and bradycardia, and is thus recommended only for a patient with an uncomplicated pregnancy. For a patient with a high-risk pregnancy, indirect or direct electronic fetal monitoring provides more accurate information on fetal status. (See *Evaluating FHR*, page 170.)

Third maneuver

Spread apart your thumb and fingers of one hand. Place them just above the patient's symphysis pubis. Bring your fingers together. If the fetus is in the vertex position and hasn't descended, you'll feel the head. If the fetus is in the vertex position and has descended, you'll feel a less distinct mass. If the fetus is in the breech position, you'll also feel a less distinct mass, which could be the feet or knees.

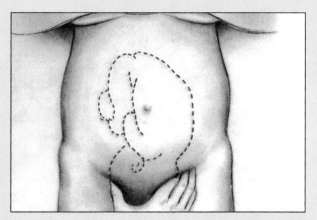

Fourth maneuver

The fourth maneuver can determine flexion or extension of the fetal head and neck. Place your hands on both sides of the lower abdomen. Apply gentle pressure with your fingers as you slide your hands downward, toward the symphysis pubis. If the head (rather than the feet or a shoulder) is the presenting fetal part, one of your hands is stopped by the cephalic prominence. The other hand descends unobstructed more deeply. If the fetus is in the vertex position, you'll feel the cephalic prominence on the same side as the small parts; if it's in the face position, it will be on the same side as the back. If the fetus is engaged, you won't be able to feel the cephalic prominence.

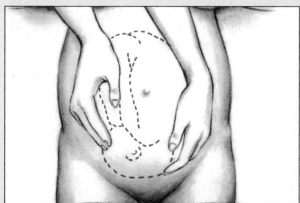

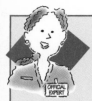

Advice from the experts

Evaluating FHR

To evaluate fetal heart rate (FHR), position the fetoscope or Doppler ultrasound stethoscope on the patient's abdomen, midway between the umbilicus and symphysis pubis for cephalic presentation, or above or at the level of the umbilicus for breech presentation. Locate the loudest heartbeats, and palpate the maternal pulse. Monitor maternal pulse and count fetal heartbeats for 60 seconds. Notify the practitioner immediately of marked changes in FHR from the baseline.

Fetoscope
A fetoscope is a modified stethoscope attached to a headpiece. A fetoscope can detect fetal heartbeats as early as 20 weeks' gestation.

Doppler ultrasound stethoscope
A Doppler ultrasound stethoscope uses ultrasound waves that bounce off the fetal heart to produce echoes or a clicking noise that reflect the rate of the fetal heartbeat. The Doppler ultrasound stethoscope can detect fetal heartbeats as early as 10 weeks' gestation, and has greater sensitivity than the fetoscope.

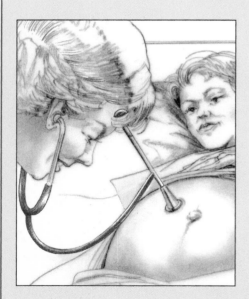

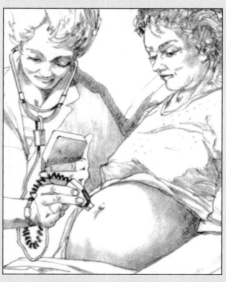

Ultrasonography

Through the use of sound waves bouncing off of internal structures, ultrasonography allows visualization of the fetus without the hazards of X-rays. Ultrasonography allows the patient to see her baby and even produces an image (called a *sonogram*) that she can show to friends and family.

In ultrasonography, sound waves bounce off internal structures to let you see the fetus.

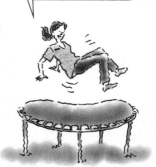

How ultra-useful!

Ultrasonography is used to:
- verify the due date and correlate it with fetus size
- evaluate the condition of the fetus through observation of fetal activity, breathing movements, and amniotic fluid volume
- determine the condition of the fetus when there's a greater than average risk of an abnormality or a greater than average concern
- rule out pregnancy by week 7 if there has been a suspected false-positive pregnancy test
- determine the cause of bleeding or spotting in early pregnancy
- locate an IUD that was in place at the time of conception
- locate the fetus before amniocentesis and during CVS
- determine the condition of the fetus if no heartbeat has been detected by week 14 with a Doppler device or if no fetal movement has occurred by week 22
- diagnose multiple pregnancy, especially if the patient has taken fertility drugs or the uterus is larger than it should be for the expected due date
- determine if abnormally rapid uterine growth is being caused by excessive amniotic fluid
- determine the condition of the placenta when deterioration might be responsible for fetal growth retardation or distress
- verify presentation and uncommon fetal or cord position before delivery.

Screen debut

Here's how it's usually done. An ultrasonic transducer that's placed on the mother's abdomen transmits high-frequency sound waves through the abdominal wall. These sound waves deflect off the fetus, bounce back to the transducer, and are transformed into a visual image on a monitoring screen.

A fluid fill-up

To prepare a patient for an abdominal ultrasound, have her drink 1 qt (1 L) of fluid 1 to 2 hours before the test. Instruct her not to void before the test because a full bladder serves as a landmark to define other pelvic organs.

A bladder-friendly version

Transvaginal ultrasonography is another type of imaging. It's well tolerated because it eliminates the need for a full bladder and is usually used during the first trimester of pregnancy. It also lets you—and the patient—see the developing fetus at a much earlier gestation.

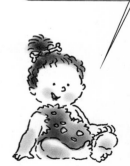

As you can imagine, I've had lots of practice posing. My first "photo op" was courtesy of a sonogram.

Fetal activity determination

The activity of the fetus (kick counts) determines its condition in utero. Daily evaluation of movement provides an inexpensive, noninvasive way of assessing fetal well-being. Decreased activity in a previously active fetus may reflect a disturbance in placental function.

As early as 7 weeks' gestation, the embryo can produce spontaneous movements; however, these movements don't become apparent to the mother until sometime between weeks 14 and 26 (but generally between weeks 18 and 22). The first noticeable movement of the fetus by the mother is called *quickening*. The acknowledgment of fetal movements may be delayed if the due date is miscalculated or if the mother doesn't recognize the sensation. A patient who has had a baby before is likely to recognize movement earlier. If the mother hasn't felt any movements by week 22, an ultrasound may be ordered to assess the condition of the fetus.

Looking for some fetal action

Fetal movements may be elicited by having the patient lie down for about an hour after having a glass of milk or another snack. The jolt of energy produced by a light snack commonly produces fetal movement. After the 28th week, patients are usually asked to monitor fetal movements twice daily—once in the morning, when activity tends to be sparser, and once in the more-active evening hours. Instruct the patient to check the clock when she's ready to start counting fetal movements. She should count movements of any kind (kicks, flutters, swishes, rolls). After she counts 10 movements, she should note the time again.

If the patient doesn't feel 10 movements after 30 minutes, she should eat another snack and then count for another 30 minutes. If the patient feels no movement or less than 10 movements after the second 30-minute period, she should contact her health care provider. The closer the patient is to her due date, the more important regular checking of fetal movements becomes. (See *Monitoring for fetal distress.*)

Maternal urinalysis

During pregnancy, the patient is monitored routinely for potential problems. Some problems may be detected by a simple urine test. The urine specimen should be obtained from the patient during her regularly scheduled visit using a clean-catch technique. The specimen is examined for bacteriuria as well as protein, glucose, and ketones. Urinalysis can detect such problems as infection and diabetes before the patient shows any signs.

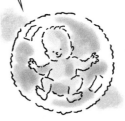

I'm kicking up a storm in here! It's just my way of letting mom know I'm doing great—and the placenta is working just fine, thank you!

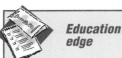

Education edge

Monitoring for fetal distress

If the patient is performing fetal activity determination, make sure that she rests during the counting period. If she's walking around or otherwise physically moving, she may not feel the movements as much as if she were at rest. If 2 hours go by without 10 movements, she should promptly contact her practitioner. Absence of fetal activity doesn't necessarily mean there's a problem but, in some cases, it indicates fetal distress. Immediate action may be needed.

Maternal serum assays

Serum assays—including those for estrogens, human placental lactogen (hPL), and human chorionic gonadotropin (hCG)—are used in addition to urinalysis to monitor the pregnant patient for problems.

Estrogens

Three major estrogens exist: estrone, estradiol, and estriol. Production of estrogens, particularly estriol, increases during pregnancy. During pregnancy, levels of estrone and estradiol increase to about 100 times their nonpregnancy levels, whereas estriol levels increase 1,000 times. Estrogen production depends on the interaction of the maternal fetal-placental unit. Estriol is secreted by the placenta into the maternal circulation and is eventually excreted in maternal urine.

The old estriol test just ain't what it used to be

In the past, a mother's urinary estriol levels were measured regularly to assess fetal and placental well-being. Today, however, estriol levels are measured only as part of the triple screen test. (For more information, see the section on the triple screen test later in this chapter.)

Salivary signs

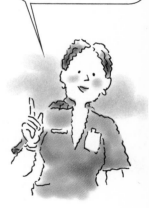

A positive SalEst test indicates that a patient is at risk for premature labor.

The SalEst test is a salivary test that measures estriol levels. For women at risk, the test is 98% accurate in ruling out premature labor and delivery. The test is performed between 22 and 36 weeks' gestation. Estriol has been found to increase 2 to 3 weeks before the spontaneous onset of labor and delivery. A positive test indicates that the patient is at risk for premature labor. With this knowledge, precautions can be taken to decrease the risk of preterm labor and maintain fetal viability.

Human placental lactogen

Also known as *human chorionic somatomammotropin*, hPL works with prolactin to prepare the breasts for lactation. It also indirectly provides energy for maternal metabolism and fetal nutrition. It facilitates the protein synthesis and mobilization that are essential for fetal growth.

Secretion of hPL is autonomous, beginning around 5 weeks' gestation and declining rapidly after delivery. According to some evidence, however, this hormone may not be essential for a successful pregnancy.

The purposes of hPL testing are to:
- assess placental function and fetal well-being (combined with measurement of estriol levels)
- aid diagnosis of hydatidiform moles and choriocarcinoma
- aid diagnosis and monitor treatment of nontrophoblastic tumors that ectopically secrete hPL.

Serial evaluation

A radioimmunoassay measures plasma hPL levels. The test may be required in high-risk pregnancies, such as those involving diabetes mellitus, hypertension, or suspected placental tissue dysfunction. Because values vary widely during the latter half of pregnancy, serial determinations over several days provide the most reliable test results.

For pregnant women, normal hPL levels slowly increase throughout pregnancy, reaching 7 mg/ml at term. Low hPL concentrations are also characteristically associated with postmaturity syndrome, intrauterine growth retardation, preeclampsia, and eclampsia. However, low hPL concentrations don't confirm fetal distress. Conversely, concentrations over 4 mg/ml after 30 weeks' gestation don't guarantee fetal well-being because elevated levels have been reported after fetal death. An hPL value above 6 mg/ml after 30 weeks' gestation may suggest an unusually large placenta, common in patients with diabetes mellitus, multiple pregnancy, and Rh isoimmunization.

Human chorionic gonadotropin

Although the precise function of hCG (a glycoprotein hormone produced in the placenta) is still unclear, it appears that hCG and progesterone maintain the corpus luteum during early pregnancy. Production of hCG increases steadily during the first trimester, peaking around 10 weeks' gestation. Levels then fall to less than 10% of first-trimester peak levels during the remainder of the pregnancy. About 2 weeks after delivery, the hormone may no longer be detectable.

The serum test for hCG, which is more sensitive and costly than the routine pregnancy test using a urine sample, provides a quantitative analysis. It's used to:
- detect pregnancy
- determine adequacy of hormonal production in high-risk pregnancies
- aid diagnosis of trophoblastic tumors, such as hydatidiform moles and choriocarcinoma
- detect tumors that ectopically secrete hCG
- monitor treatment for induction of ovulation and conception.

Leveling with you

Normal hCG levels are less than 4 IU/L. During pregnancy, hCG levels vary widely, depending partly on the number of days after the last normal menses. Elevated hCG levels indicate pregnancy; significantly higher concentrations are present in a multiple pregnancy. Low hCG levels can occur in ectopic pregnancy or pregnancy of less than 9 days. Unfortunately, hCG levels can't differentiate between pregnancy and tumor recurrence because levels are high in both conditions.

Down and out

In addition, researchers have found that a high level of hCG in a pregnant woman's blood means she's at greater risk for having a baby with Down syndrome. If conception occurs, a specific assay for hCG, commonly called the *beta-subunit assay*, may detect this hormone in the blood as soon as 9 days after ovulation. This interval coincides with the implantation of the fertilized ovum into the uterine wall. If hCG levels are indicative of Down syndrome, amniocentesis is used to confirm.

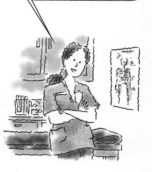

A high level of hCG in a pregnant woman's blood means she's at greater risk for having a baby with Down syndrome.

Amniocentesis

Amniocentesis is the sterile needle aspiration of fluid from the amniotic sac for analysis. This procedure is recommended when:
• the mother is older than age 35
• the couple has already had a child with a chromosomal abnormality (such as Down syndrome) or a metabolic disorder (such as Hunter's syndrome)
• the mother is a carrier of an X-linked genetic disorder, such as hemophilia, which she has a 50% chance of passing on to a son
• a parent is known to have a condition, such as Huntington's chorea, that's passed on by autosomal dominant inheritance, giving the baby a 1 in 2 chance of inheriting the disease
• both parents are carriers of an autosomal recessive inherited disorder, such as Tay-Sachs disease or sickle-cell anemia, and thus have a 1 in 4 chance of bearing an affected child
• results of triple screening tests and ultrasonography are abnormal and amniotic fluid evaluation is necessary to determine whether there's a fetal abnormality.

Oh, the uses you'll find

Amniocentesis is valuable because it can be used to:
• detect fetal abnormalities, particularly chromosomal and neural tube defects
• detect hemolytic disease of the fetus

- diagnose metabolic disorders, amino acid disorders, and mucopolysaccharidosis
- assess fetal lung maturity (the lungs are the last organs ready to function on their own)
- determine fetal age and maturity, especially fetal lung maturity
- detect the presence of meconium or blood
- measure amniotic levels of estriol and fetal thyroid hormone
- identify fetal gender.

Diagnostic second-trimester amniocentesis is usually performed between weeks 16 and 18 of pregnancy, although it may be done as early as week 14 or as late as week 20. Most tests require cells to be cultured in the laboratory and take from 24 to 35 days to complete. A few tests—such as those used to detect Tay-Sachs disease, Hunter's syndrome, and neural tube defects—can be performed immediately.

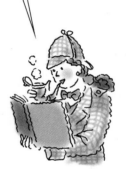

Very interesting, my dear nurses. Apparently, amniocentesis is a great detective in its own right—of fetal abnormalities, hemolytic disease, metabolic disorders, and more!

Aspiring toward aspirate

To begin, ask the patient to change into an examination gown and empty her bladder. Then explain that she'll be positioned on the examining table on her back and her body will be draped so that only her abdomen is exposed. During the test, FHR, maternal vital signs, and ultrasonography are monitored. The doctor:
- prepares the skin with antiseptic and alcohol
- injects the skin with lidocaine to numb the area
- inserts a 20G spinal needle with a stylet into the amniotic cavity
- aspirates amniotic fluid and places it in an amber or foil-covered test tube.

Generally speaking, not for general use

Complications of amniocentesis include spontaneous abortion, trauma to the fetus or placenta, bleeding, premature labor, infection, and Rh sensitization from fetal bleeding into the maternal circulation. Because of the potential severity of possible complications, amniocentesis is contraindicated as a general screening test.

Meaning in amnio

Abnormal test results or failure of the tissue cultures to grow may necessitate repetition of the test. (See *Amniotic fluid analysis findings*.)

Chorionic villi sampling

Performed between 8 and 10 weeks' gestation, CVS involves aspirating chorionic villi from the placenta for prenatal diagnosis of genetic disorders. Chorionic villi are fingerlike projections that surround the embryonic membrane and eventually give rise to the placenta. Cells obtained from the sample are of fetal—rather than

Amniotic fluid analysis findings

Amniotic fluid analysis can provide important information about the condition of the mother, fetus, and placenta. This table shows normal findings as well as abnormal findings and their implications.

Test component	Normal findings	Abnormal findings and fetal implications
Color	Clear, with white flecks of vernix caseosa in a mature fetus	Blood of maternal origin is usually harmless. "Port wine" fluid may indicate abruptio placentae. Fetal blood may indicate damage to the fetal, placental, or umbilical cord vessels.
Bilirubin	Absent at term	High levels indicate hemolytic disease of the neonate in isoimmunized pregnancy.
Meconium	Absent (except in breech presentation)	Presence indicates fetal hypotension or distress.
Creatinine	More than 2 mg/dl in a mature fetus	Decrease may indicate immature fetus (less than 37 weeks).
Lecithin-sphingomyelin ratio	More than 2 generally indicates fetal pulmonary maturity	A ratio of less than 2 indicates pulmonary immaturity and subsequent respiratory distress syndrome.
Phosphatidylglycerol	Present	Absence indicates pulmonary immaturity.
Glucose	Less than 45 mg/dl	Excessive increases at term or near term indicate hypertrophied fetal pancreas and subsequent neonatal hypoglycemia.
Alpha-fetoprotein	Variable, depending on gestation age and laboratory technique; highest concentration (about 18.5 mcg/ml) occurs at 13 to 14 weeks	Inappropriate increases indicate neural tube defects, such as spina bifida or anencephaly, impending fetal death, congenital nephrosis, or contamination of fetal blood.
Bacteria	Absent	Presence indicates chorioamnionitis.
Chromosome	Normal karyotype	Abnormal karyotype may indicate fetal sex and chromosome disorders.
Acetylcholinesterase	Absent	Presence may indicate neural tube defects, exomphalos, or other serious malformations.

maternal—origin and thus can be analyzed for fetal abnormalities. Experts believe that villi in the chorion frondosum reflect fetal chromosome, enzyme, and deoxyribonucleic acid (DNA) content. (See *A look at CVS*, page 178.)

A look at CVS

Chorionic villi sampling (CVS) is a prenatal test for quick detection of fetal chromosomal and biochemical disorders that's performed during the first trimester of pregnancy. Preliminary results may be available within 1 hour; complete results, within a few days.

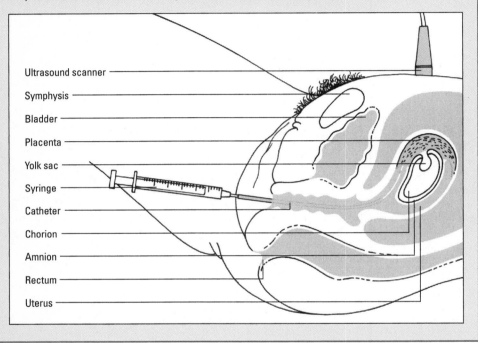

- Ultrasound scanner
- Symphysis
- Bladder
- Placenta
- Yolk sac
- Syringe
- Catheter
- Chorion
- Amnion
- Rectum
- Uterus

Trans times two

Either a transcervical or transabdominal approach can be used to obtain a CVS specimen. In transcervical sampling, a sterile catheter is introduced into the cervix using direct visualization with real-time ultrasonography. A small portion of chorionic villi is aspirated through the catheter into a syringe. In transabdominal sampling, the maternal abdomen is cleaned and an 18G to 20G needle is inserted into the chorion frondosum under ultrasound guidance. The specimen is then aspirated into a syringe. Aspirated villi are placed into a sterile medium for cytogenic analysis.

Painting a picture of the fetus

The cells from the villi normally have the same genetic and biochemical makeup as the embryo. Therefore, examining villi cells provides a complete picture of the genetic makeup of the develop-

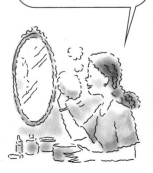

Chorionic villi sampling can provide a complete picture of the genetic "makeup" of the fetus.

ing fetus. CVS can detect fetal karyotype, hemoglobinopathies (such as sickle cell anemia, alpha-thalassemias, and some beta-thalassemias), phenylketonuria, alpha antitrypsin$_1$-deficiency, Down syndrome, Duchenne's muscular dystrophy, and factor IX deficiency. The test also identifies sex, allowing early detection of X-linked conditions in male fetuses.

Complicated matters

Test complications include failure to obtain tissue, ruptured membranes or leakage of amniotic fluid, bleeding, intrauterine infection, spontaneous abortion, contamination of the specimen, and possible Rh isoimmunization. If the patient is Rh-negative, administer RhoGAM, as ordered, to cover the risk of Rh sensitization from the procedure. Also, recent research indicates an incidence of limb malformations in neonates whose mothers have undergone CVS. However, this incidence appears to be low when CVS is performed after 10 weeks' gestation.

Many women feel physically and emotionally drained after undergoing this procedure. Advise the patient to have someone drive her home. Tell her not to make other plans for the rest of the day. Instruct her to call her practitioner with any concerns or symptoms of complications, such as fever, vaginal discharge, vaginal bleeding, or cramping.

Percutaneous umbilical blood sampling

PUBS, which is used to obtain blood samples directly from the fetal circulation, is indicated for prenatal diagnosis of inherited blood disorders, detection of fetal infection, and assessment of the acid-base status of a fetus with intrauterine growth retardation. PUBS can also be used to administer blood products or drugs directly to the fetus. Allowing for treatment of the fetus in utero, PUBS reduces the risk of prematurity and mortality for a neonate with erythroblastosis fetalis (hemolytic disease of the newborn due to Rh incompatibility).

Point of origin

In PUBS, a fine needle is passed through the mother's abdomen and uterine wall into a vessel in the umbilical cord. Ultrasonography is used for guidance. The mobility of the cord complicates the procedure. Although the cord is more stable close to the placenta—allowing for a more accurate puncture—maternal intervillous blood lakes occupy this site, creating a risk of contamination with maternal blood. The Betke-Kleihauer procedure, which is used to detect fetal cells in maternal blood, is immediately performed on the blood sample obtained to ensure that it's fetal in origin.

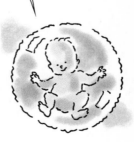

PUBS? I'm not even born yet and already I'm getting my first blood test! Let me know when it's over!

Direct access

Performed anytime after 16 weeks' gestation, PUBS can help diagnose fetal coagulopathies, hemoglobinopathies, hemophilias, and congenital infections. It also provides for rapid fetal karyotyping. Rather than analyzing amniotic fluid to detect abnormalities, PUBS directly assesses fetal blood. This is especially helpful in a patient who may have an isoimmunized pregnancy from Rh disease or another antibody sensitization.

Fetoscopy

Fetoscopy is a procedure in which a fetoscope—a telescope-like instrument with lights and lenses—is inserted into the amniotic sac, where it can view and photograph the fetus. This procedure makes it possible to diagnose, through blood and tissue sampling, several blood and skin diseases that amniocentesis can't detect. Fetoscopy is a relatively risky procedure and, because other safer techniques are becoming available to detect the same disorders, it isn't widely used.

Internal observation

Fetoscopy is typically performed at or after 16 weeks' gestation. The patient's abdomen is swabbed with antiseptic solution and numbed with a local anesthetic. Tiny incisions are made in the abdomen and uterus. Using ultrasonography to guide the instrument, a fiber-optic endoscope is passed through the incisions and into the uterus. The fetus, placenta, and amniotic fluid are observed and blood samples are taken from the junction of the umbilical cord and the placenta. A small piece of fetal or placental tissue may also be removed for examination.

The procedure carries with it a 3% to 5% chance of fetal loss. Though this risk is greater than that of other diagnostic tests, it's outweighed for some women by the benefit of discovering—and possibly treating or correcting—a defect in the fetus.

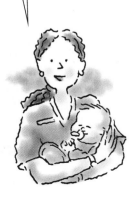

Long before this little one was born, a biophysical profile allowed assessment of his well-being as a fetus.

Biophysical profile

A biophysical profile assesses fetal well-being in the later stages of pregnancy and is used to aid in detecting central nervous system depression in the fetus. It utilizes five variables: amniotic fluid volume, fetal body movements, fetal breathing movements, fetal heart rate reactivity, and fetal muscle tone. Each variable can score a maximum of 2 points. The total score is then calculated. A score of 8 to 10 indicates a potentially healthy fetus; a score of 6 is suspicious and a score of 4 indicates that the fetus may be in jeopardy. (See *Scoring the biophysical profile.*)

Scoring the biophysical profile

Parameter	Diagnostic tool	Factor for a score of 2
Amniotic fluid volume	Ultrasound	Presence of a pocket of amniotic fluid measuring more than 1 cm in vertical diameter
Fetal breathing movements	Ultrasound	At least one episode of 30 seconds of sustained fetal breathing movements within 30 minutes of observation
Fetal heart rate reactivity	Nonstress test	Two or more fetal heart rate accelerations of at least 15 beats/minute above baseline and 15 seconds' duration occurring with fetal movement over a 20-minute period
Fetal body movements	Ultrasound	At least three separate episodes of fetal limb or trunk movement within a 30-minute observation
Fetal muscle tone	Ultrasound	Extension and then flexing of the spine or extremities at least once in 30 minutes

Blood studies

During pregnancy, blood studies are ordered to assess the mother's health, screen for maternal conditions that may endanger the fetus, detect genetic defects, and monitor fetal well-being. Initial studies include blood typing, a complete blood count (CBC) with differential, antibody screening tests, and a serologic test for syphilis and gonorrhea. Other tests may be performed to assess alpha-fetoprotein (AFP) levels, blood glucose, and other chemicals, if indicated.

Blood typing

Blood typing, including Rh factor, is performed to determine the patient's blood type and detect possible blood type incompatibilities. The patient's Rh status is also tested to determine if she's Rh-negative or Rh-positive.

Complete blood count

A CBC includes hemoglobin level, hematocrit, red blood cell (RBC) index, and platelet and white blood cell (WBC) counts.

Hemoglobin level and hematocrit help to determine the presence of anemia. The RBC index helps to classify anemia, if present. Platelet count estimates clotting ability. An elevated WBC count may indicate an infection.

Antibody screening tests

The blood studies performed during pregnancy also include antibody screening tests for Rh compatibility (indirect Coombs' test), rubella, and hepatitis B. Antibodies for varicella (chickenpox) may also be assessed.

Indirect Coombs' test

The indirect Coombs' test screens maternal blood for RBC antibodies.

A sensitive situation

This test should be performed on a patient who's Rh negative; if her fetus is Rh-positive and its blood mixes with the maternal blood during pregnancy or delivery, the woman's immune system produces antibodies against the fetus's RBCs. This antibody response is called *Rh sensitization*. Rh sensitization usually isn't a problem with the first Rh-positive fetus. However, future Rh-positive fetuses are in danger of having their RBCs destroyed by the mother's immune system. After sensitization has occurred, the fetus can develop mild to severe problems, such as Rh disease or hemolytic disease of the newborn.

If the patient doesn't show Rh sensitivity, the test is usually repeated at 28 weeks' gestation. If the titers aren't elevated, an Rh-negative woman would receive RhoGAM at this time and after any procedure that might cause placental bleeding (amniocentesis or CVS).

Rubella titer

A rubella (German measles) titer detects antibodies in maternal blood for the virus that causes rubella. If antibodies are found, the woman is immune to rubella. Most women have either had the virus as a child or have received a vaccination for rubella and, therefore, have antibodies in the blood.

Rubella exposure during pregnancy can lead to blindness, deafness, and heart defects in the fetus. If tests reveal that the patient isn't immune, she should avoid anyone who has the infection. She can't receive the vaccination while she's pregnant, but she should get the vaccine after she gives birth to provide protection during future pregnancies.

Hepatitis B

Another antibody screening test, called the *hepatic antibody surface antigen* (HbsAg) test, is used to determine if a patient has hepatitis B. In many cases, the HbsAg test is the only way to tell if a patient has hepatitis B because many people who carry the virus have no symptoms. If the patient is a carrier, she could pass this to her baby during labor or delivery.

If the patient tests positive for hepatitis B, the neonate must receive injections of hepatitis B immunoglobulin and hepatitis B vaccine immediately after birth to prevent liver damage. The neonate then receives additional doses of the vaccine at 2 to 4 months and again at 6 to 18 months.

HIV testing

HIV screening may be done for a woman who's at high risk for developing acquired immunodeficiency syndrome. This test uses an enzyme-linked immunosorbent assay on a blood sample to determine the presence of HIV antibodies. If the HIV screening test is positive, findings are confirmed by a second test—the Western blot test.

The Centers for Disease Control and Prevention (CDC) recommend that all pregnant women be tested for HIV. However, in some cases, a pregnant woman won't pursue HIV testing because she doesn't want to know if she's infected. This choice should be respected. Screening isn't mandatory in prenatal settings, but is recommended for patients who:
- have a history of I.V. drug use
- have unprotected sex
- have multiple sex partners
- have had a sexual partner who was infected with HIV or was at risk for contracting it (because he was bisexual, an I.V. drug user, or a hemophiliac)
- received a blood transfusion between 1977 and 1985.

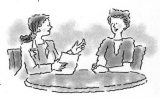

The CDC recommends that all pregnant women be tested for HIV, even if they don't think they're at risk.

Damage control

A woman who's antibody-positive for HIV may begin therapy with zidovudine (AZT) to decrease the risk of transmitting the disease to her fetus. Alternatively, the patient may choose to terminate the pregnancy to avoid giving birth to a neonate who has a high risk of developing the disease. When discussing test results with a patient, keep in mind that a positive test result or an antibody-positive result indicates that the patient has been exposed to the disease—she doesn't necessarily have the disease.

Purport support

Positive HIV screening results should be presented with tact and compassion. Results are confidential; the information should be reported only to the patient. Extra support needs to be given to the patient who tests positive because there's no known cure for the infection.

Serologic tests

The Venereal Disease Research Laboratories (VDRL) test and rapid plasma reagin (RPR) test are serologic tests for syphilis. Syphilis needs to be treated early in pregnancy, before fetal damage occurs.

Pregnant women who test positive for syphilis must receive treatment before 16 week' gestation. Untreated syphilis infection during pregnancy can cause miscarriage, premature birth, stillbirth, or birth defects.

Alpha-fetoprotein testing

AFP testing—sometimes called the *MSAFP* test or *maternal serum AFP* test—is usually used to detect neural tube defects. AFP is a protein that's secreted by the fetal liver and excreted in the mother's blood. When testing by immunoassay, AFP values are less than 15 ng/ml in nonpregnant women.

MOM's levels

The test is considered positive for an increased risk of neural tube defect when the AFP level is greater than 2.5 times the median (midpoint of levels of a group of patients at the same gestational age), or 2.5 MOM (multiples of median).

AFP testing can also indicate:
• abdominal wall defects
• esophageal and duodenal atresia
• renal and urinary tract anomalies
• Turner's syndrome
• low birth weight
• placental complications.

Congenital anomalies, such as Down syndrome, may be associated with low maternal serum AFP concentrations. Elevated maternal serum AFP levels may suggest neural tube defects or other anomalies. Maternal AFP levels rise sharply in the blood of about 90% of women carrying a fetus with anencephaly and in about 50% of those carrying a fetus with spina bifida. Definitive diagnosis requires ultrasonography and amniocentesis. High AFP levels can

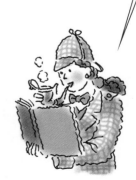

Even the best detective can use some help! AFP levels can be used to detect neural tube defects, abdominal wall defects, low birth weight, and other complications.

also indicate intrauterine death or other anomalies, such as duodenal atresia, omphalocele, tetralogy of Fallot, and Turner's syndrome.

Glucose tolerance testing

If the patient has a history of previously unexplained fetal loss, has a family history of diabetes, has previously delivered a large-for-gestational age neonate (over 4.1 kg [9 lb]), is obese, or has glycosuria, a 50-g oral 1-hour glucose-loading or glucose-tolerance test should be scheduled toward the end of the first trimester. This test is performed to rule out or confirm gestational diabetes. It's routinely done between 24 and 28 weeks' gestation to evaluate insulin-antagonistic effects of placental hormones but, in high-risk pregnancies, testing should be performed earlier. Fasting plasma glucose levels shouldn't be above 140 mg/dl.

Triple screen

The triple screen is a blood test routinely offered between weeks 15 and 20. It measures three chemicals: AFP, unconjugated estriol, and hCG.

Picking up on patterns

By detecting chemical patterns, the test predicts if there's an increased risk of bearing a child with a chromosomal abnormality or open-tube defect, including:
• Down syndrome—extra chromosome 21 that results in mental retardation
• trisomy 18—extra chromosome 18 that results in mental retardation that's much more serious than Down syndrome; the neonate usually dies within hours of birth but may live for months or, in rare cases, years
• spina bifida—fetal spine doesn't properly close; size and location of opening determine severity; surgery is required at birth; may cause paralysis
• anencephaly—the most severe type of neural tube defect in which the brain and skull don't form properly; babies are stillborn or die within a few weeks
• omphalocele and gastroschisis—improper closure of the abdominal wall; severity depends on size and location of opening; surgery may correct problem; prognosis depends upon severity.

Suggestive, not definitive

Triple screening doesn't definitively answer whether a fetus has a birth defect. It only suggests that there's a possibility for birth defects. In some cases, results appear to be abnormal because the fetus is younger or older than initially estimated. Suspicions can be confirmed by amniocentesis.

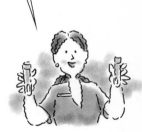

The triple screen uses chemical patterns to predict any increased risk of a chromosomal abnormality in the fetus.

Nonstress testing

Performed by a specially trained nurse, a prepartum NST evaluates fetal well-being by measuring the fetal heart response to fetal movements. Such movements produce transient accelerations in the heart rate of a healthy fetus. Usually ordered during the third trimester of pregnancy, this noninvasive screening test uses indirect electronic monitoring to record FHR and the duration of uterine contractions. It's indicated for suspected fetal distress or placental insufficiency associated with the following maternal conditions:

- diabetes mellitus
- hyperthyroidism
- chronic hypertension or gestational hypertension
- collagen disease
- heart disease
- chronic renal disease
- intrauterine growth retardation
- sickle cell disease
- Rh sensitization
- suspected postmaturity (when the woman is suspected of being past her due date)
- history of miscarriage or stillbirth
- abnormal estriol excretion.

> Relax! Nonstress testing can be used to detect fetal distress related to some serious conditions, but the test itself is stress-free.

Getting it on the record

To perform the test, the patient is placed in a semi-Fowler or lateral-tilt position with a pillow under one hip. The patient shouldn't be placed in the supine position because pressure on the maternal great vessels from the gravid uterus may cause maternal hypotension and reduced uterine perfusion. Conductive gel is applied to the abdomen and transducers are placed on the patient's abdomen to transmit and record FHR and fetal movement.

Shake it up

The patient is then instructed to depress the monitor's mark or test button when she feels the fetus move. If no spontaneous fetal movement occurs within 20 minutes, apply gentle pressure to the patient's abdomen or shake it to stimulate fetal movement.

A positive reaction

If the monitor records two FHR accelerations that exceed baseline by at least 15 beats/minute, that last longer than 15 seconds, and that occur within a 20-minute period, conclude the test. Such findings, called a *reactive NST*, indicate that an intact fetal autonomic nervous system controls FHR.

Lack of reaction

If reactive results aren't obtained, the fetus should be monitored for an additional 40 minutes. If reactive NST results still aren't obtained, a contraction stress test (CST) may be performed to more definitively assess fetal status.

Contraction stress test

The prepartum CST evaluates respiratory function of the placenta and indicates whether the fetus will be able to withstand the stress of labor. Performed by a specially trained nurse, this test uses indirect electronic monitoring to measure fetal heart response to spontaneous or oxytocin-induced uterine contractions. The CST is indicated when the NST fails to produce reactive results.

Contraindications to the CST include the following maternal conditions:
- preterm labor or preterm membrane rupture
- multiple pregnancy
- previous vertical cesarean delivery
- abruptio placentae
- placenta previa
- incompetent cervical os
- previous uterine rupture.

If the test must be performed despite the presence of one of these conditions, prepare for emergency delivery.

Places, everyone!

To perform the test, the patient is placed in a semi-Fowler or lateral-tilt position with a pillow beneath one hip. As with the NST, the supine position shouldn't be used because pressure on the maternal great vessels from the gravid uterus may cause maternal hypotension and reduced uterine perfusion.

Roll ultrasound…and action!

A tocotransducer and an ultrasound transducer are placed on the abdomen for 20 minutes to record baseline vital signs and baseline measurements of uterine contractions, fetal movements, and FHR. The contractions cause a temporary decrease in blood and oxygen flow to the fetus, which most fetuses are able to tolerate. Three contractions, each lasting 40 seconds, must occur within a 10-minute period. If the fetus's heart rate stays constant, the test is considered normal.

The lowdown on a slowdown

The fetus may experience a decelerated heart rate during the test. If 50% or more of the contractions cause FHR to decrease, the test is stopped and results are considered abnormal. If test results are abnormal, the patient should be observed for 30 minutes after the test to make sure that contractions don't continue. FHR shouldn't drop below baseline at the end of the contraction or after the contraction. This is termed *late deceleration* and can be indicative of fetal hypoxia.

The solution may be a solution

If testing fails to produce spontaneous contractions, an oxytocin solution may be prepared and infused. After three contractions are recorded, the oxytocin drip is stopped. Continue to monitor the patient for 30 minutes or until the contraction rate returns to baseline. Make sure the patient is comfortable while she waits for the results of the test.

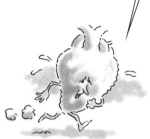

If I slow down during a CST for more than 50% of the contractions, stop the test.

Nipple stimulation contraction stress test

Nipple stimulation can induce the uterine contractions necessary for a prepartum CST by stimulating the body to produce oxytocin itself. This is a natural and practical alternative to I.V. oxytocin administration. However, this test is controversial because it has the potential to cause hyperstimulation and uncontrollable contractions.

A hands-on approach

To stimulate contractions, tell the patient to apply warm washcloths to one of her breasts and then gently roll or tug on one nipple until contractions start. If necessary, she can apply a water-soluble lubricant, such as K-Y jelly, to reduce nipple irritation. If a second contraction doesn't occur within 2 minutes of the first contraction, ask the patient to massage her nipple again. If no contractions occur after 15 minutes of stimulation, the patient may be instructed to stimulate both nipples. The patient should be instructed to discontinue stimulation when three contractions lasting 35 seconds each occur within a 10-minute period.

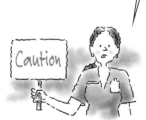

The nipple stimulation contraction stress test may cause hyperstimulation and uncontrollable contractions.

Caution

Nutritional care

Nutritional needs must also be addressed as a part of prenatal care. A pregnant woman's nutritional intake—including calories, protein, fat, vitamins, minerals, and fluid—needs to be increased to provide sufficient nutrients for her growing fetus. In most cases, the patient doesn't have to increase the quantity of food she eats; she simply needs to increase the quality of the food she eats.

Let the pyramid be your guide

A pregnant woman's food choices should be based on the food guide pyramid. When discussing nutrition with the patient, refer to servings of food rather than milligrams or percentages. (See *Food guide pyramid.*)

Food guide pyramid

Because not all foods in a food group are created equal, the U.S. Department of Agriculture makes the following recommendations for choosing foods within a food group. Pass these recommendations along to your pregnant patients.

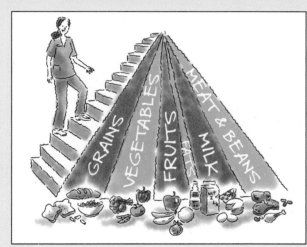

Grains

• Make half your grains whole.

• Eat at least 3 oz of whole-grain cereals, breads, crackers, rice, or pasta every day.

• 1 oz is about 1 slice of bread, about 1 cup of breakfast cereal, or ½ cup of cooked rice, cereal, or pasta.

Vegetables

• Vary your veggies.

• Eat more dark-green veggies like broccoli, spinach, and other dark leafy greens.

• Eat more orange veggies, like carrots and sweet potatoes.

• Eat more dry beans and peas, such as pinto beans, kidney beans, and lentils.

Fruits

• Focus on fruits.

• Eat a variety of fruit.

• Choose fresh, frozen, canned, or dried fruit.

• Go easy on fruit juices.

Milk

• Consume calcium-rich foods.

• Go low-fat or fat-free when you choose milk, yogurt, and other milk products.

• If you don't or can't consume milk, choose lactose-free products or other calcium sources, such as fortified foods and beverages.

• Get 3 cups every day.

Fats

• Choose most from fish, nuts, and vegetable oils.

• Limit solid fats like butter, stick margarine, shortening, and lard.

Meats & beans

• Go lean with protein.

• Choose low-fat or lean meats and poultry.

• Bake it, broil it, or grill it.

• Vary your protein routine; choose more fish, beans, peas, nuts, and seeds.

• Eat 5½ oz every day.

Adapted from U.S. Department of Agriculture. Center for Nutrition Policy and Promotion (2005). MyPyramid Mini-Poster [Online]. *http://www.mypyramid.gov/downloads/miniposter.pdf*

Education edge

Foods to avoid during pregnancy

Although several nutritional needs increase during pregnancy, other food restrictions become necessary. Tell the patient to avoid the following food products.

Alcohol

A pregnant patient shouldn't drink alcohol because alcohol crosses the placental barrier and can result in fetal alcohol syndrome (FAS). FAS can cause prenatal and postnatal growth failure, microcephaly, facial and musculoskeletal abnormalities, and mental retardation.

Caffeine

Caffeine is a central nervous system stimulant that increases heart rate, urine production in the kidneys, and secretion of acid in the stomach. Sources of caffeine include chocolate, soft drinks, tea, and coffee. A daily caffeine intake of more than 300 mg (about 4 cups of coffee) has been associated with low birth weight. Foods and beverages with caffeine should be avoided or limited. To reduce caffeine intake, suggest that the patient switch to decaffeinated beverages, such as decaffeinated tea or coffee.

Artificial sweeteners and additives

Artificial sweeteners, such as saccharin and aspartame, aren't recommended during pregnancy. According to the results of some animal studies, a large intake of saccharin may be carcinogenic. Some studies also suggest that saccharin may cross the placental barrier. Although no definitive study has been performed that indicates that aspartame crosses the placental barrier, a woman should still be advised to avoid ingesting food products with this substance during pregnancy.

A pregnant patient should also avoid foods that contain additives because the effects of many of these additives are unknown.

Cholesterol

A pregnant patient should limit her cholesterol intake. Encourage her to eat lean meats, to cook with olive oil instead of lard or butter, and to remove the skin from poultry. Even though such foods as eggs are good sources of protein, a woman who has a family history of high cholesterol shouldn't consume more than one egg per week.

> We're only going to increase your calorie intake by 300 calories. That should provide the extra energy that you need.

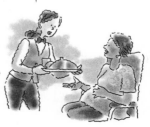

Infliction of restriction

Although certain nutritional requirements increase during pregnancy, certain restrictions also become necessary to protect the health of the baby. (See *Foods to avoid during pregnancy*.)

Calories

During the first trimester, the energy needs of a pregnant woman are essentially the same as those of a nonpregnant woman. In the second and third trimesters, however, the increased need for energy ranges from 300 to 400 calories per day. Because nutrient needs increase more than calorie needs, a pregnant woman's food choices need to be nutrient-dense. More calories (2,700 to 3,000 per day) may be needed for active, large, or nutritionally deficient women. Inadequate calorie intake can lead to protein breakdown for energy, depriving the fetus of essential protein and, possibly, resulting in ketoacidosis and neurologic defects.

Meal plan

To help a woman plan for increased calorie intake, consider her lifestyle. Many women skip meals, have erratic eating patterns, and rely on fast or convenient foods. Help the patient plan on adding calories by eating foods rich in protein, iron, and other essential nutrients rather than eating empty-calorie foods, such as pretzels and doughnuts. Suggest such snacks as carrot sticks or cheese and crackers. Encourage the patient to have these snacks on hand ahead of time to provide needed nutrients.

Ascertain weight gain

The easiest way to determine if your patient's calorie intake is adequate is to assess weight gain. The patient's weight gain pattern is as important as her total weight gain. Even if she surpasses the target weight before the end of the third trimester, encourage her not to restrict her intake—she should continue to gain weight because the fetus is growing rapidly during this time.

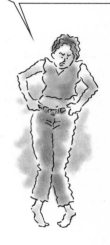

Get out the scale! Assessing weight gain is the easiest way to find out if your patient is getting enough calories in her diet.

Protein

Recommended protein intake during pregnancy increases only 10 to 15 g/day to 60 g/day total. Many pregnant women consume more than this already and don't need to increase protein intake.

You complete me

Good animal sources of protein include meat, poultry, fish, cheese, yogurt, eggs, and milk. Because the protein in these forms contains all nine essential amino acids, it's considered *complete protein*. However, lunch meats such as bologna and salami shouldn't be consumed regularly because they're high in fat and aren't typically good sources of protein.

Full of complements

The protein found in nonanimal sources doesn't contain all nine essential amino acids. Vitamin B_{12} is found exclusively in animal proteins. Therefore, a pregnant patient who excludes animal proteins from her diet may have a vitamin B_{12} deficiency. Complete protein can be obtained through nonanimal sources by cooking different protein sources together. For example, eating complementary proteins, such as beans and rice, legumes and rice, or beans and wheat together, can provide the patient with all nine essential amino acids.

Got milk?

Milk products are also rich in protein and may be consumed in various forms—buttermilk, yogurt, cheese, custards, eggnogs, and cream soups—to meet daily protein requirements. If the patient is lactose intolerant, lactose supplements may be purchased over the counter. These supplements predigest milk and make it palatable for the patient.

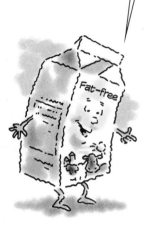

Milk products are great sources of protein, calcium, and vitamin D—which are all necessary nutrients.

Fats

Linoleic acid is an essential fatty acid that's necessary for new cell growth. It isn't manufactured in the body but can be found in such vegetable oils as safflower, corn, olive, peanut, and cottonseed. In addition, these vegetable oils are low in cholesterol compared with animal oils such as lard. They're also recommended for all adults to prevent hypercholesterolemia and atherosclerosis.

Vitamins

Requirements of fat-soluble and water-soluble vitamins increase during pregnancy to support the growth of new fetal cells. A healthy, varied diet with plenty of fruits and vegetables usually allows the pregnant patient to meet these requirements. A specially designed multivitamin supplement is usually also prescribed. The patient should be advised to take these vitamins as directed. The recommended dose shouldn't be exceeded because fat-soluble vitamins can be toxic. In addition, tell the patient not to use mineral oil as a laxative because it can prevent absorption of fat-soluble vitamins from the GI tract.

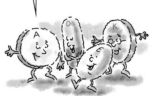

Warn your patient to take us fat-soluble vitamins only as prescribed. Too much of us can be toxic!

Restock the stores

A woman who was taking hormonal contraceptives before she became pregnant also needs to include good sources of vitamin A, vitamin B_6, and folic acid in her diet in early pregnancy because hormonal contraceptives may deplete her stores of these vitamins. Vitamin A can be found in milk, eggs, yellow fruits and vegetables, dark green fruits and vegetables, and liver; vitamin B_6, in whole grains, organ meats, brewer's yeast, blackstrap molasses, and wheat germ; folic acid, in citrus fruits, tomatoes and other vegetables, grain products, and most ready-to-eat cereals (fortified with folic acid).

Too little...

Vitamin deficiencies can cause many problems. For example:
• Vitamin D deficiency may result in the breakdown of fetal and maternal mineral bone density (vitamin D is necessary for calcium and phosphorus absorption).

...too much

Likewise, an overdose of vitamins can also cause problems:
• Vitamin A excess can result in fetal malformation and congenital anomalies. Such an excess can occur through the body's absorption of isotretinoin (Accutane), a medication for acne.
• Megadoses of vitamin C may cause withdrawal scurvy in the infant at birth.

Folic acid

Folic acid (folacin) is a water-soluble B_9 vitamin that's necessary for RBC formation. A folic acid deficiency may result in megaloblastic anemia (development of large but ineffective RBCs). If evidence of folic acid deficiency is present at the time of birth, the neonate may be affected as well. Low levels of folic acid in pregnant women have been associated with premature separation of the placenta, spontaneous abortions, and neural tube defects. Good sources of folic acid include fruits and vegetables. Prescribed prenatal vitamins, which contain a folic acid supplement of 0.4 to 1 mg, are also essential.

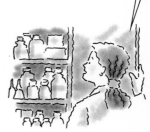

Remind the patient that all vitamins should be kept out of reach of small children because the folic acid and iron in these pills may be poisonous.

Minerals

Minerals are needed for fetal cell development. They're found in many foods, so most mineral deficiencies in pregnant women are rare. For women whose intake of minerals is below daily requirements, supplements may be necessary.

Calcium and phosphorus

Calcium and phosphorus are vital to the structure of bones and teeth. Between 1,200 and 1,500 mg of calcium and 1,200 mg of phosphorus are recommended per day during pregnancy. In the last trimester of pregnancy, fetal skeletal growth is greatest and the fetus draws calcium directly from the mother's stores. In addition, clinical trials have shown that adequate calcium intake during pregnancy lowers blood pressure and may reduce the incidence of premature births.

Because calcium and phosphorus help with tooth and bone formation in the fetus, a maternal diet high in calcium and vitamin D (a vitamin needed for calcium to enter bones) is necessary. If a woman can't drink milk or eat milk products, a daily calcium supplement may be prescribed. Inadequate calcium intake can result in diminished maternal bone density. The woman should eat foods that are high in protein to ensure adequate phosphorus intake because most foods that are high in protein are also high in phosphorus.

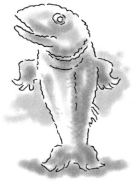

If you dine on me, iodine for you.

Iodine

The recommended daily requirement of iodine during pregnancy is 175 mg. Iodine is essential for the formation of thyroxine and proper functioning of the thyroid gland. The best sources of this mineral are ocean fish, including cod, haddock, sole, and ocean perch (Atlantic redfish).

If iodine deficiency occurs, it may result in thyroid enlargement (goiter) in the woman or fetus and, in extreme cases, can cause hypothyroidism (cretinism) in the fetus. Thyroid enlargement in the fetus at birth is serious because the increased pressure the enlarged gland places on the airway can result in early respiratory distress. If not discovered at birth, hypothyroidism may lead to cognitive impairment. In areas where water and soil are known to be iodine-deficient, women should use iodized salt and include a serving of seafood in their diet at least once per week.

Iron

The recommended daily allowance (RDA) of iron for pregnant women is 30 mg. In most cases, about one-half of this intake comes from supplements because dietary intake alone can't provide sufficient iron. Remember to tell the patient to take iron supplements with orange juice to enhance absorption. Inform her that they may cause her stools to be black and that constipation may develop if she doesn't include enough fluids and fiber in her diet.

Pumping iron

Iron is necessary to build high levels of hemoglobin, which is needed for oxygenation after the baby is born. After the 20th week of pregnancy, the fetus begins to store iron in the liver. These stores need to be adequate to last through the first 3 months of life, when intake consists mainly of milk (which is typically low in iron). The pregnant woman also needs iron to increase her RBC volume and to replace iron lost in blood at delivery.

Because the richest sources of iron are also the most expensive—organ meats, eggs, green leafy vegetables, whole grain, enriched breads, dried fruits—a woman with a low income may have trouble taking in adequate amounts of iron in her diet. Today, many cereals are iron-fortified, but even these foods may not supply the amount of iron that the patient needs.

Fluoride

Fluoride helps to form sound teeth. If the pregnant woman doesn't drink fluoridated water, supplemental fluoride may be recommended. Because large amounts of fluoride stain teeth brown, a woman shouldn't take a supplement if her water contains fluoride and she shouldn't take supplements more often than prescribed.

Sodium

Sodium is a major electrolyte that regulates fluids in the body. It helps with retention of fluid in the maternal circulation to ensure a pressure gradient for optimal exchange across the placenta. It also plays a role in maintaining the acid-base balance of blood and helps nutrients cross cell membranes.

During pregnancy and lactation, a woman's sodium metabolism (utilization) is altered by hormone activity. As a result, sodium needs are slightly higher during these times. However, there's rarely a need for additional sodium intake because a typical diet usually provides adequate amounts. Unless the patient is hypertensive or has heart disease, seasoning foods as usual is recommended during pregnancy. However, extremely salty foods, such as lunch meats and potato chips, should be avoided. Additives, such as monosodium glutamate, should also be avoided. Excessive salt intake could result in fluid retention, which strains the heart.

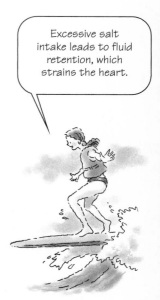

Excessive salt intake leads to fluid retention, which strains the heart.

Zinc

Zinc is necessary for synthesis of DNA and ribonucleic acid as well as cell division and growth. Zinc deficiency has been associated with preterm birth. The RDA of zinc during pregnancy is 15 mg daily. Meat, liver, eggs, seafood, and prenatal vitamins are good sources of zinc.

Fluid

Because a pregnant woman is excreting not only her own waste products but also those of her fetus, her body requires extra water to promote kidney function. In addition, fluids:

- keep skin soft
- lessen the likelihood of constipation
- rid the body of toxins and waste products
- reduce excessive swelling.

Recommended fluid intake is 2 qt (8 cups) daily. Fluid sources include juices, milk, soups, and carbonated beverages. The patient should avoid excess intake of caffeinated beverages.

Minimizing discomforts of pregnancy

Being aware of patient discomforts during pregnancy allows you to provide information on how to alleviate them. In addition, early monitoring of certain conditions can help to reduce their occurrence.

Have them share so you can provide care

A pregnant woman may not mention her concerns or discomforts unless she's specifically asked because she isn't aware of the significance of her problems or she's reluctant to take up a lot of time during a prenatal visit. Encourage the patient to discuss whatever concerns she has at her visits. Although some issues may represent minor common discomforts associated with normal pregnancy, others may be early indicators of potential problems. For example, a problem such as constipation, which the patient may consider a minor discomfort, may result in hemorrhoids, which can become a long-term problem if left to progress throughout the pregnancy.

On the other hand, a woman may see the discomforts of pregnancy as deterrents to good health. The minor discomforts of pregnancy may not seem minor to the patient, especially if they occur daily and make her wonder if she'll ever feel like herself again. You need to provide empathetic and sound advice for relieving discomforts and helping promote the overall health and well-being of a pregnant patient. (See *Dealing with pregnancy discomforts*.)

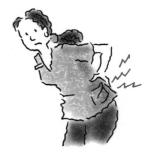

A pregnant patient should be encouraged to discuss the discomforts she's experiencing. Some discomforts can be easily allayed and others may be problematic.

Education edge

Dealing with pregnancy discomforts

This table lists common discomforts associated with pregnancy and suggestions that you can give to the patient on how to prevent and manage them.

Discomfort	Patient teaching	Discomfort	Patient teaching
Urinary frequency	• Void as necessary. • Avoid caffeine. • Perform Kegel exercises.	Nasal stuffiness	• Use a cool-mist vaporizer. • Use saline nose drops. • Avoid medicated nasal sprays because of rebound stuffiness with repeated use.
Fatigue	• Try to get a full night's sleep. • Schedule a daily rest time. • Maintain good nutrition.	Hemorrhoids	• Avoid constipation. • Set a regular time for bowel movements. • Take sitz baths with warm water as often as needed to relieve discomfort. • Apply ice packs for reduction of swelling, if preferred over heat.
Breast tenderness	• Wear a supportive bra. • Wear a bra at night if breast discomfort interferes with sleep.		
Vaginal discharge	• Wear cotton underwear. • Avoid tight-fitting pantyhose. • Bathe daily.	Varicosities	• Exercise regularly. • Rest with the legs elevated daily. • Avoid standing or sitting for long periods. • Avoid crossing the legs. • Avoid wearing constrictive knee-high stockings; wear support stockings instead. • Keep within the recommended weight range during pregnancy.
Backache	• Avoid standing for long periods. • Keep within the recommended weight range during pregnancy. • Avoid high-heeled shoes. • Bend at the knees, not the waist.		
Round ligament pain	• Slowly rise from a sitting position. • Bend forward to relieve pain. • Avoid twisting motions. • Lie on the side opposite the discomfort.	Ankle edema	• Avoid standing or sitting for long periods. • Rest with the feet elevated. • Avoid wearing garments that constrict the lower extremities.
Constipation	• Increase fiber intake in the diet. • Set a regular time for bowel movements. • Drink more fluids, including water and fruit juices (unless contraindicated). Avoid caffeinated drinks.	Leg cramps	• Straighten the leg and dorsiflex the ankle. • Avoid pointing the toes. • Rest frequently with legs elevated.

First trimester

Although a pregnant woman may be excited about pregnancy and childbirth, the many discomforts that occur during the first trimester can take away from the joyful feelings of motherhood. Such discomforts are usually accepted as an expected part of pregnancy. However, there are ways to ease discomforts and prevent further complications. You should pass this information along to your patient as necessary.

Nausea and vomiting

Nausea and vomiting are the most common discomforts during the first trimester. Although these symptoms are commonly referred to as *morning sickness*, they can last all day for some women. Nausea and vomiting rarely interfere with proper nutrition enough to harm the developing fetus.

At least 50% of women experience nausea normally during pregnancy. Medications are rarely prescribed to relieve nausea because they may adversely effect on the fetus.

Queasiness cause

Although a specific cause of nausea during pregnancy hasn't been determined, it has been suggested that nausea is the body's reaction to the high levels of hCG that occur during the first trimester. Other possible contributors to nausea include the rapid stretching of the woman's uterine muscles, the relative relaxation of the muscle tissue in the digestive tract (making digestion less efficient), excess acid in the stomach, and the woman's enhanced sense of smell. (See *Reducing nausea*.)

Nausea and vomiting are considered abnormal if:
- the patient is losing weight instead of gaining it.
- the patient hasn't gained the projected amount of weight for a particular week of pregnancy.
- lost meals are unable to be made up for during some time of the day.
- signs of dehydration, such as little urine output, are present.
- nausea lasts past the 12th week of pregnancy.
- the patient vomits more than once daily.

To prevent potential complications, such as hyperemesis gravidarum (severe nausea and vomiting during pregnancy that result in dehydration and loss of at least 10 lb [4.5 kg]), inform the patient's practitioner if these signs and symptoms occur. (For more information on hyperemesis gravidarum, see the discussion in chapter 6, High-risk pregnancy.)

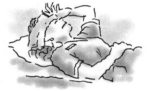

At least half of pregnant women experience the joys of nausea!

Education edge

Reducing nausea

To help the patient relieve nausea during pregnancy, give her these tips:
• Before getting out of bed in the morning, eat a high-carbohydrate food, such as saltines, melba toast, or other crackers.
• Eat small, frequent meals rather than large, infrequent ones.
• Avoid greasy and highly seasoned foods.
• Delay breakfast (or dinner, if experiencing evening nausea) until nausea passes. Make up for missed meals at another time to maintain nutrition.
• Avoid sudden movements and fatigue, which are known to increase nausea.
• If breakfast is usually eaten late in the morning, eat a snack before bedtime to help avoid long periods between meals.
• Buy a wrist acupressure band (available at travel stores), which may help to reduce motion sickness.
• Sip carbonated beverages, water, or herbal decaffeinated tea.
• Take a walk outside or take deep breaths through an open window to inhale fresh air.

Nasal stuffiness

Nasal stuffiness is common during pregnancy and may persist during all three trimesters. Estrogen contributes to vasocongestion and makes the nasal mucosa more friable, possibly leading to epistaxis.

Urinary frequency

Urinary frequency occurs in the first trimester because of increasing blood volume and an increased GFR. It may last for about 3 months and disappears in midpregnancy, when the uterus rises above the bladder. It commonly returns again in late pregnancy as the fetal head presses against the bladder.

If a patient reports urinary frequency, ask her if she has experienced burning or pain on urination or if she has noticed blood in her urine—both signs of a UTI. After infection is ruled out, focus on teaching the patient ways to alleviate discomfort. Suggest to the patient that she reduce the amount of caffeine she drinks, if applicable. She can also perform Kegel exercises to help strengthen the pelvic muscles so that the feeling of urgency is less noticeable later in pregnancy. Kegel exercises also help with urinary control.

Breast tenderness

Breast tenderness is commonly noticed early in pregnancy and may be most noticeable when the patient is exposed to cold air. For most women, tenderness is minimal and transient. Many are aware of it but aren't distressed by it.

If breast tenderness causes the patient discomfort, recommend that she wear a bra with wide shoulder straps for support and dress warmly to avoid cold drafts (if cold increases symptoms). Wearing a bra at night may help if breast discomfort is preventing her from getting a good night's sleep. If actual pain exists, suspect the presence of an underlying condition, such as nipple fissures or mastitis.

Fatigue

Fatigue is common early in pregnancy and may be caused by the body's increased metabolic requirements. Fatigue can also intensify morning sickness; for example, if the patient becomes too tired, she may not eat properly. If she remains on her feet without at least one break during the day, the risk of varicosities and thromboembolitic complications increases.

Putting fatigue to rest

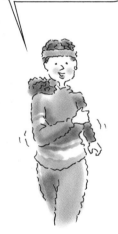

Balancing sedentary activities with physical activities can help reduce fatigue during pregnancy.

Increasing the amount of rest and sleep may relieve the patient's fatigue. During prenatal visits, ask her whether she manages to take at least one short rest period every day. Modifying her routine to allow rest periods is advised. If the patient has a sedentary job inside or outside of the home, she needs to increase her activity, such as by walking or using a treadmill. By balancing rest and exercise, she can reduce her fatigue.

A modified Sims' position with the top leg forward is a good resting position. This puts the weight of the fetus on the bed, not on the woman, and allows good circulation to the lower extremities.

Increased vaginal discharge

Leukorrhea is another discomfort of pregnancy. It's a whitish, viscous vaginal discharge or an increase in the amount of normal vaginal secretions. It's caused by the high estrogen levels and increased blood supply to the vaginal epithelium and cervix that occur during pregnancy. A woman who's uncomfortable about discussing this part of her body or who associates vaginal infections with poor hygiene or STDs may be reluctant to mention an irritating vaginal discharge. Be sure to ask every patient at prenatal visits whether they're experiencing this problem.

Deterring discharge

Tell the patient that a daily bath or shower can help wash away accumulated secretions and prevent vulvar excoriation. Warn her not to douche; this is contraindicated throughout pregnancy. She can also use perineal pads to control discharge; she shouldn't use tampons, however, because they promote stasis of secretions, which can lead to infection. Wearing cotton underwear and sleeping without underwear are helpful in reducing moisture and possible excoriation. Tell the patient that she should avoid tight-fitting underwear and pantyhose to prevent yeast infections.

Advise the patient to contact her practitioner if there's a change in the color, odor, or character of the discharge. This could indicate infection. Vulvar pruritus (itching of the vulva) also needs evaluation because this sign also strongly indicates infection. Caution the patient not to self-treat vaginal infections during pregnancy because such preparations as metronidazole (Flagyl) may harm the fetus.

Second and third trimesters

Although the patient may be focused on bonding with the fetus, she must be reminded to report any discomforts she has to ensure that nothing serious is occurring. In addition, at the midpoint of pregnancy, review with the patient precautionary measures that help prevent constipation, varicosities, and hemorrhoids and discuss with her the new symptoms that may occur.

Indigestion

Indigestion may be caused by large amounts of progesterone and estrogen, which tend to relax smooth muscle tissue throughout the body—including the GI tract. This causes food to move through the system more slowly and may result in bloating and indigestion. This slowdown is beneficial because it allows for better absorption of nutrients into the bloodstream and subsequently into the fetus's system.

> Indigestion and heartburn may result when the relaxation of smooth muscle tissue and the cardiac sphincter cause food processing to slow down.

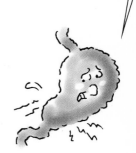

Feeling the burn

Heartburn results when the cardiac sphincter relaxes, allowing food and digestive juices to back up from the stomach into the esophagus. This irritates the lining, causing a burning sensation. This problem may increase later in pregnancy because of the pressure of the fetus on the mother's internal organs. (See *Relieving heartburn and indigestion*, page 202.)

If measures fail to relieve symptoms, a low-sodium antacid or other OTC medication that's safe to use during pregnancy may be recommended. Sodium or sodium bicarbonate solutions should be avoided because they can exacerbate heartburn.

Ankle edema

Most women experience some swelling of the ankles and feet during late pregnancy, most noticeably at the end of the day. It may result from reduced blood circulation in the lower extremities caused by uterine pressure and general fluid retention. The patient may become aware of it if she takes off her shoes and then can't get them back on again comfortably. As long as proteinuria and hypertension aren't present, ankle edema is a normal occurrence.

To help relieve edema, tell the patient to rest in a left side-lying position; this increases the GFR. Sitting for half an hour in the afternoon and again in the evening with the legs elevated should also help. Tell the patient to avoid constricting panty girdles or knee-high stockings because these garments impede lower-extremity circulation and venous return.

Don't discount a report of lower-extremity edema until you're certain the woman doesn't exhibit signs of proteinuria, edema of other nondependent parts, or sudden weight increase that's indicative of gestational hypertension.

Varicose veins

Varicose veins are tortuous veins that commonly appear during pregnancy. They develop because the weight of the distended uterus puts pressure on the veins returning blood from the lower extremities. This causes blood to pool in the vessels, and the veins become engorged, inflamed, and painful. Varicose veins are common in women with a family history and in women who have a large fetus or multiple pregnancies. Sitting for prolonged periods with the legs dependent also promotes venous stasis.

Simple Sims'

Resting in Sims' position for 15 to 20 minutes twice daily is a good preventive measure against varicose veins. Advise the patient to avoid sitting with her legs crossed or her knees bent and to avoid wearing constrictive knee-high hose or garters. Elastic medical support stockings, such as TEDS, should be used to relieve varicose veins and should be applied before the patient arises in the morning to be most effective. Alternating exercise with rest periods is also effective in alleviating varicose veins. The patient should be advised to break up periods of sitting or standing with a walk at least twice daily. Vitamin C may also be helpful in reducing the size of varicose veins because it's involved in forming col-

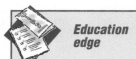

Education edge

Relieving heartburn and indigestion

To decrease the incidence of heartburn and indigestion in the pregnant patient, advise her to:

• avoid gaining too much weight (this puts excess pressure on the stomach)

• avoid wearing clothing that's tight around the abdomen and waist

• eat frequent, small meals instead of three large ones

• eat slowly and chew thoroughly

• avoid highly seasoned foods, fried and fatty foods, processed meats, chocolate, coffee, alcohol, carbonated beverages, and spearmint or peppermint

• avoid smoking

• avoid bending at the waist

• sleep with her head elevated about 6″ (15 cm).

lagen and endothelium for blood vessels. Ask at prenatal visits whether fresh fruit is included in the woman's diet.

Surgical removal of varicose veins isn't recommended during pregnancy. In most cases, they improve on their own after delivery, usually by the time prepregnancy weight is reached.

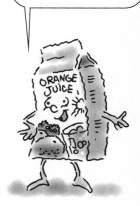

Vitamin C may help reduce the size of varicose veins.

Hemorrhoids

Hemorrhoids are varicosities of the rectal veins. They occur commonly in pregnancy because the bulk of the growing uterus puts pressure on the veins. Measures taken early in pregnancy to prevent their occurrence are key to reducing their incidence as well as severity.

Resting in a modified Sims' position daily helps to reduce the discomfort of hemorrhoids. Tell the patient to assume a knee-chest position at the end of the day to reduce pressure on rectal veins. Because this position can result in light-headedness, advise the patient to start by doing this for only a few minutes and gradually increasing to 10 to 15 minutes. Stool softeners may be recommended as well as application of witch hazel or cold compresses to help relieve pain.

Constipation

As pregnancy progresses, the growing uterus presses against the bowel and slows peristalsis, resulting in constipation and sometimes flatulence. Prescribed oral iron supplements also contribute to constipation. Reinforce the need for the supplements to build fetal iron stores but also help the woman to find a method to relieve or prevent constipation.

Advise the patient not to use home remedies, such as mineral oil and enemas. Mineral oil interferes with the absorption of fat-soluble vitamins (A, D, E, and K), which are necessary for fetal growth. Enemas might initiate labor through their action. OTC laxatives and all drugs are contraindicated during pregnancy unless specifically prescribed or authorized by the patient's health care provider. (See *Preventing constipation*.)

If the patient experiences excessive flatulence, recommend that she avoid gas-forming foods, such as cabbage and beans. In addition, if dietary measures and regular bowel evacuation fail, a stool softener (such as docusate sodium [Colace] and evacuation suppositories (such as glycerin) may be prescribed.

Backache

As pregnancy advances, a lumbar lordosis occurs and postural changes necessary to maintain balance may lead to backache.

Education edge

Preventing constipation

When teaching the pregnant patient about preventing constipation, include these tips:
• Encourage her to evacuate her bowels regularly.
• Advise her to increase the amount of roughage in her diet by eating raw fruits, bran, and vegetables.
• Instruct her to drink extra amounts of water daily.

Backache can also be an initial sign of bladder or kidney infection. To determine the cause of the patient's backache, assess the manner in which she walks, determine what type of shoes she wears, and obtain a detailed account of her symptoms.

To help alleviate pain, instruct the patient to wear shoes with low to moderate-height heels. Such shoes reduce the amount of spinal curvature necessary to maintain an upright posture. Advise the patient to walk with her pelvis tilted forward. This helps to alleviate back pain by putting pelvic support under the weight of the uterus. Local heat and a firmer mattress (or a board placed under the mattress) can help to relieve discomfort. Pelvic rocking or tilting can also be beneficial. To avoid back strain, advise the patient to squat—not bend over—to lift objects and to hold objects close to the body when lifting.

Tell the patient not to take muscle relaxants or analgesics (as well as other medications) for back pain without first consulting her practitioner. Generally, acetaminophen (Tylenol) is considered safe and effective for relieving this type of pain during pregnancy.

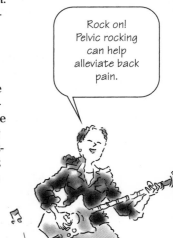

Rock on! Pelvic rocking can help alleviate back pain.

Leg cramps

Decreased serum calcium, increased serum phosphorus, and interference with circulation commonly cause muscle cramps of the lower extremities during pregnancy. The pain may be extreme and the intensity of the contraction frightening. Make sure to ask the patient at prenatal visits if she's having leg cramps. If leg cramps are a problem, provide her with information on techniques for relieving discomfort.

Extend and elevate

The best way to relieve symptoms is to have the patient lie on her back momentarily and extend the involved leg while keeping her knee straight and dorsiflexing the foot until the pain is gone. Elevating the lower extremities frequently during the day to improve circulation and avoiding full leg extension, such as stretching with the toes pointed, may also be beneficial.

If the woman is having frequent leg cramps, her practitioner may prescribe aluminum hydroxide gel (Amphojel) to bind phosphorus in the intestinal tract, lowering it in the circulation. Lowering milk intake to only a pint daily and supplementing this with calcium lactate may also help to reduce her phosphorus level.

Light-headedness

Light-headedness in the first trimester may be caused by a blood supply that inadequately fills the rapidly expanding circulatory system. During the second trimester, the pressure of the expanding uterus on maternal blood vessels may cause it. Faintness can occur anytime the patient rises from a sitting or prone position (postural hypotension) because the blood suddenly shifts away from the brain when blood pressure drops rapidly. Advise the patient to get up slowly in these situations.

Light-headedness may also be the result of low glucose levels caused by skipping meals. Carrying fruit or crackers to snack on is helpful to quickly increase glucose levels.

If the patient feels faint, advise her to lie down with her legs elevated or sit down and place her head between her knees until faintness subsides. She should also report to her practitioner any light-headedness because it can be a sign of severe anemia or another illness and should be evaluated.

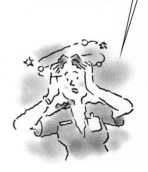

Lying down and elevating the legs helps to relieve light-headedness.

Shortness of breath

As the expanding uterus puts pressure on the diaphragm, the lungs may compress, causing dyspnea (shortness of breath). This may be more noticeable to the patient on exertion or during the night, when her body is flat.

Sitting upright and allowing the weight of the uterus to fall away from the diaphragm can help relieve the problem. As pregnancy progresses, the patient may require two or more pillows to sleep on at night to avoid dyspnea.

Always question the patient about shortness of breath at prenatal visits to be certain the sensation isn't continuous. Constant shortness of breath may indicate cardiac problems or a respiratory tract infection.

Insomnia

Insomnia is common during pregnancy. It's difficult for a pregnant women to rest physically because her large abdomen makes it difficult to get comfortable, and mentally because she has a lot on her mind. In cases of insomnia, it's helpful to review stress-reduction and relaxation techniques to help the patient get in the frame of mind for a good night's sleep. In addition, a comfortable bed and pillows to support the head, back, and abdomen are helpful. Eating a light snack before bedtime and avoiding caffeine after noontime is also beneficial. If the patient naps during the day, suggest shortening the nap and trying to stay up later to promote better sleep at night. If measures fail, suggest that the patient get out of bed and read, knit, or do a favorite activity until she's drowsy and able to fall asleep.

Abdominal discomfort and Braxton Hicks contractions

A woman may experience uncomfortable feelings of abdominal pressure early in pregnancy. A woman with a multiple pregnancy may notice this throughout pregnancy. The patient can relieve this pressure by putting gentle pressure on the uterine fundus or by standing with her arms crossed in front.

Pain around the round ligaments

When a woman stands up quickly, she may experience a pulling pain in the right or left lower abdomen from tension on the round ligaments. It can be very sharp and frightening and may be prevented by always rising slowly from a lying to a sitting position or from a sitting to a standing position. Keep in mind that round ligament pain may simulate the abrupt pain that occurs with ruptured ectopic pregnancy. The patient's description of the pain needs to be evaluated carefully.

As early as the 12th week of pregnancy, the uterus periodically contracts and relaxes again. These contractions, termed *Braxton Hicks contractions,* usually aren't noticeable early in pregnancy. In middle and late pregnancy, the contractions become stronger, causing the woman to tense and possibly feel minimal pain, similar to a hard menstrual cramp. These feelings are normal and aren't a sign of beginning labor.

Be certain the woman understands that a rhythmic pattern of contractions, characteristic of labor, shouldn't be mistaken for Braxton Hicks contractions.

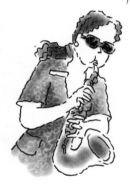

I've got rhythm, but a rhythmic pattern of contractions is characteristic of labor.

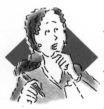

Quick quiz

1. A pregnant patient who's older than age 35 is at greater risk for having:

    A.   a low-birth-weight infant.
    B.   a preterm infant.
    C.   gestational hypertension.
    D   placenta previa.

Answer: D. Expectant mothers who are older than age 35 are at risk for placenta previa, hydatidiform mole, and vascular, neoplastic, and degenerative diseases. They're also at risk for having fraternal twins or infants with genetic abnormalities, especially Down syndrome.

2. Which familial factor is most likely to cause discomfort during pregnancy?

    A.   Anemia

    B.   Varicose veins

    C.   Cancer

    D.   Colitis

Answer: B. Varicose veins are an inherited weakness in blood vessel walls that become evident during pregnancy and can cause the patient discomfort.

3. A patient reports that the first day of her last normal menses was January 7. The calculated EDD is:

    A.   October 14.

    B.   April 14.

    C.   September 31.

    D.   April 7.

Answer: A. Based on information obtained in the patient's menstrual history, you can calculate the patient's EDD using Nägele's rule: Take the first day of the last normal menses, subtract 3 months, and then add 7 days.

4. A patient has had two previous pregnancies, has had no abortions or miscarriages, delivered two full-term neonates, and is currently pregnant. Using GTPAL, you would consider this woman a:

    A.   3-2-0-2-0.

    B.   3-2-0-0-2.

    C.   2-3-0-0-2.

    D.   3-2-0-2-2.

Answer: B. This woman would be considered a 3-2-0-0-2. G is the total number of pregnancies (3). T is the number of pregnancies that end at term (38 weeks or later), which totals 2. P is for preterm, the number of pregnancies that ended after 20 weeks and before the end of 37 weeks' gestation, which is 0 for this patient. A is the number of pregnancies that ended in spontaneous or induced abortions, which is 0 for this patient. L is the number of living children.

5. Normal FHR is:

    A.   110 to 150 beats/minute.

    B.   120 to 160 beats/minute.

    C.   130 to 170 beats/minute.

    D.   140 to 180 beats/minute.

Answer: B. Normal FHR usually ranges from 120 to 160 beats/minute.

6. Triple screening combines data from which prenatal tests?
   A.   Ultrasound, amniocentesis, and serum estriol
   B.   Serum hPL, serum estriol, and urinalysis
   C.   Serum hCG, serum estriol, and urinalysis
   D.   MSAFP, serum hCG, and unconjugated estriol

Answer: D. Triple screening combines data from MSAFP, hCG, and unconjugated estriol.

7.   A pregnant patient who's fatigued is likely to be more comfortable in which position?
   A.   Modified Sims'
   B.   Supine with legs elevated
   C.   Supine with head elevated
   D.   Sitting upright with legs elevated

Answer: A. A good resting position is a modified Sims' position with the top leg forward. This puts the weight of the fetus on the bed, not on the woman, and allows good circulation in the lower extremities.

Scoring

☆☆☆   If you answered all seven questions correctly, wow! You've sailed through prenatal care!

☆☆   If you answered five or six questions correctly, great job! You have smooth seas ahead!

☆   If you answered fewer than five questions correctly, don't go overboard! Forge ahead after a quick review!

High-risk pregnancy

Just the facts

In this chapter, you'll learn:

♦ factors that contribute to high-risk pregnancy

♦ ways to identify high-risk situations based on key assessment findings

♦ appropriate treatments for high-risk pregnancies

♦ relevant nursing interventions for high-risk pregnancies.

A look at high-risk pregnancy

Most women progress through pregnancy without serious problems. They enter pregnancy in good health and give birth to healthy neonates. However, problems sometimes develop that put a woman and her fetus in jeopardy. These problems may result from a chronic illness in the mother, a complication that develops during the pregnancy, or an external factor that impacts the health and well-being of the mother or the fetus.

Mother + fetus = one

Keep in mind that the health of a woman and her fetus are interdependent. Changes in the woman's health may affect fetal health, and changes in fetal health may affect the mother's physical and emotional health.

Group effort

Rarely is just one risk factor responsible for a high-risk pregnancy. Several factors can work together to contribute to a high-risk situation. For example, a pregnant adolescent is considered at higher risk; however, it isn't simply her age that places her in this category. Rather, her age is an indication of other factors that contribute to increased risk. First, as a pregnant adolescent, she

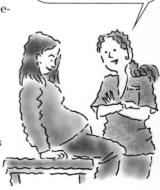

You can depend on it! The health of a woman and her fetus are interdependent.

faces a developmental crisis. In addition, adolescents in general tend to lack proper nutrition, adequate support, and knowledge—all contributors to increased risk. Moreover, such conditions as iron deficiency anemia, gestational hypertension, and preterm labor occur more commonly in adolescents than in older women.

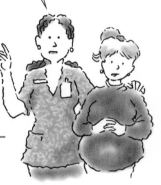

High-risk conditions such as iron deficiency anemia, gestational hypertension, and preterm labor are more common in adolescent pregnancies.

Maternal age

Reproductive risks increase among adolescents younger than age 15 and women older than age 35. The adolescent patient faces serious risks, including increased incidence of low-birth-weight and preterm neonates, anemia, labor dysfunction, and cephalo-pelvic disproportion. Expectant mothers older than age 35 are at risk for placenta previa, hydatidiform mole, and vascular, neoplastic, and degenerative diseases. They're also at risk for having fraternal twins or infants with genetic abnormalities, especially Down syndrome.

Maternal parity

Maternal parity may place a pregnant woman at high risk. For example, a multigravida who has had five or more pregnancies lasting at least 20 weeks is considered high-risk. In addition, if the current pregnancy occurs within 3 months of the last delivery, the pregnancy is considered high-risk.

Maternal obstetric and gynecologic history

Many factors in the mother's obstetric and gynecologic history can place a pregnancy at high risk. These factors may include:
- two or more premature deliveries or spontaneous abortions
- one or more stillbirths at term
- one or more neonates born with gross anomalies
- pelvic inadequacy or abnormal shaping
- cervical incompetency
- uterine incompetency, position, or structural anomalies
- history of multiple pregnancy, placental anomalies, amniotic fluid abnormalities, or poor weight gain
- history of gestational diabetes, gestational hypertension, or infection
- history of delivering a postterm neonate
- history of dystocia, precipitous delivery, cervical or vaginal lacerations caused by labor and delivery, cephalopelvic disproportion, hemorrhage during labor and delivery, or retained placenta
- lack of previous prenatal care.

In addition, a pregnancy that occurs within 3 years of menarche indicates an increased risk of maternal mortality and morbidity. Such a pregnancy also places the patient at risk for delivering a neonate who's small for gestational age.

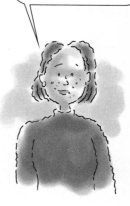

Getting pregnant within 3 years of menarche increases the risk of maternal mortality and morbidity. No thanks!

Maternal medical history

Medical problems can cause complications during pregnancy. For example, abdominal trauma may lead to premature rupture of membranes (PROM) or abruptio placentae. Severe cardiac disease can adversely affect placental perfusion, thus jeopardizing fetal nutrition. As a result, the neonate may be born with a low birth weight. Gestational hypertension, which commonly develops in women with essential hypertension, renal disease, or diabetes, increases the risk of abruptio placentae.

Insulin influx

Diabetes can worsen during pregnancy and harm the mother and fetus. Because pregnant women typically develop insulin resistance, women with diabetes need increased amounts of insulin during pregnancy. The fetus of a woman with diabetes tends to be large because the increased insulin production needed to counteract the overload of glucose from the mother stimulates fetal growth. This, in turn, can lead to problems of cephalopelvic disproportion and dystocia for the mother.

Gravida aggravations

Stomach displacement by the gravid uterus, along with cardiac sphincter relaxation and decreased GI motility caused by increased progesterone, may aggravate symptoms of peptic ulcer disease such as gastric reflux. Also, the increase in blood volume and cardiac output associated with pregnancy can exhaust a patient with underlying cardiac disease.

The increase in blood volume and cardiac output associated with pregnancy can be quite taxing on me!

Maternal lifestyle

Lifestyle and occupation can adversely affect a pregnancy. Make the patient aware that what she consumes and what she's exposed to can seriously affect her pregnancy. For example, taking over-the-counter and prescription drugs can be detrimental to the fetus. In addition, cigarette smoking is associated with intrauterine growth retardation and low-birth-weight neonates. Exposure to toxic substances, such as lead, organic solvents, radiation, and carbon monoxide, can also lead to fetal malformations.

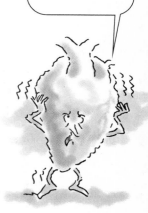

Substance sabotage

Substance use or abuse of drugs or alcohol is another cause of fetal anomalies. After birth, the neonate may experience withdrawal. Substance abuse may also interfere with the pregnant woman's ability to obtain adequate nutrition, which can adversely affect fetal growth. Additionally, if the substance abuse involves injection, the pregnant woman is at risk for infection with hepatitis B and human immunodeficiency virus (HIV).

Nourish to flourish

Adequate nutrition is especially vital during pregnancy. Inadequate nutrition can lead to a deficiency of iron, folic acid, or protein. Iron deficiency anemia during pregnancy is associated with low fetal birth weight and preterm birth. Folic acid deficiency is associated with neural tube defects. Protein deficiency can lead to poor development of the fetus and growth restriction.

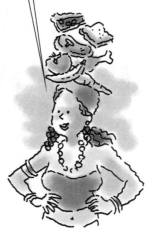

Food, glorious food! Adequate nutrition is especially vital during pregnancy.

Cultural background

Several genetic disorders are associated with specific cultures. For example, sickle cell anemia occurs primarily in persons of African and Mediterranean descent. Tay-Sachs disease is about 100 times more common in people of Eastern European Jewish (Ashkenazi) ancestry than in the general population.

Faith and the fetus

A woman's religious practices may also affect her health during pregnancy and could predispose her to complications. For example, an Amish woman may not be immunized against rubella. If the woman is exposed, her fetus is at risk for congenital anomalies. Seventh-Day Adventists traditionally exclude dairy products from their diets, which may conflict with the woman's need for additional calcium for fetal bone growth.

Family history

Certain conditions and disorders that contribute to high-risk pregnancy are familial. For example, a family history of multiple births, congenital diseases or deformities, or mental disability may place a pregnancy at higher risk.

Don't forget Dad

Some fetal congenital anomalies may be traced to the father's exposure to environmental hazards. The father's blood type and Rh status are also important because isoimmuniza-

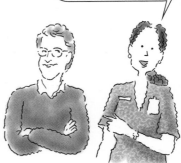

It isn't just mom. Dad also plays a role in fetal congenital anomalies; specifically related to his exposure to environmental hazards and his blood type and Rh status.

tion in the fetus may occur if the father is Rh positive, the mother is Rh negative, and the fetus is Rh positive.

On the home front

The family environment is also important in determining whether a pregnancy is high-risk. A history of battering or abuse, a lack of support persons, inadequate housing, or lack of adequate finances can increase risk during pregnancy.

Abruptio placentae

Abruptio placentae—also called *placental abruption*—occurs when the placenta separates from the uterine wall prematurely, usually after 20 weeks' gestation, producing hemorrhage. This disorder may be classified according to the degree of placental separation and the severity of maternal and fetal symptoms.

More births, more risk

Abruptio placentae is most common in multigravidas—usually in women over age 35—and is a common cause of bleeding during the second half of pregnancy. The fetal prognosis depends on its gestational age and the amount of blood lost. The maternal prognosis is good if hemorrhage can be controlled.

What causes it

The cause of abruptio placentae is unknown. Predisposing factors include:
• traumatic injury such as a direct blow to the uterus
• placental site bleeding caused by a needle puncture during amniocentesis
• chronic hypertension or gestational hypertension, which raises pressure on the maternal side of the placenta
• multiparity (more than 5)
• short umbilical cord
• dietary deficiency
• smoking
• pressure on the venae cavae from an enlarged uterus. (See *Understanding abruptio placentae,* page 214.)

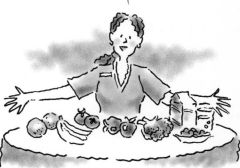

Dietary deficiency is thought to be a predisposing factor in abruptio placentae. So, encourage your patient to eat up!

Understanding abruptio placentae

With abruptio placentae, lack of resiliency or abnormal changes in uterine vasculature cause blood vessels at the placental bed to rupture spontaneously. Hypertension and an enlarged uterus that can't contract sufficiently to seal off the torn blood vessels further complicate the situation. As a result, bleeding continues unchecked, potentially shearing off part or all of the placenta.

External versus internal

About 80% of bleeding is external (marginal), meaning that a peripheral portion of the placenta separates from the uterine wall. The bleeding is internal (concealed) if the central portion of the placenta becomes detached and the still-intact peripheral portions trap the blood. This occurs in about 20% of cases.

Effects of bleeding

As blood enters the muscle fibers, detached and still-intact peripheral portions of the placenta trap the blood. Complete relaxation of the uterus becomes impossible. Uterine tone and irritability increase. If bleeding into the muscle fibers is profuse, the uterus turns blue or purple and the accumulated blood prevents its normal contractions after delivery (known as *Couvelaire uterus* or *uteroplacental apoplexy*).

What to look for

Abruptio placentae produces a wide range of signs and symptoms, depending on the extent of placental separation and the amount of blood lost from maternal circulation. In addition to the major complications of abruptio placentae—hemorrhage and shock—it may also cause renal failure, pituitary necrosis (Sheehan's syndrome), disseminated intravascular coagulation (DIC), and maternal and fetal death.

Three degrees of separation

Three degrees of separation can occur with abruptio placentae.

Mild abruptio placentae (marginal separation) develops gradually and produces mild to moderate bleeding, vague lower abdominal discomfort, mild to moderate abdominal tenderness, and uterine irritability. Fetal heart tones remain strong and regular.

Moderate abruptio placentae (about 50% placental separation) may develop gradually or abruptly and produces continuous abdominal pain, moderate dark red vaginal bleeding, a tender uterus that remains firm between contractions, barely audible or irregular and bradycardic fetal heart tones and, possibly, signs of shock. Labor typically starts within 2 hours and usually proceeds rapidly.

Severe abruptio placentae (70% placental separation) develops abruptly and causes agonizing, unremitting uterine pain (de-

Placental separation in abruptio placentae

Here are descriptions and illustrations of the three degrees of placental separation in abruptio placentae.

Mild separation
Mild separation begins with small areas of separation and internal bleeding (concealed hemorrhage) between the placenta and uterine wall.

Moderate separation
Moderate separation may develop abruptly or progress from mild to extensive separation with external hemorrhage.

Severe separation
With severe separation, external hemorrhage occurs, along with shock and, possibly, fetal cardiac distress.

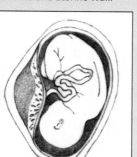 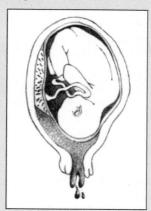 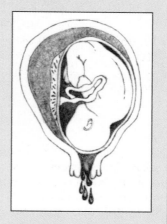

scribed as tearing or knifelike); a boardlike, tender uterus; moderate vaginal bleeding; rapidly progressive shock; and absence of fetal heart tones (related to fetal cardiac distress). (See *Placental separation in abruptio placentae.*)

As abruptio placentae becomes more severe, I'm at greater risk for cardiac distress.

What tests tell you

Vaginal examination (in preparation for emergency cesarean delivery) and ultrasonography are performed to rule out placenta previa. Decreased hemoglobin levels and platelet counts support the diagnosis. Periodic assays for fibrin split products aid in monitoring the progression of abruptio placentae and in detecting DIC. Differential diagnosis excludes placenta previa, ovarian cysts, appendicitis, and degeneration of leiomyomas.

How it's treated

Treatment of abruptio placentae focuses on assessing, controlling, and restoring the amount of blood lost; delivering a viable neonate; and preventing coagulation disorders.

First things first!

Immediate measures for treatment of abruptio placentae include:
- starting an I.V. infusion (through a large-bore catheter) of lactated Ringer's solution to combat hypovolemia
- placing a central venous pressure (CVP) line and urinary catheter to monitor fluid status
- drawing blood for hemoglobin level, hematocrit, coagulation studies, and typing and crossmatching
- external electronic fetal monitoring and monitoring of maternal vital signs and vaginal bleeding
- administering blood replacement as necessary.

Delivery details

After the severity of abruption has been determined and fluid and blood have been replaced, prompt cesarean delivery is necessary if the fetus is in distress or if heavy bleeding continues. If the fetus isn't in distress, monitoring continues.

Because of possible fetal blood loss through the placenta, a pediatric team should be ready at delivery to assess and treat the neonate for shock, blood loss, and hypoxia. If placental separation is severe and no signs of fetal life are present, vaginal delivery may be performed unless it's contraindicated by uncontrolled hemorrhage or other complications.

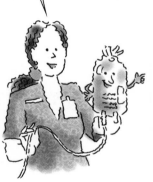

One of the top priorities for treating abruptio placentae is to start an I.V. infusion of lactated Ringer's solution.

What to do

- Assess the patient's extent of bleeding and monitor fundal height every 30 minutes for changes. Count the number of perineal pads used by the patient, weighing them as needed to determine the amount of blood loss.
- Monitor maternal blood pressure, pulse rate, respirations, CVP, intake and output, and amount of vaginal bleeding every 10 to 15 minutes.
- Begin electronic fetal monitoring to assess fetal heart rate (FHR) continuously.
- Have equipment for emergency cesarean delivery readily available.
- If vaginal delivery is elected, provide emotional support during labor. Because of the neonate's prematurity, the mother may not

receive analgesics during labor and may experience intense pain. Reassure the patient of her progress through labor, and keep her informed of the fetus's condition.

• Prepare the patient and her family for the possibility of an emergency cesarean delivery of a premature neonate and the changes to expect in the postpartum period. Offer emotional support and an honest assessment of the situation.

• Tactfully discuss the possibility of neonatal death. Tell the mother that the neonate's survival depends primarily on gestational age, the amount of blood lost, and associated hypertensive disorders. Assure her that frequent monitoring and prompt management greatly reduce the risk of death.

• Encourage the patient and her family to verbalize their feelings.

• Help the patient and her family develop effective coping strategies. Refer them for counseling if necessary.

Cardiac disease

The pregnant woman with preexisting cardiac disease is considered high-risk. Despite improvements in early identification and management of cardiac problems, these disorders contribute to complications in approximately 1% of pregnancies.

Rating the risk

The type and extent of the woman's cardiac disease determine whether she can successfully complete a pregnancy. Guidelines developed by the New York Heart Association are commonly used to predict a pregnancy's outcome. These guidelines categorize pregnancy based on the degree of compromise. (See *Cardiac disease classification*, page 218.)

What causes it

The most common underlying cause of cardiac disease in pregnancy involves congenital anomalies, such as atrial septal defect and coarctation of the aorta that hasn't been corrected. Valvular disease caused by rheumatic fever or Kawasaki disease may also be an underlying problem. Moreover, with an increase in the number of women becoming pregnant at an older age, the incidences of ischemic cardiac disease and myocardial infarction are increasing.

Many women have more birthdays under their belts when they decide to have children. That's why the incidence of cardiac disease is increasing in pregnant women.

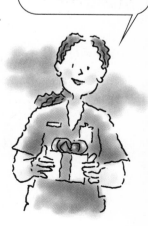

Cardiac disease classification

Here are the New York Heart Association's guidelines for classifying the degree of compromise in a pregnant woman with cardiac disease. Typically, a woman with Class I or II cardiac disease can complete a pregnancy and delivery without major complications. A woman with Class III cardiac disease usually must maintain complete bed rest during the pregnancy. A woman with Class IV cardiac disease is a poor candidate for pregnancy and should be strongly urged to avoid becoming pregnant.

Class	Description
I	*Uncompromised*—The woman has unrestricted physical activity. Ordinary physical activity causes no discomfort, cardiac insufficiency, or anginal pain.
II	*Slightly compromised*—The woman has a slight limitation on physical activity. Ordinary activity causes excess fatigue, palpitations, dyspnea, or anginal pain.
III	*Markedly compromised*—The woman has a moderate or marked limitation on physical activity. With less than ordinary activity, she experiences excessive fatigue, palpitations, dyspnea, or anginal pain.
IV	*Severely compromised*—The woman can't engage in any physical activity without experiencing discomfort. Cardiac insufficiency or anginal pain occurs even at rest.

Adapted with permission from Criteria Committee of the New York Heart Association. *Nomenclature and Criteria for Diagnosis of Diseases of the Heart and Great Vessels*, 9th ed. Boston: Little, Brown, & Co., 1994:253-256.

On rare occasion

Peripartal cardiomyopathy (cardiac disease that manifests primarily with pregnancy) is rare. Although the exact cause is unknown, it's believed to result from the effects of pregnancy on the circulatory system. In many cases, previously undiagnosed cardiac disease is the cause.

What to look for

Signs and symptoms of cardiac disease in a pregnant woman depend on the type and severity of the underlying disease. Primarily, these signs and symptoms are those associated with heart failure. (See *The weaker weeks*.) Fetal signs of maternal cardiac disease are nonspecific—such as abnormally low FHR and fetal growth retardation—so diagnosis depends mainly on maternal signs and symptoms.

The weaker weeks

The most dangerous time for a pregnant woman with cardiac disease and her fetus is between weeks 28 and 32 of gestation. During this time, blood volume peaks and the woman's heart may be unable to compensate adequately for the increase. As a result, cardiac decompensation can occur, causing the woman's cardiac output to drop, possibly to such an extent that perfusion to vital organs, including the placenta, is significantly affected. Consequently, oxygen and nutrients aren't delivered in adequate amounts to the cells, including those of the fetus.

Failure to the left

Left-sided heart failure occurs with such conditions as mitral valve disorder and congenital coarctation of the aorta. Common signs and symptoms are those associated with pulmonary hypertension and pulmonary edema and may include:

- decreased systemic blood pressure
- productive cough with blood-streaked sputum
- tachypnea
- dyspnea on exertion, progressing to dyspnea at rest
- tachycardia
- orthopnea
- paroxysmal nocturnal dyspnea
- edema.

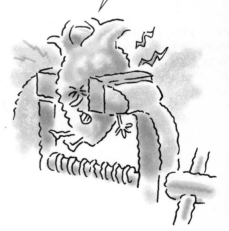

I've got coarctation to the left of me, defects to the right. Here I am, stuck in the middle.

Failure to the right

Right-sided heart failure can occur in a woman with a congenital heart defect, such as atrial and ventricular septal defect and pulmonary valve stenosis. Signs and symptoms may include:

- hypotension
- jugular vein distention
- liver and spleen enlargement
- ascites
- dyspnea and pain.

My, oh, myocardial failure

For the woman with peripartal cardiac disease, signs and symptoms typically reflect myocardial failure. Shortness of breath, chest pain, and edema are common. Cardiomegaly also may occur.

What tests tell you

An electrocardiogram (ECG) may show cardiac changes in the mother but may be less accurate later in pregnancy as the enlarged uterus pushes the diaphragm upward and displaces the heart. Echocardiography shows cardiomegaly. If the mother's cardiac decompensation has reached the point of placental insufficiency and incompetency, late decelerations during fetal monitoring may indicate fetal distress. Ultrasonography may show growth retardation.

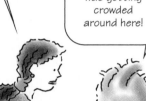

How it's treated

Treatment focuses on ensuring the health and safety of the mother and fetus. Commonly, more frequent prenatal visits are scheduled, such as every 2 weeks and then every week during the last month, to achieve this goal.

Minor adjustments

If the woman was taking cardiac medications before becoming pregnant, the medications are typically continued during pregnancy. However, maintenance doses may need to be increased to aid in compensating for the increased blood volume associated with pregnancy.

The deal with other drugs

If the patient required digoxin (Lanoxin) before her pregnancy, she can continue use during pregnancy without risk. Even if she wasn't taking digoxin before her pregnancy, she may require it to help increase or strengthen her cardiac output as her pregnancy advances. The effects on pregnancy of propranolol (Inderal), a beta-adrenergic blocker commonly used for cardiac arrhythmias, aren't known; however, the drug doesn't appear to cause fetal abnormalities. The effects of nitroglycerin (Nitro-quick), a compound commonly prescribed for angina, are also unknown; however, the drug appears to be safe. A woman who's taking heparin for venous thromboembolitic disease shouldn't take any after labor begins. If the woman has had a valve replacement and is receiving warfarin (Coumadin) therapy, warfarin—which is associated with an increase in fetal anomalies—is discontinued and heparin is used instead.

Prophylactic tactics

For women with valvular or congenital cardiac disease, some practitioners may begin prophylactic antibiotic therapy near to the patient's expected due date to prevent the development of possible subacute bacterial endocarditis secondary to bacterial invasion from the placental site into the bloodstream. If the woman was taking prophylactic antibiotics to prevent a recurrence of rheumatic fever before becoming pregnant, they're continued during pregnancy.

Rest for the weary

Another key area of treatment is rest. A pregnant woman with cardiac disease requires more rest than the average pregnant woman. In addition, practitioners commonly recommend complete bed rest for the woman after gestational week 30 to ensure the fetus is carried to term or at least to week 36.

A weighty subject

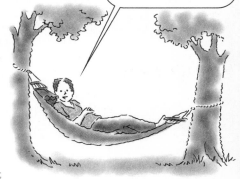

The prescription for pregnant women with cardiac disease is complete bed rest after week 30. Unfortunately, there's no such prescription for nurses!

Maintaining good nutrition is an important component of ensuring a healthy mother and fetus. For the woman with cardiac disease, it's especially important that weight gain be balanced to ensure that the nutritional needs of the mother and fetus are met, while also ensuring that the mother's heart isn't overburdened. As a general practice, salt intake may be limited; however, it shouldn't be severely restricted because sodium is needed for fluid volume. Prenatal vitamins are essential to help ensure adequate iron intake and avoid anemia, which reduces the blood's capacity to carry oxygen. The pregnant woman with cardiac disease and her fetus need as much oxygen as possible, so anemia must be avoided.

What to do

• Assess maternal vital signs and cardiopulmonary status closely for changes; question the patient about increased shortness of breath, palpitations, or edema; monitor FHR for changes.
• Monitor weight gain throughout pregnancy. Assess for edema and note any pitting.
• Explain signs and symptoms of worsening disease and tell the patient to report them immediately.
• Reinforce use of prescribed medications to control cardiac disease. Explain possible adverse reactions to these medications and instruct the patient to report these reactions immediately.
• Anticipate the need for increased doses of maintenance medications; explain to the patient the rationale for this increase.
• Assess the woman's nutritional pattern. Work with her to develop a feasible meal plan. Stress the need for prenatal vitamins.
• Assess FHR and ultrasound results to monitor fetal growth.

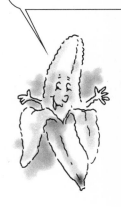

Weight gain should meet the nutritional needs of the mother and fetus but shouldn't overburden mom's heart.

• Encourage frequent rest periods throughout the day. Discuss measures for pacing activities and conserving energy.
• Advise the woman to immediately report signs and symptoms of infection, such as upper respiratory or urinary tract infection (UTI), to prevent overtaxing the heart.
• Advise the woman to rest in the left lateral recumbent position to prevent supine hypotension and provide the best possible oxygen exchange to the fetus; if necessary, use semi-Fowler's position to relieve dyspnea.
• Prepare the woman for labor, anticipating the use of epidural anesthesia to avoid overtaxing the patient's heart.
• Monitor FHR, uterine contractions, and maternal vital signs closely for changes during labor.
• Assess vital signs closely after delivery. Anticipate anticoagulant and cardiac glycoside therapy immediately after delivery for the woman with severe heart failure.
• Encourage ambulation, as ordered, as soon as possible after delivery.
• Anticipate administration of prophylactic antibiotics, if not already ordered, after delivery to prevent subacute bacterial endocarditis.

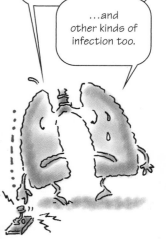

Don't wait! A pregnant woman with cardiac disease should immediately report signs of upper respiratory tract infection...

...and other kinds of infection too.

Diabetes mellitus

Diabetes mellitus is a metabolic disorder characterized by hyperglycemia (elevated serum glucose level) resulting from lack of insulin, lack of insulin effect, or both. It's a disorder of carbohydrate, protein, and fat metabolism.

Three general classifications are recognized.

Type 1 diabetes (absolute insulin insufficiency) usually occurs before age 30, although it may occur at any age. The patient is typically thin and requires exogenous insulin and dietary management to achieve control.

Type 2 diabetes (insulin resistance with varying degrees of insulin secretory defects) usually occurs in obese adults after age 40. It's treated with diet and exercise in combination with various antidiabetic drugs, although treatment may also include insulin therapy.

Gestational diabetes (diabetes that emerges during pregnancy) typically develops during the middle of the pregnancy when insulin resistance is most apparent.

Losing balance

Diabetes affects approximately 2% to 5% of all pregnancies. The overall challenge associated with diabetes and pregnancy is controlling the balance between glucose levels and insulin requirements. Poor glucose control can adversely affect the mother, the fetus, or both. The risk of gestational hypertension and infection (most commonly candidal infections) is higher in pregnant women with diabetes. Moreover, continued fetal consumption of glucose may lead to maternal hypoglycemia, especially between meals and during the night. Additionally, polyhydramnios (increased amount of amniotic fluid) may occur because of increased fetal urine production caused by fetal hyperglycemia.

Neonates who are born to mothers with poorly controlled diabetes typically are large, possibly more than 4.5 kg (10 lb). This large size may complicate labor and delivery, necessitating a cesarean birth. The risks of congenital anomalies, spontaneous abortions, and stillbirths also increase in women with poorly controlled or uncontrolled diabetes.

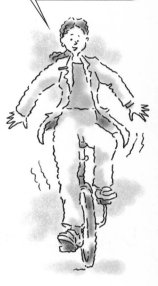

Mom and baby can be adversely affected by poor glucose control. The key is to maintain balance between glucose levels and insulin.

What causes it

Evidence indicates that diabetes has various causes, including:
- heredity
- environment (infection, diet, exposure to toxins and stress)
- lifestyle in genetically susceptible persons.

Unwanted relative

Although the cause of type 1 diabetes isn't known, scientists believe that the tendency to develop diabetes may be inherited and related to viruses. In persons with a supposed genetic predisposition to type 1 diabetes, a triggering event (possibly infection with a virus) spurs the production of autoantibodies that destroy the pancreas's beta cells. The destruction of beta cells causes insulin secretion to decrease or ultimately stop. When more than 90% of the beta cells have been destroyed, the subsequent insulin deficiency leads to hyperglycemia, enhanced lipolysis (decomposition of fat), and protein catabolism.

Impaired, inappropriate…

Type 2 diabetes is a chronic disease caused by one or more of these factors:
- impaired insulin production
- inappropriate hepatic glucose production
- peripheral insulin receptor insensitivity
- history of gestational diabetes
- stress.

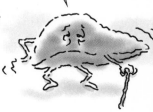

Please excuse my inappropriate behavior; specifically, my inappropriate glucose production. I'm truly sorry about the type 2 diabetes.

...and intolerant

Gestational diabetes occurs when a woman who hasn't been previously diagnosed with diabetes shows glucose intolerance during pregnancy. Of those women who don't have diabetes when they become pregnant, approximately 3% develop gestational diabetes. It isn't known whether gestational diabetes results from inadequate insulin response to carbohydrates, excessive insulin resistance, or both. Identifiable risk factors include:

• obesity
• history of delivering large neonates (usually more than 4.5 kg [10 lb]), unexplained fetal or perinatal loss, or evidence of congenital anomalies in previous pregnancies
• age older than 25
• family history of diabetes.

What to look for

The signs and symptoms noted in the pregnant woman with diabetes are the same as those for any person with diabetes. Common signs and symptoms include hyperglycemia, glycosuria, and polyuria. Dizziness and confusion may be related to hyperglycemia. In addition, the woman may experience an increased incidence of monilial infections. Hydramnios may be present along with poor FHR and variability arising from inadequate tissue (placental) perfusion.

The woman with type 1 or 2 diabetes may also exhibit signs and symptoms related to microvascular and macrovascular changes, such as peripheral vascular disease, retinopathy, nephropathy, and neuropathy.

What tests tell you

All women are screened for gestational diabetes during pregnancy. Testing typically occurs between weeks 24 and 28 and may be repeated at week 32 if the woman is obese or older than age 40. If the woman has risk factors for gestational diabetes, this screening takes place at the first prenatal visit and again between weeks 24 and 28.

The glucose challenge

Screening involves an oral glucose challenge test (a test that obtains a fasting plasma glucose level) using a 100-g glucose load. One hour after ingestion, a venous blood sample is obtained. If the glucose level is greater than 180 mg/dl, the woman is scheduled for a 3-hour glucose tolerance test using a 100-g glucose load. Two

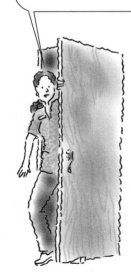

Come one, come all! During pregnancy, all women are screened for gestational diabetes.

Glucose challenge values in pregnancy

Here are normal values for pregnant patients taking the oral glucose challenge test to determine risk of diabetes. These values are determined after a 100-g glucose load. Normal blood glucose levels should remain between 90 and 120 mg/dl. If a pregnant woman's plasma glucose value exceeds these levels, she should be treated as a potential diabetic.

Test type	Pregnancy glucose level (mg/dl)
Fasting	95
1 hour	180
2 hour	155
3 hour	140

abnormal levels or a fasting glucose level greater than 95 mg/dl confirms a diagnosis of gestational diabetes. (See *Glucose challenge values in pregnancy*.)

If the woman is known to have diabetes, serial blood glucose monitoring and measurement of glycosylated hemoglobin levels are used to determine the degree of glucose control.

How it's treated

Any woman with diabetes, whether preexisting or gestational, requires more frequent prenatal visits to ensure optimal control of glucose levels, minimizing the risks to the woman and her fetus. Additionally, treatment focuses on balancing rest with exercise and maintaining adequate nutrition for fetal growth and control of blood glucose levels.

Ideally, the woman with preexisting diabetes should consult with her practitioner before becoming pregnant to ensure the best possible health for herself and her fetus. At that time, blood glucose levels can be assessed closely and medication adjustments can be made to ensure optimal regulation before she becomes pregnant.

Pregnant women with diabetes will rack up lots of frequent-flier miles! Frequent prenatal visits are needed to keep glucose under control.

Crucial calories

Nutritional therapy is crucial in the treatment of women with diabetes. Typically, an 1,800- to 2,200-calorie diet is prescribed for the pregnant woman with diabetes. Alternatively, caloric requirements may be calculated at 35 kcal/kg of ideal body weight. The caloric requirement is usually divided among three meals and three snacks, allowing the calories to be distributed throughout the day in an attempt to maintain constant glucose levels.

Additional dietary recommendations include reduced saturated fat and cholesterol and increased dietary fiber. Carbohydrates should make up more than half of daily caloric intake, with protein and fat supplying the remainder. The goal is to allow a weight gain of approximately 25 to 30 lb (11.3 to 13.6 kg) so that the neonate doesn't grow too large and vaginal delivery remains a possibility.

> Nutrition is the star of the show when it comes to ensuring a healthy pregnancy for a woman with diabetes.

Adjust, reduce, increase

For the woman with preexisting diabetes, insulin adjustments are necessary. Early in pregnancy, insulin may be reduced because of the increased utilization of glucose by the fetus for growth. However, later in pregnancy, an increase in insulin typically occurs because of an increase in the woman's metabolism. Insulin therapy dosages and types are highly individualized. A continuous subcutaneous insulin infusion via a pump may be ordered to maintain constant blood glucose levels. The woman with gestational diabetes may require insulin if diet therapy doesn't adequately control blood glucose levels.

Check 1: Glucose levels

To assist with blood glucose control, fingerstick blood glucose monitoring is important. For the woman with preexisting diabetes, typically this monitoring is performed daily, possibly as often as four times per day. For women with gestational diabetes, however, blood glucose monitoring may be performed only weekly. Regardless of monitoring frequency, the goal is to obtain fasting blood glucose levels below 95 mg/dl and 2-hour postprandial values below 120 mg/dl.

Check 2: Eyes and urinary tract

Throughout the pregnancy, follow-up monitoring is performed. A urine culture may be done each trimester to detect UTIs that produce no symptoms. Ophthalmic examination is done at each trimester for the woman with preexisting diabetes and at least once during the pregnancy for the woman with gestational diabetes. Retinal changes may develop or progress during pregnancy.

Check 3: The fetus

Because the risk of fetal complications is high, fetal monitoring is crucial. A serum alpha-fetoprotein (AFP) level may be done at 15 to 17 weeks' gestation to assess for neural tube defects. Ultrasonography may be done at 18 to 20 weeks to detect gross abnormalities, and then be repeated at 28 weeks and again at 36 to 38 weeks to determine fetal growth, amniotic fluid volume, placental location, and biparietal diameter. At 36 weeks, the woman may undergo an amniocentesis to assess the lecithin-sphingomyelin ratio, an indicator of fetal maturity.

Preferred delivery route

In the past, delivery occurred at approximately week 37 of gestation via cesarean birth. More recently, however, vaginal delivery has become the preferred route of delivery. During labor, uterine contractions and FHR are monitored continuously. The mother's glucose level is regulated with I.V. infusions of regular insulin based on blood glucose levels that are obtained hourly.

What to do

- Carefully monitor the woman's weight gain, blood glucose levels, and nutritional intake as well as fetal growth parameters throughout pregnancy.
- Review results of fingerstick blood glucose monitoring; assess for signs and symptoms of hypoglycemia and hyperglycemia.
- Assist with scheduling of follow-up laboratory studies, including glycosylated hemoglobin levels and urine studies as necessary.
- Encourage the patient to maintain a consistent exercise program and explain the benefits of eating certain snacks before exercise. (See *Preventing hypoglycemia during exercise.*)
- Instruct the woman in all aspects of managing diabetes, including insulin administration techniques, self-monitoring, nutrition, and danger signs and symptoms. (See *Teaching topics for pregnant patients with diabetes*, page 228.)
- Arrange for a consult with a dietitian.
- Assist with preparations for labor, including explanations about possible labor induction and required monitoring.
- Closely assess the woman in the postpartum period for changes in blood glucose levels and insulin requirements. Typically, the woman with preexisting diabetes will require no insulin in the immediate postpartum period (because insulin resistance is gone), and won't return to her prepregnancy insulin requirements for

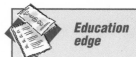

Education edge

Preventing hypoglycemia during exercise

Hypoglycemia during exercise is a common problem for patients with diabetes but there's an easy solution for a careful patient.

The problem

During exercise, the muscles increase their uptake of glucose, causing blood glucose levels to decrease. This effect can last up to 12 hours after exercise. In addition, if the woman injects insulin into the extremity involved in exercise, the insulin is released more quickly. As a result, blood glucose levels decrease even more dramatically, causing hypoglycemia.

The solution

To prevent hypoglycemia, encourage the patient with diabetes to eat a snack consisting of a protein or a complex carbohydrate before she exercises, and to maintain a consistent exercise pattern each day.

Education edge

Teaching topics for pregnant patients with diabetes

Be sure to cover these topics when teaching a pregnant patient with diabetes.
- Insulin type and dosage
- Insulin syringe preparation and injection technique or insulin pump use and care
- Sites to use (Most women prefer not to use the abdomen as an injection site.)
- Site rotation (Insulin is absorbed more slowly from the thigh than from the upper arm.)
- Blood glucose monitoring technique, including frequency of monitoring and desired glucose levels
- Nutritional plan, including suggestions for appropriate foods to include and avoid

- Consistent exercise regimen
- Signs and symptoms of urinary tract and monilial infections, including the need to report one immediately
- Signs and symptoms of hypoglycemia and hyperglycemia
- Measures to prevent and manage hypoglycemia and hyperglycemia
- Fetal monitoring methods, including fetal movement count and follow-up testing
- Preparations for labor and delivery
- Care after delivery

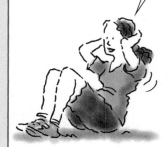

Encourage the pregnant patient with diabetes to maintain a consistent exercise program.

several days. The woman with gestational diabetes usually exhibits normal blood glucose levels within 24 hours after delivery, requiring no further insulin or diet therapy.
- Encourage the patient with gestational diabetes to keep all follow-up appointments so that glucose testing can be performed to detect possible type 2 diabetes.

Ectopic pregnancy

Ectopic pregnancy is the implantation of a fertilized ovum outside the uterine cavity. It most commonly occurs in the fallopian tube but may occur in other sites as well. (See *Sites of ectopic pregnancy*.)

Ectopic pregnancy occurs in 1 of every 200 White women and about 1 of every 120 nonwhite women. The prognosis for the patient is good with prompt diagnosis, appropriate surgical intervention, and control of bleeding. Rarely, in cases of abdominal implantation, the fetus may survive to term. Usually, only one in three women who experience an ectopic pregnancy give birth to a live neonate in a subsequent pregnancy. Rupture of the tube causes life-threatening complications, including hemor-

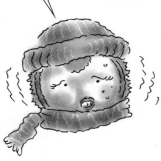

Brrr! What am I doing outside the uterine cavity? It must be ectopic pregnancy.

Sites of ectopic pregnancy

In most women with ectopic pregnancy, the ovum implants in the fallopian tube, either in the imbria, ampulla, or isthmus. Other possible sites of implantation include the interstitium, tubo-ovarian ligament, ovary, abdominal viscera, and internal cervical os.

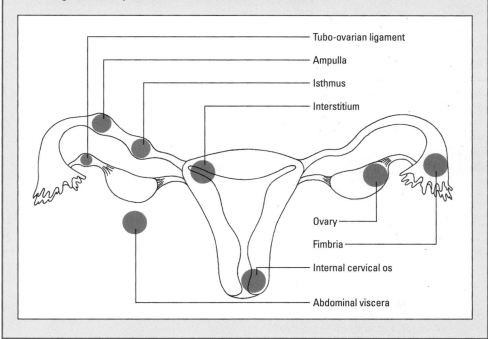

Tubo-ovarian ligament

Ampulla

Isthmus

Interstitium

Ovary

Fimbria

Internal cervical os

Abdominal viscera

rhage, shock, and peritonitis. Infertility results if the uterus, both fallopian tubes, or both ovaries are removed.

What causes it

Conditions that prevent or slow the fertilized ovum's passage through the fallopian tube into the uterine cavity include:
• endosalpingitis, an inflammatory reaction that causes folds of the tubal mucosa to agglutinate, narrowing the tube
• diverticula (blind pouches that cause tubal abnormalities)
• tumors pressing against the tube
• previous surgery, such as tubal ligation or resection, or adhesions from previous abdominal or pelvic surgery
• transmigration of the ovum from one ovary to the opposite tube resulting in delayed implantation.

Ectopic pregnancy may also result from congenital defects in the reproductive tract or ectopic endometrial implants in the tubal mucosa. Additional factors include sexually transmitted tubal infections as well as intrauterine devices that cause irritation of the cellular lining of the uterus and the fallopian tubes.

What to look for

Symptoms of ectopic pregnancy are sometimes similar to those of a normal pregnancy, making diagnosis difficult. Mild abdominal pain may occur, especially in cases of abdominal pregnancy. Typically, the patient reports amenorrhea or abnormal menses (in cases of fallopian tube implantation), followed by slight vaginal bleeding and unilateral pelvic pain over the mass. During a vaginal examination, the patient may report extreme pain when the cervix is moved and the adnexa is palpated. The uterus feels boggy and is tender. The patient may complain of lower abdominal pain precipitated by activities that increase abdominal pressure, such as a bowel movement.

No time to waste

If the tube ruptures, the patient may complain of sharp lower abdominal pain, possibly radiating to the shoulders and neck. This condition is an emergency situation that requires immediate transport to a clinic or hospital.

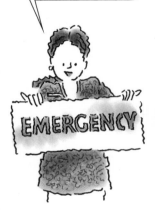

Complaints of sharp lower abdominal pain indicate tube rupture, a medical emergency!

What tests tell you

Differential diagnosis is necessary to rule out intrauterine pregnancy, ovarian cyst or tumor, pelvic inflammatory disease (PID), appendicitis, and spontaneous abortion. The following tests confirm ectopic pregnancy:
• Serum pregnancy test results show an abnormally low level of human chorionic gonadotropin (hCG) that remains lower than that in a normal intrauterine pregnancy when the test is repeated in 48 hours.
• Real-time ultrasonography performed after a positive serum pregnancy test detects intrauterine pregnancy or ovarian cyst.
• Culdocentesis (aspiration of fluid from the vaginal cul-de-sac) detects free blood in the peritoneum. This test is performed if ultrasonography detects the absence of a gestational sac in the uterus.
• Laparoscopy, performed if culdocentesis is positive, may reveal pregnancy outside the uterus.

How it's treated

If culdocentesis shows blood in the peritoneum, laparotomy and salpingectomy (excision of the fallopian tube) are indicated, possibly preceded by laparoscopy to remove the affected fallopian tube and control bleeding. Patients who wish to have children can undergo microsurgical repair of the fallopian tube. The ovary is saved, if possible; however, ovarian pregnancy requires oophorectomy. Interstitial pregnancy may require hysterectomy. Abdominal pregnancy requires a laparotomy to remove the fetus, except in rare cases, when the fetus survives to term or calcifies undetected in the abdominal cavity.

See ya, cells

Nonsurgical management of ectopic pregnancy involves oral administration of methotrexate (Folex), a chemotherapeutic drug and folic acid inhibitor that stops cell reproduction. The drug destroys remaining trophoblastic tissue, thus avoiding the need for laparotomy.

Support, in short

Supportive treatment includes whole blood or packed red blood cells (RBCs) to replace excessive blood loss, broad-spectrum I.V. antibiotics for sepsis, supplemental iron (either oral or I.M.), and a high-protein diet. Grief counseling for the loss of a child is also recommended.

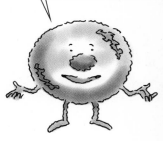

Methotrexate stops cell reproduction in ectopic pregnancy.

What to do

- Ask the patient the date of her last menses, and obtain serum hCG levels as ordered.
- Assess vital signs, and monitor vaginal bleeding for extent of fluid loss.
- Check the amount, color, and odor of vaginal bleeding; monitor perineal pad count.
- Withhold food and fluid orally in anticipation of possible surgery; prepare the patient for surgery as indicated.
- Assess for signs and symptoms of hypovolemic shock secondary to blood loss from tubal rupture. Monitor closely for decreased urine output, which suggests fluid volume deficit.
- Administer blood transfusions, as ordered, and provide emotional support.
- Record the location and character of the pain, and administer analgesics as ordered.
- Determine if the patient is Rh-negative. If she is, administer $Rh_0(D)$ immune globulin (human), also known as *RhoGAM*, as ordered after treatment or surgery.

- Provide a quiet, relaxing environment and encourage the patient and her partner to express their feelings of fear, loss, and grief. Help the patient to develop effective coping strategies.
- To prevent recurrent ectopic pregnancy from diseases of the fallopian tube, urge the patient to get prompt treatment of pelvic infections.
- Inform patients who have undergone surgery involving the fallopian tubes or those with confirmed PID that they're at increased risk for another ectopic pregnancy.
- Refer the patient to a grief counselor or support group.

Folic acid deficiency anemia

Folic acid deficiency anemia is a common, slowly progressive, megaloblastic (involving enlarged RBCs) form of anemia. Folic acid, or folacin, is a B vitamin needed for RBC formation and deoxyribonucleic acid (DNA) synthesis. It's also thought to play a role in preventing neural tube defects in the developing fetus.

Folic acid deficiency anemia is a risk factor in approximately 1% to 5% of pregnancies, becoming most apparent during the second trimester. It's believed to be a risk factor contributing to early spontaneous abortion and abruptio placentae.

Folic folly

Folic acid is found in most body tissues. It acts as a coenzyme in metabolic processes. Although its body stores are relatively small, folic acid can be found in most well-balanced diets. Even so, folic acid is water-soluble and is affected by heat, so it's easily destroyed by cooking. Moreover, about 20% of folic acid intake is excreted unabsorbed. Insufficient intake—typically less than 50 mcg/day—usually results in folic acid deficiency anemia within 4 months.

> There's plenty of folic acid in a well-balanced diet, but this important B vitamin is easily destroyed by cooking, and 20% is excreted unabsorbed.

What causes it

Alcohol abuse, which suppresses the metabolic effects of folic acid, is probably the most common cause of folic acid deficiency anemia. During pregnancy, folic acid deficiency anemia occurs most commonly in women with multiple pregnancy, probably because of the increased fetal demand for folic acid. Folic acid deficiency anemia is also seen in women who have underlying hemolytic illness that results in rapid destruction and production of RBCs. In addition, certain drugs—such as phenytoin (Dilantin), an anticonvulsant agent that interferes with folate absorption, and hormonal contraceptives—have a role in folic acid deficiency anemia.

What to look for

The main symptom of folic acid deficiency anemia is a history of severe, progressive fatigue. Associated findings include shortness of breath, palpitations, diarrhea, nausea, anorexia, headaches, forgetfulness, and irritability. The impaired oxygen-carrying capacity of the blood from lowered hemoglobin levels may produce complaints of weakness and light-headedness.

Assessment may reveal generalized pallor and jaundice. The patient may also appear wasted. Cheilosis (cracks in the corners of the mouth) and glossitis (inflammation of the tongue) may be present. Neurologic impairment is present only if the folic acid deficiency anemia is associated with a vitamin B_{12} deficiency.

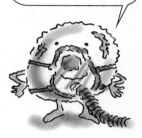

Got oxygen? In folic acid deficiency anemia, the blood's oxygen-carrying capacity is impaired. No wonder I feel light-headed!

What tests tell you

Typically, blood studies reveal:
- macrocytic RBCs
- decreased reticulocyte count
- increase mean corpuscular volume
- abnormal platelet count
- decreased serum folate levels (below 4 mg/ml).

How it's treated

During pregnancy, treatment consists primarily of folic acid supplements. Supplements may be given orally or parenterally (for patients who are severely ill, have malabsorption, or can't take oral medication). In addition, a diet high in folic acid is urged. Many patients respond favorably to a well-balanced diet.

Many patients with folic acid deficiency anemia respond favorably to a well-balanced diet.

What to do

- Strongly urge women trying to become pregnant to take a vitamin supplement or eat foods rich in folic acid. (See *Foods high in folic acid,* page 234.)
- Instruct the pregnant woman in the use of prescribed folic acid supplements and the need to continue taking them throughout pregnancy.

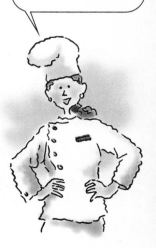

Education edge

Foods high in folic acid

If your patient is planning to become pregnant or is pregnant, encourage her to eat these foods high in folic acid to help prevent folic acid deficiency anemia:
- asparagus
- beef liver
- broccoli
- green leafy vegetables such as collards
- mushrooms
- oatmeal
- peanut butter
- red beans
- wheat germ
- whole wheat bread.

- Assist with planning a well-balanced diet that includes meals and snacks that are high in folic acid.
- Encourage the woman to eat or drink a rich source of vitamin C at each meal to enhance absorption of folic acid.
- Administer a folic acid supplement as ordered throughout pregnancy, and assess for patient compliance. (See *Vitamin use*.)
- If the patient has severe anemia and requires hospitalization, plan activities, rest periods, and diagnostic tests to conserve energy. Monitor pulse rate often; if tachycardia occurs, the patient's activities are too strenuous.
- Monitor the patient's complete blood count (CBC), platelet count, and serum folate levels as ordered.
- Assess maternal vital signs and FHR as indicated.

Gestational hypertension

Gestational hypertension, previously called *pregnancy-induced hypertension*, is a potentially life-threatening disorder that typically develops after 20 weeks' gestation. It occurs most commonly in nulliparous women. Currently, gestational hypertension and its complications are the most common cause of maternal and fetal death in developed countries.

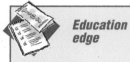

Education edge

Vitamin use

Prenatal vitamins are prescribed to prevent folic acid deficiency because over-the-counter (OTC) multivitamins generally don't contain adequate amounts of folic acid for pregnancy. Compliance may be an issue if the patient doesn't have the money to pay for the prescription supplements or lacks understanding of their role in preventing folic acid deficiency. Patients may substitute OTC vitamins, thinking they're just as effective as prescription vitamins. At prenatal visits, be sure to ask if the patient is taking her prescribed vitamins, and stress the importance of using prescription supplements during pregnancy.

To seize or not to seize

Gestational hypertension can be classified as preeclampsia or eclampsia. Preeclampsia, the nonconvulsive form of the disorder, is marked by the onset of hypertension after 20 weeks' gestation. It develops in about 7% of pregnancies and may be mild or severe. The incidence is significantly higher in patients from low socio-economic groups. Eclampsia, the convulsive form, occurs between 24 weeks' gestation and the end of the first postpartum week. The incidence increases among nulliparous women, women with multiple pregnancy, and women with a history of vascular disease.

About 5% of women with preeclampsia develop eclampsia; of these, about 15% die of eclampsia or its complications. The incidence of fetal mortality is high because of the increased incidence of premature delivery.

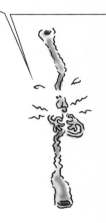

Preexisting vascular disease may contribute to gestational hypertension.

Complicating the situation

Generalized arteriolar vasoconstriction associated with gestational hypertension is thought to produce decreased blood flow through the placenta and maternal organs. This can result in intrauterine growth retardation (or restriction), placental infarcts, and abruptio placentae. Hemolysis, elevated liver enzyme levels, and a low platelet count (HELLP syndrome) are associated with severe preeclampsia. Other possible complications include stillbirth of the neonate, seizures, coma, premature labor, renal failure, and hepatic damage in the mother.

What causes it

Although the exact cause of gestational hypertension is unknown, systemic peripheral vasospasm occurs and affects every organ system. (See *Changes associated with gestational hypertension*, page 236.) Geographic, ethnic, racial, nutritional, immunologic, and familial factors may contribute to preexisting vascular disease that, in turn, may contribute to the disorder's occurrence. Age is also a factor; adolescents and primiparas older than age 35 are at higher risk for preeclampsia.

Other possible causes include potential toxic sources (such as autolysis of placental infarcts), autointoxication, uremia, maternal sensitization to total proteins, and pyelonephritis.

What to look for

The classic triad of symptoms in women with gestational hypertension is hypertension, proteinuria, and edema. A patient with mild preeclampsia typically reports a sudden weight gain of more

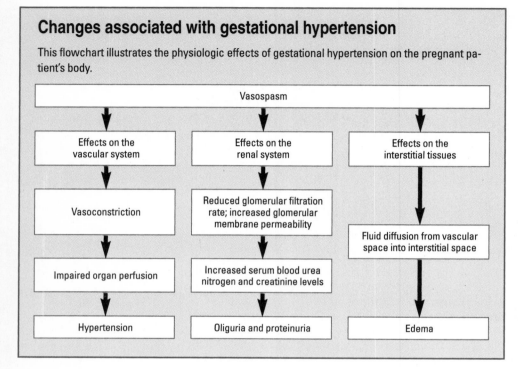

Changes associated with gestational hypertension

This flowchart illustrates the physiologic effects of gestational hypertension on the pregnant patient's body.

Vasospasm

Effects on the vascular system → Vasoconstriction → Impaired organ perfusion → Hypertension

Effects on the renal system → Reduced glomerular filtration rate; increased glomerular membrane permeability → Increased serum blood urea nitrogen and creatinine levels → Oliguria and proteinuria

Effects on the interstitial tissues → Fluid diffusion from vascular space into interstitial space → Edema

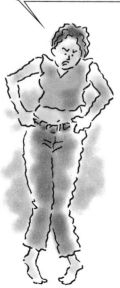

Sudden weight gain during the second or third trimester is a typical finding in a woman with gestational hypertension. So, what's my excuse?

than 3 lb (1.4 kg) per week in the second trimester or more than 1 lb (0.5 kg) per week during the third trimester. The patient's history reveals hypertension, as evidenced by high blood pressure readings (140 mm Hg or more systolic, or an increase of 30 mm Hg or more above the patient's normal systolic pressure, measured on two occasions, 6 hours apart; and 90 mm Hg or more diastolic, or an increase of 15 mm Hg or more above the patient's normal diastolic pressure, measured on two occasions, 6 hours apart). Further examination may reveal generalized edema, especially of the face. Palpation may reveal pitting edema of the legs and feet. Deep tendon reflexes may indicate hyperreflexia.

As preeclampsia worsens, the patient may demonstrate oliguria (urine output of 400 ml/day or less), blurred vision caused by retinal arteriolar spasms, epigastric pain or heartburn, irritability, and emotional tension. She may also complain of a severe frontal headache.

Pressure, spasm, hemorrhage—oh my!

In severe preeclampsia, blood pressure readings increase to 160/110 mm Hg or higher on two occasions, 6 hours apart, during bed rest. Ophthalmoscopic examination may reveal vascular spasm, papilledema, retinal edema or detachment, and arteriovenous nicking or hemorrhage.

Enter eclampsia

The onset of seizures signifies eclampsia. The patient with eclampsia may appear to cease breathing, then suddenly take a deep, gasping breath and resume breathing. The patient may then lapse into a coma, lasting a few minutes to several hours. When waking from the coma, the patient may have no memory of the seizure. Mild eclampsia may involve more than one seizure; severe eclampsia, up to 20 seizures.

Kicked up a notch

In eclampsia, physical examination findings are similar to those in preeclampsia, but more severe. Systolic blood pressure may increase to 180 mm Hg or even to 200 mm Hg. Marked edema may be present; some patients, however, don't show visible signs of edema.

What tests tell you

A differential diagnosis is used to distinguish the disorder from viral hepatitis, idiopathic thrombocytopenia, cholecystitis, hemolytic uremic syndrome, peptic ulcer, neuroangiopathic syndrome, appendicitis, renal calculi, pyelonephritis, and gastroenteritis. Laboratory test findings reveal proteinuria (more than 300 mg/24 hours [1+] with preeclampsia, and 5 g/24 hours [5+] or more with severe eclampsia). Test results may also suggest HELLP syndrome. Additionally, ultrasonography, stress and nonstress tests, and biophysical profiles are used to evaluate fetal well-being.

How it's treated

Adequate nutrition, good prenatal care, and control of preexisting hypertension during pregnancy help decrease the incidence and severity of preeclampsia. However, if preeclampsia does develop, early recognition and prompt treatment can prevent progression to eclampsia.

Suppress the progress

Therapy for patients with preeclampsia is intended to stop the disorder's progression and ensure fetal survival. Some practitioners advocate the prompt inducement of labor, especially if the patient is near term; others follow a more conservative approach. Therapy may include:

When it comes to preeclampsia, priority one is to stop its progression to ensure fetal survival.

- complete bed rest in the preferred left lateral recumbent position to enhance venous return
- administration of antihypertensive drugs, such as methyldopa (Aldomet) and hydralazine (Apresoline)
- administration of magnesium to promote diuresis, reduce blood pressure, and prevent seizures if blood pressure fails to respond to bed rest and antihypertensives (persistently rising above 160/100 mm Hg) or central nervous system irritability increases.

Plan B

If these measures fail to improve the patient's condition, or if fetal life is endangered (as determined by stress or nonstress tests and biophysical profiles), cesarean delivery or labor induction with Pitocin may be required. If the woman develops seizures, emergency treatment consists of immediate I.V. administration of magnesium, and oxygen therapy along with electronic fetal monitoring. After the patient's condition stabilizes, cesarean delivery may be indicated.

What to do

- Monitor the patient regularly for changes in blood pressure, pulse rate, respiratory rate, FHR, vision, level of consciousness, and deep tendon reflexes as well as headache unrelieved by medication. Report changes immediately. Assess these signs and symptoms before administering medications. (See *Emergency interventions for gestational hypertension.*)

Advice from the experts

Emergency interventions for gestational hypertension

When caring for a patient with gestational hypertension, be prepared to perform these nursing interventions.
- Observe for signs of fetal distress by closely monitoring the results of stress and nonstress tests.
- Keep emergency resuscitative equipment and anticonvulsant drugs readily available in case of seizures and cardiac or respiratory arrest.
- Maintain a patent airway and have oxygen readily available.
- Carefully monitor the I.V. infusion of magnesium sulfate, observing for signs and symptoms of toxicity, such as absence of patellar reflexes, flushing, muscle flaccidity, decreased urine output, a significant drop in blood pressure (more than 15 mm Hg), and respiratory rate less than 12 breaths/minute.
- Keep calcium gluconate readily available at the bedside to counteract the toxic effects of magnesium sulfate.
- Prepare for emergency cesarean delivery if indicated.
- Maintain seizure precautions to protect the patient from injury. Never leave an unstable patient unattended.

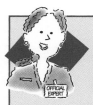

Advice from the experts

Administering magnesium sulfate safely

If your patient requires I.V. magnesium therapy, use caution when administering the drug because magnesium toxicity may occur. Follow these guidelines to ensure the patient's safety during administration.

• Always administer the drug as a piggyback infusion so that it can be discontinued immediately if the patient develops signs and symptoms of toxicity.

• Obtain a baseline serum magnesium level before initiating therapy and monitor levels frequently thereafter.

• Keep in mind that for I.V. magnesium to be effective as an anticonvulsant, serum magnesium levels should be between 5 and 8 mg/dl. Levels above 8 mg/dl indicate toxicity and place the patient at risk for respiratory depression, cardiac arrhythmias, and cardiac arrest.

• Assess the patient's patellar reflex. If the patient has received epidural anesthesia, test the biceps or triceps reflex. Diminished or hypoactive reflexes suggest magnesium toxicity.

• Assess for ankle clonus (alternating contractions and relaxations of the muscles) by rapidly dorsiflexing the patient's ankle three times, then removing your hand and observing the foot's movement. If no further motion is noted, ankle clonus is absent; if the foot continues to move involuntarily, clonus is present. Moderate (three to five movements) or severe (six or more movements) suggests possible magnesium toxicity.

• Have calcium gluconate readily available at the patient's bedside. Anticipate administering this antidote for I.V. magnesium.

• If the woman is receiving I.V. magnesium sulfate, administer the loading dose over 15 to 30 minutes and then maintain the infusion at a rate of 1 to 2 g/hour. (See *Administering magnesium sulfate safely*.)

• Monitor the extent and location of edema. Elevate affected extremities to promote venous return. Avoid constricting pantyhose, slippers, and bed linens.

• Assess fluid balance by measuring intake and output and checking daily weight. Insert an indwelling urinary catheter, if necessary, to provide a more accurate measurement of output.

• Provide a quiet, darkened room, limit visitation by friends and family members until the patient's condition stabilizes, and enforce complete bed rest.

• Provide emotional support for the patient and her family. Encourage them to verbalize their feelings. If the patient's condition requires preterm delivery, point out that infants of mothers with gestational hypertension are usually small for gestational age but sometimes fare better than other premature infants of the same weight, possibly because they have developed adaptive responses to stress in utero.

• Encourage the patient to eat a well-balanced, high-protein diet; limit high-sodium foods, include high-fiber foods, and

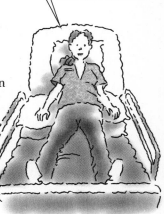

Patients with gestational hypertension should avoid constricting bed linens, so keep 'em loose!

drink at least eight 8-oz glasses of noncaffeinated beverages each day.

• Teach the patient to report signs and symptoms that indicate worsening gestational hypertension, which include headache, vision disturbances (blurring, flashes of light, "spots" before the eyes), GI symptoms (nausea, pain), worsening edema (especially of the face and fingers), and a noticeable decrease in urine output.

• Teach the woman the importance of keeping her prenatal appointments, which will be more frequent because she has gestational hypertension.

• Help the patient and her family develop effective coping strategies.

• Prepare to administer betamethasone I.M. as indicated.

Gestational trophoblastic disease

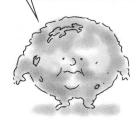

As trophoblast cells deteriorate, they fill with fluid. I'm pretty full already!

Gestational trophoblastic disease, also called *hydatidiform mole* or *molar pregnancy*, is the rapid deterioration of trophoblastic villi cells. Trophoblast cells are located in the outer ring of the blastocyst (the structure that develops around the third or fourth day after fertilization) and eventually become part of the structure that forms the placenta and fetal membranes. As trophoblast cells begin to deteriorate, they fill with fluid. The cells become edematous, appearing as grapelike clusters of vesicles. As a result of these cell abnormalities, the embryo fails to develop past the early stages.

Leading to bleeding

Gestational trophoblastic disease is a major cause of second trimester bleeding. It's also associated with choriocarcinoma (a fast-growing, highly invasive malignant tumor that develops in the uterus), which is why early detection is important.

All or some

Chromosomal analysis helps classify gestational trophoblastic disease as a complete or partial mole. A complete mole is characterized by swelling and cystic formation of all trophoblastic cells. No fetal blood is present. If an embryo does develop, it's most likely only 1 to 2 mm in size and will probably die early in development. This form is associated with the development of choriocarcinoma.

A partial mole is characterized by edema of some of the trophoblastic villi with some of the normal villi. Fetal blood may be present in the villi, and an embryo up to the size of 9 weeks' gestation may be present. Typically, a partial mole has 69 chromosomes in which there are 3 chromosomes for every one pair.

Hard to recognize

Gestational trophoblastic disease is reported to occur in about 1 in every 2,000 pregnancies. Recent research indicates that the incidence would be much higher if all cases of the disorder were identified. Some cases aren't recognized because the pregnancy is aborted early and the products of conception aren't available for analysis. The incidence is higher in women from low socioeconomic groups, older women, and multiparous women. The incidence is highest in Asian women, especially those from Southeast Asia.

What causes it

The cause of gestational trophoblastic disease is unknown. Several unconfirmed theories relate gestational trophoblastic disease to chromosomal abnormalities, hormonal imbalances, or deficiencies in protein and folic acid. About one-half of patients with choriocarcinoma have had a preceding molar pregnancy. In the remaining patients, the disease is usually preceded by a spontaneous or induced abortion, an ectopic pregnancy, or a normal pregnancy.

What to look for

A patient with gestational trophoblastic disease may report vaginal bleeding, ranging from brownish red spotting to bright red hemorrhage. She may report passing tissue that resembles grape clusters. Her history may also include hyperemesis, lower abdominal cramps (such as those that accompany spontaneous abortion), and signs and symptoms of preeclampsia.

On inspection, a uterus that's exceptionally large for the patient's gestational date is detected. Vaginal examination may reveal grapelike vesicles in the vagina. Palpation may detect ovarian enlargement caused by cysts. Auscultation of the uterus may reveal the absence of fetal heart tones that had been noted at a previous visit.

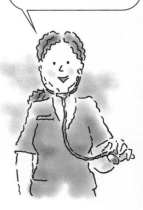

Hmmm...an exceptionally large uterus, presence of grapelike vesicles, and absence of fetal heart tones. Sounds like gestational trophoblastic disease.

What tests tell you

Differential diagnosis is necessary to rule out normal pregnancy, imminent spontaneous abortion, uterine leiomyomas, multiple pregnancy, and incorrect gestational date. These diagnostic test results suggest the presence of gestational trophoblastic disease:

• Radioimmunoassay detects extremely elevated hCG levels for early pregnancy.
• Histologic examination confirms the presence of vesicles.
• Ultrasonography performed after the third month shows grape-like clusters instead of a fetus.
• Amniography (a procedure that introduces a water-soluble dye into the uterus) reveals the absence of a fetus. (This test is done only when the diagnosis is in question.)
• Doppler ultrasonography shows the absence of fetal heart tones.
• Hemoglobin level and hematocrit, RBC count, prothrombin time, partial thromboplastin time, fibrinogen levels, and hepatic and renal function findings are abnormal.
• White blood cell (WBC) count and erythrocyte sedimentation rate (ESR) are increased.

How it's treated

Gestational trophoblastic disease necessitates uterine evacuation by dilatation and suction curettage. Labor induction with oxytocin (Pitocin) or prostaglandins is contraindicated because of the increased risk of hemorrhage.

Postoperative treatment varies, depending on the amount of blood lost and complications. If no complications develop, hospitalization is usually brief and normal activities can be resumed quickly as tolerated.

Monitoring for malignancy

Because of the possibility that choriocarcinoma will develop following gestational trophoblastic disease, scrupulous follow-up care is essential. Such care includes monitoring hCG levels weekly until titers are negative for 3 consecutive weeks, then monthly for 6 months, then every 2 months for the next 6 months.

Follow-up also includes monthly chest X-rays to check for lung metastasis until hCG titers are negative. Chest X-rays are then obtained once every 2 months for 1 year. Contraceptive methods are used to prevent another pregnancy until at least 1 year after all titers and X-ray findings are negative.

Ounce of prevention

Prophylactic chemotherapy with methotrexate or actinomycin-D (Cosmegen) after evacuation of the uterus has been successful in preventing malignant gestational trophoblastic disease. Chemotherapy and irradiation are used for metastatic choriocarcinoma.

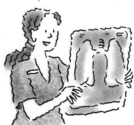

There's no sign of lung metastasis and hCG titers are negative. This patient hasn't developed choriocarcinoma.

What to do

• Assess the patient's vital signs to obtain a baseline for future comparison.
• Preoperatively, observe for signs of complications, such as hemorrhage and uterine infection, and vaginal passage of vesicles. Save any expelled tissue for laboratory analysis.
• Prepare the patient for surgery.
• Postoperatively monitor vital signs and fluid intake and output, and check for signs of hemorrhage.
• Encourage the patient and her family to express their feelings about the disorder. Offer emotional support and help them through the grieving process.
• Help the patient and her family develop effective coping strategies. Refer them to a mental health professional for additional grief and loss counseling if needed.
• Assist with obtaining baseline information—including a pelvic examination, chest X-ray, and serum hCG levels—and with ongoing monitoring. (See *Monitoring hCG levels.*)
• Stress the need for regular monitoring (hCG levels and chest X-rays) to detect malignant changes.
• Instruct the patient to report new symptoms promptly (for example, hemoptysis, cough, suspected pregnancy, nausea, vomiting, and vaginal bleeding).
• Explain to the patient that she must use contraceptives to prevent pregnancy for at least 1 year after hCG levels return to normal and her body reestablishes regular ovulation and menstrual cycles.

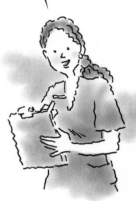

Explain to the patient the importance of reporting new symptoms promptly.

Monitoring hCG levels

When evaluating serum human chorionic gonadotropin (hCG) levels in a woman previously diagnosed with gestational trophoblastic disease, gradually declining levels suggest no further disease. However, if hCG levels plateau three times or increase at any time during the monitoring period, suspect the development of a malignancy.

HELLP syndrome

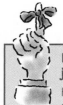
HELLP is an acronym that stands for **h**emolysis, **e**levated **l**iver enzymes, and **l**ow **p**latelets. HELLP syndrome is a category of gestational hypertension that involves changes in blood components and liver function.

Temporary HELLP

HELLP syndrome develops in 12% of women with gestational hypertension. It can occur in primigravidas and multigravidas. When it occurs, maternal and infant mortality is high; approximately one-fourth of women and one-third of infants die from this disorder. However, after birth, laboratory results return to normal—usually within 1 week—and the mother experiences no further problems.

What causes it

Although the exact cause of HELLP is unknown, theories have been proposed about the development of its signs and symptoms. Hemolysis is believed to result because RBCs are damaged by their travel through small, impaired blood vessels. Elevated liver enzymes are believed to result from obstruction in liver flow by fibrin deposits. Low platelets are believed to be the result of vascular damage secondary to vasospasm. Women with severe preeclampsia are at high risk for developing HELLP syndrome.

What to look for

Typically, the patient complains of pain, most commonly in the right upper quadrant, epigastric area, or lower chest. Additional signs and symptoms include nausea, vomiting, general malaise, and severe edema. The right upper quadrant may be tender on palpation because of a distended liver. In addition, the woman exhibits signs and symptoms of preeclampsia.

What tests tell you

Laboratory studies reveal:
• hemolysis of RBCs (appearing fragmented and irregular on a peripheral blood smear)
• thrombocytopenia (a platelet count below 100,000/mm^3)
• elevated levels of alanine aminotransferase and serum aspartate aminotransferase.

How it's treated

Treatment involves intensive care management for the woman and her fetus. Drug therapy, such as with magnesium sulfate, is instituted to reduce blood pressure and prevent seizures. Transfusions of fresh frozen plasma or platelets may be used to reverse thrombocytopenia. Delivery of the fetus may occur vaginally or by cesarean birth and generally resolves the condition.

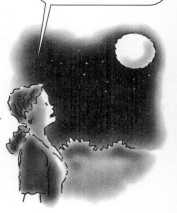

A quiet, dimly lit environment with limited visitors reduces the risk of seizures.

What to do

• Assess maternal vital signs and FHR frequently; be alert for signs and symptoms of complications, including hemorrhage, hypoglycemia, hyponatremia, subcapsular liver hematoma, and renal failure.
• Maintain a quiet, calm, dimly lit environment to reduce the risk of seizures; limit visitation.
• Avoid palpating the abdomen because this increases intra-abdominal pressure, which could lead to rupture of a subcapsular liver hematoma.
• Institute bleeding precautions, and monitor the patient for signs and symptoms of bleeding. Administer blood transfusions and medications as ordered.
• If the patient develops hypoglycemia, expect to administer I.V. dextrose solutions.
• Prepare the patient for delivery; explain all events and procedures being done; assist with evaluations for fetal maturity.
• Be aware that because of the increased risk of bleeding due to thrombocytopenia the woman may not be a candidate for epidural anesthesia.
• Assess the patient carefully throughout labor and delivery for possible hemorrhage.

HIV infection

HIV is the organism that causes acquired immunodeficiency syndrome (AIDS). Considered a sexually transmitted disease (STD), HIV infection can have serious implications for a pregnant woman and her fetus.

Women on the rise

Currently, women are the fastest growing segment of the population infected with HIV. Research also shows that women are diagnosed with HIV infection later in the course of the disease than men are. HIV infection and AIDS are considered the third leading cause of death in women between ages 25 and 45. Approximately 2 out of every 100 women giving birth are HIV-positive.

Don't lose hope

Nevertheless, studies demonstrate that pregnancy doesn't accelerate progression of the infection in the mother. In addition, women who stay healthy during pregnancy reduce the risk of transmitting the virus to the fetus because the placenta provides a barrier to disease transmission. Even so, if HIV is contracted concurrently or close to the time of conception or the mother suffers from disorders that affect placental health (such as infections unrelated to HIV or complications of advanced HIV infection [malnutrition]), the placenta may not be an effective barrier.

Suspending transmission

Before advances in drug therapy, the risk of a neonate becoming infected via maternal virus transmission ranged from 25% to 35%. However, with appropriate antiviral drug therapy during and after pregnancy, the rate of possible infection has dropped to nearly 5%. Unfortunately, if infection occurs in the fetus or neonate, it progresses more quickly than in an adult.

What causes it

HIV infection is caused by a retrovirus that targets helper T-cells containing the CD4+ antigen (cells that regulate normal immune response). The virus integrates itself into the cells' genetic make-up, causing cellular dysfunction that disrupts immune response. This makes patients vulnerable to opportunistic infections.

HIV is transmitted in several ways:
- through sexual intercourse
- through contact with infected blood
- across the placenta to the fetus during pregnancy (in cases of active disease, medication noncompliance, and placental inflammation)
- through contact during labor and delivery
- through breast milk.

For women, heterosexual contact and use of injectable drugs are the two major modes of HIV transmission. Other risk factors for contracting HIV include:
- a history of multiple sexual partners (either in the patient or her partner)
- having bisexual partners
- use of injectable drugs by the patient's partner
- blood transfusions (rare).

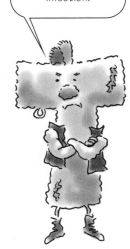

I'm a target for the retrovirus that causes HIV infection.

What to look for

Signs and symptoms of HIV infection include lymphadenopathy, bacterial pneumonia, fevers, night sweats, weight loss, dermatologic problems, thrush, thrombocytopenia, and diarrhea. In addition, women commonly experience severe vaginal yeast infections that are difficult to treat.

Other manifestations specific to women may include:
- abnormal Papanicolaou tests
- frequent human papilloma virus infections
- frequent and recurrent bacterial vaginosis, trichomonas, and genital herpes infections
- severe PID.

Pneumocystis carinii pneumonia is the most common opportunistic infection associated with female HIV infection. Cervical cancer ranks second in prevalence. Kaposi's sarcoma may also occur in women, although it's rare.

What tests tell you

In some cases, a woman doesn't know that she's HIV-positive until it's discovered at a prenatal visit, after pregnancy has begun. Positive results from two enzyme-linked immunosorbent assays that are then further confirmed by the Western Blot test classify a woman as HIV-positive. Positive status means that the woman has developed antibodies to the virus after having been exposed. In addition, a CD4+ T-cell count of less than 200 cells/µl and the presence of one or more opportunistic infections confirm the diagnosis.

Load up on viral load

Viral load testing measures the level of HIV in the blood. Although blood levels don't reflect all possible areas of HIV infection, research suggests that these levels effectively demonstrate virus levels throughout the body. This testing relies on the detection of ribonucleic acid (RNA) in HIV molecules. This RNA is responsible for replication of the virus. Scientists have a good idea of what some parts of HIV RNA look like. With this image, they can find HIV RNA in the blood of a potentially infected person. Two techniques are used to detect HIV RNA strands in a blood sample:

Branched-chain DNA sets off a chemical reaction in the HIV RNA; the RNA gives off light and the amount of light is measured to determine the levels of HIV RNA in a sample.

The quantitative polymerase chain reaction technique encourages the HIV RNA to replicate in a test tube. This replica-

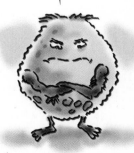

Viral load measures HIV levels in the bloodstream, which effectively indicates levels throughout the body.

tion makes it easier to measure the amount of HIV RNA that was originally in the blood sample.

How it's treated

The Centers for Disease Control and Prevention recommend treating the pregnant woman who's HIV-positive with combination antiretroviral therapy. This treatment is aimed at reducing the mother's viral load and minimizing the risk of transmitting the infection to the fetus.

Risky delivery

Cesarean delivery provides the lowest risk of HIV transmission from mother to fetus—lowest if performed before labor begins or membranes are ruptured (usually at 37 weeks' gestation). If vaginal delivery is unavoidable, episiotomy is contraindicated as is amniocentesis and fetal monitoring via scalp electrodes. For every hour of labor after membranes rupture, the risk of transmission from mother to fetus increases by 2%.

When breast isn't best

Risk of transmission during breast-feeding depends on the mother's health, including her nutritional and immune status and viral load, as well as the length of time the child nurses at each feeding and whether the mother breast-feeds exclusively. In addition, the duration of breast-feeding impacts the likelihood of transmission. About 15% of infected mothers who breast-feed for 24 months or longer transmit the infection to their neonates.

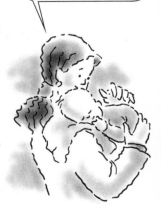

Mothers with HIV who breast-feed increase the risk of transmission to their infants.

Shutting the door on opportunity

Zidovudine (AZT) and didanosine (Videx) are used to slow progression of opportunistic infections such as *P. carinii* pneumonia, the most common. These drugs are given orally during pregnancy, I.V. during labor, and then to the neonate in syrup form. Co-trimoxazole (Bactrim) is also used but may be teratogenic in early pregnancy. Additionally, sulfamethoxazole (Gantanol) may cause increased bilirubin levels in the neonate if administered late in pregnancy.

What to do

• Provide emotional support and guidance for the woman who's HIV-positive and considering pregnancy.
• Institute standard precautions when caring for the mother throughout the pregnancy, after delivery, and when caring for the neonate.

- Teach the pregnant woman measures to minimize the risk of virus transmission.
- Allow the pregnant woman who's HIV-positive to verbalize her feelings; provide support.
- Monitor CD4+ T-cell counts and viral loads as indicated.
- Assess the patient for signs and symptoms of opportunistic infections, such as *P. carinii* pneumonia (fever, dry cough, chest discomfort, fatigue, shortness of breath on exertion and later at rest) and Kaposi's sarcoma (slightly raised, painless lesions on the skin or oral mucous membranes that are reddish or purple in fair-skinned patients and bluish or brown in dark-skinned patients; painful swelling, especially in the lower legs; nausea, vomiting, and bleeding if the GI tract is involved; difficulty breathing if the lungs are involved).
- Encourage the patient to keep prenatal follow-up appointments to evaluate the status of her pregnancy.
- Administer antiretroviral therapy as ordered, and instruct the patient about this regimen. Assist with scheduling medications and evaluate for compliance on return visits.
- Institute measures during labor and delivery to minimize the fetus's risk of exposure to maternal blood or body fluids. Avoid the use of internal fetal monitors, scalp blood sampling, forceps, and vacuum extraction to prevent the creation of an open lesion on the fetal scalp.
- Advise the mother that breast-feeding isn't recommended because of the risk of transmitting the virus.
- Delay blood sampling and injections in the neonate until maternal blood has been removed with the first bath.
- Educate the mother about the mode of HIV transmission and safer sex practices.

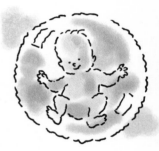

Special precautions must be taken during pregnancy to reduce my risk of contracting HIV.

Hyperemesis gravidarum

Unlike the transient nausea and vomiting that's normally experienced until about the 12th week of pregnancy, hyperemesis gravidarum is severe and unremitting nausea and vomiting that persists after the first trimester. It usually occurs with the first pregnancy and commonly affects women with conditions that produce high levels of hCG, such as gestational trophoblastic disease or multiple pregnancy.

This disorder occurs in about 7 out of 1,000 pregnancies in Blacks and in about 16 out of 1,000 pregnancies in Whites. The prognosis is usually good. However, if untreated, hyperemesis gravidarum produces substantial weight loss, starvation with ketosis and acetonuria, dehydration with subsequent fluid and electrolyte imbalance (hypokalemia), and acid-base disturbances (acidosis and alkalosis). Retinal, neurologic, and renal damage may also occur.

What causes it

The specific cause of hyperemesis gravidarum is unknown. Possible causes include pancreatitis (elevated serum amylase levels are common), biliary tract disease, decreased secretion of free hydrochloric acid in the stomach, decreased gastric motility, drug toxicity, inflammatory obstructive bowel disease, and vitamin deficiency (especially B_6). In some patients, this disorder may be related to psychological factors.

What to look for

The patient typically complains of unremitting nausea and vomiting. The vomitus initially contains undigested food, mucus, and small amounts of bile. Later, it contains only bile and mucus. Finally, the vomitus includes blood and material that resembles coffee grounds.

Enough is enough!

The patient may report thirst, hiccups, oliguria, vertigo, and headache as well as substantial weight loss and eventual emaciation caused by persistent vomiting. She may appear confused or delirious. Lassitude, stupor and, possibly, coma may occur. Additional findings may include:
• pale, dry, waxy and, possibly, jaundiced skin with decreased skin turgor
• dry, coated tongue
• subnormal or elevated temperature
• rapid pulse
• fetid, fruity breath (from acidosis).

> Unremitting nausea and vomiting should be enough! But there's more— headache, weight loss, vertigo, lassitude, and so on, and so on... Stop me any time!

What tests tell you

Diagnostic tests are used to rule out other disorders, such as gastroenteritis, cholecystitis, peptic ulcer, and pancreatic or liver disorders, which produce similar clinical effects. Differential diagnosis also rules out gestational trophoblastic disease, hepatitis, inner ear infection, food poisoning, emotional problems, and eating disorders.

Urine test results show ketonuria and slight proteinuria. The following results of serum analysis support a diagnosis of hyperemesis gravidarum:

- decreased protein, chloride, sodium, and potassium levels
- increased blood urea nitrogen levels
- elevated hemoglobin levels
- elevated WBC count.

How it's treated

The patient with hyperemesis gravidarum may require hospitalization to correct electrolyte imbalances and prevent starvation. I.V. infusions are used to maintain nutrition until the patient can tolerate oral feedings.

Infuse while you snooze—and snack

An infusion of 3,000 ml of I.V. fluid over 24 hours will usually cause a reduction in symptoms. Oral fluids and food are usually withheld until there's no vomiting for 24 hours, after which clear liquids can be initiated. Metoclopramide (Reglan) or ondansetron (Zofran) may be administered to control vomiting. This infusion can be performed at the mother's home in the presence of a visiting nurse. The patient progresses slowly to a clear liquid diet, then a full liquid diet and, finally, small, frequent meals of high-protein solid foods. A midnight snack helps stabilize blood glucose levels. Parenteral vitamin supplements and potassium replacements are used to help correct deficiencies.

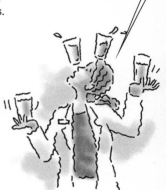

When a patient with hyperemesis gravidarum can tolerate oral feedings, she'll start with a clear liquid diet.

Easy does it

If persistent vomiting jeopardizes the patient's health, antiemetic medications may be prescribed. Note, however, that no drug has been approved by the FDA for the treatment of nausea and vomiting during pregnancy. Therefore, any antiemetic must be prescribed with caution and the benefits must outweigh the risks to the patient and her fetus. Meclizine (Antivert) and diphenhydramine (Benadryl) may be prescribed. More commonly, however, a continuous I.V. infusion of Reglan is administered through a portable I.V. pump worn under the patient's clothes. The latter treatment is highly successful.

After vomiting stops and the patient's electrolyte balance has been restored, the pregnancy usually continues without recurrence of hyperemesis gravidarum. Most patients feel better as they begin to regain normal weight, but some continue to vomit throughout the pregnancy, requiring extended treatment and total parenteral nutrition. If appropriate, some patients may benefit from consultations with clinical nurse specialists, psychologists, or psychiatrists.

What to do

- Administer I.V. fluids as ordered until the patient can tolerate oral feedings.
- Monitor fluid intake and output, vital signs, skin turgor, daily weight, serum electrolyte levels, and urine for ketones; anticipate the need for electrolyte replacement therapy.
- Provide frequent mouth care.
- Consult a dietitian to provide a diet high in dry, complex carbohydrates. Suggest decreased liquid intake during meals. Provide company and encourage diversionary conversation at mealtime.
- Instruct the patient to remain upright for 45 minutes after eating to decrease reflux.
- Suggest that the patient eat two or three dry crackers before getting out of bed in the morning to alleviate nausea.
- Provide reassurance and a calm, restful atmosphere. Encourage the patient to discuss her feelings about her pregnancy and the disorder.
- Help the patient develop effective coping strategies. Refer her to a mental health professional for additional counseling if necessary (hyperemisis may be an extreme response to psychosocial problems). Refer her to the social service department for help in caring for other children at home if appropriate.
- Teach the patient protective measures to conserve energy and promote rest. Include relaxation techniques, fresh air and moderate exercise (if tolerated), and activities scheduled appropriately to prevent fatigue.

Iron deficiency anemia

Iron deficiency anemia is a disorder in which hemoglobin synthesis is deficient and the body's capacity to transport oxygen is impaired. A common disease worldwide, iron deficiency anemia affects 10% to 30% of the adult population of the United States. It's the most common anemia during pregnancy, affecting up to one-fourth of all pregnancies. Iron deficiency anemia during pregnancy is associated with low fetal birth weight and preterm birth.

What causes it

During pregnancy, maternal iron stores are used for fetal RBC production, thus causing an iron deficiency in the mother. In addition, many women have deficient iron stores when they enter pregnancy because of factors such as a diet low in iron (inadequate intake), heavy menses (blood loss), or misguided weight-reduction

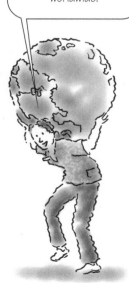

Iron deficiency anemia is common worldwide.

programs. Iron stores also tend to be low in women who have fewer than 2 years between pregnancies and in those from low socioeconomic communities. Other possible causes of iron deficiency anemia include:

- iron malabsorption
- intravascular hemolysis–induced hemoglobinuria or paroxysmal nocturnal hemoglobinuria
- mechanical trauma to RBCs caused by a prosthetic heart valve or vena caval filter.

No iron, no hemoglobin, no oxygen

Iron deficiency anemia is considered a microcytic, hypochromic anemia, meaning that inadequate iron intake results in smaller RBCs that contain less hemoglobin. Cells that aren't as large and rich in hemoglobin as they should be affect the proper transport of oxygen.

> Adequate iron intake helps me grow rich with hemoglobin so I can properly transport oxygen.

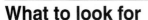

What to look for

Typically, the signs and symptoms exhibited by a pregnant woman with iron deficiency anemia are the same as those for any patient with this disorder. They tend to develop gradually and may include fatigue, listlessness, pallor, and exercise intolerance. Some women develop pica (eating of substances such as ice or starch) in response to the body's need for increased nutrients. If the anemia is severe or prolonged, other signs and symptoms may include:

- dyspnea on exertion
- inability to concentrate
- susceptibility to infection
- tachycardia
- coarsely ridged, spoon-shaped, brittle, thin nails
- sore, red, burning tongue
- sore, dry skin in the corners of the mouth.

What tests tell you

Diagnosis of iron deficiency anemia must not precede exclusion of other causes of anemia, such as thalassemia minor, cancer, and chronic inflammatory, hepatic, or renal disease. Blood studies (serum iron, total iron-binding capacity, ferritin levels) and assessment of iron stores in bone marrow may confirm iron deficiency anemia. However, the results of these tests can be misleading because of complicating factors, such as infection, blood transfusion, or use of iron supplements. Characteristic blood test results for women include:

- low hemoglobin (less than 10 g/dl)

- low hematocrit (less than 33%)
- low serum iron (less than 30 mcg/dl) with high binding capacity (greater than 400 mcg/dl)
- low serum ferritin (less than 100 mg/dl)
- low RBC count with microcytic and hypochromic cells (in early stages, RBC count may be normal)
- decreased mean corpuscular hemoglobin (less than 30 g/dl) in severe anemia
- depleted or absent iron stores (identified by specific staining) and hyperplasia of normal precursor cells (identified by bone marrow studies).

How it's treated

Preventing iron deficiency anemia with prescription prenatal vitamins is the primary goal. However, if iron deficiency anemia does develop, an iron supplement (such as ferrous sulfate or ferrous gluconate) is prescribed. Additionally, patients should be advised to eat a well-balanced diet that includes foods high in vitamins and iron.

I.V. Fe

If the woman's anemia is severe or she can't comply with the prescribed oral therapy, parenteral iron may be prescribed. Because total-dose I.V. infusion of supplemental iron is painless and requires fewer injections, it's usually preferred to I.M. administration. In pregnant patients with severe anemia, total-dose infusion of iron dextran in normal saline solution is given over 1 to 8 hours. A test dose of 0.5 ml I.V. is given first to help minimize the risk of allergic reaction.

What to do

- Instruct the patient to use prenatal vitamins as prescribed.
- If the patient is hospitalized, administer oral iron with an acid, such as orange juice, to enhance absorption; for outpatients, advise women to take prescribed iron supplements with orange juice or a vitamin C supplement.
- Monitor the patient's CBC and serum iron and ferritin levels regularly.
- Assess the family's dietary habits for iron intake, noting the influence of childhood eating patterns, cultural food preferences, and family income on adequate nutrition.
- Monitor the woman's vital signs, especially heart rate, noting tachycardia, which suggests that her activities are too strenuous.
- Evaluate for signs and symptoms of decreased perfusion to vital organs (such as dyspnea, chest pain, and dizziness) and symptoms of neuropathy (such as tingling in the extremities).

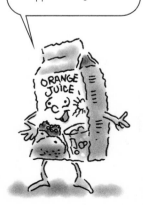

Just a glass full of OJ helps the iron supplement go down!

- Assess FHR at each visit; if the patient is hospitalized, monitor FHR at least every 4 hours.
- Provide frequent rest periods to decrease physical exhaustion. Assist the patient with planning activities so that she has sufficient rest between them.
- If the anemia is severe, expect to administer oxygen, as ordered, to help prevent and reduce hypoxia.
- Administer iron supplements as ordered. Use the Z-track injection method when administering iron I.M. to prevent skin discoloration, scarring, and irritating iron deposits in the skin. (See *Z-track injection for iron.*)

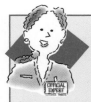

Advice from the experts

Z-track injection for iron

When administering iron using the I.M. route, use the Z-track injection method to displace the skin. This technique blocks the needle pathway after an injection, thereby preventing discomfort and tissue irritation secondary to drug leakage into subcutaneous tissue. To perform a Z-track injection, follow these steps.

- Place your finger on the skin surface, and pull the skin and subcutaneous layers out of alignment with the underlying muscle. You should move the skin approximately ½" (1 cm).

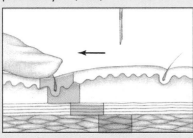

- Insert the needle at a 90-degree angle at the site where you initially placed your finger.

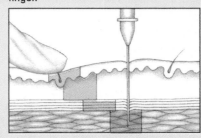

- Aspirate for blood return; if none appears, inject the drug slowly.
- Wait 10 seconds and then withdraw the needle slowly.

- Remove your finger from the skin surface, letting the layers return to normal, thus sealing the needle track. The needle track (as shown by the dotted line in the illustration below) is now broken at the junction of each tissue layer, trapping the drug in the muscle.

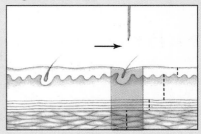

- Don't massage the site or allow the patient to wear a tight-fitting garment over the site because doing so could force medication into the subcutaneous tissue.
- Encourage the patient to walk or move about in bed to facilitate drug absorption from the injection site.

Education edge

Teaching topics on iron supplements

Be sure to cover the following topics when teaching your pregnant patient about iron supplements.
• Reinforcement of the practitioner's explanation of the anemia
• Prescribed treatments and possible complications
• Need for continuing therapy—even if the patient feels better—because replacement of iron stores takes time
• Foods that interfere with absorption, such as milk and antacids
• Foods that enhance absorption, such as citrus juices and foods containing vitamin C
• Administration guidelines, including using a straw when taking the liquid form to prevent staining the teeth, and taking iron on an empty stomach (if possible) with a vitamin C-rich food or with food if gastric irritation occurs
• Need to report adverse effects of iron therapy, such as nausea, vomiting, diarrhea, and constipation (dosage adjustment or supplemental stool softeners may be necessary)
• Change in stool appearance
• Components of a nutritionally balanced diet, including red meats, green vegetables, eggs, whole wheat, iron-fortified bread, and milk
• Intake of high-fiber foods to prevent constipation
• Infection prevention measures
• Need to report signs and symptoms of infection, such as fever and chills
• Need for regular checkups and compliance with prescribed treatments

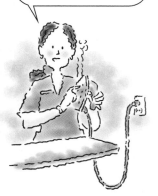

It takes time to restock the iron stores. That's why patients should be encouraged to stick with their treatment, even when they're feeling better.

• If the patient receives iron I.V., monitor the infusion rate carefully. Stop the infusion and begin supportive treatment immediately if the patient shows signs of an allergic reaction. Also, watch for dizziness and headache and for thrombophlebitis around the I.V. site.
• Assist with planning a well-balanced diet with an increased intake of foods high in vitamins and iron. Consult a nutrition therapist as indicated.
• Provide patient teaching about therapy. (See *Teaching topics on iron supplements*.) Offer suggestions for intake of high-fiber foods to prevent possible constipation from iron therapy; also warn the patient that the medication may cause stools to appear black and tarry.

Isoimmunization

Isoimmunization, also called *Rh incompatibility*, refers to a condition in which the pregnant woman is Rh-negative but her fetus is Rh-positive. This condition, if left untreated, can lead to hemolytic disease in the neonate. Isoimmunization develops in about 7% of all pregnancies in the United States. Before the development of RhoGAM, this condition was a major cause of kernicterus (nerve cell deterioration) and neonatal death.

What causes it

During her first pregnancy, an Rh-negative woman may become sensitized to Rh antigens by:
• being exposed to Rh-positive fetal blood antigens inherited from the father
• receiving alien Rh antigens from a blood transfusion, causing agglutinins (antibodies in the patient's blood) to develop
• receiving inadequate doses of $Rh_o(D)$ or failing to receive $Rh_o(D)$ after significant fetal-maternal leakage from abruptio placentae.

Subsequent pregnancy with an Rh-positive fetus provokes increasing amounts of maternal agglutinating antibodies to cross the placental barrier, attach to Rh-positive cells in the fetus, and cause hemolysis and anemia. To compensate for this, the fetus steps up the production of RBCs, and erythroblasts (immature RBCs) appear in the fetal circulation. Extensive hemolysis results in the release of large amounts of unconjugated bilirubin, which the liver can't conjugate and excrete, causing hyperbilirubinemia and hemolytic anemia. (See *Pathogenesis of Rh isoimmunization,* page 258.)

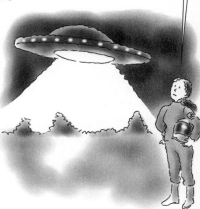

> Alien Rh antigens from a blood transfusion may sensitize an Rh-negative woman to Rh antigens during her first pregnancy. It's a close encounter of the Rh kind!

What to look for

Typically, the pregnant woman doesn't exhibit signs or symptoms of this disorder. The fetus—and subsequently the neonate—are affected.

What tests tell you

At the first prenatal visit, an anti-D antibody titer should be performed on all women with Rh-negative blood. If the results are normal (titer is 0) or the titer is minimal (a ratio below 1:8), the test will be repeated at week 28. No therapy is needed at this time.

A sensitive situation

An anti-D antibody titer of 1:16 or greater indicates Rh sensitization. Titer monitoring continues every 2 weeks for the remainder of the pregnancy.

Pathogenesis of Rh isoimmunization

Rh isoimmunization progresses throughout pregnancies in Rh-negative mothers who give birth to Rh-positive neonates. The illustrations below outline the process of isoimmunization.

A non-pregnant woman has Rh-negative blood.	She becomes pregnant with an Rh-positive fetus. Normal antibodies appear.	Placental separation occurs.	After delivery, the mother develops anti–Rh-positive antibodies.	With the next Rh-positive fetus, antibodies enter fetal circulation, causing hemolysis.

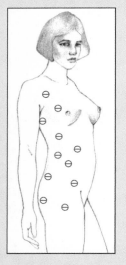 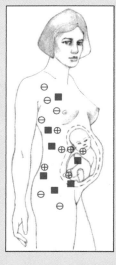 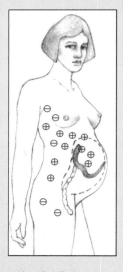 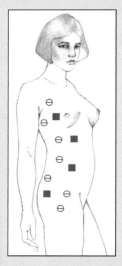 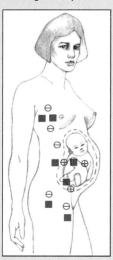

⊖ Rh– blood   ⊕ Rh+ blood   ■ Normal antibodies

Amniocentesis is performed to evaluate the status of the fetus. During amniocentesis, the fluid density of the amniotic fluid is determined using spectrophotometry. The results are plotted on a graph and correlated with gestational age to determine the extent of involvement and the amount of bilirubin present. Amniotic fluid analysis may show increased bilirubin levels (indicating possible hemolysis) and increased anti-Rh titers.

Radiologic studies may show edema and, in those with hydrops fetalis (edema of the fetus), the halo sign (edematous, elevated subcutaneous fat layers).

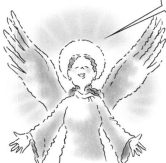

Believe me, I'm no angel! The halo sign refers to edematous, elevated subcutaneous fat layers from hydrops fetalis.

How it's treated

Treatment focuses on preventing Rh isoimmunization by administering RhoGAM to any unsensitized Rh-negative woman as soon as possible after the birth of an Rh-positive neonate or after spontaneous or elective abortion. In addition, screening for Rh isoimmunization or irregular antibodies is indicated for the following patients:
• Rh-negative women during their first prenatal visit and at 24, 28, 32, and 36 weeks' gestation
• Rh-positive women with a history of transfusion, a neonate with jaundice, stillbirth, cesarean birth, induced abortion, placenta previa, or abruptio placentae.

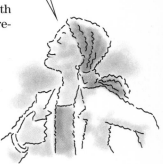

I'm positive that RhoGAM should be administered to an unsensitized Rh-negative woman as soon as possible after delivery of an Rh-positive neonate.

Towering titer

If the pregnant woman's Rh antibody titer is high, she may be given high doses of gamma globulin to help reduce fetal involvement; the goal is to interfere with the rapid destruction of fetal RBCs. The fetus may receive a blood transfusion in utero via an injection of RBCs directly into a vessel in the fetal cord or instillation in the fetal abdomen via amniocentesis. After birth, the neonate may receive an exchange transfusion to remove hemolyzed RBCs and replace them with healthy blood cells.

Bilirubin levels in amniotic fluid are monitored for early delivery intervention or intrauterine fetal transfusion if needed. Repeated transfusions may be needed in the neonate.

What to do

• Assess all pregnant women for possible Rh incompatibility.
• Expect to administer RhoGAM I.M., as ordered, to Rh-negative women at 28 weeks' gestation and after transfusion reaction, ectopic pregnancy, spontaneous or induced abortion, or during the second and third trimesters to patients with abruptio placentae, placentae previa, or amniocentesis. (See *Administering RhoGAM*, page 260.)
• Assist with intrauterine transfusion as indicated; before intrauterine transfusion, obtain a baseline FHR through electronic monitoring and explain the procedure and its purpose to the patient. Afterward, carefully observe the mother for uterine contractions and fluid leakage from the puncture site. Monitor FHR for tachycardia or bradycardia.
• Prepare the woman for a planned delivery, usually 2 to 4 weeks before term date depending on maternal history, serologic tests, and amniocentesis.

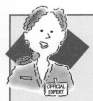

Advice from the experts

Administering RhoGAM

$Rh_o(D)$ immune globulin (human), also known as *RhoGAM,* is a concentrated solution of immune globulin containing $Rh_o(D)$ antibodies. I.M. injection of RhoGAM keeps the Rh-negative mother from producing active antibody responses and forming anti-$Rh_o(D)$ to Rh-positive fetal blood cells and endangering future Rh-positive fetuses.

RhoGAM is administered to an Rh-negative mother after abortion, ectopic pregnancy, delivery of a neonate with $Rh_o(D)$-positive blood and cord blood that's direct Coombs' negative, accidental transfusion of Rh-positive blood, amniocentesis, abruptio placentae, or abdominal trauma. It's given within 72 hours to prevent future maternal sensitization. Administration at approximately 28 weeks' gestation can also protect the fetus of an Rh-negative mother.

RhoGAM is given I.M. into the gluteal site. When administering RhoGAM, the same steps are followed as for any I.M. injection. However, be sure to include these steps:
• Check the vial's identification numbers with another nurse, and sign the triplicate form that comes with the RhoGAM.
• Attach the top copy to the patient's chart.
• Send the remaining two copies, along with the empty RhoGAM vial, to the laboratory or blood bank.
• Give the woman a card indicating her Rh-negative status, and instruct her to carry it with her or keep it in a convenient location.

• Assist with labor induction, if indicated, from 34 to 38 weeks' gestation. During labor, monitor the fetus electronically; obtain capillary blood scalp sampling to determine acid-base balance. An indication of fetal distress necessitates immediate cesarean delivery.
• Administer RhoGAM within 72 hours of delivery to prevent complications in subsequent pregnancies.
• Provide emotional support to the patient and her family; encourage them to express their fears concerning possible complications of treatment.

Multiple pregnancy

Multiple pregnancy, or *multiple gestation*, refers to a pregnancy involving more than one fetus. It's considered a complication of pregnancy because the woman's body must adjust to the effects of carrying multiple fetuses.

Baby boom

The increased use of fertility drugs has lead to a more than 50% rise in the incidence of multiple pregnancy. For example, births of triplets (or more) is 100 times more common now than in 1978. about 68,000 sets of twins—monozygotic (identical) or dizygotic

Types of twins

There are two types of twins: monozygotic and dizygotic.

Monozygotic

Monozygotic (identical) twins begin with one ovum and one spermatozoan. In the process of fusion, or in one of the first cell divisions, the zygote divides into two identical individuals. Single-ovum twins usually have one placenta, one chorion, two amnions, and two umbilical cords. The twins are always the same sex.

Dizygotic

Dizygotic, (fraternal) twins are the result of the fertilization of two separate ova by two separate spermatozoa. Double-ova twins have two placentas, two chorions, two amnions, and two umbilical cords. The twins may be of the same or different sex.

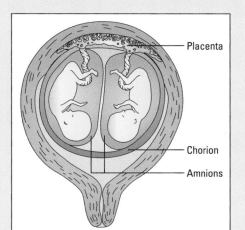

Placenta

Chorion

Amnions

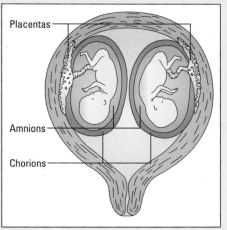

Placentas

Amnions

Chorions

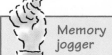

Memory jogger

To remember the difference between monozygotic (identical) and dizygotic (fraternal) twins, picture the "i" in "identical" as the Roman numeral one (I). One egg fertilized by one spermatozoan makes an Identical twin.

(fraternal)—were born in 1978; this increased to about 104,000 in 1997. (See *Types of twins.*)

Multiple pregnancies may be single-ovum conceptions (monozygotic twins) or multiple-ova conceptions (dizygotic twins and greater). Naturally occurring multiple pregnancies are more common in nonwhites than in Whites. The higher a woman's parity and age, the more likely she is to have a multiple pregnancy. Inheritance, based on the mother's family pattern, also appears to play a role in natural dizygotic twinning.

Double, triple, or quadruple the risks

The risks of such complications as gestational hypertension, hydramnios, placenta previa, preterm labor, and anemia are higher in women with multiple pregnancy. Additionally, postpartum bleeding is more common because the uterus is stretched more.

Multiple pregnancies also tend to end before normal term, meaning that the fetuses are at risk for premature birth.

It's a twin thing

With twins, the risk of congenital anomalies, such as spinal cord defect, is higher. The incidence of velamatous cord insertion (the cord inserted into the fetal membranes) is also higher and increases the risk of bleeding during delivery due to a torn cord. With monozygotic twins, fetuses share the placenta, which may lead to a condition known as twin-to-twin transfusion. In this condition, one fetus overgrows while the other undergrows. Additionally, if a single amnion is present, the umbilical cords can become knotted or twisted, leading to fetal distress or difficulty with birth.

Best to be first

In addition, the second fetus (twin B) is at more risk for birth-related complications, such as umbilical cord prolapse, malpresentation, and abruptio placentae.

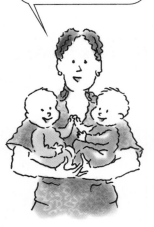

The risk of congenital anomalies is higher with twins than with single births.

What causes it

Multiple pregnancy is the result of the fertilization of one ova forming one zygote that divides into two identical zygotes, or the simultaneous fertilization of two or more ova. The increasing use of fertility drugs has led to a rise in the number of multiple pregnancies because these drugs stimulate the ovaries to release multiple ova to increase chances of fertilization.

What to look for

When the uterus begins to grow at a rate faster than usual, a multiple pregnancy is suspected. In addition, the woman may report that with quickening she feels fluttering actions at different areas of her abdomen rather than at one specific and consistent spot. She also may report an increased amount of fetal activity than expected for the date. Auscultation may reveal multiple sets of fetal heart sounds.

The woman may report an increase in fatigue and backache. Resting or sleeping may be difficult because of the increased discomfort and fetal activity level. Appetite and intake may decrease because the enlarging uterus is compressing her stomach.

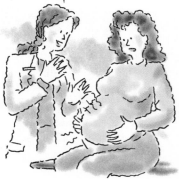

If you're experiencing this much fetal activity at this stage of your pregnancy, you may be expecting more than one baby!

What tests tell you

Diagnostic test results that help determine multiple pregnancy may include:
- elevated AFP levels
- evidence of multiple gestational sacs on ultrasound and, possibly, evidence of multiple amniotic sacs early in pregnancy.

A multiple gestation pregnancy puts the patient at risk for preterm labor and PROM.

How it's treated

Multiple gestation pregnancies put the mother at risk for developing many complications of pregnancy, such as preterm labor, intrauterine growth retardation, PROM, gestational hypertension, and abruptio placentae. Treatment centers on complications that may arise. In addition, the patient may be ordered to go on complete bed rest for a period of her pregnancy to prevent such complications as preterm labor. Depending on the number of fetuses, their gestational age, and their position, the manner of delivery will vary. Vaginal delivery is possible for a mature twin gestation at term when both twins are in the head down, or *vertex*, position. If the first, or *presenting*, twin is vertex and the second is breech, it's possible to proceed with a vaginal birth; however, because this situation is more complicated, a cesarean delivery would most probably be the method of choice.

What to do

Other than more frequent monitoring, nursing care for the woman with multiple pregnancy is similar to that for any pregnancy.
- Help the woman understand her current condition and stress the need for close, frequent follow-up visits.
- Encourage frequent rest periods throughout the day to help relieve fatigue.
- Urge the woman to rest in the side-lying position to prevent supine hypotension syndrome.
- Monitor maternal vital signs, weight gain, and fundal height at every visit.
- Assess FHR and position at every visit.
- Arrange for follow-up testing, such as ultrasounds and non-stress-test monitoring, as well as 24-hour fetal monitoring if the patient is on complete bed rest for the third trimester of her pregnancy.

• Urge the woman to comply with her prenatal vitamin regimen and to eat a well-balanced diet high in vitamins and iron.
• Explain danger signs and symptoms to report immediately, especially those related to preterm labor.
• Provide emotional support to the woman and her family; allow the pregnant woman to verbalize her fears and anxieties about the pregnancy and fetuses. Correct any misconceptions that the woman verbalizes.
• During labor, provide separate electronic fetal monitoring for each fetus.
• Maintain the patient in the side-lying position to aid breathing during labor.
• Be alert for hypotonic labor, which might necessitate labor augmentation or cesarean delivery.
• At delivery, have all medication readily accessible for each neonate.
• During delivery, make sure that one nurse is available for each neonate and one for the mother; in most cases, an anesthesiologist and a pediatrician or a neonatal nurse practitioner should be present in anticipation of maternal or neonatal problems.

Placenta previa

Placenta previa occurs when the placenta implants in the lower uterine segment, obstructing the internal cervical os and failing to provide as much nourishment as implantation in the fundus would supply. The placenta tends to spread out, seeking the blood supply it needs, and it becomes larger and thinner than normal. Hemorrhage occurs as the internal cervical os effaces and dilates, tearing the uterine vessels. One of the most common causes of bleeding during the second half of pregnancy, this disorder occurs in about 1 in 200 pregnancies and more commonly in multigravidas than primigravidas. If the patient has heavy bleeding and is then diagnosed with placenta previa, the pregnancy may be terminated.

It's a cover-up!

The placenta may cover all or part of the internal cervical os, or it may gradually overlap the os as the cervix dilates. Complete obstruction is known as *total, complete,* or *central placenta previa.* Partial obstruction is known as *incomplete* or *partial placenta previa.* When a small placental edge is felt through the maternal os, the placenta previa is referred to as *low marginal.* (See *Three types of placenta previa.*) Obstruction that occurs as the cervix dilates is caused by marginal implantation or a low-lying placenta.

Three types of placenta previa

There are three basic types of placenta previa: low marginal, partial, and complete.

Low marginal
In low-marginal placenta previa, a small placental edge can be felt through the maternal os.

Partial
In partial placenta previa, the placenta partially caps the internal os.

Complete
In complete placenta previa, the placenta completely covers the internal os.

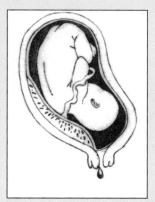 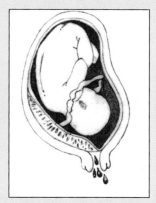 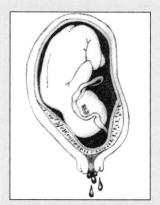

The apparent degree of placenta previa may depend largely on the extent of cervical dilation at the time of examination. Maternal prognosis is good if hemorrhage can be controlled. Fetal prognosis depends on gestational age and the amount of blood lost.

What causes it

The specific cause of placenta previa is unknown. Factors that may affect the site of the placenta's attachment to the uterine wall include:
- defective vascularization of the decidua
- multiple pregnancy (the placenta requires a larger surface for attachment)
- previous uterine surgery
- multiparity
- advanced maternal age.

What to look for

Typically, a patient with placenta previa reports the onset of painless, bright red vaginal bleeding after the 20th week of pregnancy.

Such bleeding, beginning before the onset of labor, tends to be episodic; it starts without warning, stops spontaneously, and resumes later.

About 7% of patients with placenta previa are asymptomatic. In these women, ultrasound examination reveals the disorder incidentally.

Palpation may reveal a soft, nontender uterus. Abdominal examination using Leopold's maneuvers reveals various malpresentations because the placenta's abnormal location has interfered with descent of the fetal head. Minimal descent of the fetal presenting part may indicate placenta previa. The fetus remains active, however, with good heart tones audible on auscultation.

What tests tell you

A differential diagnosis is necessary to exclude genital lacerations, excessive bloody show, abruptio placentae, and cervical lesions. Laboratory studies may reveal decreased maternal hemoglobin levels (due to blood loss).

Ultrasound is most sound

Transvaginal ultrasonography is used to determine placental position. Radiologic tests, such as femoral arteriography, retrograde catheterization, or radioisotope scanning or localization, may be done to locate the placenta. However, these tests have limited value, are risky, and are usually performed only when ultrasound is unavailable.

Cesarean-ready

Pelvic examination should be performed only in a surgical suite or a birthing room that's equipped for cesarean birth in the event that hemorrhage necessitates immediate delivery.

How it's treated

Treatment of placenta previa focuses on assessing, controlling, and restoring blood loss; delivering a viable neonate; and preventing coagulation disorders. Immediate therapy includes:
• starting an I.V. infusion using a large-bore catheter
• drawing blood for hemoglobin levels, hematocrit, typing, and crossmatching
• initiating external electronic fetal monitoring
• monitoring maternal blood pressure, pulse rate, and respirations
• assessing the amount of vaginal bleeding.

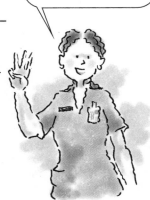

Treatment of placenta previa focuses on controlling and restoring blood loss, delivering the neonate, and preventing coagulation disorders.

When the bun's not done

If the fetus is premature (following determination of the degree of placenta previa and necessary fluid and blood replacement), treatment consists of careful observation to allow the fetus more time to mature. If clinical evaluation confirms complete placenta previa, the patient is usually hospitalized because of the increased risk of hemorrhage. As soon as the fetus is sufficiently mature, or in cases of severe hemorrhage, immediate cesarean delivery may be necessary. Vaginal delivery is considered only when the bleeding is minimal and the placenta previa is marginal, or when the labor is rapid.

Have hands on hand

Because of possible fetal blood loss through the placenta, a pediatric team should be on hand during such a delivery to immediately assess and treat neonatal shock, blood loss, and hypoxia.

What to do

• If the patient with placenta previa shows active bleeding, continuously monitor her blood pressure, pulse rate, respirations, CVP, intake and output, and amount of vaginal bleeding in the fetus; continuously monitor the FHR and rhythm.
• Anticipate the need for electronic fetal monitoring, and assist with application as indicated.
• Have oxygen readily available in case fetal distress occurs. (Many facilities will administer oxygen continuously in labor and delivery to increase the amount of oxygen delivered to the fetus.) Evidence of fetal distress includes bradycardia, tachycardia, or late or variable decelerations.
• If the patient is Rh-negative, administer RhoGAM after every bleeding episode.
• Institute complete bed rest.
• Prepare the patient and her family for a possible cesarean delivery and the birth of a preterm neonate. Thoroughly explain postpartum care so the patient and her family know which measures to expect.
• If the fetus isn't mature, expect to administer an initial dose of betamethasone (Celestone) I.M. to aid in promoting fetal lung maturity. Explain that additional doses may be given again in 24 hours and, possibly, 1 to 2 weeks.
• Provide emotional support during labor. Because of the fetus's prematurity, the patient may not be given analgesics, so labor pain may be intense. Reassure her of her

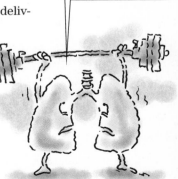

I.M. betamethasone will help me grow big and strong.

progress throughout labor, and keep her informed of the fetus's condition.
• If the patient's bleeding ceases and she's to return home on bed rest, anticipate the need for a referral for home care.
• Assess for signs of infection (fever, chills). The patient is at increased risk for infection because of the proximity of vaginal organisms to the placenta and the susceptibility of the placental environment to the growth of microorganisms.
• Teach the patient to identify and report signs of placenta previa (bleeding, cramping) immediately.
• During the postpartum period, monitor the patient for signs of hemorrhage and shock caused by the uterus's diminished ability to contract.
• Tactfully discuss the possibility of neonatal death. Tell the mother that the neonate's survival depends primarily on gestational age, the amount of blood lost, and associated hypertensive disorders. Assure her that frequent monitoring and prompt management greatly reduce the risk of death.
• Encourage the patient and her family to verbalize their feelings, and help them develop effective coping strategies. Refer them for counseling if necessary.

Premature labor

Premature labor, also known as *preterm labor,* is the onset of rhythmic uterine contractions that produce cervical changes after fetal viability but before fetal maturity. It usually occurs between weeks 20 and 37 of gestation. Between 5% and 10% of pregnancies end prematurely; about 75% of neonatal deaths result from premature labor.

Weighing in

Fetal prognosis depends on birth weight and length of gestation. Fetuses born before 26 weeks' gestation and weighing less than 737 g (1 lb, 10 oz) have a survival rate of about 10%. Fetuses born at 27 to 28 weeks' gestation and weighing between 737 g (1 lb, 10 oz) and 992 g (2 lb, 3 oz) have a survival rate of more than 50%. Those born after 28 weeks' gestation and weighing 992 g (2 lb, 3 oz to 2 lb) to 1,219 g (2 lb, 11 oz) have a 70% to 90% survival rate.

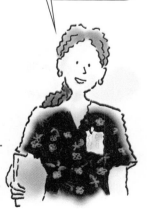

In premature labor, fetal prognosis depends on birth weight and length of gestation.

What causes it

Causes of premature labor include PROM (in 30% to 50% of cases), gestational hypertension, chronic hypertensive vascular disease, hydramnios, multiple pregnancy, placenta previa, abruptio placentae, incompetent cervix, abdominal surgery, trauma, structural anomalies of the uterus, infections (such as group B streptococci), and fetal death.

What to look for

The patient reports the onset of rhythmic uterine contractions, possible rupture of membranes, passage of the cervical mucus plug, and a bloody discharge. Her history indicates that she's in week 20 to 37 of pregnancy. Vaginal examination shows cervical effacement and dilation.

What tests tell you

Premature labor is confirmed by the combined results of prenatal history, physical examination, presenting signs and symptoms, and ultrasonography (if available), showing the position of the fetus in relation to the mother's pelvis.

How it's treated

Treatment is designed to suppress preterm labor when tests show immature fetal pulmonary development, cervical dilation of less than 4 cm, and the absence of factors that contraindicate continuation of pregnancy. Such treatment consists of bed rest and, when necessary, tocolytic drug therapy.

> Steps to prevent premature labor begin with good prenatal care, nutrition, and proper rest.

Prevention first

Taking steps to prevent premature labor is important. This requires good prenatal care, adequate nutrition, and proper rest. Inserting a purse-string suture (cerclage) to reinforce an incompetent cervix at 14 to 18 weeks' gestation may prevent premature labor in a patient with a history of incompetent cervix.

In some patients, premature labor is prevented with at-home tocolytic drug therapy (either orally or through an I.V. infusion pump). Women at risk who are treated at home can have their contractions monitored via telephone hookup.

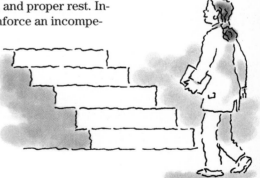

Slow to a stop

Several types of drug therapy may be used to stop the patient's contractions. Magnesium sulfate is typically the first drug of choice. It acts as a central nervous system (CNS) depressant, resulting in the slowing and cessation of contractions. A beta-adrenergic agent such as terbutaline (Brethine) is used to stimulate beta-2 receptors, thus inhibiting the contractility of uterine smooth muscle. Brethine is the most widely used drug for tocolysis.

Indomethacin (Indocin), a prostaglandin synthesis inhibitor, may be given, but its use has been associated with premature closure of ductus arteriosus if given after 34 weeks' gestation.

Weighing the risks

Sometimes preterm delivery is the lesser risk if maternal factors, such as intrauterine infection, abruptio placentae, placental insufficiency, and severe preeclampsia, jeopardize the fetus. Fetal problems, particularly isoimmunization and congenital anomalies, can become more perilous as pregnancy nears term and may require preterm delivery.

Treatment and delivery require intensive team effort. The fetus's health requires continuous assessment through fetal monitoring.

Close at hand

Ideally, treatment of active premature labor should take place in a perinatal intensive care center, where the staff is specially trained to handle this situation. In such settings, the neonate can remain close to his parents. (Community hospitals commonly lack the facilities for special neonatal care and transfer the neonate alone to a perinatal center.)

Sedatives and narcotics, which may harm the fetus, shouldn't be used. Although morphine (Duramorph) and meperidine (Demerol) have little effect on uterine contractions, they depress CNS function and may cause fetal respiratory depression; therefore, they should be administered in the smallest doses possible and only when absolutely necessary.

Amniotomy (rupture of the amniotic fluid membranes) is avoided, if possible, to prevent cord prolapse or damage to the fetus's tender skull. Adequate hydration is maintained with I.V. fluids.

What to do

• Closely observe the patient in premature labor for signs of fetal or maternal distress and provide comprehensive supportive care.

Advice from the experts

Administering terbutaline

I.V. terbutaline (Brethine) may be ordered for a woman in premature labor. When administering this drug, follow these steps.

• Obtain baseline maternal vital signs, fetal heart rate (FHR), and laboratory studies, including hematocrit, and serum glucose and electrolyte levels.

• Institute external monitoring of uterine contractions and FHR.

• Prepare the drug with lactated Ringer's solution instead of dextrose in water to prevent additional glucose load and hyperglycemia.

• Administer the drug as an I.V. piggyback infusion into a main I.V. solution so that the drug can be discontinued immediately if adverse effects occur.

• Use microdrip tubing and an infusion pump to ensure an accurate flow rate.

• Expect to adjust the infusion flow rate every 10 minutes until contractions cease or adverse effects become problematic.

• Monitor maternal vital signs every 15 minutes while the infusion rate is increased and every 30 minutes thereafter until contractions cease; monitor FHR every 15 to 30 minutes.

• Auscultate breath sounds for evidence of crackles or changes; be alert for complaints of dyspnea and chest pain.

• Monitor for maternal pulse rate greater than 120 beats/minute, blood pressure less than 90/60 mm Hg, or persistent tachycardia or tachypnea, chest pain, dyspnea, or abnormal breath sounds, which may indicate developing pulmonary edema. Notify the practitioner immediately.

• Watch for fetal tachycardia or late or variable decelerations in FHR pattern because these could indicate possible uterine bleeding or fetal distress necessitating emergency birth.

• Monitor intake and output closely, every hour during the infusion and every 4 hours thereafter.

• Expect to continue the infusion for 12 to 24 hours after contractions have ceased. Administer the first dose of oral therapy 30 minutes before discontinuing the I.V. infusion.

• Teach the patient how to take the oral Brethine, and stress the importance of continuing therapy until 37 weeks' gestation or fetal lung maturity has been confirmed by amniocentesis. Alternatively, if the patient is prescribed subcutaneous terbutaline therapy via a continuous pump, teach her how to use the pump.

• Teach the woman how to measure her pulse rate before each dose of oral terbutaline, or at the recommended times with subcutaneous therapy; instruct the patient to call the practitioner if her pulse rate is over 120 beats/minute or if she experiences palpitations or extreme nervousness.

• Make sure the patient maintains bed rest during attempts to suppress premature labor.

• Administer medications as ordered. (See *Administering terbutaline.*)

• Give sedatives and analgesics sparingly because they may be harmful to the fetus. Minimize the need for these drugs by provid-

ing comfort measures, such as frequent repositioning and good perineal and back care.
• Monitor blood pressure, pulse rate, respirations, FHR, and uterine contraction pattern when administering a beta-adrenergic stimulant, sedative, or narcotic. Minimize adverse reactions by keeping the patient in a side-lying position as much as possible to ensure adequate placental perfusion.
• Administer fluids as ordered to ensure adequate hydration.
• Assess deep tendon reflexes frequently when administering magnesium sulfate. Monitor the neonate for signs of magnesium toxicity, including neuromuscular and respiratory depression.
• During active premature labor, remember that the preterm fetus has a lower tolerance for the stress of labor and is more likely to become hypoxic than a full-term fetus. If necessary, administer oxygen to the patient through a nasal cannula. Encourage the patient to lie on her left side or sit up during labor; this position prevents vena caval compression, which can cause supine hypotension and subsequent fetal hypoxia.
• Observe fetal response to labor through continuous monitoring. Prevent maternal hyperventilation; use a rebreathing bag as necessary. Continually reassure the patient throughout labor to help reduce her anxiety.
• Prepare to administer I.M. betamethasone as indicated.
• Help the patient proceed through labor with as little analgesia and anesthesia as possible. To minimize fetal CNS depression, avoid administering an analgesic when delivery seems imminent. Monitor fetal and maternal response to local and regional anesthetics.
• Anticipate that the patient may have an extended hospitalization if the neonate is delivered before 34 weeks' gestation.

Premature rupture of membranes

PROM is a spontaneous break or tear in the amniotic sac before onset of regular contractions. It results in progressive cervical dilation. This common abnormality of parturition occurs in nearly 10% of all pregnancies longer than 20 weeks' gestation; more than 80% of neonates are mature. Labor usually starts within 24 hours.

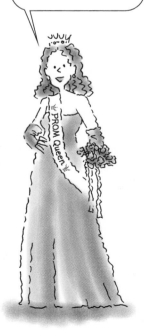

You definitely don't want an invitation to this PROM! It stands for premature rupture of membranes.

In labor limbo

The latent period (between membrane rupture and labor onset) is generally brief when membranes rupture near term. When the neonate is premature, the latent period is prolonged, which increases the risk of mortality from maternal infection (amnionitis, endometritis), fetal infection (pneumonia, septicemia), and prematurity.

If membranes rupture when the fetus isn't near term, the neonate is then at increased risk for mortality from maternal infection (amnionitis, endometritis), fetal infection (pneumonia, septicemia), and prematurity.

Mom's PROM problems

Maternal complications associated with PROM include:
- endometritis
- amnionitis
- septic shock and death if amnionitis goes untreated.

Baby's PROM predicament

Neonatal complications of PROM include:
- increased risk of respiratory distress syndrome
- asphyxia
- pulmonary hypoplasia
- congenital anomalies
- malpresentation
- cord prolapse
- severe fetal distress that can result in neonatal death.

What causes it

Although the cause of PROM is unknown, malpresentation and a contracted pelvis commonly accompany the rupture.

Usual suspects

Predisposing factors include:
- lack of proper prenatal care
- poor nutrition and hygiene
- smoking
- incompetent cervix
- increased intrauterine tension from hydramnios or multiple gestation
- reduced amniotic membrane tensile strength
- uterine infection.

What to look for

Typically, PROM causes blood-tinged amniotic fluid containing vernix caseosa particles to gush or leak from the vagina. Maternal fever, fetal tachycardia, and foul-smelling vaginal discharge indicate infection.

What tests tell you

Differential diagnosis is used to exclude urinary incontinence or vaginal infection as the underlying cause. Passage of amniotic fluid confirms the rupture. Slight fundal pressure or Valsalva's maneuver may expel fluid through the cervical os. Physical examination is performed to determine if multiple pregnancy is involved. Abdominal palpation (Leopold's maneuvers) determines fetal presentation and size. Patient history and physical examination findings determine gestational age.

Diagnosis of PROM is confirmed by the following test results:

- Alkaline pH of fluid collected from the posterior fornix turns Nitrazine paper deep blue. (The presence of blood can give a false-positive result.) Staining the fluid with Nile blue sulfate reveals two categories of cell bodies. Blue-stained bodies represent sheath fetal epithelial cells; orange-stained bodies originate in sebaceous glands. Incidence of prematurity is low when more than 20% of cells stain orange.
- If fluid is amniotic, a smear of the fluid placed on a slide and allowed to dry takes on a fernlike pattern (because of the high sodium and protein content of amniotic fluid). Verification of amniotic fluid leakage confirms PROM.
- Vaginal probe ultrasonography allows visualization of the amniotic sac to detect tears or ruptures.

Blood-tinged amniotic fluid is a sure sign of PROM.

How it's treated

Treatment of PROM depends on fetal age and the risk of infection. In a term pregnancy, if spontaneous labor and vaginal delivery don't result within a relatively short time (usually within 24 hours after the membranes rupture), induction of labor with oxytocin usually follows; then, if induction fails, cesarean delivery is performed. Cesarean hysterectomy may be recommended with gross uterine infection.

Heed the signs

Management of a preterm pregnancy of less than 34 weeks is controversial. Treatment of preterm pregnancy between 28 and 34 weeks includes hospitalization and observation for signs of infection (such as maternal leukocytosis or fever and fetal tachycardia) while the fetus matures.

Suspect infect? Induce to reduce

If the presence of infection is suspected, baseline cultures and sensitivity tests are appropriate. If these tests confirm infection, labor must be induced, followed by I.V. administration of an antibiotic. A culture of gastric aspirate or a swabbing from the neonate's ear may also be done, as antibiotic therapy may be indicated for him as well. During such a delivery, resuscitative equipment must be readily available to manage neonatal distress.

What to do

- Prepare the patient for a vaginal examination. Before physically examining a patient who's suspected of having PROM, explain all diagnostic tests and clarify any misunderstandings she may have.
- During the exam, stay with the patient and offer reassurance.
- Provide sterile gloves and sterile lubricating jelly. Don't use iodophor antiseptic solution because it discolors Nitrazine paper and makes pH determination impossible.
- After the examination, provide proper perineal care.
- Send fluid specimens to the laboratory promptly because bacteriologic studies require immediate evaluation.
- Anticipate administering prophylactic antibiotics to the woman who's positive for streptococcal B infection to reduce the risk of this infection in the neonate.
- If labor starts, observe the contractions and monitor vital signs every 2 hours.
- Watch for signs and symptoms of maternal infection (fever, abdominal tenderness, changes in amniotic fluid such as purulence and foul odor) and fetal tachycardia. Fetal tachycardia may precede maternal fever. Report such signs and symptoms immediately.
- Perform patient teaching. (See *Teaching about PROM.*)
- Encourage the patient and her family to express their feelings and concerns related to the fetus's health and survival.
- Tell the patient to record fetal kick counts and to report fewer than 10 kicks in a 12-hour period. A decrease in fetal kick counts may indicate fetal distress.
- Tell the patient to report uterine contractions, reduced fetal activity, or signs of infection (fever, chills, foul-smelling discharge).

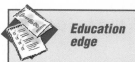

Education edge

Teaching about PROM

Here are some guidelines to follow when teaching a patient about premature rupture of membranes (PROM).

- Inform the patient about PROM, including its signs and symptoms, during the early stages of pregnancy.
- Make sure the patient understands that amniotic fluid doesn't always gush; it sometimes leaks slowly in PROM.
- Stress the importance of immediately reporting PROM (prompt treatment may prevent dangerous infection).
- Warn the patient not to engage in sexual intercourse, douche, or take a tub bath after her membranes rupture.
- Advise the patient to refrain from orgasm and breast stimulation after rupture of membranes, which can stimulate uterine contractions.
- Tell the patient to report to the practitioner a temperature above 100.4° F (38° C), which may indicate the onset of infection.

Sexually transmitted diseases

STDs are those conditions spread through sexual contact with an infected partner. Although all STDs can be serious, certain STDs place the pregnant woman at greater risk for problems because of their potential effect on the pregnancy, fetus, or neonate. (See *Selected STDs and pregnancy*.)

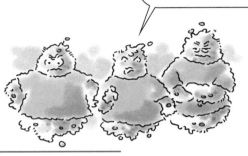

Some STDs can cause serious problems for the pregnant patient.

What causes it

STDs can be caused by infection with various organisms, including:
- fungi
- bacteria
- protozoa
- parasites
- viruses.

What to look for

The signs and symptoms exhibited by the patient with an STD typically involve some type of vaginal discharge or lesion. Vulvar or vaginal irritation, such as itching and pruritus, commonly accompany the discharge or lesion.

How it's treated

Treatment focuses on the underlying causative organism. Typically, antimicrobial or antifungal agents are prescribed.

Preventing the spread

In addition, education about the mode of transmission and safer sex practices are important to prevent the spread of infection.

What to do

- Explain the mode of transmission of the STD and instruct the patient in measures to reduce the risk of transmission.
- Administer drug therapy, as ordered, and teach the patient about the drug therapy regimen. Advise her to comply with therapy, completing the entire course of medication even if she feels better.

(Text continues on page 280.)

Selected STDs and pregnancy

This chart lists some common sexually transmitted diseases (STDs) along with their causative organisms and assessment findings, appropriate treatments for pregnant patients, and special considerations.

STD	Causative organism	Assessment findings	Treatment	Special considerations
Chlamydia	*Chlamydia trachomatis*	• Commonly produces no symptoms; suspicion raised if partner treated for nongonococcal urethritis • Heavy, gray-white vaginal discharge • Painful urination • Positive vaginal culture using special chlamydial test kit	• Amoxicillin (Amoxil)	• Screening for infection at first prenatal visit because it's one of the most common types of vaginal infection seen during pregnancy • Repeated screening in the third trimester if the woman has multiple sexual partners • Doxycycline (Vibramycin)—drug of choice for treatment if the woman isn't pregnant—contraindicated during pregnancy due to association with fetal long-bone deformities • Concomitant testing for gonorrhea due to high incidence of concurrent infection • Possible premature rupture of the membranes, preterm labor, and endometritis in the postpartum period resulting from infection • Possible development of conjunctivitis or pneumonia in neonate born to mother with infection present in the vagina
Condyloma acuminata	Human papillomavirus	• Discrete papillary structures that spread, enlarge, and coalesce to form large lesions; increase in size during pregnancy • Possible secondary ulceration and infection with foul odor	• Topical application of trichloroacetic acid or bichloroacetic acid to lesions • Lesion removal with laser therapy, cryocautery, or knife excision; lesions left in place during pregnancy unless bothersome and removed during the postpartum period	• Serious infections associated with the development of cervical cancer later in life

(continued)

Selected STDs and pregnancy *(continued)*

STD	Causative organism	Assessment findings	Treatment	Special considerations
Genital herpes	Herpes simplex virus, type 2	• Painful, small vesicles with erythematous base on vulva or vagina rupturing within 1 to 7 days to form ulcers • Low-grade fever • Dyspareunia • Positive viral culture of vesicular fluid • Positive enzyme-linked immunosorbent assay	• Acyclovir (Zovirax) orally or in ointment form	• Reduction or suppression of symptoms, shedding, or recurrent episodes only with drug therapy (not a cure for infection) • Abstinence urged until vesicles completely heal • Primary infection transmission possible across the placenta, resulting in congenital infection • Transmission to neonate possible at birth if active lesions are present in the vagina or on the vulva (can be fatal) • Cesarean delivery recommended if patient has active lesions
Gonorrhea	*Neisseria gonorrhoeae*	• May not produce symptoms • Yellow-green vaginal discharge • Male partner who experiences severe pain on urination and purulent, yellow penile discharge • Positive culture of vaginal, rectal, or urethral secretions	• Cefixime (Suprax) as a one-time I.M. injection	• Associated with spontaneous miscarriage, preterm birth, and endometritis in the postpartum period • Treatment of sexual partners required to prevent reinfection • Major cause of pelvic infectious disease and infertility • Severe eye infection leading to blindness in the neonate (ophthalmia neonatorum) if infection present at birth
Group B streptococci infection	Spirochete	• Usually no symptoms	• Broad-spectrum penicillin such as ampicillin	• Occurs in as many as 15% to 35% of pregnant women • May lead to urinary tract infection, intra-amniotic infection leading to preterm birth, and postpartum endometritis • Screening for all pregnant women recommended by The Centers for Disease Control and Prevention at 35 to 38 weeks' gestation

Selected STDs and pregnancy (continued)

STD	Causative organism	Assessment findings	Treatment	Special considerations
Group B streptococci infection (continued)				• Infection rate of approximately 40% to 70% in neonates of actively infected mothers due to placental transfer or direct contact with the organisms at birth, possibly leading to severe pneumonia, sepsis, respiratory distress syndrome, or meningitis
Syphilis	Treponema pallidum	• Painless ulcer on vulva or vagina (primary syphilis) • Hepatic and splenic enlargement, headache, anorexia, and maculopapular rash on the palms of the hands and soles of the feet occurring about 2 months after initial infection (secondary syphilis) • Cardiac, vascular, and central nervous system changes occurring after an undetermined latent phase (tertiary syphilis) • Positive Venereal Disease Research Laboratory serum test; confirmed with positive rapid plasma reagin and fluorescent treponemal antibody absorption tests • Dark-field microscopy positive for spirochete	• Penicillin G benzathine (Bicillin L-A) I.M. (single dose)	• Possible transmission across placenta after approximately 18 weeks' gestation, leading to spontaneous miscarriage, preterm labor, stillbirth, or congenital anomalies • Standard screening for syphilis at the first prenatal visit, screening at 36 weeks' gestation for women with multiple partners, and possible rescreening at beginning of labor (with neonates subsequently tested for congenital syphilis using a sample of cord blood) • Jarisch-Herxheimer reaction (sudden hypotension, fever, tachycardia, and muscle aches) after medication administration, lasting for about 24 hours, and then fading because spirochetes are destroyed

(continued)

Selected STDs and pregnancy *(continued)*

STD	Causative organism	Assessment findings	Treatment	Special considerations
Trichomoniasis	Single-cell protozoa	• Yellow-gray, frothy, odorous vaginal discharge • Vulvar itching, edema, and redness • Vaginal secretions on a wet slide treated with potassium hydroxide positive for organism	• Topical clotrimazole (Gyne-Lotrimin) instead of metronidazole (Flagyl) because of the latter drug's possible teratogenic effects if used during the first trimester of pregnancy	• Possibly associated with preterm labor, premature rupture of membranes, and postcesarean infection • Treatment of partner required, even if asymptomatic

• Urge the patient to refrain from sexual intercourse until the active infection is completely gone.

• Instruct the patient to have her partner arrange to be examined so that treatment can be initiated, thus preventing the risk of reinfection.

• Provide comfort measures to reduce vulvar and vaginal irritation; encourage the woman to keep the vulvar area clean and dry and to avoid using strong soaps, creams, or ointments unless prescribed.

• Suggest the use of cool or tepid sitz baths to relieve itching.

• Encourage the woman to wear cotton underwear and avoid tight-fitting clothing as much as possible.

• Instruct the patient in safer sex practices, including the use of condoms and spermicides such as nonoxynol 9.

• Encourage follow-up to ensure complete resolution of the infection (if possible).

Sickle cell anemia

Sickle cell anemia is a congenital hematologic disease that causes impaired circulation, chronic ill health, and premature death. It results from an inherited mutation in the formation of hemoglobin, the blood component that carries oxygen to body tissues. Patients who suffer from this disease inherit the sickling gene from both parents, although some parents may be only carriers and don't experience symptoms. If both parents are carriers, chances are that one in four of their children will be affected. (See *Sickle cell anemia and race*.)

Viral blockage

The sickle cell trait doesn't appear to influence the course of pregnancy; however, women with the trait tend to experience bacteriuria (which commonly produces no symptoms), which leads to pyelonephritis. Sickle cell anemia can threaten the woman's life if such vital blood vessels as those to the liver, kidneys, heart, lungs, or brain become blocked. During pregnancy, placental circulation may become blocked, causing low fetal birth weight and, possibly, fetal death.

What causes it

Sickle cell anemia results from homozygous inheritance of an autosomal recessive gene that produces a defective hemoglobin molecule (hemoglobin S). The defect is caused by a structural change in the gene that encodes the beta chain of hemoglobin. The amino acid valine is substituted for glutamic acid in the sixth position of the beta chain, causing the hemoglobin's structure to change.

Hemoglobin S causes RBCs to become sickle-shaped. The sickle cells start to build up in the capillaries and smaller blood vessels, making the blood more viscous. Normal circulation is impaired, causing pain, tissue infarctions, and swelling. The level of oxygen deficiency in sickle cell anemia and the factors that trigger a sickle cell crisis differ in each patient. (See *Sickle cell crisis*, page 282.)

Sickle cell trait, which results from heterozygous inheritance of this gene, causes few or no symptoms. However, people with this trait are carriers who may pass the gene to their offspring.

What to look for

The disease begins to manifest in the later part of the first year of life. Signs and symptoms include unusual swelling of the fingers and toes, chronic anemia, pallor, fatigue, and decreased appetite. Signs and symptoms of sickle cell crisis include severe abdominal pain, muscle spasms, leg pains, painful and swollen joints, fever, vomiting, hematuria, seizures, stiff neck, coma, and paralysis.

What tests tell you

Diagnosis of sickle cell anemia is based on:
• positive family history and presence of typical clinical features

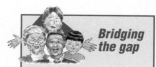

Bridging the gap

Sickle cell anemia and race

Sickle cell anemia is an inherited disease that's most common in people of African or Mediterranean descent. About 1 in 10 Blacks carries the abnormal gene, and 1 in every 400 to 600 Black children has sickle cell anemia.

It's a family affair—unfortunately. Sickle cell trait is passed on from parents.

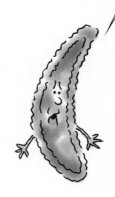

Sickle cell crisis

Infection, exposure to cold, high altitudes, overexertion, or other situations that cause cellular oxygen deprivation may trigger a sickle cell crisis. The deoxygenated, sickle-shaped red blood cells stick to the capillary wall and one another, blocking blood flow and causing cellular hypoxia. The crisis worsens as tissue hypoxia and acidic waste products cause more sickling and cell damage. With each new crisis, organs and tissues (especially the kidneys and spleen) are slowly destroyed.

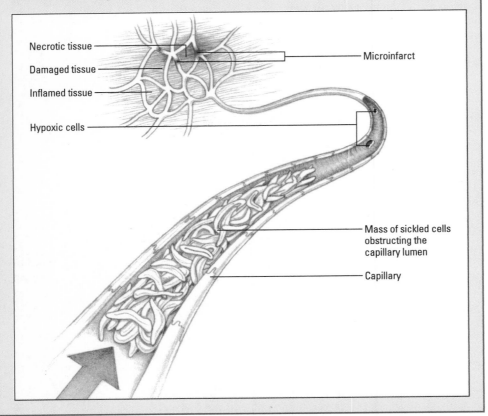

Necrotic tissue
Damaged tissue
Inflamed tissue
Hypoxic cells
Microinfarct
Mass of sickled cells obstructing the capillary lumen
Capillary

- hemoglobin electrophoresis revealing hemoglobin S
- stained blood smear showing sickled cells
- hemoglobin level of 6 to 8 mg/dl or less, possibly decreasing to as low as 5 to 6 mg/dl during a crisis
- decreased RBC count and ESR
- increased indirect bilirubin level (during a crisis)
- clean-catch urine specimen positive for bacteria.

How it's treated

Although sickle cell anemia can't be cured, treatments can alleviate symptoms and prevent painful crises. A pregnant woman who's considered at risk for this disease but hasn't been tested should be screened for sickle cell anemia at the first prenatal visit.

Drugs for bugs

Anti-infectives (such as low-dose oral penicillin) and certain vaccines (such as polyvalent pneumococcal vaccine and *Haemophilus influenzae* B vaccine) can minimize complications of sickle cell disease and transfusion therapy. Analgesics may be used to relieve the pain of crisis.

Selected supplements

For pregnant women, it's crucial to maintain adequate fluid intake and administer folic acid supplements. Iron supplements typically aren't prescribed because the woman's cells can't absorb iron in the usual manner; taking supplements can lead to iron overload.

Sickle stock exchange

Periodic exchange transfusions throughout the pregnancy may be used to replace sickle cells with normal cells. This procedure also helps reduce the high levels of bilirubin produced from the breakdown of RBCs.

What to do

- Monitor the patient's CBC regularly.
- Assess the patient's hydration status. Monitor her intake and output, and check for signs of dehydration.
- Urge the woman to drink at least eight 8-oz glasses of fluid each day.
- Monitor the patient's vital signs and the FHR as indicated. Monitor weight gain, and assess fundal height for changes indicating adequate fetal growth.
- Assess the patient for signs and symptoms of sickle cell crisis and chronic complications. Administer analgesics and I.V. fluids as ordered if crisis develops.
- Expect to administer hypotonic saline solution I.V. for fluid replacement because the kidneys have difficulty concentrating urine to remove large amounts of fluid.
- Obtain a clean-catch urine specimen for culture to assess for possible bacteriuria.

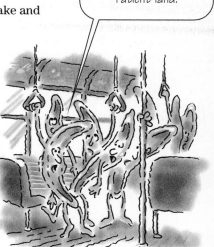

Thanks to periodic exchange transfusions, we're on a one-way trip out of Patient-land.

• Assess lower extremities for venous pooling. Encourage the woman to avoid standing for long periods and to rest in a chair with her legs elevated or in a side-lying position to promote venous return to the heart.
• Prepare the patient for ultrasound at 16 to 24 weeks' gestation and for weekly nonstress tests beginning at approximately 30 weeks' gestation.
• Be aware that blood flow velocity tests may be ordered to evaluate blood flow through the uterus and placenta. Reduced blood flow may suggest intrauterine growth retardation.
• Anticipate the patient's desire to determine if the fetus has the disease. Assist with percutaneous umbilical blood sampling to obtain a sample for RBC electrophoresis.
• Watch for signs and symptoms of infection, such as fever, chills, and purulent drainage.
• Assess the patient's respiratory status. Perform regular respiratory assessments, including auscultation of breath sounds. Expect to administer oxygen if sickle cell crisis develops.
• Provide comfort and emotional support to the patient and her family.
• Assist with measures to maintain hydration during labor and delivery.

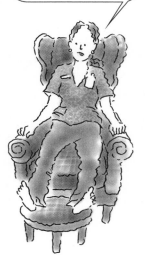

Ah, that feels better! Resting in a chair with the legs elevated promotes venous return to the heart.

Spontaneous abortion

Abortion refers to the spontaneous (occurring without medical intervention) or therapeutically induced expulsion of the products of conception from the uterus before fetal viability (fetal weight of less than 496.1 g [17½ oz] and gestation of fewer than 20 weeks). Up to 15% of all pregnancies and about 30% of first pregnancies end in spontaneous abortion (miscarriage). At least 75% of spontaneous abortions occur during the first trimester. (See *Types of spontaneous abortion.*)

What causes it

Spontaneous abortion may result from abnormal fetal, placental, or maternal factors.

Small flaws

When caused by fetal factors, spontaneous abortion usually occurs at 6 to 10 weeks' gestation. Such factors include defective embryologic development from abnormal chromosome division

Types of spontaneous abortion

Spontaneous abortions occur without medical intervention and in various ways.

• In *complete abortion,* the uterus passes all products of conception. Minimal bleeding usually accompanies complete abortion because the uterus contracts and compresses the maternal blood vessels that feed the placenta.

• *Habitual abortion* refers to the spontaneous loss of three or more consecutive pregnancies.

• In *incomplete abortion,* the uterus retains part or all of the placenta. Before 10 weeks' gestation, the fetus and placenta are usually expelled together; after the 10th week, they're expelled separately. Because part of the placenta may adhere to the uterine wall, bleeding continues. Hemorrhage is possible because the uterus doesn't contract and seal the large vessels that feed the placenta.

• In *inevitable abortion,* the membranes rupture and the cervix dilates. As labor continues, the uterus expels the products of conception.

• In *missed abortion,* the uterus retains the products of conception for 2 months or more after the fetus has died. Uterine growth ceases; uterine size may even seem to decrease. Prolonged retention of the dead products of conception may cause coagulation defects such as disseminated intravascular coagulation.

• In *septic abortion,* infection accompanies abortion. This may occur with spontaneous abortion but usually results from a lapse in sterile technique during therapeutic abortion.

• In *threatened abortion,* bloody vaginal discharge occurs during the first half of pregnancy. About 20% of pregnant women have vaginal spotting or actual bleeding early in pregnancy. Of these, about 50% abort.

(the most common cause of fetal death), faulty implantation of the fertilized ovum, and failure of the endometrium to accept the fertilized ovum.

Poor placenta performance

When placental factors are responsible, spontaneous abortion usually occurs around the 14th week, when the placenta takes over the hormone production needed to maintain the pregnancy. Placental factors include premature separation of the normally implanted placenta, abnormal placental implantation, and abnormal platelet function.

Maternal mechanical difficulties

When caused by maternal factors, spontaneous abortion usually occurs between weeks 11 and 19. Such factors include maternal infection, severe malnutrition, and abnormalities of the reproductive organs (especially incompetent cervix, in which the cervix dilates painlessly and without blood in the second trimester). Other maternal factors include endocrine problems (such as thyroid dysfunction and lowered estriol secretion), trauma (including any type of surgery that requires manipulation of the pelvic organs), ABO blood group incompatibility and Rh isoimmunization, and drug ingestion.

What to look for

Prodromal symptoms of spontaneous abortion include a pink discharge for several days or a scant brown discharge for several weeks before the onset of cramps and increased vaginal bleeding. For a few hours, the cramps intensify and occur more frequently; then, the cervix dilates for expulsion of uterine contents. If the entire contents are expelled, cramps and bleeding subside. However, if contents remain, cramps and bleeding continue.

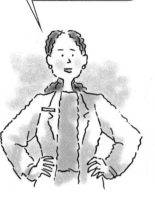

If the uterine contents are expelled completely during spontaneous abortion, cramps and bleeding subside. Cramps and bleeding continue if there are remnants in the uterus.

What tests tell you

Diagnosis of spontaneous abortion is based on evidence of expulsion of uterine contents, vaginal examination, and laboratory studies. If the blood or urine contains hCG, pregnancy is confirmed; decreased hCG levels suggest spontaneous abortion. Vaginal examination determines the size of the uterus and whether that size is consistent with the stage of the pregnancy. Expelled tissue cytology provides evidence of products of conception. Laboratory tests reflect decreased hemoglobin levels and hematocrit from blood loss. Ultrasonography confirms the presence or absence of fetal heartbeats or an empty amniotic sac.

Decreased hCG levels suggest spontaneous abortion.

How it's treated

An accurate evaluation of uterine contents is necessary before planning treatment. Spontaneous abortion can't be stopped, except in those cases attributed to an incompetent cervix. Control of severe hemorrhage requires hospitalization. Severe bleeding requires transfusion with packed RBCs or whole blood. Initially, I.V. administration of oxytocin stimulates uterine contractions. If there are remnants in the uterus, the preferred treatment is dilatation and vacuum extraction or dilatation and curettage.

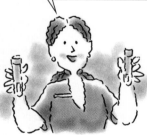

The Rh factor

After an abortion, an Rh-negative female with a negative indirect Coombs' test should receive RhoGAM to prevent future Rh isoimmunization.

Unfortunate habit

Habitual abortion can result from an incompetent cervix. Treatment involves surgical reinforcement of the cervix (cerclage) about 14 to 16 weeks after the patient's last menses. A few weeks before the estimated delivery date, the sutures are removed and the patient waits for the onset of labor. An alternative procedure—used particularly for women wanting to have more children—involves leaving the sutures in place and delivering the neonate by cesarean birth.

What to do

- Don't allow bathroom privileges because the patient may expel uterine contents without knowing it. After she uses the bedpan, inspect the contents carefully for intrauterine material.
- Note the amount, color, and odor of vaginal bleeding. Save all pads the patient uses for evaluation.
- Place the patient's bed in Trendelenburg's position as ordered.
- Administer analgesics and oxytocin as ordered.
- Assess vital signs every 4 hours for 24 hours (or more frequently depending on the extent of bleeding).
- Monitor urine output closely.
- Provide good perineal care by keeping the area clean and dry.
- Check the patient's blood type and administer RhoGAM as ordered.
- Provide emotional support and counseling during the grieving process; refer to patient and her family to loss or grief counselors as appropriate.
- Encourage the patient and her partner to express their feelings. Some couples may want to talk to a member of the clergy or, depending on their religion, may wish to have the fetus baptized.
- Help the patient and her partner develop effective coping strategies.
- Explain all procedures and treatments to the patient and provide teaching about aftercare and follow-up. (See *After spontaneous abortion*, page 288.)

Education edge

After spontaneous abortion

If your patient experiences a spontaneous abortion, be sure to include these instructions in your teaching plan.

• Expect vaginal bleeding or spotting to continue for several days.

• Immediately report bleeding that lasts longer than 8 to 10 days, or bleeding that's excessive or appears as bright red blood.

• Watch for signs of infection, such as a temperature higher than 100° F (37.8° C) and foul-smelling vaginal discharge.

• Gradually increase daily activities to include whatever tasks are comfortable to perform, as long as the activities don't increase vaginal bleeding or cause fatigue.

• Abstain from sexual intercourse for approximately 2 weeks.

• Use a contraceptive when you and your partner resume intercourse.

• Avoid the use of tampons for 1 to 2 weeks.

• Schedule a follow-up visit with the practitioner in 2 to 4 weeks.

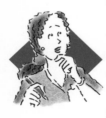

Quick quiz

1. The risks for a pregnant woman with cardiac disease and her fetus are greatest between gestation weeks:

    A.   8 and 12.

    B.   16 and 24.

    C.   28 and 32.

    D.   36 and 40.

Answer: C. Although the risks for the pregnant woman with cardiac disease and her fetus are always present, the most dangerous time is between weeks 28 and 32, when blood volume peaks and the woman's heart may be unable to compensate adequately for this change.

2. Screening for gestational diabetes in women is usually performed at:

    A.   4 to 8 weeks' gestation.

    B.   12 to 16 weeks' gestation.

    C.   24 to 28 weeks' gestation.

    D.   32 to 36 weeks' gestation.

Answer: C. All women are typically screened for gestational diabetes at 24 to 28 weeks' gestation.

3. The ovum of an ectopic pregnancy most commonly lodges in the:
    A.   fallopian tube.
    B.   abdominal viscera.
    C.   ovary.
    D.   cervical os.

Answer: A. The most common site of an ectopic pregnancy is the fallopian tube, either in the fimbria, ampulla, or isthmus.

4. After a spontaneous abortion, a woman who's Rh-negative would be given:
    A.   magnesium sulfate.
    B.   RhoGAM.
    C.   terbutaline.
    D.   betamethasone.

Answer: B. A woman who's Rh-negative would receive RhoGAM after a spontaneous abortion to reduce the risk of possible isoimmunization of the fetus in a future pregnancy.

5. A major factor contributing to the increased incidence of multiple pregnancy is:
    A.   increased use of fertility drugs.
    B.   women becoming pregnant at a younger age.
    C.   previous pregnancy.
    D.   underlying iron deficiency anemia.

Answer: A. The increased use of fertility drugs has led to a doubling of the incidence of multiple pregnancy.

6. Assessment of a woman with placenta previa would most likely reveal:
    A.   absence of fetal heart tones.
    B.   boardlike abdomen.
    C.   painless, bright red vaginal bleeding.
    D.   signs of shock.

Answer: C. A patient with placenta previa would most likely report the onset of painless, bright red vaginal bleeding after week 20 of gestation.

7. The drug of choice for a treating a pregnant woman with chlamydia is:

    A.   doxycycline (Vibramycin).
    B.   azithromycin (Zithromax).
    C.   acyclovir (Zovirax).
    D.   miconazole (Monistat).

Answer: B. Chlamydia infection in the pregnant woman is treated with azithromycin or amoxicillin.

Scoring

☆☆☆ If you answered all seven questions correctly, congratulations! You've labored long and hard to optimize your knowledge!

☆☆ If you answered five or six questions correctly, great job! You've delivered the goods on this labor-intensive topic.

☆ If you answered fewer than five questions correctly, don't belabor the matter. Give the material a quick review and keep on kickin'!

Labor and birth

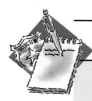

Just the facts

In this chapter, you'll learn:

♦ types of fetal presentations and positions

♦ ways in which labor can be stimulated

♦ signs and symptoms of labor

♦ stages and cardinal movements of labor

♦ nursing responsibilities during labor and birth, including ways to provide comfort and support.

A look at labor and birth

Labor and birth is physically and emotionally straining for a woman. As the patient's body undergoes physical changes to help the fetus pass through the cervix, she may also feel discomfort, pain, panic, irritability, and loss of control. To ensure the safest outcome for the mother and child, you must fully understand the stages of labor as well as the factors affecting its length and difficulty. With an understanding of the labor and birth process, you'll be better able to provide supportive measures that promote relaxation and help increase the patient's sense of control.

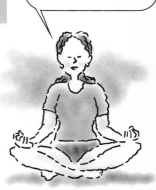

Meditate on this: Relaxation is key during labor and birth.

Fetal presentation

Fetal presentation is the relationship of the fetus to the cervix. It can be assessed through vaginal examination, abdominal inspection and palpation, sonography, or auscultation of fetal heart tones. By knowing the fetal presentation, you can anticipate which part of the fetus will first pass through the cervix during delivery.

How long and how hard

Fetal presentation can affect the length and difficulty of labor as well as how the fetus is delivered. For example, if the fetus is in a breech presentation (the fetus's soft buttocks are presenting first), the force exerted against the cervix by uterine contractions is less than it would be if the fetus's firm head presented first. The decreased force against the cervix decreases the effectiveness of the uterine contractions that help open the cervix and push the fetus through the birth canal.

Presenting difficulties

Sometimes, the fetus's presenting part is too large to pass through the mother's pelvis or the fetus is in a position that's undeliverable. In such cases, cesarean birth may be necessary. In addition to the usual risks associated with surgery, an abnormal fetal presentation increases the risk of complications for the mother and fetus.

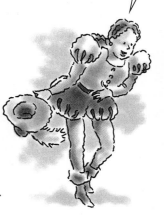

Hail Caesar! Cesarean birth may be necessary when the fetus's presenting part is too large to pass through the mother's pelvis.

Factors determining fetal presentation

The primary factors that determine fetal presentation during birth are fetal attitude, lie, and position.

Fetal attitude

Fetal attitude (degree of flexion) is the relationship of the fetal body parts to one another. It indicates whether the presenting parts of the fetus are in flexion or extension.

Complete flexion

The most common fetal attitude is *complete flexion*. This attitude results in a vertex (top of the head) presentation of the fetus through the birth canal. Commonly called "the fetal position," complete flexion is the traditional attitude referred to when describing a fetus in utero.

Tucked, folded, and crossed

In complete flexion, the head of the fetus is tucked down onto the chest, with the chin touching the sternum. The fetus's arms are folded over the chest with the elbows flexed. The lower legs are crossed, and the thighs are drawn up onto the abdomen. The calf of each leg is pressed against the thigh of the opposite leg.

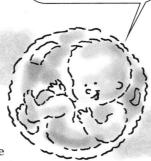

Hey mom! For once, I bet you won't mind me giving you some attitude.

All about attitude

Complete flexion is the ideal attitude for gestation and birth because the fetus occupies as little space as possible in the uterus. Birth of a fetus in complete flexion is easier because the smallest anteroposterior diameter of the fetal skull is presented to pass through the pelvis first.

Moderate flexion

Moderate flexion (military position) is the second most common fetal attitude. It tends to result in a sinciput (forehead) presentation through the birth canal. Many fetuses assume this attitude early in labor but convert to complete flexion as labor progresses.

Ten-hut!

In moderate flexion, the head of the fetus is slightly flexed but held straighter than in complete flexion. The chin doesn't touch the chest. This attitude is commonly called the *military position* because the straightness of the head makes the fetus appear to be at attention.

Low rank of difficulty

The birth of a fetus in moderate flexion usually isn't difficult because the second smallest anteroposterior diameter of the skull is presented through the pelvis first.

Partial extension

Partial extension is an uncommon fetal attitude that results in a brow presentation through the birth canal. The head of the fetus is extended, with the head pushed slightly backward so that the brow becomes the first part of the fetus to pass through the pelvis during birth. Partial extension of the fetus can make birth difficult because the anteroposterior diameter of the skull may be the same size as or larger than the opening in the woman's pelvis.

Complete extension

Complete extension is a relatively rare and abnormal fetal attitude that results in a face presentation through the birth canal. This attitude occurs in an average of 1 in 500 births.

Extended and arched

In complete extension, the head and neck of the fetus are hyperextended and the occiput touches the fetus's upper back. The back is usually arched, which increases the degree of hyperextension. The occipitomental diameter of the head presents first to pass through the pelvis. Commonly, this skull diameter is too large

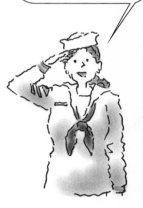

Give a salute to the military position—moderate flexion where the fetal head looks as if it's at attention.

to pass through the pelvis. About 12% to 20% of patients with a fetus in complete extension require cesarean birth.

Complete extension may be caused by:
- oligohydramnios (less than normal amniotic fluid)
- neurologic abnormalities
- multiparity
- a large abdomen with decreased uterine tone
- a nuchal cord with multiple coils around the fetus's neck
- fetal malformation (found in up to 60% of cases).

Fetal lie

The relationship of the fetal spine to the maternal spine is referred to as *fetal lie*. Fetal lie can be described as longitudinal, transverse, or oblique.

Longitudinal lie

When the fetal spine is parallel to the maternal spine, the fetus is in a longitudinal lie. This means that the fetus is lying vertically (top to bottom) in the uterus. Approximately 99% of fetuses are in longitudinal lie at the onset of labor.

Heads or tails?

Longitudinal lie can be further classified as *cephalic* or *breech*. In cephalic longitudinal lie, an area of the fetal head—determined by attitude and position—is the presenting part. In a breech longitudinal lie, the fetal buttocks or foot (possibly feet) is the presenting part.

Transverse lie

When the fetal spine and the maternal spine are at 90-degree angles to each other, the fetus is in transverse lie. This means that the fetus is lying horizontally (side to side) in the uterus. Transverse lie is considered abnormal, and it occurs in less than 1% of deliveries. If labor progresses while the fetus is in transverse lie, the presenting part may be a shoulder, iliac crest, hand, or elbow.

Oblique lie

When the fetal spine and the maternal spine are at 45-degree angles to each other—midway between the transverse and the longitudinal lies—the fetus is in an oblique lie. This lie is rare and is considered abnormal if the fetus remains in this position after the onset of labor.

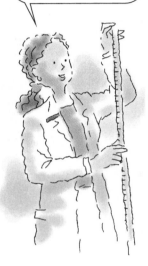

It all measures up! A cesarean birth may be necessary if the fetus is in complete extension because occipitomental skull diameter makes it impossible for the fetus to pass through the pelvis.

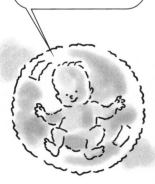

I wouldn't lie to you. When I'm in line with my mom's spine, I'm in longitudinal lie.

Fetal position abbreviations

Here's a list of abbreviations, organized according to variations in presentation, that are used when documenting fetal position.

Vertex presentations (occiput)	Breech presentations (sacrum)	Face presentations (mentum)	Shoulder presentations (acromion process)
LOA, left occipitoanterior	LSaA, left sacroanterior	LMA, left mentoanterior	LAA, left scapuloanterior
LOP, left occipitoposterior	LSaP, left sacroposterior	LMP, left mentoposterior	LAP, left scapuloposterior
LOT, left occipitotransverse	LSaT, left sacrotransverse	LMT, left mentotransverse	RAA, right scapuloanterior
ROA, right occipitoanterior	RSaA, right sacroanterior	RMA, right mentoanterior	RAP, right scapuloposterior
ROP, right occipitoposterior	RSaP, right sacroposterior	RMP, right mentoposterior	
ROT, right occipitotransverse	RSaT, right sacrotransverse	RMT, right mentotransverse	

Fetal position

Fetal position is the relationship of the presenting part of the fetus to a specific quadrant of the mother's pelvis. It's important to define fetal position because it influences the progression of labor and whether surgical intervention is needed.

Spelling it out

Fetal position is defined using three letters. The first letter designates whether the presenting part is facing the woman's right (R) or left (L) side. The second letter or letters refer to the presenting part of the fetus: the occiput (O), mentum (M), sacrum (Sa), or scapula or acromion process (A). The third letter designates whether the presenting part is pointing to the anterior (A), posterior (P), or transverse (T) section of the mother's pelvis. The occiput typically presents first when the fetus is in the vertex fetal presentation; the mentum, in face presentation; the sacrum, in breech presentation; and the scapula or acromion process, in shoulder presentation.

The most common fetal positions are left occiput anterior (LOA) and right occiput anterior (ROA). (See *Fetal position abbreviations.*)

Duration determinant

Commonly, the duration of labor and birth is shortest when the fetus is in the LOA or ROA position. When the fetal position is posterior, such as left occiput posterior (LOP), labor tends to be longer and more painful for the woman because the fetal head puts pressure on her sacral nerves. (See *Determining fetal position,* page 296.)

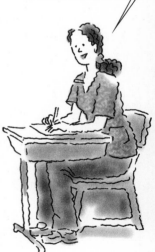

I love writing letters. Like LOA—meaning an ideal fetal position!

Determining fetal position

Fetal position is determined by the relationship of a specific presenting part (occiput, sacrum, mentum [chin], or sinciput [deflected vertex]) to the four quadrants (anterior, posterior, right, or left) of the maternal pelvis. For example, a fetus whose occiput (O) is the presenting part and who's located in the right (R) and anterior (A) quadrant of the maternal pelvis is identified as ROA.

These illustrations show the possible positions of a fetus in vertex presentation.

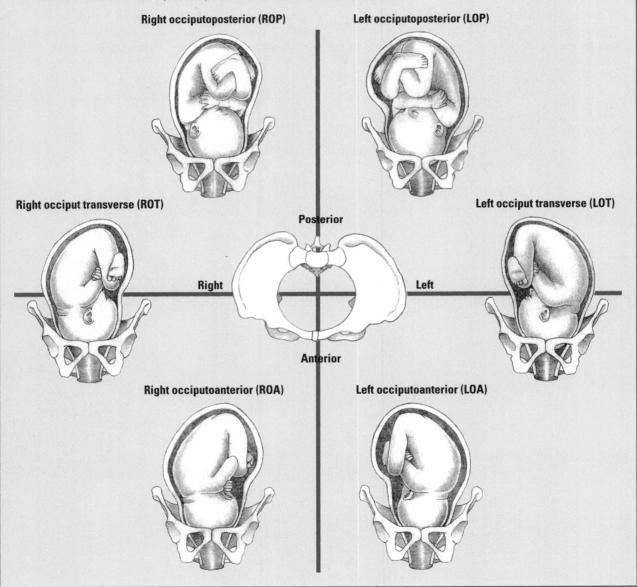

Right occiputoposterior (ROP)

Left occiputoposterior (LOP)

Right occiput transverse (ROT)

Left occiput transverse (LOT)

Posterior

Right   Left

Anterior

Right occiputoanterior (ROA)

Left occiputoanterior (LOA)

Types of fetal presentation

Fetal presentation refers to the part of the fetus that presents into the birth canal first. It's determined by fetal attitude, lie, and position. Fetal presentation should be determined in the early stages of labor in case an abnormal presentation endangers the mother and the fetus. (See *Classifying fetal presentation*, pages 298 and 299.)

The four main types of fetal presentation are:

- cephalic
- breech
- shoulder
- compound.

Cephalic presentation

When the fetus is in cephalic presentation, the head is the first part to contact the cervix and expel from the uterus during delivery. About 95% of all fetuses are in cephalic presentation at birth.

The four types of cephalic presentation are vertex, brow, face, and mentum (chin).

Vertex

In the vertex cephalic presentation, the most common presentation overall, the fetus is in a longitudinal lie with an attitude of complete flexion. The parietal bones (between the two fontanels) are the presenting part of the fetus. This presentation is considered optimal for fetal descent through the pelvis.

Brow

In brow presentation, the fetus's brow or forehead is the presenting part. The fetus is in a longitudinal lie and exhibits an attitude of moderate flexion. Although this isn't the optimal presentation for a fetus, few suffer serious complications from the delivery. In fact, many brow presentations convert to vertex presentations during descent through the pelvis.

Face

The face type of cephalic presentation is unfavorable for the mother and the fetus. In this presentation, the fetus is in a longitudinal lie and exhibits an attitude of partial extension. Because the face is the presenting part of the fetal head, severe edema and facial distortion may occur from the pressure of uterine contractions during labor.

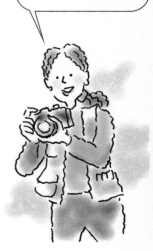

Picture this. Vertex presentation is considered optimal for delivery.

Classifying fetal presentation

Fetal presentation may be broadly classified as cephalic, shoulder, compound, or breech. Almost all births are cephalic presentations. Breech births are the second most common type.

Cephalic

In the cephalic, or head-down, presentation, the position of the fetus may be further classified by the presenting skull landmark, such as vertex, brow, sinciput, or mentum (chin).

Vertex

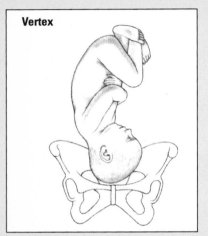

Brow

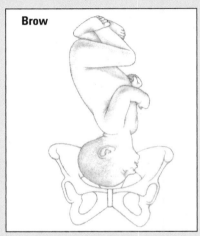

Sinciput

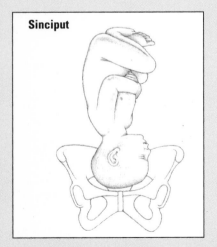

Mentum

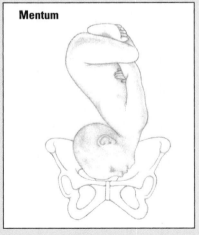

Shoulder

Although a fetus may adopt one of several shoulder presentations, examination can't differentiate among them; thus, all transverse lies are considered shoulder presentations.

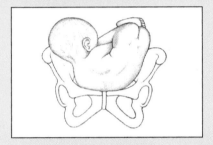

Compound

In compound presentation, an extremity prolapses alongside the major presenting part so that two presenting parts appear in the pelvis at the same time.

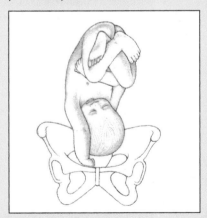

Classifying fetal presentation *(continued)*

Breech

In the breech, or head-up, presentation, the position of the fetus may be further classified as *frank,* where the hips are flexed and knees remain straight; *complete,* where the knees and hips are flexed; *kneeling,* where the knees are flexed and the hips remain extended; and *incomplete,* where one or both hips remain extended and one or both feet or knees lie below the breech; or *footling,* where one or both feet extend below the breech.

Frank

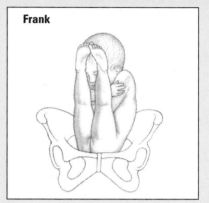

Complete

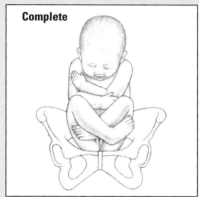

Footling

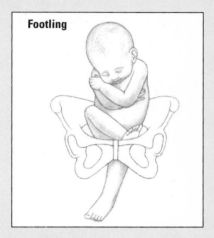

Kneeling

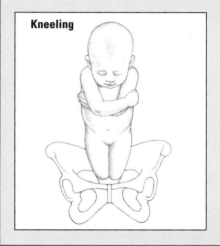

Incomplete

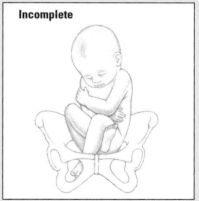

Faced with potential complications

If labor is allowed to progress, careful monitoring of both the fetus and the mother is necessary to reduce the risk of compromise. Labor may be prolonged and ineffective in some instances, and vaginal birth may not be possible because the presenting part has a larger diameter than the pelvic outlet. Attempts to manually convert the face presentation to a more favorable position are rarely successful and are associated with high perinatal mortality and maternal morbidity.

Mentum

The mentum, or chin, type of cephalic presentation is also unfavorable for the mother and the fetus. In this presentation, the fetus is in a longitudinal lie with an attitude of complete extension. The presenting part of the fetus is the chin, which may lead to severe edema and facial distortion from the pressure of the uterine contractions during labor. The widest diameter of the fetal head is presenting through the pelvis because of the extreme extension of the head. If labor is allowed to progress, careful monitoring of both the fetus and the mother is necessary to reduce the risk of compromise. Labor is usually prolonged and ineffective. Vaginal delivery is usually impossible because the fetus can't pass through the ischial spines.

> Let's face it. For fetuses in the mentum cephalic presentation, pressure from uterine contractions may cause severe edema and facial distortion.

Breech presentation

Although 25% of all fetuses are in breech presentation at week 30 of gestation, most turn spontaneously at 32 to 34 weeks' gestation. However, breech presentation occurs at term in about 3% of births. Labor is usually prolonged with breech presentation because of ineffective cervical dilation caused by decreased pressure on the cervix and delayed descent of the fetus.

It gets complicated

In addition to prolonging labor, the breech presentation increases the risk of complications. In the fetus, cord prolapse; anoxia; intracranial hemorrhage caused by rapid molding of the head; neck trauma; and shoulder, arm, hip, and leg dislocations or fractures may occur. Complications that may occur in the mother include perineal tears and cervical lacerations during delivery and infection from premature rupture of the membranes.

How will I know?

A breech presentation can be identified by abdominal and cervical examination. The signs of breech presentation include:
• fetal head is felt at the uterine fundus during an abdominal examination
• fetal heart tones are heard above the umbilicus
• soft buttocks or feet are palpated during a cervical examination.

Once, twice, three types more

The three types of breech presentation are complete, frank, and incomplete.

Complete breech

In a complete breech presentation, the fetus's buttocks and the feet are the presenting parts. The fetus is in a longitudinal lie and is in complete flexion. The fetus is sitting crossed-legged and both legs are drawn up (hips flexed) with the anterior of the thighs pressed tightly against the abdomen; the lower legs are crossed with the calves pressed against the posterior of the thighs; and the feet are tightly flexed against the outer aspect of the posterior thighs. Although considered an abnormal fetal presentation, complete breech is the least difficult of the breech presentations.

Frank breech

In a frank breech presentation, the fetus's buttocks are the presenting part. The fetus is in a longitudinal lie and is in moderate flexion. Both legs are drawn up (hips flexed) with the anterior of the thighs pressed against the body; the knees are fully extended and resting on the upper body with the lower legs stretched upward; the arms may be flexed over or under the legs; and the feet are resting against the head. The attitude is moderate.

Incomplete breech

In an incomplete breech presentation, also called a *footling breech*, one or both of the knees or legs are the presenting parts. If one leg is extended, it's called a *single-footling breech* (the other leg may be flexed in the normal attitude); if both legs are extended, it's called a *double-footling breech*. The fetus is in a longitudinal lie. At least one of the thighs and one of the lower legs are extended with little or no hip flexion.

Perhaps expect prolapse

A footling breech is the most difficult of the breech deliveries. Cord prolapse is common in a footling breech because of the space created by the extended leg. A cesarean birth may be necessary to reduce the risk of fetal or maternal mortality.

Shoulder presentation

Although common in multiple pregnancies, the shoulder presentation of the fetus is an abnormal presentation that occurs in less than 1% of deliveries. In this presentation, the shoulder, iliac crest, hand, or elbow is the presenting part. The fetus is in a transverse lie, and the attitude may range from complete flexion to complete extension.

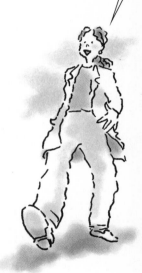

Don't be defeated by a complete breech, where the presenting parts of the fetus are the buttocks and the feet.

Lacking space and support

In the multiparous woman, shoulder presentation may be caused by the relaxation of the abdominal walls. If the abdominal walls are relaxed, the unsupported uterus falls forward, causing the fetus to turn horizontally. Other causes of shoulder presentation may include pelvic contraction (the vertical space in the pelvis is smaller than the horizontal space) or placenta previa (the low-lying placenta decreases the vertical space in the uterus).

Early identification and intervention are critical when the fetus is in a shoulder presentation. Abdominal and cervical examination and sonography are used to confirm whether the mother's abdomen has an abnormal or distorted shape. Attempts to turn the fetus may be unsuccessful unless the fetus is small or preterm. A cesarean delivery may be necessary to reduce the risk of fetal or maternal death.

> Ahem! A compound presentation compounds the difficulty of birth because an extremity presents with the major presenting part. Whew! There, I said it.

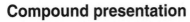

Compound presentation

In a compound presentation, an extremity presents with another major presenting part, usually the head. In this type of presentation, the extremity prolapses alongside the major presenting part so that they present simultaneously.

Engagement

Engagement occurs when the presenting part of the fetus passes into the pelvis to the point where, in cephalic presentation, the biparietal diameter of the fetal head is at the level of the mid-pelvis (or at the level of the ischial spines). Vaginal and cervical examinations are used to assess the degree of engagement before and during labor.

A good sign

Because the ischial spines are usually the narrowest area of the female pelvis, an engagement indicates that the pelvic inlet is large enough for the fetus to pass through (because the widest part of the fetus has already passed through the narrowest part of the pelvis).

Floating away

In the primipara, nonengagement of the presenting part at the onset of labor may indicate a complication, such as cephalopelvic disproportion, abnormal presentation or position, or an abnormality of the fetal head. The nonengaged presenting part is described as *floating*. In the multipara, nonengagement is common at the onset of labor; however, the presenting part quickly becomes engaged as labor progresses.

Station

Station is the relationship of the presenting part of the fetus to the mother's ischial spines. If the fetus is at station 0, the fetus is considered to be at the level of the ischial spines. The fetus is considered engaged when it reaches station 0.

Grand central stations

Fetal station is measured in centimeters. The measurement is called *minus* when it's above the level of the ischial spines and *plus* when it's below that level. Station measurements range from −1 to −3 cm (minus station) and +1 to +4 cm (plus station).

A crowning achievement

When the station is measured at +4 cm, the presenting part of the fetus is at the perineum—commonly known as *crowning*. (See *Assessing fetal engagement and station*.)

Advice from the experts

Assessing fetal engagement and station

During a cervical examination, you'll assess the extent of the fetal presenting part into the pelvis. This is referred to as *fetal engagement*.

After you have determined fetal engagement, palpate the presenting part and grade the fetal station (where the presenting part lies in relation to the ischial spines of the maternal pelvis). If the presenting part isn't fully engaged into the pelvis, you won't be able to assess station.

Station grades range from −3 (3 cm above the maternal ischial spines) to +4 (4 cm below the maternal ischial spines, causing the perineum to bulge). A zero grade indicates that the presenting part lies level with the ischial spines.

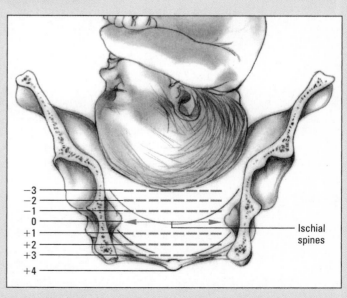

A look at labor stimulation

For some patients, it's necessary to stimulate labor. The stimulation of labor may involve induction (artificially starting labor) or augmentation (assisting a labor that started spontaneously).

Although induction and augmentation involve the same methods and risks, they're performed for different reasons. Many high-risk pregnancies must be induced because the safety of the mother or fetus is in jeopardy. Medical problems that justify induction of labor include preeclampsia, eclampsia, severe hypertension, diabetes, Rh sensitization, prolonged rupture of the membranes (over 24 hours), and a postmature fetus (a fetus that's 42 weeks' gestation or older). Augmentation of labor may be necessary if the contractions are too weak or infrequent to be effective.

Conditions for labor stimulation

Before stimulating labor, the fetus must be:
• in longitudinal lie (the long axis of the fetus is parallel to the long axis of the mother)
• engaged
• in cephalopelvic proportion (the fetal head can pass through the pelvis).

The ripe type

In addition to the above fetal criteria, the mother must have a ripe cervix before labor is induced. A ripe cervix is soft and supple to the touch rather than firm. Softening of the cervix allows for cervical effacement, dilation, and effective coordination of contractions. Using Bishop's score, you can determine whether a cervix is ripe enough for induction. (See *Bishop's score.*)

> Here's something interesting. A ripe cervix allows for effacement and dilation.

When it isn't so great to stimulate

Stimulation of labor should be done with caution in women age 35 and older and in those with grand parity or uterine scars.

Labor shouldn't be stimulated if:
• vaginal birth is too risky.
• stimulation of the uterus increases the risk of such complications as placenta previa, abruptio placenta, uterine rupture, and decreased fetal blood supply caused by the increased intensity or duration of contractions.
• multiple pregnancy is involved.
• the woman has an active genital herpes infection.

Bishop's score

Bishop's score is a tool that you can use to assess whether a woman is ready for labor. A score ranging from 0 to 3 is given for each of five factors: cervical dilation, length (effacement), consistency, position, and station.

 If the woman's score exceeds 8, the cervix is considered suitable for induction.

Factor	Score
Cervical dilation	
• Cervix dilated < 1 cm	0
• Cervix dilated 1 to 2 cm	1
• Cervix dilated 2 to 4 cm	3
• Cervix dilated > 4 cm	2
Cervical length (effacement)	
• Cervical length > 4 cm (0% effaced)	0
• Cervical length 2 to 4 cm (0% to 50% effaced)	1
• Cervical length 1 to 2 cm (50% to 75% effaced)	2
• Cervical length < 1 cm (> 75% effaced)	3
Cervical consistency	
• Firm cervical consistency	0
• Average cervical consistency	1
• Soft cervical consistency	2
Cervical position	
• Posterior cervical position	0
• Middle or anterior cervical position	1
Zero station notation (presenting part level)	
• Presenting part at ischial spines −3 cm	0
• Presenting part at ischial spines −1 cm	1
• Presenting part at ischial spines +1 cm	3
• Presenting part at ischial spines +2 cm	2

Modifiers

Add 1 point to score for:
• Preeclampsia
• Each prior vaginal delivery

Subtract 1 point from score for:
• Postdates pregnancy
• Nulliparity
• Premature or prolonged rupture of membranes

Adapted with permission from Bishop, E.H. "Pelvic Scoring for Elective Induction," *Obstetrics and Gynecology* 24:266-68, August 1964.

- evidence of fetal distress exists.
- the fetus is in an unusual presentation (such as a footling breech presentation).
- the uterus is unusually large (which increases the risk of uterine rupture).

Methods of labor stimulation

If labor is to be induced or augmented, one method or a combination of methods may be used. Methods of labor stimulation include breast stimulation, amniotomy, oxytocin administration, and ripening agent application.

Breast stimulation

In breast stimulation, the nipples are massaged to induce labor. Stimulation results in the release of oxytocin, which causes contractions that sometimes result in labor.

The patient or her partner can help with breast stimulation by:
- applying a water-soluble lubricant to the nipple area (to prevent irritation)
- gently rolling the nipple through the patient's clothing.

Too much, too soon?

One drawback of breast stimulation is that the amount of oxytocin being released by the woman's body can't be controlled. In some cases (rarely), too much oxytocin leads to excessive uterine stimulation (hyperstimulation, or tetanic contractions), which impairs fetal or placental blood flow, causing fetal distress.

Amniotomy

Amniotomy (artificial rupturing of the membranes) is performed to augment or induce labor when the membranes haven't ruptured spontaneously. This procedure allows the fetal head to contact the cervix more directly, thus increasing the efficiency of contractions. Amniotomy is virtually painless for both the mother and the fetus because the membranes don't have nerve endings.

System requirements

To perform amniotomy, the fetus must be in the vertex presentation with the fetal head at -2 station or lower. In addition, the mother must have a Bishop's score of at least 8.

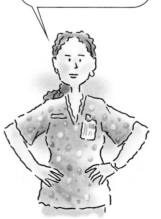

Amniotomy allows the fetal head to contact the cervix more directly, increasing the efficiency of contractions.

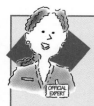

Advice from the experts

Complications of amniotomy

Umbilical cord prolapse—a life-threatening complication of amniotomy—is an emergency that requires immediate cesarean birth to prevent fetal death. It occurs when amniotic fluid, gushing from the ruptured sac, sweeps the cord down through the cervix. Prolapse risk is higher if the fetal head isn't engaged in the pelvis before rupture occurs.

Cord prolapse can lead to cord compression as the fetal presenting part presses the cord against the pelvic brim. Immediate action must be taken to relieve the pressure and prevent fetal anoxia and fetal distress. Here are some options:
• Insert a gloved hand into the vagina and gently push the fetal presenting part away from the cord.

• Place the woman in Trendelenburg's position to tilt the presenting part backward into the pelvis and relieve pressure on the cord.
• Administer oxygen to the mother by face mask to improve oxygen flow to the fetus.

If the cord has prolapsed to the point that it's visible outside the vagina, don't attempt to push the cord back in. This can add to the compression and may cause kinking. Cover the exposed portion with a compress soaked with sterile saline solution to prevent drying, which could result in atrophy of the umbilical vessels.

Let it flow, let it flow, let it flow

During amniotomy, the woman is placed in a dorsal recumbent position. An amniohook (a long, thin instrument similar to a crochet hook) is inserted into the vagina to puncture the membranes. If puncture is properly performed, amniotic fluid gushes out.

Persevere if it isn't clear

Normal amniotic fluid is clear. Bloody or meconium-stained amniotic fluid is considered abnormal and requires careful, continuous monitoring of the mother and fetus. Bloody amniotic fluid may indicate a bleeding problem. Meconium-stained amniotic fluid may indicate fetal distress. If the fluid is meconium-stained, note whether the staining is thin, moderate, thick, or particulate.

Prolapse potential

Amniotomy increases the risk to the fetus because there's a possibility that a portion of the umbilical cord will prolapse with the amniotic fluid. Fetal heart rate (FHR) should be monitored during and after the procedure to make sure that umbilical cord prolapse didn't occur. (See *Complications of amniotomy*.)

Oxytocin administration

Synthetic oxytocin (Pitocin) is used to induce or augment labor. It may be used in patients with gestational hypertension, prolonged gestation, maternal diabetes, Rh sensitization, premature or prolonged rupture of membranes, and incomplete or inevitable abortion. Oxytocin is also used to evaluate for fetal distress after 31 weeks' gestation and to control bleeding and enhance uterine contractions after the placenta is delivered.

Oxytocin is always administered I.V. with an infusion pump. Throughout administration, FHR and uterine contractions should be assessed and monitored to ensure that they're occurring in a 20-minute span.

> Oxytocin is always administered I.V. with an infusion pump.

Nursing interventions

Here's how to administer oxytocin:
- Start a primary I.V. line.
- Insert the tubing of the administration set through the infusion pump, and set the drip rate to administer the oxytocin at a starting infusion rate of 0.5 to 1 mU/minute. The maximum dosage of oxytocin is 20 to 40 mU/minute. Typically, the recommended labor-starting dosage is 10 units of oxytocin in 100 ml isotonic solution to run at 0.5 to 1 mU/minute, with the maximum dosage being 20 to 40 mU.

Piggyback ride

- The oxytocin solution is then piggybacked to the primary I.V. line.
- If a problem occurs, such as decelerations of FHR or fetal distress, stop the piggyback infusion immediately and resume the primary line.

Immediate action

- Because oxytocin begins acting immediately, be prepared to start monitoring uterine contractions.
- Increase the oxytocin dosage as ordered—but never increase the dose more than 1 to 2 mU/minute every 15 to 60 minutes. Typically, the dosage continues at a rate that maintains a regular pattern (uterine contractions occur every 2 to 3 minutes).

If more is in store

- Before each increase, be sure to assess contractions, maternal vital signs, fetal heart rhythm, and FHR. If you're using an external fetal monitor, the uterine activity strip or grid should show contractions occurring every 2 to 3 minutes. The contractions should last for about 60 seconds and be followed by uterine relaxation. If you're using an internal fetal monitor, look for an optimal baseline value ranging from 5 to 15 mm Hg. Your goal is to verify uterine relaxation between contractions.
- Assist with comfort measures, such as repositioning the patient on her other side, as needed.

Following through

• Continue assessing maternal and fetal responses to the oxytocin.

• Review the infusion rate to prevent uterine hyperstimulation. To manage hyperstimulation, discontinue the infusion and administer oxygen. (See *Complications of oxytocin administration.*)

• To reduce uterine irritability, try to increase uterine blood flow. Do this by changing the patient's position and increasing the infu-

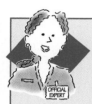

Advice from the experts

Complications of oxytocin administration

Oxytocin can cause uterine hyperstimulation. This, in turn, may progress to tetanic contractions, which last longer than 2 minutes. Signs of hyperstimulation include contractions that are less than 2 minutes apart and last 90 seconds or longer, uterine pressure that doesn't return to baseline between contractions, and intrauterine pressure that rises over 75 mm Hg.

What else to watch for

Other potential complications include fetal distress, abruptio placentae, uterine rupture, and water intoxication. Water intoxication, which can cause maternal seizures or coma, can result because the antidiuretic effect of oxytocin causes decreased urine flow.

Stop signs

Watch for the following signs of oxytocin administration complications. If any indication of any potential complications exists, stop the oxytocin administration, administer oxygen via face mask, and notify the doctor immediately.

Fetal distress

Signs of fetal distress include:
• late decelerations
• bradycardia.

Abruptio placentae

Signs of abruptio placentae include:
• sharp, stabbing uterine pain
• pain over and above the uterine contraction pain
• heavy bleeding
• hard, boardlike uterus.

Also watch for signs of shock, including rapid, weak pulse; falling blood pressure; cold and clammy skin; and dilation of the nostrils.

Uterine rupture

Signs of uterine rupture include:
• sudden, severe pain during a uterine contractions
• tearing sensation
• absent fetal heart sounds.

Also watch for signs of shock, including rapid, weak pulse; falling blood pressure; cold and clammy skin; and dilation of the nostrils.

Water intoxication

Signs and symptoms of water intoxication include:
• headache and vomiting (usually seen first)
• hypertension
• peripheral edema
• shallow or labored breathing
• dyspnea
• tachypnea
• lethargy
• confusion
• change in level of consciousness.

sion rate of the primary I.V. line. After hyperstimulation resolves, resume the oxytocin infusion per your facility's policy.

Ripening agent application

If a woman's cervix isn't soft and supple, a ripening agent may be applied to it to stimulate labor. Drugs containing prostaglandin E_2—such as dinoprostone (Cervidil, Prepidil, Prostin E2)—are commonly used to ripen the cervix. These drugs initiate the breakdown of the collagen that keeps the cervix tightly closed.

The ripening agent can be:
- applied to the interior surface of the cervix with a catheter or suppository.
- applied to a diaphragm that's then placed against the cervix.
- inserted vaginally.

Additional doses may be applied every 3 to 6 hours; however, two or three doses are usually enough to cause ripening. The woman should remain flat after application to prevent leakage of the medication.

Success half the time

The success of this labor stimulation method varies with the agent used. After just a single application of a ripening agent, about 50% of women go into labor spontaneously and deliver within 24 hours. Those women who don't go into labor require a different method of labor stimulation.

Prostaglandin should be removed before amniotomy. Use this drug with caution in women with asthma, glaucoma, and renal or cardiac disease.

Not to be ignored

While the ripening agent is applied, carefully monitor the patient's uterine activity. If uterine hyperstimulation occurs or if labor begins, the prostaglandin agent should be removed. The patient should also be monitored for adverse effects of prostaglandin application, including headache, vomiting, fever, diarrhea, and hypertension. FHR should be monitored continuously for at least 30 minutes after each application and up to 2 hours after vaginal insertion.

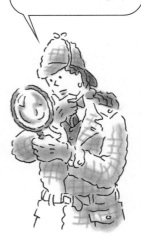

Ah ha! As I suspected, prostaglandin application may cause uterine hyperstimulation. Monitor the patient's uterine activity.

Onset of labor

True labor begins when the woman has bloody show, her membranes rupture, and she has painful contractions of the uterus that cause effacement and dilation of the cervix. The actual mechanism that triggers this process is unknown.

Before the onset of true labor, preliminary signs appear that indicate the beginning of the birthing process. Although not considered to be a true stage of labor, these signs signify that true labor isn't far away.

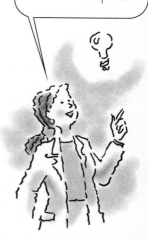

To illuminate, lightening is the descent of the fetal head into the pelvis.

Preliminary signs and symptoms of labor

Preliminary signs and symptoms of labor include lightening, increased level of activity, Braxton Hicks contractions, and ripening of the cervix. Subjective signs, such as restlessness, anxiety, and sleeplessness, may also occur. (See *Labor: True or false?*)

Lightening

Lightening is the descent of the fetal head into the pelvis. The uterus lowers and moves into a more anterior position, and the contour of the abdomen changes. In primiparas, these changes commonly occur about 2 weeks before birth. In multiparas, these changes can occur on the day labor begins or after labor starts.

Advice from the experts

Labor: True or false?

Use this chart to help differentiate between the signs and symptoms of true labor and those of false labor.

Signs and symptoms	True labor	False labor
Cervical changes	Cervix softens and dilates	No cervical dilation or effacement
Level of discomfort	Intense	Mild
Location of contractions	Start in the back and spread to the abdomen	Abdomen or groin
Uterine consistency when palpated	Hard as a board; can't be indented	Easily indented with a finger
Regularity of contractions	Regular with increasing frequency and duration	Irregular; no discernible pattern; tends to decrease in intensity and frequency with activity
Frequency and duration of contractions affected by position or activity	No	Yes
Ruptured membranes	Possible	No

More pressure here, less pressure there

Lightening increases pressure on the bladder, which may cause urinary frequency. In addition, leg pain may occur if the shifting of the fetus and uterus increases pressure on the sciatic nerve. The mother may also notice an increase in vaginal discharge because of the pressure of the fetus on the cervix. However, breathing becomes easier for the woman after lightening because pressure on the diaphragm is decreased.

Increased level of activity

After having endured increased fatigue for most of the third trimester, it's common for a woman to experience a sudden increase in energy before true labor starts. This phenomenon is sometimes referred to as "nesting" because, in many cases, the woman directs this energy toward last-minute activities, such as organizing the baby's room, cleaning and straightening her home, and preparing other children in the household for the new arrival.

A built-in energy source

The woman's increase in activity may be caused by a decrease in placental progesterone production (which may also be partly responsible for the onset of labor) that results in an increase in the release of epinephrine. This epinephrine increase gives the woman extra energy for labor.

Braxton Hicks contractions

Braxton Hicks contractions are mild contractions of the uterus that occur throughout pregnancy. They may become extremely strong a few days to a month before labor begins, which may cause some women, especially a primipara, to misinterpret them as true labor. Several characteristics, however, distinguish Braxton Hicks contractions from labor contractions.

Patternless

Braxton Hicks contractions are irregular. There's no pattern to the length of time between them and they vary widely in their strength. They gradually increase in frequency and intensity throughout the pregnancy, but they maintain an irregular pattern. In addition, Braxton Hicks contractions can be diminished by increasing activity or by eating, drinking, or changing position. Labor contractions can't be diminished by these activities.

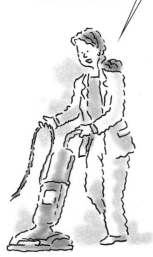

Experiencing an increased energy level before true labor starts can induce a different kind of labor—like cleaning house.

Bon appetit! Eating can help calm Braxton Hicks contractions.

Painless

Braxton Hicks contractions are commonly painless—especially early in pregnancy. Many women feel only a tightening of the abdomen in the first or second trimester. If the woman does feel pain from these contractions, it's felt only in the abdomen and the groin—usually not in the back. This is a major difference from the contractions of labor.

No softening or stretching

Probably the most important differentiation between Braxton Hicks contractions and true labor contractions is that Braxton Hicks contractions don't cause progressive effacement or dilation of the cervix. The uterus can still be indented with a finger during a contraction, which indicates that the contractions aren't efficient enough for effacement or dilation to occur.

Ripening of the cervix

Ripening of the cervix refers to the process in which the cervix softens to prepare for dilation and effacement. It's thought to be the result of hormone-mediated biochemical events that initiate breakdown of the collagen in the cervix, thus causing it to soften and become flexible. As the cervix ripens, it also changes position by tipping forward in the vagina.

Ripening of the cervix doesn't produce outwardly observable signs or symptoms. The ripeness of the cervix is determined during a pelvic examination, usually in the last weeks of the third trimester.

Signs of true labor

Signs of true labor include uterine contractions, show, and spontaneous rupture of membranes.

Uterine contractions

The involuntary uterine contractions of true labor help effacement and dilation of the uterus and push the fetus through the birth canal. Although uterine contractions are irregular when they begin, as labor progresses they become regular with a predictable pattern.

Early contractions occur anywhere from 5 to 30 minutes apart and last about 30 to 45 seconds. The interval between the contractions allows blood flow to resume to the placenta, which supplies oxygen to the fetus and removes waste products. As labor progresses, the contractions increase in frequency, duration, and intensity. During the transition phase of the first stage of labor—when contractions reach their maximum intensity, frequency, and duration—they each last 60 to 90 seconds and recur every 2 to 3 minutes.

Sweeping waves

Uterine contractions are painful and wavelike—they build and recede—beginning in the lower back and moving around to the abdomen and, possibly, the legs. They're stronger in the upper uterus than in the lower uterus so they can push the fetus downward and allow for dilation. These contractions cause a palpable hardening of the uterus that can't be indented with a finger.

Efface it!

Most important, the uterine contractions of labor cause progressive effacement and dilation of the cervix. As labor progresses, a visible bulging of intact membranes can be observed.

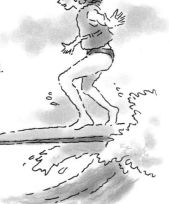

Uterine contractions are like, wavelike, you know? Awesome!

Show

Bloody show occurs as the cervix thins and begins to dilate, allowing passage of the mucus plug that seals the cervical canal during pregnancy. Mucus from the plug mixes with blood from the cervical capillaries because of the pressure of the fetus on the canal and other changes in the cervix. Consequently, show may appear pinkish, blood-tinged, or brownish. Occasionally, in primiparas it may be passed up to 2 weeks before labor begins.

Spontaneous rupture of membranes

Twenty-five percent of all labors begin with spontaneous rupture of the membranes. The membranes—consisting of the amniotic and chorionic membranes—cover the fetal surface of the placenta and form a sac that contains and supports the fetus and the amniotic fluid. This fluid, produced by the amniotic membrane, acts as a cushion throughout gestation, protects the fetus from temperature changes, protects the umbilical cord from pressure, and is believed to aid in fetal muscular development by allowing the fetus to move freely.

Fluid facts

Spontaneous rupture of the membranes may occur as a sudden gush of fluid or as a steady or intermittent, slow leakage of fluid. Rupture isn't painful because the membranes don't have a nerve supply. Even though much of the amniotic fluid is lost when the membranes rupture, the fetus is still protected. The amniotic

(Text continues on page 315.)

The pregnant woman

As a result of hormonal activity, the breasts may double in size during pregnancy. During this time, fatty tissue is largely replaced by glandular tissue and the mammary glands become capable of secreting milk.

During the third trimester, the fundus reaches the xiphoid process. In addition, the uterus remains oval in shape. Its muscular walls become progressively thinner as it enlarges. In some women, the uterus becomes large enough that the maternal umbilicus everts and protrudes.

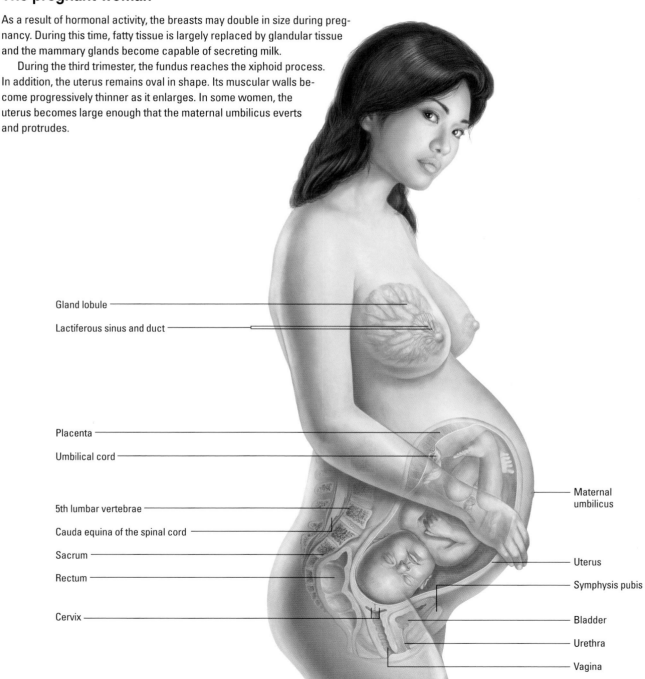

Gland lobule

Lactiferous sinus and duct

Placenta

Umbilical cord

5th lumbar vertebrae

Cauda equina of the spinal cord

Sacrum

Rectum

Cervix

Maternal umbilicus

Uterus

Symphysis pubis

Bladder

Urethra

Vagina

Conditions for cesarean birth

A cesarean birth is removal of the fetus through an abdominal incision. It's a surgical procedure that's performed in certain instances when a vaginal birth would pose a problem to either the mother or the fetus. Conditions that may necessitate cesarean birth include fetal malpresentation, cephalopelvic disproportion (CPD), placenta previa, selected cases of abruptio placentae, and umbilical cord prolapse. A cesarean birth may also be performed in cases of fetal distress.

Fetal malpresentation

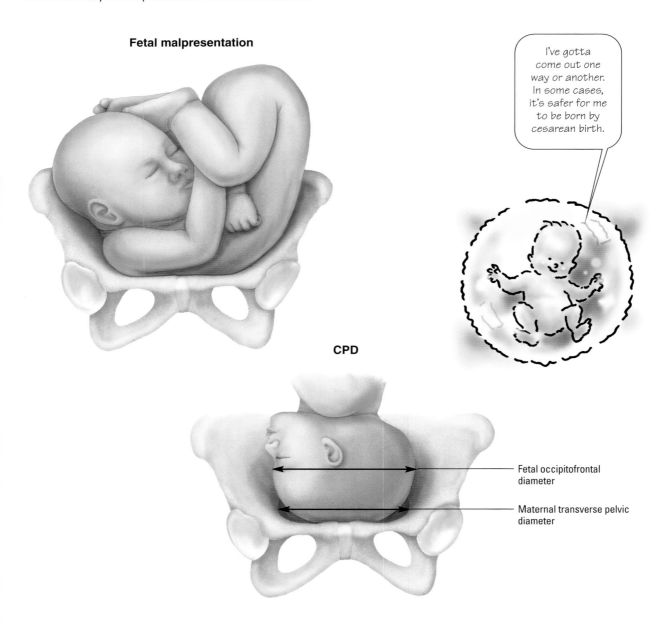

I've gotta come out one way or another. In some cases, it's safer for me to be born by cesarean birth.

CPD

Fetal occipitofrontal diameter

Maternal transverse pelvic diameter

Placenta previa

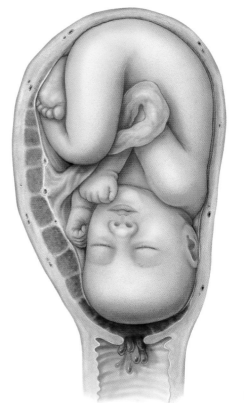

Abruptio placentae

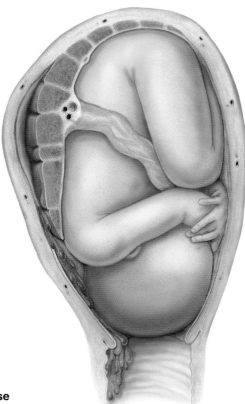

Umbilical cord prolapse

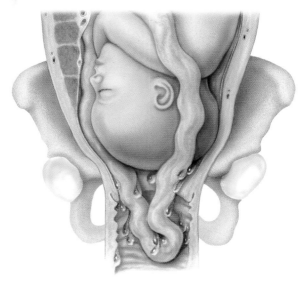

Fetal circulation

Because fetal lungs don't function until after birth, fetal blood is oxygenated by the placenta. Fetal circulation differs from neonatal circulation in that three shunts bypass the liver and the lungs and separate the systemic and pulmonary circulation.
These shunts include:
• ductus venosus—circulatory pathway that allows blood to bypass the liver
• foramen ovale—opening in the interstitial septum that directs blood from the right atrium to the left atrium
• ductus arteriosus—tubular connection that shunts blood away from the pulmonary circulation.
   Because of these shunts, the umbilical vein carries oxygenated blood and the umbilical arteries carry deoxygenated blood.

To head

To arm

Superior vena cava

Foramen ovale

Right atrium

Right lung

Inferior vena cava

Portal vein

Umbilical vein

From placenta

To placenta

Umbilical arteries

Aorta

Ductus arteriosus

Left atrium

Left lung

Aorta

Liver

Ductus venosus

To leg

membrane continues to produce more fluid that surrounds and protects the fetus until it's delivered.

Color-coded

The amniotic fluid that's lost after the rupture of the membranes should be odorless and clear. Colored fluid usually indicates a problem. Yellow fluid indicates that the amniotic fluid is bilirubin-stained from the breakdown of red blood cells, which may be caused by blood incompatibility. Green fluid indicates meconium staining, possibly from a breech presentation or fetal anoxia, and needs immediate evaluation.

Rupture or be ruptured

If a woman's membranes haven't ruptured spontaneously before the transition phase of the first stage of labor, they may rupture when the cervix becomes fully dilated at 10 cm or amniotomy may be performed. Membrane rupture shortens the duration of labor and aids in the dilation of the cervix. Membranes that remain intact delay full dilation and lengthen the duration of labor because the amniotic fluid cushions the pressure of the fetal head against the cervix, preventing the contractions from exerting their full impact.

A little premature

Premature rupture of membranes (rupture that occurs more than 24 hours before labor begins) is associated with a risk of infection and umbilical cord prolapse.

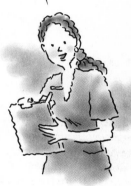

Intact membranes inhibit dilation of the cervix.

Stages of labor

Labor is typically divided into four stages:

☝ The first stage, when effacement and dilation occur, begins with the onset of true uterine contractions and ends when the cervix is fully dilated.

✌ The second stage, which encompasses the actual birth, begins when the cervix is fully dilated and ends with the delivery of the fetus.

🤟 The third stage, also called the *placental stage*, begins immediately after the neonate is delivered and ends when the placenta is delivered.

🖐 The fourth stage begins after delivery of the placenta. During this stage, homeostasis is reestablished.

First stage

The first stage of labor begins with the onset of contractions and ends when the cervix is dilated to 10 cm (full dilation). It's divided into three phases: latent, active, and transition.

Latent phase

The latent phase of labor begins with the onset of regular contractions. Usually, the contractions during this phase are mild. They last about 20 to 40 seconds and recur every 5 to 30 minutes. Initially, the contractions may vary in intensity and duration, but they become consistent within a few hours.

Waiting for dilation

The latent phase lasts about 6 hours in the primipara and 4½ hours in the multipara and ends when rapid cervical dilation begins. During this phase, the cervix dilates from 0 to 3 cm and becomes fully effaced; however, there's minimal fetal descent through the pelvis. The contractions usually cause little discomfort if the woman remains relaxed and continues to walk around.

Lasting longer than expected?

Premature analgesia administration, poor fetal position, cephalo-pelvic disproportion, and a cervix that hasn't softened sufficiently may increase the duration of the latent phase.

Keep her calm, moving, or voiding

Nursing care during the latent phase is mainly supportive. Provide the woman with a calm environment and psychological support for the conflicting emotions—such as excitement, anxiety and, possibly, depression—that she's experiencing. Give a clear liquid diet or ice chips as tolerated, and encourage the woman to move and empty her bladder frequently. Be sure to involve the woman's partner or support person in her care as much as possible.

Technical stuff

Obtain the required blood sample and urine specimen, monitor the woman's vital signs, monitor FHR, and explain and initiate electronic monitoring or intermittent auscultation of fetal heart tones, as ordered.

It's all about timing and intensity

During the latent phase, start timing the frequency and length of the contractions and assessing their intensity. To time the frequency of contractions, gently rest a hand on the woman's abdomen at the fundus of the uterus. Count from the beginning of one contrac-

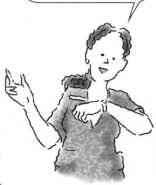

During the latent phase, start timing the frequency and length of contractions. OK? Ready, set go!

tion to the beginning of the next. Begin timing at the start of the gradual tensing and upward rising of the fundus (initially, these sensations may not be felt by the woman); end timing when the uterus has fully relaxed.

Do you feel a nose, a chin, or a forehead?

The intensity of contractions can be determined by assessing the uterus. With mild contractions, the uterus is minimally tense. It may be easily indented with a fingertip and feel similar to pressing on the tip of the nose. With moderate contractions, the uterus feels firmer. It can't be indented with a finger, and it feels similar to pressing on the chin. With strong contractions, the uterus feels extremely hard. It can't be indented—even with firm pressure—and it feels similar to pressing on the forehead.

Active phase

During the active phase of labor, the release of show increases and the membranes may rupture spontaneously. The contractions are stronger, each lasting about 40 to 60 seconds and recurring about every 3 to 5 minutes. The increased strength of the contractions commonly causes pain. Cervical dilation occurs more rapidly, increasing from about 3 to 7 cm, and the fetus begins to descend through the pelvis at an increased rate.

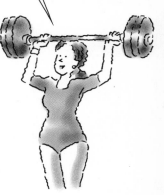

The strength of contractions increases in the active phase of labor.

Whole lot of changing going on

The active phase is an emotionally charged time for the woman. She may be feeling excitement as well as fear. The woman also undergoes many systemic changes. (See *Systemic changes in the active phase of labor*, page 318.)

How long must this go on?

The active phase of labor lasts about 3 hours in a primipara and 2 hours in a multipara. If analgesics are given at this time, they won't slow labor. Poor fetal position and a full bladder may prolong this phase.

Shower her with comfort and support

Nursing care during the active phase focuses on the psychological status of the woman as well as her physical care. Expect the woman to have mood swings and difficulty coping. Offer support, and encourage the woman to use proper breathing techniques. In addition, continue to involve the woman's partner or labor support person in her care. Placing the woman in an upright or side-lying position may provide additional comfort.

Other nursing measures that may be necessary include:
• monitoring I.V. fluids, as ordered, to maintain fluid balance
• monitoring intake and output

Systemic changes in the active phase of labor

This chart shows the systemic changes that occur during the active phase of labor.

System	Change
Cardiovascular	• Increased blood pressure • Increased cardiac output • Supine hypotension
Respiratory	• Increased oxygen consumption • Increased rate • Possible hyperventilation leading to respiratory alkalosis, hypoxia, and hypercapnia (if breathing isn't controlled)
Neurologic	• Increased pain threshold and sedation caused by endogenous endorphins • Anesthetized perineal tissues caused by constant intense pressure on nerve endings
GI	• Dehydration • Decreased motility • Slow absorption of solid food • Nausea • Diarrhea
Musculoskeletal	• Diaphoresis • Fatigue • Backache • Joint pain • Leg cramps
Endocrine	• Decreased progesterone level • Increased estrogen level • Increased prostaglandin level • Increased oxytocin level • Increased metabolism • Decreased blood glucose
Renal	• Difficulty voiding • Proteinuria (1+ normal)

• monitoring vital signs
• auscultating FHR every 30 minutes for a low-risk patient and every 15 minutes for a high-risk patient
• performing perineal care frequently to reduce the risk of infection, especially after each voiding and bowel movement.

Transition phase

During the transition phase, contractions reach maximum intensity. They each last 60 to 90 seconds, and they occur every 2 to 3 minutes. The cervix dilates from about 7 to 10 cm to become fully dilated and effaced. If the membranes aren't already ruptured, they usually rupture when the woman is 10 cm dilated and the remainder of the mucus plug is expelled from the cervix.

The transition phase peaks when cervical dilation slows slightly at 9 cm. This slowdown signifies the end of the first stage of labor. For multiparas, birth may be imminent at this time.

What she's feeling

When in the transition phase, the woman may experience intense pain or discomfort as well as nausea and vomiting. She may also experience intense mood swings and feelings of anxiety, panic, irritability, and loss of control because of the intensity and duration of contractions.

What you're doing

Nursing care during the transition phase includes monitoring vital signs and FHR, encouraging proper breathing techniques, and administering medications, as ordered. Arrange for a nurse to be with the woman at all times because there's a possibility that birth is imminent. Make sure to provide emotional support to the woman and her partner or support person during this time.

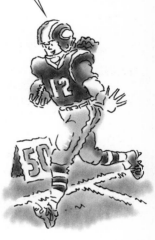

Contractions reach maximum intensity during the transition phase of labor. I'm at maximum intensity ALL the time.

Second stage

The second stage of labor starts with full dilation and effacement of the cervix and ends with the delivery of the neonate. It lasts about 1 to 3 hours for the primipara and 30 to 60 minutes for the multipara. During the second stage, the frequency of the contractions slows to about one every 3 to 4 minutes; however, they continue to last 60 to 90 seconds and are accompanied by the uncontrollable urge to push or bear down. The decreased frequency of the contractions gives the woman a chance to rest.

Vigilance!

During the second stage of labor (including pushing), auscultate FHR every 15 minutes for a low-risk patient and every 5 minutes for a high-risk patient.

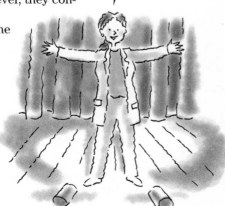

All the world's a stage, and although the second stage of labor ends with delivery of the neonate, there are still two stages yet to go!

Movin' out

Whereas the previous stage of labor primarily involved thinning and opening of the uterus, the second stage involves moving the fetus through the birth canal and out of the body.

As the uterine contractions work to accomplish this movement, the fetus pushes on the internal side of the perineum, causing the perineum to bulge and become tense. The fetal scalp becomes visible at the opening to the vagina (called *crowning*). The vaginal opening changes from a slit to an oval and then to a circle. The circular opening then gradually increases in size to allow the fetus's head to emerge. The combination of involuntary uterine contractions and the mother pushing with her abdominal muscles helps the fetus proceed through the cardinal movements of labor and expel from the body.

The physiologic changes that began in the first stage of labor continue throughout the second stage. In addition, the mother's oxytocin level increases, which helps to intensify the contractions.

Cardinal movements of labor

The cardinal movements of labor are fetal position changes that occur during the second stage of labor. They help the fetus pass through the birth canal. These movements are necessary because of the size of the fetal head in relation to the irregularly shaped pelvis. Specific, deliberate, and precise, the various movements allow the smallest diameter of the fetus to pass through the corresponding diameter of the woman's pelvis. (See *Cardinal movements of labor*.)

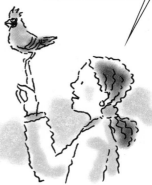

Cardinal movements are fetal position changes that occur during the second stage of labor and help the fetus pass through the birth canal.

Descent

Descent, the first of the cardinal movements, is the downward movement of the fetus. It's determined when the biparietal diameter of the head passes the ischial spines and moves into the pelvic inlet.

May the forces be with you

Descent progresses intermittently with contractions and occurs because of several forces:
• direct pressure on the fetus by the contracting uterine fundus
• pressure of the amniotic fluid
• contraction of the abdominal muscles (fetal pressure on the mother's sacral nerves causes her to experience an uncontrollable need to push)
• extension and straightening of the fetal body.

Cardinal movements of labor

These illustrations show the fetal movements that occur during the cardinal movements of labor.

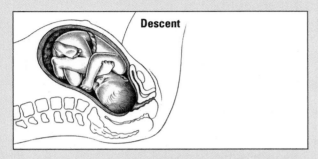

Descent

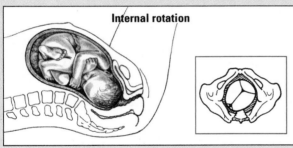

Internal rotation

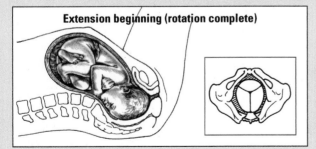

Extension beginning (rotation complete)

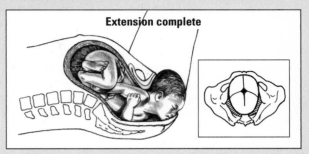

Extension complete

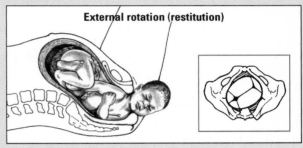

External rotation (restitution)

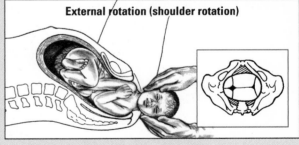

External rotation (shoulder rotation)

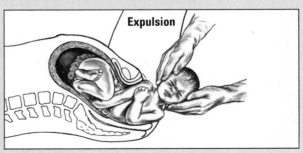

Expulsion

Making contact

Full descent is accomplished when the fetal head passes beyond the dilated cervix and contacts the posterior vaginal floor.

Flexion

Flexion, the second of the cardinal movements, occurs during descent. It's caused by the resistance of the fetal head against the pelvic floor. The combined pressure from this resistance and uterine and abdominal muscle contractions forces the head of the fetus to bend forward so that the chin is pressed to the chest. This allows the smallest diameter of the fetal head to descend through the pelvis.

A different angle

Flexion causes the presenting diameter to change from occipitofrontal (nasal bridge to the posterior fontanel) to suboccipitobregmatic (posterior fontanel to subocciput) in an occiput anterior position. If the fetus is an occiput posterior position, flexion is incomplete and the fetus has a larger presenting diameter, which can prolong labor.

Internal rotation

The fetal head typically enters the pelvis with its anteroposterior head diameter in a transverse (right to left) position. This position is beneficial when entering the pelvis because the diameter at the pelvic inlet is widest from right to left. However, if the head remains in the transverse position, the shoulders are in a position where they're too wide to pass through the pelvic inlet.

Shifting toward the same plane

To allow the shoulders to pass through the pelvic inlet, the fetal head rotates about 45 degrees as it meets the resistance of the pelvic floor. With the head rotated, the anteroposterior diameter of the head is in the anteroposterior plane of the pelvis (front to back), which places the widest part of the shoulders in line with the widest part of the pelvic inlet and outlet. At this point, the face of the fetus is usually against the woman's back and the back of the fetal head is against the front of the woman's pelvis.

Extension

Extension occurs after the internal rotation is complete. As the head passes through the pelvis, the occiput emerges from the vagina and the back of the neck stops under the symphysis pubis (pubic arch). Further descent is temporarily halted because the fetus's shoulders are too wide to pass through the pelvis or under the pubic arch.

Pivotal movements

With the back of the fetal neck resting against the pubic arch, the arch acts as a pivot. The upward resistance from the pelvic floor causes the head to extend. As this occurs, the brow, nose, mouth, and chin are born.

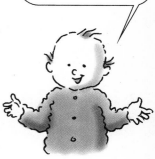

I turned out all right. I turned to fit through the pelvic inlet, then turned again to fit through the pelvic outlet and under the pubic arch.

External rotation

External rotation (also called *restitution*) is necessary because the shoulders, which previously turned to fit through the pelvic inlet, must now turn again to fit through the pelvic outlet and under the pubic arch.

Return the fetus to the transverse position...

After the head is born, the face, which is facing down after the completion of extension, is turned to face one of the mother's inner thighs. The head rotates about 45 degrees, returning the anteroposterior head diameter to the transverse (right to left) position assumed during descent.

...and prepare for shoulder delivery

The anterior shoulder (closest to the front of the mother) is delivered first with the possible assistance of downward flexion on the head. After the anterior shoulder is delivered, a slight upward flexion may be necessary to deliver the posterior shoulder.

Weighing in

During external rotation, a neonate who weighs more than 4.5 kg (9.9 lb) has a greater likelihood of experiencing shoulder dystocia than one who weighs less. Shoulder dystocia occurs when lack of room for passage causes the shoulders to stop at the pelvic outlet. Commonly, shoulder dystocia is resolved by sharply flexing the maternal thighs against the maternal abdomen. This movement reduces the angle between the sacrum and the spine and allows the shoulders to pass through; however, the neonate may sustain some injury to the brachial plexus.

Look Ma! I've been expulsed! Aren't I wonderful?!

Expulsion

After delivery of the shoulders, the remainder of the body is delivered quickly and easily. Termed *expulsion*, this step signifies the end of the second stage of labor.

Third stage

The third stage of labor, also called the *placental stage*, occurs after delivery of the neonate and ends with the delivery of the placenta. It consists of two phases: placental separation and placental expulsion. This stage of labor is important because a placenta that remains in place may cause hemorrhage, shock, infection, or even death.

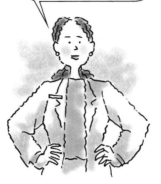

The placenta may cause hemorrhage, shock, infection, or death if it isn't delivered.

From round to discoid

After the neonate has been delivered, uterine contractions commonly stop for several minutes. During this time, the uterus is a round mass located below the level of the umbilicus that feels firm to the touch. When contractions resume, the uterus takes on a discoid shape until the placenta has separated from the uterus.

Thirty minutes or less

The duration of the third stage varies widely. It may last from several minutes to up to 30 minutes.

Placental separation

Separation of the placenta from the uterus occurs after the uterus resumes contractions. Uterine contractions continue to occur in the wavelike pattern that they assumed throughout the other stages of labor; however, in the other stages, the fetus exerted pressure on the placenta during contractions, which prevented the placenta from separating prematurely. When the fetus is no longer in the uterus, the uterine walls contract on an almost empty space. Nothing exerts reverse pressure on the placenta. As a result, the placenta folds and begins to separate from the uterine wall. This separation causes bleeding that further pushes the placenta away from the uterine wall, ultimately causing the placenta to fall to the upper vagina or lower uterine segment.

Ready to roll

Signs that the placenta has separated and is ready to be delivered include:
- absence of cord pulse
- lengthening of the umbilical cord
- sudden gush of vaginal blood
- change in the shape of the uterus.

Separating from the center...

Approximately 80% of all separated placentas are Schultze's placentas. A Schultze's placenta starts to separate at the center and folds onto itself. It delivers with the fetal surface exposed and appears shiny and glistening from the fetal membranes.

...or the edge

A Duncan placenta separates at the edges, then slides down the surface of the uterus and delivers with the maternal surface exposed. It appears red, raw, and irregular because of the ridges that separate the blood collection spaces.

Placental expulsion

Natural bearing down by the mother or gentle pressure on the fundus of the contracting uterus (Credé's maneuver) aids in the delivery of the placenta. To avoid possible eversion (turning inside out) of the uterus, which can result in gross hemorrhage, never exert pressure on the uterus when it isn't contracted. Manual removal of the placenta may be indicated if it doesn't deliver spontaneously.

Check it out

After delivery, examine the placenta to make sure it's intact and normal in appearance and weight. This helps determine whether any has been retained in the uterus. The placenta is usually one sixth the weight of the infant.

Additional layers

An outer area of decidua (the lining of the uterus) is expelled at the same time as the placenta. The remainder of the decidua separates into two layers:

the superficial layer that's shed in the lochia during the postpartum period

the basal layer that remains in the uterus to regenerate new endothelium.

Blood volume matters

Normal bleeding occurs until the uterus contracts with enough force to seal the blood collection spaces. A blood loss of 300 to 500 ml should be expected. Blood loss exceeding 500 ml may indicate a cervical tear or a problem at the episiotomy site. It may also indicate that the uterus isn't contracting properly because of retained placenta or a full bladder.

Commonly, after the placenta is delivered, the mother is given I.V. oxytocin (Pitocin) or I.M. methylergonovine (Methergine) to increase uterine contractions and minimize bleeding; however, these drugs shouldn't be given if the mother's blood pressure is increased because they cause vasoconstriction and hypertension.

Memory jogger

To help remember which type of placenta is which, think "Shiny Schultze's" and "Dirty Duncan." The Schultze's placenta is shiny from the fetal membrane. The Duncan placenta exposes the maternal side and appears red and dirty with an irregular surface.

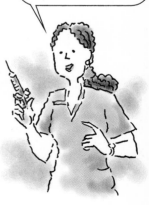

Not to needle you, but remember: Neither Pitocin nor Methergine should be administered if the mother's blood pressure is increased because they can cause vasodilation and hypertension.

Fourth stage

The fourth stage of labor occurs immediately after the delivery of the placenta. It usually lasts for about 1 to 4 hours, and it initiates the postpartum period. During this stage, the woman should be monitored closely because her body has just undergone many changes.

Risks associated with the fourth stage of labor include hemorrhage, bladder distention, and venous thrombosis. Oxygen, type O-negative blood or blood tested for compatibility, and I.V. fluids must be available for 2 to 3 hours after delivery.

Inspect and repair

Initially, the cervix and vagina are inspected to check for and repair lacerations that may have occurred during birth. If an episiotomy was performed, the incision is sutured. Keep in mind that a woman who delivered without the aid of an anesthetic requires a local anesthetic for this procedure; a woman who received regional or local anesthesia during the birth probably won't need additional medication. When suturing is complete, the woman's legs should be lowered from the stirrups. Make sure the legs are lowered simultaneously to prevent back injury.

Monitoring mommy

Monitor the woman's vital signs every 15 minutes for a minimum of 1 hour, then as ordered. Expect the woman's pulse, respirations, and blood pressure to be slightly increased at this time because of the birth process, excitement, and oxytocin administration. In addition, the woman may experience a normal chill and shaking sensation shortly after the birth. This is common and may be caused by excess epinephrine production during labor or the sudden release of pressure on the pelvic nerves.

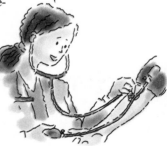

After delivery, the woman's pulse, respirations, and blood pressure will be slightly increased.

The incredible shrinking uterus

After delivery, the uterus gradually decreases in size and descends into its prepregnancy position in the pelvis—a process known as *involution*. To evaluate this process, palpate the uterine fundus and determine uterine size, degree of firmness, and rate of descent (which is measured in fingerbreadths above or below the umbilicus). Involution normally begins immediately after delivery, when the firmly contracted uterus lies almost at the umbilicus. If the woman is breast-feeding, the release of natural oxytocics should help to maintain or stimulate contraction of the uterus. If it doesn't remain contracted, gently massage the uterus or administer medications as ordered.

Void to avoid interference

Encourage the woman to void because a full bladder interferes with uterine contractions that work to compress the open blood vessels at the placental site. If these blood vessels are allowed to bleed freely, hemorrhage may occur. Observe the amount, color, and consistency of the lochia and watch for its absence, which may indicate that a clot is blocking the cervical os. Sudden heavy bleeding could result if a change of position dislodges the clot.

Clot watch

Pregnant and postpartum women have higher fibrinogen levels, which increase the possibility of clot formation. A woman has an additional risk of clot formation if she has varicose veins or a history of thrombophlebitis or if she had a cesarean delivery. Monitor closely for signs of venous thrombosis, especially if the duration of labor was abnormally long or if the woman was confined to bed for an extended period.

Ongoing support

Be sure to take the following steps as well:
• Offer emotional support as needed to the mother and her partner or labor support person.
• Perform perineal care, and apply a clean perineal pad as needed.
• Offer a regular diet as soon as the patient requests food (sometimes this request is made shortly after delivery).
• Encourage full ambulation as soon as possible.
• Provide comfort measures, such as a clean gown and a warmed blanket.

Nursing procedures

Nursing procedures performed during labor and delivery include uterine contraction palpation, continuous external electronic monitoring, internal electronic monitoring, intermittent FHR monitoring, and cervical examination.

Uterine contraction palpation

External uterine palpation can tell you the frequency, duration, and intensity of contractions and the relaxation time between them. The character of contractions varies with the stage of labor and the body's response to labor-inducing drugs, if administered. As labor advances, contractions become more intense, occur more often, and last longer. In some patients, labor progresses rapidly, preventing the patient from entering a health care facility.

To palpate uterine contractions:

• Review the patient's admission history to determine the onset, frequency, duration, and intensity of contractions. Also, note where contractions feel strongest or exert the most pressure.
• Describe the procedure to the patient.
• Assist the patient into a comfortable side-lying position.
• Drape the patient with a sheet.
• Place the palmar surface of your fingers on the uterine fundus, and palpate lightly to assess contractions. Each contraction has three phases: increment (rising), acme (peak), and decrement (letting down or ebbing).

How fast?

• To assess frequency, time the interval between the beginning of one contraction and the beginning of the next.

How long?

• To assess duration, time the period from when the uterus begins tightening until it begins relaxing.

How hard?

• To assess intensity, press your fingertips into the uterine fundus when the uterus tightens. During mild contractions, the fundus indents easily; during moderate contractions, the fundus indents less easily; during strong contractions, the fundus resists indenting.
• Determine how the patient copes with discomfort by assessing her breathing and relaxation techniques.
• Assess contractions in low-risk patients every 30 minutes in the latent phase, every 15 to 30 minutes in the active phase, and every 15 minutes in the transition phase. More frequent assessments are required for high-risk patients. High-risk fetal status assessments should also occur every 30 minutes during the latent phase, every 15 minutes during the active phase, and every 5 minutes in the second stage. (See *Contraction without relaxation.*)

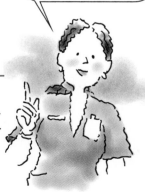

Continuous external fetal monitoring is a noninvasive way to assess contractions and fetal heart rate.

Continuous external electronic monitoring

Continuous external electronic monitoring is an indirect, noninvasive procedure. Two devices, an ultrasound transducer and a tocotransducer, are placed on the mother's abdomen to evaluate fetal well-being and uterine contractions during labor. These devices are held in place with an elastic stockinette or by using plastic or soft straps.

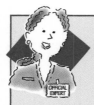

Advice from the experts

Contraction without relaxation

If any contraction lasts longer than 90 seconds and isn't followed by uterine muscle relaxation, or if the relaxation period is less than 1 minute between contractions, notify the doctor. This may indicate hyperstimulation of the uterus or tetanic contractions. When the uterus doesn't relax, or the relaxation period is less than 1 minute, uteroplacental blood flow is interrupted, which can lead to fetal hypoxia and fetal distress.

If you determine that the patient's contractions last longer than 90 seconds or if the relaxation period is less than 1 minute, follow these steps:

• Discontinue the oxytocin infusion to stop uterine stimulations (if the patient is receiving oxytocin).
• Make sure that the patient is lying on her left side; this increases uteroplacental perfusion.
• Administer oxygen via face mask to increase fetal oxygenation.
• Notify the doctor or nurse-midwife immediately.

Two readings, one printout

The ultrasound transducer transmits high-frequency sound waves aimed at the fetal heart. The tocotransducer, in turn, responds to the pressure exerted by uterine contractions and simultaneously records the duration and frequency of the contractions. (See *Applying continuous external monitoring devices*, page 330.) The monitoring apparatus traces FHR and uterine contraction data onto the same printout paper.

Continuous external fetal monitoring is used for most women, especially those with a high-risk pregnancy or oxytocin-induced labor.

Monitoring FHR and uterine contractions

Here are the steps you should take when monitoring FHR and uterine contractions:
• Explain the procedure to the patient, and make sure that she has signed a consent form, if required by your facility.
• Label the monitoring strip with, or enter into the computer, the patient's identification number or birth date, her name, the date, maternal vital signs and position, the paper speed, and the number of the strip paper.
• Assist the patient to the semi-Fowler or left-lateral position with her abdomen exposed, and palpate the abdomen to locate the fundus—the area of greatest muscle density in the uterus.

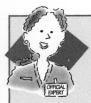

Advice from the experts

Applying continuous external monitoring devices

To ensure clear tracings that define fetal status and labor progress, be sure to precisely position continuous external monitoring devices. These devices include an ultrasound transducer and a tocotransducer.

Fetal heart monitor

Palpate the uterus to locate the fetus's back, and place the ultrasound transducer, which reads the fetal heart rate, over the site where the fetal heartbeat sounds the loudest. Then tighten the belt. Use the fetal heart tracing on the monitor strip to confirm the transducer's position.

Tocotransducer

A tocotransducer records uterine motion during contractions. Place the tocotransducer over the uterine fundus where it contracts, either midline or slightly to one side. Place your hand on the fundus, and palpate a contraction to verify proper placement. Secure the tocotransducer's belt; then adjust the pen set so that the baseline values read between 5 and 15 mm Hg on the monitor strip.

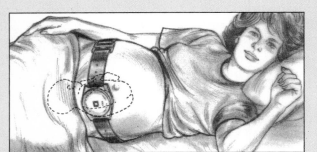

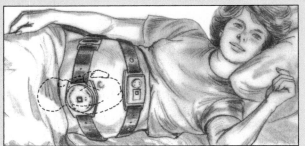

Buckle up and get tracing

    • Using transducer straps or a stockinette binder, secure the tocotransducer over the fundus.
    • Adjust the pen set tracer controls so that the baseline values read between 5 and 15 mm Hg on the monitor strip or as indicated by the model.

Goo for good contact

    • Apply conduction gel to the ultrasound transducer, and use Leopold's maneuvers to palpate the fetal back, through which fetal heart tones resound most audibly.
    • Start the monitor, and apply the ultrasound transducer directly over the site having the strongest heart tones.
    • Activate the control that begins the printout.
    • Observe the tracings to identify the frequency and duration of uterine contractions, but palpate the uterus to determine the intensity of the contractions.

Compare and contract

- Note the baseline FHR, and assess periodic accelerations or decelerations from the baseline. Compare the FHR patterns with those of the uterine contractions.
- Move the tocotransducer and the ultrasound transducer to accommodate changes in maternal or fetal position. Readjust both transducers every hour, and assess the patient's skin for reddened areas caused by the pressure of the monitoring device.
- Clean the ultrasound transducer periodically with a damp cloth to remove dried conduction gel, and apply fresh gel as necessary.
- If the patient reports discomfort in the position that provides the clearest signal, try to obtain a satisfactory 5- or 10-minute tracing with the patient in this position before assisting her to a more comfortable position.

Internal electronic monitoring

Internal monitoring, also called *direct monitoring*, is an invasive procedure that uses a spiral electrode attached to the presenting fetal part (usually the scalp). This electrode detects the fetal heartbeat and transmits it to the monitor, which converts the signals to a fetal electrocardiogram (ECG) waveform. This helps assess fetal response to uterine contractions, measures intrauterine pressure, tracks labor progress, and allows evaluation of short- and long-term FHR variability.

Without a tracing

Internal monitoring is indicated for high-risk pregnancies. However, it can be performed only if the amniotic sac has ruptured, the cervix is dilated at least 2 cm, and the presenting part of the fetus is at at least the –1 station. Maternal complications of internal fetal monitoring may include uterine perforation and intrauterine infections. Fetal complications may include abscess, hematoma, and infection.

An intrauterine pressure catheter may be used if external uterine monitoring doesn't provide satisfactory information. It may also be necessary in high-risk pregnancies or if the patient is obese.

Monitoring uterine contractions

Follow these steps when monitoring uterine contractions:
- Make sure that the patient understands the procedure and that she signs a consent form, if required by your facility.
- Label the printout paper with the patient's identification number or name, her birth date, the date, the paper speed, and the number on the monitor strip.

- Help the patient into a lithotomy position.

Cable connection

- Attach the connection cable to the uterine activity outlet on the monitor, and zero the catheter with a gauge on the distal end of the catheter.
- Cover the patient's perineum with a sterile drape, and clean the perineum with antiseptic solution, according to your facility's policy.
- The doctor will perform a vaginal examination, insert the catheter into the uterine cavity until it advances to the black line, and secure the catheter with hypoallergenic tape to the patient's inner thigh.

Strip tips

- You'll need to observe the monitoring strip to verify proper placement and a clear tracing. Periodically evaluate the strip to determine the amount of pressure exerted with each contraction. Note all such data on the strip and the patient's medical record. (See *Applying an internal electronic fetal monitor.*)

Advice from the experts

Applying an internal electronic fetal monitor

During internal electronic fetal monitoring, a spiral electrode monitors the fetal heart rate (FHR) and an internal catheter monitors uterine contractions.

Monitoring FHR
The spiral electrode is inserted after a cervical examination that determines the position of the fetus. As shown below, the electrode is attached to the presenting fetal part, usually the scalp or buttocks.

Monitoring uterine contractions
The intrauterine catheter is inserted up to a premarked level on the tubing and then connected to a monitor that interprets uterine contraction pressures.

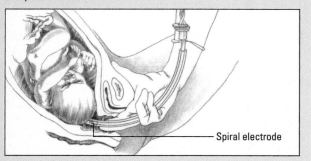

Spiral electrode

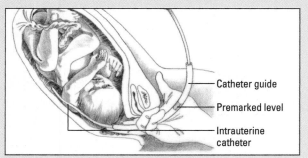

Catheter guide

Premarked level

Intrauterine catheter

Monitoring FHR

Follow these steps when monitoring FHR:
• Help the patient into the lithotomy position so the practitioner can perform a cervical examination.
• After identifying the presenting fetal part and level of descent, the practitioner applies a fetal scalp electrode to the fetal scalp.
• Attach the internal fetal scalp electrode to a cable from the monitor. Then secure the electrode to the mother's body.
• Finally, observe the FHR. (See *Reading a fetal monitor strip*.)

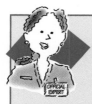

Advice from the experts

Reading a fetal monitor strip

Presented in two parallel recordings, the fetal monitor strip records the fetal heart rate (FHR) in beats per minute in the top recording and uterine activity (UA) in millimeters of mercury (mm Hg) in the bottom recording. You can obtain information on fetal status and labor progress by reading the strips horizontally and vertically.

Reading horizontally on the FHR or the UA strip, each small block represents 10 seconds. Six consecutive small blocks, separated by a dark vertical line, represent 1 minute. Reading

vertically on the FHR strip, each block represents an amplitude of 10 beats/minute. Reading vertically on the UA strip, each block represents 5 mm Hg of pressure.

Assess the baseline FHR (the "resting" heart rate) between uterine contractions when fetal movement diminishes. This baseline FHR (normal range: 120 to 160 beats/minute) pattern serves as a reference for subsequent FHR tracings produced during contractions.

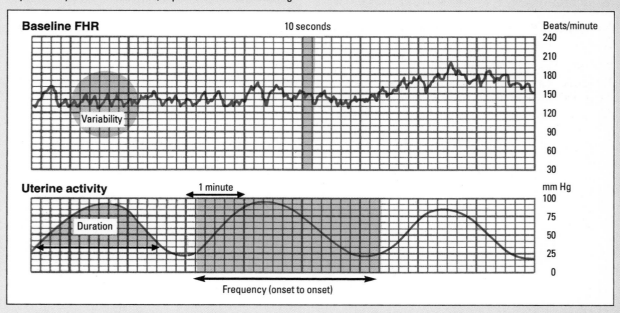

Check and compare

- Check the baseline FHR, and assess periodic accelerations or decelerations from the baseline. Compare the FHR pattern with the uterine contraction pattern. Note the interval between the onset of deceleration and uterine contractions, the interval between the lowest level of an FHR deceleration and the peak of a uterine contraction, and the range of FHR deceleration.
- Check for FHR variability, which is a measure of fetal oxygen reserve and neurologic integrity and stability. (See *Understanding fetal heart rate variability.*)
- Interpret FHR and uterine contractions at regular intervals. Guidelines of the Association of Women's Health, Obstetric, and Neonatal Nurses specify that high-risk patients need continuous FHR monitoring, whereas low-risk patients should have FHR auscultated every 30 minutes after a contraction during the first stage of labor and every 15 minutes after a contraction during the second stage. First, determine the baseline FHR within 10 beats/minute; then assess the degree of baseline variability. Identify changes such as decelerations (early late, variable, or mixed) and nonperiodic changes such as a sinusoidal pattern. (See *Identifying baseline FHR irregularities.*) If vaginal delivery isn't imminent (within 30 minutes) and fetal distress patterns are identified, cesarean birth is necessary.

Understanding fetal heart rate variability

Fetal heart rate (FHR) is the fluctuation of the baseline FHR of at least 2 cycles per minute. This fluctuation represents the interaction between the sympathetic and parasympathetic nervous systems of the fetus. The constant interactions between these systems results in a moment-to-moment change in the FHR. It signals that both nervous systems are working. This interaction can be termed as *absent, minimal, moderate,* or *marked* and is determined by the beats per minute (bpm).

Variability	Amplitude range
Absent	Undetectable
Minimal	> undetectable ≤ 5 bpm
Moderate	6 to 25 bpm
Marked	> 25 bpm

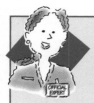

Advice from the experts

Identifying baseline FHR irregularities

When monitoring fetal heart rate (FHR), you need to be familiar with irregularities that may occur, their possible causes, and nursing interventions to take. Here's a guide to these irregularities.

Irregularity	Possible causes	Clinical significance	Nursing interventions
Baseline tachycardia FHR > 160 beats/minute	• Early fetal hypoxia • Maternal fever • Parasympathetic agents, such as atropine and scopolamine • Beta-adrenergics, such as ritodrine and terbutaline • Amnionitis (inflammation of inner layer of fetal membrane, or amnion) • Maternal hyperthyroidism • Fetal anemia • Fetal heart failure • Fetal arrhythmias	Persistent tachycardia without periodic changes doesn't usually adversely affect fetal well-being, especially when associated with maternal fever. However, tachycardia is an ominous sign when associated with late decelerations, severe variable decelerations, or lack of variability.	• Intervene to alleviate the cause of fetal distress, and provide supplemental oxygen as ordered. Also administer I.V. fluids as prescribed. • Discontinue oxytocin infusion to reduce uterine activity. • Turn the patient onto her left side and elevate her legs. • Continue to observe FHR. • Document interventions and outcomes. • Notify the practitioner; further medical intervention may be necessary.
Baseline bradycardia FHR < 160 beats/minute	• Late fetal hypoxia • Beta-adrenergic blockers, such as propranolol, and anesthetics • Maternal hypotension • Prolonged umbilical cord compression • Fetal congenital heart block	Bradycardia with good variability and no periodic changes doesn't signal fetal distress if FHR remains higher than 80 beats/minute. However, bradycardia caused by hypoxia and acidosis is an ominous sign when associated with loss of variability and late decelerations.	• Intervene to correct the cause of fetal distress. Administer supplemental oxygen as ordered. Start an I.V. line and administer fluids as prescribed. • Discontinue oxytocin infusion to reduce uterine activity. • Turn the patient onto her left side and elevate her legs. • Continue observing FHR. • Document interventions and outcomes. • Notify the practitioner; further medical intervention may be necessary.

(continued)

Identifying baseline FHR irregularities *(continued)*

Irregularity	Possible causes	Clinical significance	Nursing interventions
Early decelerations beats/minute 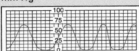 mm Hg 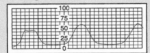	• Fetal head compression	Early decelerations are benign, indicating fetal head compression at dilation of 4 to 7 cm.	• Reassure the patient that the fetus isn't at risk. • Observe FHR. • Document the frequency of decelerations.
Late decelerations beats/minute 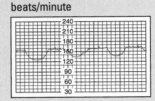 mm Hg 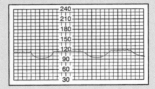	• Uteroplacental circulatory insufficiency (placental hypoperfusion) caused by decreased intervillous blood flow during contractions or a structural placental defect such as abruptio placentae • Uterine hyperactivity caused by excessive oxytocin infusion • Maternal hypotension • Maternal supine hypotension	Late decelerations indicate uteroplacental circulatory insufficiency and may lead to fetal hypoxia and acidosis if the underlying cause isn't corrected.	• Turn the patient onto her left side to increase placental perfusion and decrease contraction frequency. • Increase the I.V. fluid rate to boost intravascular volume and placental perfusion, as prescribed. • Administer oxygen by mask to increase fetal oxygenation as ordered. • Assess for signs of the underlying cause, such as hypotension or uterine tachysystole. • Take other appropriate measures such as discontinuing oxytocin as prescribed. • Document interventions and outcomes. • Notify the practitioner; further medical intervention may be necessary.

Identifying baseline FHR irregularities (continued)

Irregularity	Possible causes	Clinical significance	Nursing interventions
Variable decelerations beats/minute 240 210 180 150 120 90 60 30 mm Hg 100 75 50 25 0	• Umbilical cord compression causing decreased fetal oxygen perfusion	Variable decelerations are the most common deceleration pattern in labor because of contractions and fetal movement.	• Help the patient change position. No other intervention is necessary unless you detect fetal distress. • Assure the patient that the fetus tolerates cord compression well. Explain that cord compression affects the fetus the same way that breath-holding affects her. • Assess the deceleration pattern for reassuring signs: a baseline FHR that isn't increasing, short-term variability that isn't decreasing, abruptly beginning and ending decelerations, and decelerations lasting less than 50 seconds. If assessment doesn't reveal reassuring signs, notify the practitioner. • Start I.V. fluids and administer oxygen by mask at 10 to 12 L/minute, as prescribed. • Document interventions and outcomes. • Discontinue oxytocin infusion to decrease uterine activity.

Intermittent fetal heart rate monitoring

Intermittent FHR monitoring is the periodic auscultation of FHR by either fetoscope or a handheld Doppler device. Because the Doppler is more sensitive to fluctuations in FHR, it's more commonly used.

Up and about

Intermittent FHR monitoring allows the patient to ambulate during the first stage of labor. Because auscultation isn't done until after a contraction, this type of monitoring doesn't document how the fetus is responding to the stress of labor as well as continuous FHR monitoring does.

Because the Doppler is more sensitive to fluctuations in FHR, it's more commonly used in intermittent FHR monitoring.

Limited

Intermittent FHR monitoring can detect FHR baseline and rhythm as well as changes from the baseline; however, it can't detect variability in FHR as documented by electronic fetal monitoring.

Baseline

To establish the baseline FHR, auscultate FHR for a full minute after a contraction has ended. Then auscultate FHR for 30 seconds and multiply by two to get the full-minute rate. This type of auscultation can be done until a change in the patient's condition occurs, such as the onset of bleeding or rupture of amniotic fluid membranes. Assess FHR more frequently after the patient ambulates, after cervical examination, or after pain medication administration. Auscultate FHR every 30 minutes during labor for a low-risk patient and every 15 minutes for a high-risk patient.

Risky business

For patients whose pregnancy is considered high-risk—because of an increased risk for prenatal death, cerebral palsy, or neonatal encephalopathy and the use of oxygen for labor induction or augmentation—continuous electronic fetal monitoring is recommended.

Cervical examination

During first-stage labor, a cervical examination may be done to assess cervical dilation and effacement; membrane status; and fetal presentation, position, and engagement. If the patient has excessive vaginal bleeding, which may signal placenta previa, cervical examination is contraindicated.

Only practitioners and specially trained nurses can perform cervical examinations. In early labor, perform the cervical examination between contractions, focusing on the extent of cervical dilation and effacement. At the end of first-stage labor, perform the examination during a contraction to focus on assessing fetal descent.

Get into position

Follow these steps during cervical examination:
- Explain the procedure to the patient.
- Ask the patient to empty her bladder.
- Use Leopold's maneuvers to identify the fetal presenting part and position.
- Help the patient into a lithotomy position. Place a linen-saver pad under the patient's buttocks.

• Put on sterile gloves, and lubricate the index and middle fingers of your examining hand with sterile water or sterile water-soluble lubricant. If the membranes are ruptured, use an antiseptic solution.

Breathe and release

• Ask the patient to relax by taking several deep breaths and slowly releasing the air.
• Insert your lubricated fingers (palmar surface down) into the vagina. Keep your uninserted fingers flexed to avoid the rectum.
• Palpate the cervix, noting its consistency. The cervix gradually softens throughout pregnancy, reaching a buttery consistency before labor begins. (See *Cervical effacement and dilation.*)
• After identifying the presenting fetal part and position and evaluating dilation, effacement, engagement, station, and membrane status, gently withdraw your fingers.

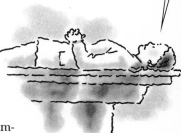

A cervical exam works best when the patient is relaxed. Take a moment to help her breathe deeply.

Cervical effacement and dilation

As labor advances, so do cervical effacement and dilation, promoting delivery. During effacement, the cervix shortens and its walls become thin, progressing from 0% effacement (palpable and thick) to 100% effacement (fully indistinct, or effaced, and paper thin). Full effacement obliterates the constrictive uterine neck to create a smooth, unobstructed passageway for the fetus.

At the same time, dilation occurs. This progressive widening of the cervical canal—from the upper internal cervical os to the lower external cervical os—advances from 0 to 10 cm. As the cervical canal opens, resistance decreases. This further eases fetal descent.

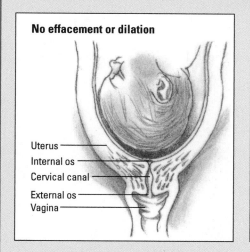

No effacement or dilation

Uterus
Internal os
Cervical canal
External os
Vagina

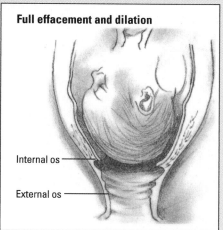

Full effacement and dilation

Internal os

External os

- Help the patient clean her perineum, and change the linen-saver pad, as necessary.

Flood zone

If the amniotic membrane ruptures during the examination, record FHR and time and describe the color, odor, and approximate amount of fluid. If FHR becomes unstable, determine fetal station and check for umbilical cord prolapse. After the membranes rupture, perform the cervical examination only when labor changes significantly to minimize the risk of introducing intrauterine infection.

Comfort and support issues

Labor and birth usually involve a significant amount of discomfort and can be emotionally draining for the woman. Comfort and support measures, such as prenatal education, planning, and the presence of a birthing partner or coach, can promote relaxation and decrease or eliminate the need for analgesia or anesthesia during labor and birth.

Expect the unexpected

Although it's helpful for the woman to make decisions about the issue of pain relief during labor before the actual event, advise the woman to keep an open mind. She should be aware of the other acceptable pain relief options available in case the situation changes during labor and birth. Sometimes, it may be necessary to take the decision regarding pain relief out of the woman's hands—for example, in cases of cesarean birth. No matter what method of pain relief is used, the woman should feel comfortable with it and it should be medically safe.

To provide comfort and support to the woman during labor and birth, you must understand sources of pain, pain perception and how it affects the woman's response to relief measures, cultural and familial influences on responses to pain, and different approaches to relieving pain.

Sources of pain

The pain experienced during labor and birth comes from several sources.

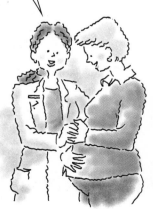

To decrease the need for analgesia or anesthesia during labor and birth, try using appropriate comfort and support measures.

Uterine contractions

The contraction of the uterine muscles is a prominent source of pain during labor and birth. Like the heart, stomach, and intestine, the uterus is part of an involuntary muscle group. Although most muscles of this type don't cause pain when they contract, uterine contractions do. During a contraction, the blood vessels constrict, which reduces the blood supply to the uterine and cervical cells, causing temporary hypoxia or anoxia and pain. As labor progresses and contractions increase in intensity and duration, the blood supply to the cells decreases further, thus increasing the pain.

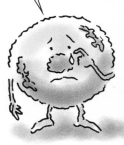

Hey! Where'd everybody go? When contractions increase in intensity and duration, the blood supply to cells decreases.

Dilation

Dilation and stretching of the cervix and lower uterine segment also cause pain during labor. Similar to the intestinal pain caused by accumulated gas in the bowel, this pain increases as the dilation increases.

Distention

Distention of the vagina and perineum to accommodate passage of the fetal head also causes pain during labor. As the fetal head is delivered, an episiotomy or possible tearing of the perineum intensifies this pain.

Pressure on adjacent organs

Another source of pain during labor is the pressure of the presenting part on the adjacent organs, such as the bladder, urethra, or lower colon. This varies depending on the position of the fetus.

Tension

Tension also contributes to pain during labor and birth. The woman's anticipation of pain and her inability to relax commonly cause tension or constriction of the voluntary muscles, including the muscles of the abdominal wall. Tense abdominal muscles increase the pressure on the uterus by preventing the uterus from rising with the contractions.

Pain perception

Pain is a subjective symptom that's unique to each individual who experiences it. What may be slight discomfort to one person may be intense, unbearable pain to another. Only the woman who's experiencing the pain can describe it or know its extent. When assessing the woman in labor, watch for signs of pain, such as increased respiratory and pulse rates, clenched fists, facial tenseness, and flushed or pale areas of the skin.

Under the influence of endorphins

Many factors influence how pain is perceived. A woman's pain threshold (the amount of pain perceived at a given time) may be influenced by her level of endorphins, the opiate-like substances that are produced by the body in response to pain.

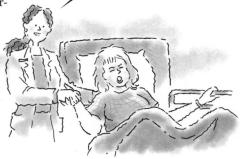

Ouch! Pain is subjective. Each patient's experience during labor and birth will be unique, just like her!

If you expect it, pain will come

Expectations of pain can also affect how pain is perceived. A woman who expects the pain of labor to be the most horrible pain she has ever experienced commonly becomes increasingly tense with each contraction and episode of pain, which can intensify her overall perception of the pain.

Too tired and weak for distractions

Fatigue, nutritional status, and sleep deprivation can also affect pain perception. A tired or malnourished individual has less energy than a rested one and can't focus on distraction strategies.

Mind games

Psychological factors, including fear, anxiety, body image, self-concept, and feelings of having no control over the situation, also affect a woman's pain perception. In addition, memories of previous childbirth experiences affect how the labor pains of the current pregnancy are perceived.

More pieces to the pain puzzle

Other factors that influence pain perception during labor include the intensity of labor, pelvic size and shape, and the interventions of caregivers (which can be a positive or negative influence on pain perception).

Cultural influences on pain

Individuals tend to react to pain in ways that are acceptable to their culture and family. Commonly learned through previous experience and conditioning, some women react to pain by becoming silent and avoiding interaction with other individuals; others may scream, verbalize their feelings of distress, or become verbally abusive to other individuals. Make sure that you determine the level of comfort each woman desires to receive and the manner in which she chooses to express her discomfort. (See *How certain cultures handle pain.*)

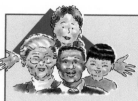

Bridging the gap

How certain cultures handle pain

Cultural and familial influences play a role in how a woman expresses, or represses, pain as well as whether she uses pharmacologic methods of pain relief. If her family views childbirth as a natural process or function for the female in the family unit, the woman is less likely to outwardly react to labor pains and she's less likely to require pharmacologic methods of pain relief. For example:

• Middle Eastern women are verbally expressive during labor and commonly cry out and scream loudly; in addition, many refuse pain medication.

• Samoan women believe they shouldn't express any pain verbally because they believe the pain must simply be endured. They may also refuse pain medication.

• Filipino women lie quietly during labor.

• Vietnamese, Laotian, and other women of Southeast Asian descent believe that crying out during labor is shameful and that pain during labor must be endured.

• Hispanic women are taught by *pateras* (midwives) to endure pain and to keep their mouths closed during labor because to cry out would cause the uterus to rise and retard labor.

Nonpharmacologic pain relief

Most nonpharmacologic pain relief methods are based on the gate control theory of pain, which poses that local physical stimulation can interfere with pain stimuli by closing a hypothetical gate in the spinal cord, thus blocking pain signals from reaching the brain. Nonpharmacologic pain relief methods may be used as the only method of pain management during labor and delivery, or they may be used in conjunction with pharmacologic interventions. Be flexible when a woman chooses an alternative method of pain relief, and provide support and reassurance if she finds that the method she has chosen isn't working effectively.

Nonpharmacologic pain relief methods include various relaxation techniques, breathing techniques, heat and cold application, counterpressure, transcutaneous electrical nerve stimulation (TENS), hypnosis, acupuncture and acupressure, and yoga.

Relaxation techniques

Most childbirth education classes teach relaxation techniques to their students. Relaxation turns the woman's focus away from the pain, which reduces tension. The reduced tension leads to a perceived decrease in pain, which then further reduces tension, thus breaking the pain cycle.

You're getting sleepy. Relaxation techniques take focus away from the pain.

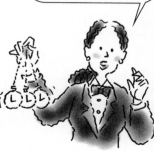

Let the sound take you away...

Relaxation techniques include positioning, focusing and imagery, therapeutic touch and massage, music therapy, and the support of a birthing partner or coach. Many women find these techniques helpful in the early stages of labor, even if they later decide that they need supplemental analgesia or anesthesia. Usually, the amount of pharmacologic assistance that's needed is reduced when used in conjunction with relaxation techniques.

Positioning

Part of the relaxation process involves positioning. The woman should be taught to shift her position during labor until she finds the one that's most comfortable for her. Commonly, the position of the fetus and its presenting part determines the most comfortable position for the mother. For example, a woman with a fetus in an occiput posterior position usually experiences intense back pain during labor. A change from a back- or side-lying position to one on her hands and knees with her head lower than her hips usually helps to ease this pain. Left side-lying position provides the greatest perfusion of blood to the mother's organs and to the placenta, so it's the position of choice no matter what the fetal position is.

Focusing and imagery

Focusing is a relaxation technique that's used to keep the sensory input perceived during the contraction from reaching the pain center in the cortex of the brain. During contractions, the woman concentrates intently on an object that has special meaning or appeal to her, such as a photograph.

Picture this

In imagery (also known as *visualization*), the woman concentrates on a mental image of a person, place, or thing. The woman may picture herself on a beach with the waves crashing on shore, in a forest or meadow with the sound of rustling leaves or singing birds, or near a stream or river with the sound of the water flowing by.

> When using imagery, the woman mentally places herself in a relaxing environment.

Stop, hey, what's that sound?

The sounds the woman hears during this process are an important part of effective imagery because they help her stay concentrated on the image. She may want to use an item such as a music box playing her favorite tune to help her visualize her image. If a person participating in the delivery is included in the woman's visualization, the individual should speak softly and offer words of comfort. The person could also sing or read a favorite poem to the woman.

Zip the lip

You shouldn't talk to the woman or ask her questions when she's using focusing or imagery techniques because the dialogue could break her concentration and allow the painful stimuli to cross into the brain. An exception should be made if a coach or other support person is assisting her in maintaining her concentration by providing verbal cues. (See *Using imagery during contractions*.)

Therapeutic touch and massage

Therapeutic touch is based on the premises that the body contains energy fields that lead to either good or ill health and that the hands can be used to redirect the energy fields that lead to pain. Touching and massage actually offer a distraction that directs the woman's focus from the pain to the action of the hands. Although not well documented, it's also believed that touch and massage cause the release of endorphins that block the perception of pain.

Music therapy

As an adjunct to relaxation, focusing, and imagery, it's usually helpful for the woman to have her favorite music available during labor and delivery. Listening to her favorite tunes usually helps the woman throughout the focusing or imagery process. It also acts as a form of diversion. Al-

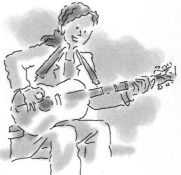

You won't strike a wrong chord when playing music to divert attention from the pain of labor and delivery.

Education edge

Using imagery during contractions

Teach your patient about using imaging techniques by telling her to follow these steps:
• Begin with a deep cleansing breath.
• Close your eyes.
• Relax every part of your body: head and neck, shoulders, arms, hands, fingers, chest, back, stomach, hips, bottom, legs, feet, and toes.
• Picture a place in your mind where you feel warm and safe. The place could be your home, a place you remember from your childhood, or a place that reminds you of peacefulness, such as a warm sandy beach or a quiet meadow. Keep these details in your mind so that when a contraction gets closer, you can focus on this image and have all the details in place.
• Slowly breathe with the contraction.
• When the contraction ends, take a deep cleansing breath and return to reality.
• Open your eyes.

though it's recommended that the music be soft and soothing, many women find greater distraction from dance or rock and roll rhythms. It may also be used in conjunction with breathing exercises; however, depending on the rhythm, music may serve to disrupt an established breathing pattern, rather than support it.

Birthing partner or coach

Having a capable birthing partner or coach to provide support during labor and delivery is one of the most important factors in making the birth experience a positive one. The presence of a birthing partner can alleviate the woman's anxiety and increase her self-esteem and feelings of control over the experience, which can effectively reduce the pain or at least increase her ability to deal with it. The birthing partner or coach may be the woman's husband, partner, parent, sibling, or friend. The most important factor in choosing a support person is determining who will provide the most effective coaching and support without being influenced on an emotional level.

Doula on duty

Sometimes, a woman doesn't have someone close to her who can take on birthing partner responsibilities. In such cases, the woman may use a *doula*, an independent contractor with or without formal medical training who provides support during labor and delivery. As effective as a traditional support person, the doula can help increase the woman's self-esteem and decrease the use of pharmacologic pain relief. Using a doula as a birthing partner or coach doesn't prevent the woman's partner or the baby's father from being present, providing emotional support, or participating in the birth of the child.

Breathing techniques

Breathing techniques are an important part of nonpharmacologic pain relief and are taught in most childbirth preparation classes. They distract the woman from the pain of the contractions and also help to relax the abdominal muscles. When a woman is focusing on slow-paced, rhythmic breathing, she's less likely to concentrate on the pain she's experiencing.

Easing pain one breath at a time

The most common breathing technique used is the Lamaze method. Originally developed in Russia and based on Pavlov's conditioning studies, the Lamaze method was popularized by Ferdinand Lamaze, a French physician. The method incorporates the theory that women can learn to use controlled breathing to reduce

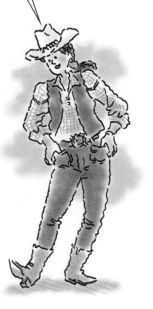

Howdy pardner! A birthing partner helps alleviate anxiety during labor and delivery.

the pain felt during labor through the use of stimulus-response conditioning.

In Lamaze, the woman is encouraged to direct her attention to a focal point, such as a spot on the wall, at the first sign of a contraction. This focus creates a visual stimulus that goes directly to the woman's brain. The woman then takes a deep cleansing breath, which is followed by rhythmic breathing. During the contraction, the woman's partner provides a series of commands or verbal encouragements to provide an auditory stimulus to her brain.

Relief at your fingertips

The rhythmic breathing is followed by effleurage (a light fingertip massage) that the woman or her partner performs on the abdomen or thighs. The massage introduces a tactile stimulus that goes directly to her brain, calming the nerves and promoting relaxation. The rate of effleurage is slow and remains constant, even though the rate of breathing may change. (See *Effective effleurage patterns*, page 348.)

It isn't too late to educate

If a woman hasn't attended childbirth preparation classes and hasn't received instruction in breathing and relaxation techniques, the techniques can be taught to her while she's in the early stages of labor. Although techniques learned under these circumstances usually aren't as effective, they may at least help to delay the use of analgesics.

Breathing on so many levels

Different levels of breathing are used depending on the intensity of the contractions. The woman's coach assists in determining the level of breathing by resting a hand on her abdomen or watching a contraction monitor. As the strength of the contraction changes, the coach calls out the key words that act as commands to the woman.

At the start and finish of each breathing exercise, the woman takes a cleansing breath—she breathes in slowly and deeply and then exhales in the same manner. This decreases the chance of hyperventilation during rapid breathing and also helps to maintain adequate oxygen supply for the fetus.

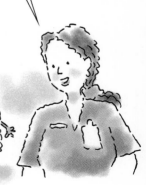

Ahhh! A cleansing breath decreases the chance of hyperventilation and helps maintain the fetus's oxygen supply.

First level

At the first level, the woman uses slow chest breathing. These full respirations

Effective effleurage patterns

Effleurage is a light fingertip massage that the woman or her partner performs on her abdomen or thighs during contractions. This illustration shows the tracing patterns used for effleurage.

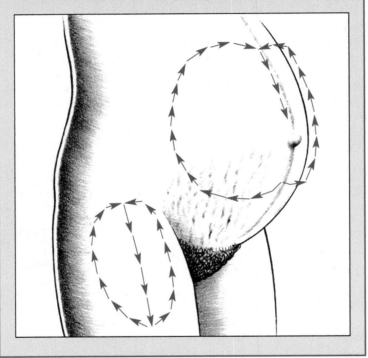

should be done at a rate of 6 to 12 breaths/minute. The woman is instructed to use this level of breathing for early contractions.

Second level

At the second level, breathing should be heavy enough so that the rib cage expands but light enough so that the diaphragm barely moves. The rate of respirations is up to 40 breaths/minute. The second level of breathing is recommended when cervical dilation is 4 to 6 cm.

Third level

The third level involves shallow, sternal breathing at a rate of 50 to 70 breaths/minute. As the respirations become faster, the exhalation must be a little stronger than the inhalation to promote good air exchange and prevent hyperventilation. The woman can achieve a stronger exhalation than inhalation if she practices saying "out" with each exhalation. The woman should use this level of breathing for contractions that occur during the transition phase of labor. To help prevent the oral mucosa from drying out during such rapid breathing, instruct the woman to keep the tip of her tongue against the roof of her mouth.

Fourth level

At the fourth level, the woman should use a "pant-blow" pattern of breathing by taking three or four quick breaths in and out and then forcefully exhaling. The breathing pattern is "hee-hee-hee-hoo" (shallow breath, shallow breath, shallow breath, long exhalation). This type of breathing is often referred to as "choo-choo" breathing because it sounds like a train.

Fifth level

At the fifth level, the woman should perform continuous chest panting. Breaths are shallow and occur at about 60 breaths/minute. This type of breathing can be used during strong contractions or during the second stage of labor to prevent the woman from pushing before full dilation.

"Choo-choo" breathing can engineer some relief from labor pain.

Heat and cold application

Heat application to the lower back is considered effective in reducing labor pain. A heating pad, moist compress, warm shower, or tub bath can significantly aid relaxation if the membranes are still intact. Applying a cool washcloth to the woman's forehead and providing ice chips to relieve dry mouth are other measures that can increase the woman's comfort level.

Counterpressure

Counterpressure is the application of firm or forceful pressure, using the heel of the hand or fist, to the woman's lower back or sacrum during a contraction. It relieves back pain during labor by countering the pressure of the fetus against the mother's back.

The amount of force applied varies, depending on the patient. Some women prefer considerable force during a contraction, whereas others prefer firm support on the back. The exact spot for applying pressure also varies from woman to woman and may change throughout the labor. If the partner is using considerable force on the back, suggest that he hold the front of the woman's hipbone to help maintain his balance.

Transcutaneous electrical nerve stimulation

TENS is the stimulation of large-diameter neural fibers via electric currents to alter pain perception. Although not documented as being a significant factor in reducing the pain caused by uterine contractions, TENS may be effective in reducing the extreme back pain that some women have during contractions.

Hypnosis

Hypnosis, though used infrequently, can provide a satisfactory method of pain relief for the woman who follows hypnotic suggestions. The woman must meet with the hypnotherapist several times during her pregnancy for evaluation and conditioning. If it's determined that she's a good candidate for this method of pain relief, she's given a posthypnotic suggestion that she'll experience either reduced pain during labor or no pain at all.

Acupuncture and acupressure

Acupuncture and acupressure are also methods of pain relief that are sometimes used during labor. Acupuncture is the stimulation of key trigger points with needles. It isn't necessary for the trigger points to be near the affected organ because their activation causes the release of endorphins, which reduce the perception of pain. Acupressure is finger pressure or massage at the same trigger points. Holding and squeezing the hand of a woman in labor may trigger the point most commonly used for acupuncture and acupressure during labor.

Yoga

Yoga uses a series of deep breathing exercises, body stretching postures, and meditation to promote relaxation, slow the respiratory rate, lower blood pressure, improve physical fitness, reduce stress, and ease anxiety. It may help reduce the pain of labor through the ability to relax the body and possibly through the release of endorphins that may occur.

Pharmacologic pain relief

Pharmacologic pain relief during labor includes analgesia and regional or local anesthesia. These approaches differ in the degree to which pain sensation is decreased. The main goals of using medication during labor are to relax the woman and relieve her discomfort without having a significant effect on her contractions, her pushing efforts, or the fetus.

The right amount at the right time

Almost all medications given during labor have an effect on the fetus because they cross the placental barrier, so it's important to give as little medication as possible. It's also important that medications be given at the proper time. When given after 5 cm dilation in a primipara or after 3 cm dilation in a multipara, medications can speed the progress of labor because the woman can focus on working with the contractions rather than against them. If given too early in labor, medications can slow or stop the contractions. If given within 1 hour of birth, the neonate is likely to experience neuromuscular, respiratory, and cardiac depression after delivery.

Know your drugs

The nurse must be familiar enough with anesthetic and analgesic agents to answer a patient's questions, assist the anesthesiologist and obstetrician, and identify adverse maternal, fetal, and neonatal effects quickly.

Opioids

Opioids are commonly used during labor because they significantly reduce pain. Common anesthetic agents used during labor are such opioids as meperidine (Demerol), butorphanol (Stadol), nalbuphine (Nubain), and fentanyl (Sublimaze). Some opioids have additional effects that are beneficial during labor, such as relaxing the cervix, which facilitates dilation. However, opioids depress the central nervous system of the fetus, which may lead to respiratory depression. In a preterm neonate or one who's already compromised in some way, this could be fatal.

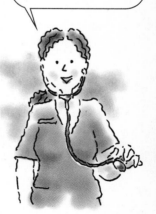

Now hear this. Opioids may cause respiratory depression in the fetus.

Labor's feel-good drug

Meperidine is commonly used to relieve labor pains because of its sedative and antispasmodic actions. It also gives the mother feelings of well-being and euphoria, while helping to relax the cervix. Meperidine is given when the mother is more than 3 hours from birth so that there's less risk of respiratory depression in the fetus.

Given in so many ways

Meperidine can be given I.V., I.M., or intrathecally (injected into the subarachnoid space of the spinal cord), although the intrathecal route isn't successful in all women. This drug may also be self-administered by the woman during labor with the use of a patient-controlled analgesic pump.

In on the action

When given I.M., meperidine usually begins to act within 30 minutes; when administered I.V., it acts within 5 minutes. Its effects last approximately 3 to 4 hours. The possible maternal or fetal adverse effects from meperidine are central nervous system depression, nausea, vomiting, respiratory depression, and maternal hypotension.

More and more

Other opioids that are given I.V. or I.M. during labor to provide pain relief include Nubain and Stadol. These drugs also pose a possible risk of respiratory depression in the neonate, and most slow labor if given too early.

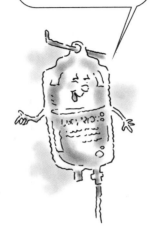

I'm just hanging around looking for some action—like taking care of labor pains.

Regional anesthesia

Regional anesthesia is used to block specific nerve pathways that pass from the uterus to the spinal cord. It relieves pain by making the nerve unable to conduct pain sensations. This form of anesthesia allows the woman to be completely awake, aware of what's happening, and—depending on the region anesthetized—aware of contractions, which gives her the opportunity to push at the appropriate time.

Regional results

Although regional anesthetics aren't injected into the maternal circulatory system, they still can produce adverse effects in the neonate, such as flaccidity, bradycardia, hypotension, and convulsions; however, these effects aren't as common or severe as with systemic anesthetics.

Lumbar epidural anesthesia is the method of regional anesthesia most frequently used for labor and delivery. An estimated 60% of laboring women in the United States receive epidural anesthesia for pain relief. A less commonly used method is spinal anesthesia, used primarily for cesarean deliveries and in emergency situations.

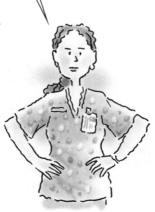

Regional anesthesia makes the nerves unable to conduct pain sensations.

Lumbar epidural anesthesia

Lumbar epidural anesthesia (also known as an *epidural block*) is the injection of an opioid medication, such as fentanyl (Sublimaze), bupivacaine (Marcaine), or a lidocaine-like drug (along with an opioid, such as fentanyl or morphine, to decrease the amount of motor blockage incurred). The medication is injected through a needle or catheter into the epidural space (the vacant space just outside the membrane in the lumbar region containing the cerebrospinal fluid that bathes the spinal column and brain).

A closer look at epidural anesthesia

This illustration shows the placement of the epidural catheter used for injecting pain-relieving medication into the epidural space. This process anesthetizes the nerves that carry pain signals from the uterus and perineum to the brain.

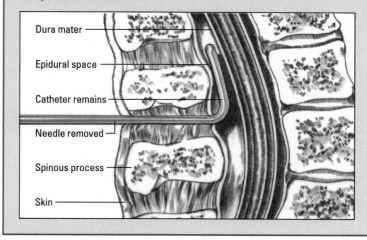

When the drug is administered into this space, it anesthetizes the nerves that carry pain signals from the uterus and perineum to the brain, thus dulling or eliminating the perception of pain for the woman. Women with preexisting medical conditions, such as heart disease, diabetes, and gestational hypertension, tend to choose this method because it makes labor almost pain-free, which can reduce physical and emotional stress. (See *A closer look at epidural anesthesia.*)

The down side, part one

Lumbar epidural anesthesia is relatively safe, but it can lower the woman's blood pressure, which can decrease the flow of blood to the uterus and the placenta. Before receiving lumbar epidural anesthesia, the woman should receive 500 to 1,000 ml of an I.V. solution, such as lactated Ringer's solution, to help prevent hypotension. Avoid administering a glucose solution because of the risk of causing rebound hypoglycemia in the neonate.

Jacking up the pressure

If the woman does become hypotensive, treatment may include placement in the left side-lying position, oxygen administration, increased I.V. fluids, and administration of a medication, such as ephedrine, to elevate blood pressure. Monitor FHR closely during periods of maternal hypotension. Fetal distress can occur as a result of reduced blood flow to the placenta from hypotension.

The down side, part two

Lumbar epidural anesthesia can also slow labor if it's given before the cervix is 5 cm dilated. It may also diminish the woman's ability to push because she's unaware of the contractions, which may result in the need for forceps-assisted delivery, vacuum extraction, or cesarean birth.

How it's done

Lumbar epidural anesthesia is administered by an anesthesiologist or nurse-anesthetist. The woman is placed on her side or in a sitting position with her back straight. This position is necessary because a back in flexion increases the possibility that the needle will pass through the epidural space into the subarachnoid space.

After the lumbar region of the woman's back is cleaned with an antiseptic and a local anesthetic is injected, a special needle is passed through the L3-L4 space into the epidural space. A catheter is then passed through the needle into the epidural space and taped in place on the skin. The needle is withdrawn, and a syringe is attached to the end of the catheter to create a closed system.

Test the waters

A small dose of the anesthetic is injected through the catheter, and the woman is observed to make sure that the catheter is in the proper position and the desired effect is obtained. When this is ascertained, the initial dose of the anesthetic is given. The anesthetic takes effect within 10 to 15 minutes and lasts from 40 minutes to 2 hours. An infusion pump is used and the anesthetic is infused at a slow, continuous rate. Close observation of the woman is necessary to avoid a toxic reaction from too much anesthetic.

Step up to the baseline

Here's what you should do during the procedure:
• Perform baseline vital signs and assess FHR before the epidural is initiated.
• If your facility requires that the patient be placed on a continuous ECG monitor, apply the leads and obtain a baseline ECG.
• Monitor the patient for signs of adverse reactions to the narcotic, such as a change in sedation level, respiratory depression, or itching. Also monitor the patient for adverse effects of the local anesthetic, which may include numbness in the arms, hands, or around mouth; ringing in the ears; seizure activity; nausea and vomiting; and metallic taste.

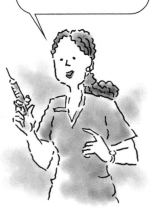

A small dose of anesthetic is injected through the catheter before the initial dose. This verifies catheter placement and patient response.

- Once you've determined that the patient isn't experiencing adverse reactions to the test, monitor maternal vital signs every 5 minutes for 20 minutes, then every 15 minutes for 45 minutes, and then every 30 minutes for the duration of the epidural and labor, or according to your facility's protocol.

Ins and outs

- Monitor the woman's intake and output because the woman can't feel the sensations associated with a full bladder. Encourage the woman to void at least once every 2 hours, and regularly palpate for bladder distention.
- Monitor FHR and observe for fetal distress, which can result from maternal hypotension.

Spinal anesthesia

With spinal anesthesia, a local anesthetic is injected into the cerebrospinal fluid in the subarachnoid space at the third or fourth lumbar interspace. Recently, the use of spinal anesthesia has significantly declined, having been replaced by lumbar epidural anesthesia. Currently, spinal anesthesia is used almost exclusively for cesarean birth.

For spinal anesthesia administration, place the woman in a side-lying or sitting position with her head bent forward and her back flexed as much as possible. If she's lying down, make sure that her head and upper body are higher than her abdomen and legs so that the anesthetic doesn't rise too high in the spinal canal.

The down side

As with epidural anesthesia, hypotension is a possible adverse effect of spinal anesthesia. Preventive measures should be taken before injecting anesthetic, and the woman should be closely monitored afterward.

Other disadvantages of spinal anesthesia include the possibility of a spinal headache, the risk of transient complete motor paralysis, increased incidence and degree of hypotension, and urine retention.

Local anesthesia

Local anesthesia is used only for pain relief during the actual birth of the fetus because it doesn't provide relief from the pain of contractions. It's used for a vaginal delivery when there isn't time for other types of anesthesia, after labor pain was relieved by the use of opioids (which can't be given within 1 hour of the birth), or when a woman

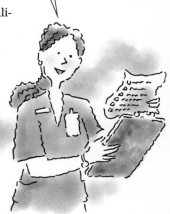

Local anesthesia is used only for pain relief during the actual birth of the fetus because it doesn't provide relief from the pain of contractions.

who was using nonpharmacologic pain relief during labor needs more relief during birth.

For when labor keeps going and going and going

In most cases, the pressure of the fetal head on the perineum causes a natural anesthesia, making local anesthesia administration unnecessary. However, after hours of exhaustive labor, many women need this relief, especially if an episiotomy is to be performed.

Local infiltration

Local infiltration is the injection of a local anesthetic (usually lidocaine) into the superficial perineal nerves. It's commonly used in preparation for or before suturing an episiotomy; however, anesthesia with this method isn't as effective as a pudendal block. (See *Local infiltration location.*)

There are no significant risks to local infiltration except rare allergic reactions and inadvertent intravascular injections. However, some practitioners believe that injection may weaken the perineal tissue and increase the likelihood of tearing.

Local infiltration location

Local infiltration is the injection of a local anesthetic (usually lidocaine [Xylocaine]) into the superficial perineal nerves. This illustration shows the location of the injection.

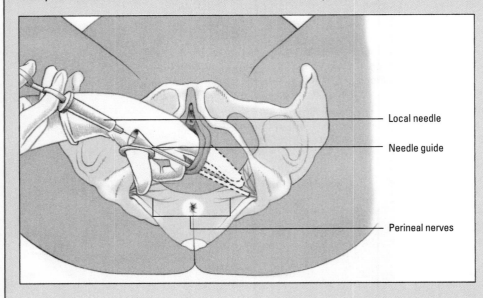

Nursing interventions

Nursing interventions during labor and delivery focus on providing the woman comfort and support. Here's what you should do:
• To promote the woman's comfort and general body cleanliness, advise her to take a warm shower or, if her membranes haven't ruptured, a Jacuzzi or a tub bath. If she can't walk, perform a sponge or bed bath with meticulous perineal care.
• To increase the woman's comfort and reduce the risk of infection, change her gown and sheets whenever they become soiled. Also be sure to change the disposable underpad, especially after a cervical examination. Wipe the woman's face and neck with a cool, clean washcloth, especially during the transition phase of labor.

Comforts of home

• To increase the woman's feelings of comfort and well-being, advise her to use her own toiletries, if available.
• To maintain throat and mouth moisture, offer the woman frequent sips of water or allow her to suck on some ice, hard candy, or a washcloth saturated with ice water. Provide mouth care during labor, and encourage the woman to brush her teeth or use mouthwash to freshen her breath.
• To moisturize and heal dry, cracked lips, help the woman to apply lip balm or petroleum jelly to her lips.
• To give the woman a sense of control over her pain, teach her about the possible causes of back pain during labor and the coping strategies that she can use.
• To help the woman relax during labor, teach her to use relaxation techniques and slow, paced breathing (not less than one-half the normal respiratory rate) between contractions.
• To help maintain relaxation during the later part of labor and to prevent hyperventilation, advise her to increase her respiratory rate (not more than twice the normal rate) and to modify her breathing pattern during contractions.

Under pressure

• To reduce the woman's pain and promote her comfort, show her partner how to apply firm counterpressure with the heel of one hand to the sacral area.
• To prevent feelings of helplessness during a difficult labor, encourage the woman to let her partner know the amount and location of counterpressure that relieves the most pain. Feedback allows the partner to relieve pain most effectively.

- To allow the pressure of the fetus to fall away from the patient's back, help the woman assume a side-lying, upright forward-leaning, or hands-and-knees position.
- To promote the woman's comfort and further anterior rotation of the fetus (if the fetus is in the occiput posterior position), help the patient change positions at least every 30 minutes—from side-lying to hands-and-knees to the opposite side-lying positions.
- To reduce back discomfort, apply a warm, moist towel, an ice bag, or a covered rubber glove filled with ice chips to the woman's lower back.

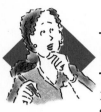

Quick quiz

1. Which option isn't a primary factor in determining the presentation of the fetus during birth?
    A.   Fetal attitude
    B.   Fetal heart rate
    C.   Fetal lie
    D.   Fetal position

Answer: B. The primary factors that determine fetal presentation are fetal attitude, lie, and position.

2. In the LOA and ROA fetal positions, the presenting part is the:
    A.   olecranon.
    B.   chin.
    C.   occiput.
    D.   buttocks.

Answer: C. The occiput is the presenting part in the LOA and ROA fetal positions.

3. Which drug is a common ripening agent?
    A.   Dinoprostone (Cervidil)
    B.   Oxytocin (Pitocin)
    C.   Fentanyl (Sublimaze)
    D.   Butorphanol tartrate (Stadol)

Answer: A. Cervidil is commonly used to ripen the cervix. The drug initiates the breakdown of the collagen that keeps the cervix tightly closed.

4. Transition is part of which stage of labor?
A. First stage
B. Second stage
C. Third stage
D. Fourth stage

Answer: A. The first stage of labor is divided into three phases: latent, active, and transition.

5. In which order do the cardinal movements of labor occur?
A. Flexion, extension, internal rotation, external rotation, descent, expulsion
B. Descent, flexion, internal rotation, extension, external rotation, and expulsion
C. Descent, internal rotation, flexion, external rotation, extension, expulsion
D. Descent, extension, internal rotation, flexion, external rotation, expulsion

Answer: B. The cardinal movements of labor occur in this order: descent, flexion, internal rotation, extension, external rotation, and expulsion.

6. Which sign isn't a sign of true labor?
A. Bloody show
B. Painful uterine contractions
C. Lightening
D. Rupture of the membranes

Answer: C. Lightening is a preliminary sign of labor—not a sign of true labor.

7. Before the administration of an epidural anesthetic, the woman should receive 500 to 1,000 ml of which I.V. solution?
A. Normal saline solution
B. Dextrose 5% in water (D_5W)
C. D_5W in lactated Ringer's solution
D. Lactated Ringer's solution

Answer: D. Lactated Ringer's solution should be administered before a woman receives epidural anesthesia.

8. Which uncommon fetal attitude results in a brow presentation?
A. Partial extension
B. Complete extension
C. Moderate flexion
D. Complete flexion

Answer: A. Partial extension is an uncommon fetal attitude that results in a brow presentation through the birth canal.

Scoring

☆☆☆ If you answered all eight questions correctly, terrific! You certainly delivered the goods on that challenge.

☆☆ If you answered six or seven questions correctly, great! Your laboring paid off.

☆ If you answered fewer than six questions correctly, keep your head up. You'll present well in the next quiz.

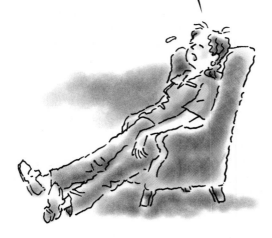

Exhausted after laboring through Labor and birth? Take a breather, and then let's move on to the next exciting chapter, Labor and birth complications.

8

Complications of labor and birth

Just the facts

In this chapter, you'll learn:

♦ various complications that can occur with labor and birth

♦ ways to assess and detect problems occurring with labor and birth

♦ treatment and management of various complications.

A look at complications

Although labor usually proceeds without problems, about 8% of births involve complications. A problem can arise at any point in the labor process and can involve uterine contractions, the fetus, or the birth canal.

Stress stinks, honesty works

Emotional support is essential for the mother and her birthing partner during labor and birth. Even when labor and birth progress normally, the process is stressful and usually lengthy. It's important to periodically assure the laboring woman that everything is going well and that she and the fetus are fine, as appropriate. When a complication arises, stress increases and honesty and sincerity remain just as important.

The importance of being careful

Because complications can occur at any point in the process, the mother and fetus need to be carefully monitored. Careful monitoring of the mother and fetus is important for several reasons. A malpositioned fetus is a major factor in birth complications. Nurses can be instrumental in identifying a malpositioned fetus by using Leopold's maneuvers and helping avoid complications. For example, early detection of signs and symptoms of uterine rupture can help decrease maternal morbidity during labor. When working

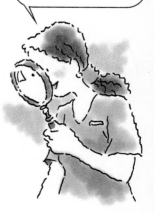

Identifying a malpositioned fetus by using Leopold's maneuvers is one thing a nurse can do to help avoid complications.

with a monitoring device, be sure to explain its importance to the patient and her partner. (See *Tips for continuous electronic monitoring*.)

C is for "complication"

In addition to problems arising from the condition of the mother or fetus, medical interventions to prevent or manage complications can cause other problems. One of the most invasive of these interventions is cesarean birth, in which a surgical incision is made in the abdominal and uterine walls for delivery of the neonate. Because this procedure is commonly performed, many times as a result of other complications, it's listed below with other birth complications.

Amniotic fluid embolism

Amniotic fluid embolism occurs as rarely as 1 in 8,000 births. Occurring during labor or during the postpartum period, amniotic fluid embolism happens when amniotic fluid is forced into an open maternal uterine blood sinus due to some defect in the membranes themselves or after membrane rupture or partial premature separation of the placenta. Solid particles then enter the maternal circulation and travel to the lungs, causing pulmonary embolism. Amniotic fluid embolism isn't preventable and requires prompt intervention and lifesaving treatment.

What causes it

The exact cause of amniotic fluid embolism is unknown, but possible risk factors include:
• oxytocin administration
• abruptio placentae
• polyhydramnios.

How it's detected

Signs of amniotic fluid embolism are dramatic. The woman, who's commonly in strong labor when the problem occurs, may sit up suddenly and grasp her chest. She may also complain of a sharp pain in her chest and an inability to breathe. In assessment, her color markedly pales and then turns the typical bluish gray associated with pulmonary embolism and lack of blood flow to the lungs.

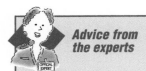

Tips for continuous electronic monitoring

When applying an external electronic fetal and uterine monitoring device, remember to explain monitoring and why it must be used to the woman in labor to ensure compliance with the technology. Also, to avoid causing the patient distraction and stress, explain in advance that the alarms may sound even when everything is going smoothly.

Don't forget
When reading the monitor pattern, remember:
• to assess the mother and fetus to verify what the various patterns suggest
• that the woman may move as a result of pain or a desire to adjust her position
• that patient movement may result in artifacts on the tracings that require monitor adjustment.

What to do

Prognosis of the mother and fetus depends on the size of the emboli and the skill and speed of the emergency interventions. Immediate management of this complication includes oxygen administration by face mask or cannula. Because vital organs are deprived of oxygen supply due to the emboli, within minutes the woman develops cardiopulmonary arrest, necessitating cardiopulmonary resuscitation (CPR). Even so, CPR may be ineffective because, despite providing oxygen transport to organs, it does nothing to remove the emboli. If the emboli aren't removed, blood can't circulate to the lungs. Death may occur within minutes.

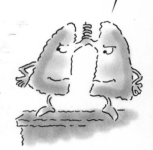

Yikes! If the emboli aren't removed, I don't get the blood I need, and death can occur.

Here are some other facts you should consider:
• Even if the initial insult (the emboli) is resolved, disseminated intravascular coagulation (DIC) is highly likely from the presence of particles in the bloodstream, further complicating the patient's condition.
• If the patient survives initial emergency procedures, she'll need continued management (such as endotracheal intubation) to maintain pulmonary function and therapy with fibrinogen to counteract DIC.
• Prompt transfer to the intensive care unit (ICU) is necessary.
• The prognosis for the fetus is guarded because reduced placental perfusion results from the severe drop in maternal blood pressure.
• The fetus may be delivered immediately by cesarean birth or vaginally using forceps.

Cephalopelvic disproportion

A narrowing, or *contraction*, of the birth canal, which can occur at the inlet, midpelvis, or outlet, causes a disproportion between the size of the fetal head and the pelvic diameters, or cephalopelvic disproportion (CPD). CPD results in failure of labor to progress.

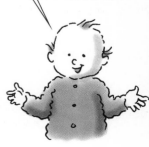

CPD means the fetal head can't fit through the mommy's pelvis. It's like trying to fit a square peg through a round hole.

Primary problems

Malpositioning can occur because the fetus's head isn't engaged in the pelvis. Malpositioning can lead to further complications. For example, if membranes rupture, the risk of cord prolapse increases significantly.

What causes it

A small pelvis is a major contributing factor in CPD. The small size of the pelvis may be the result of rickets in the early life of the mother, a genetic predisposition, or a pelvis that isn't fully matured in a young adolescent.

A perfect fit

In primigravidas, the fetal head normally engages with the pelvic brim at weeks 36 to 38 of gestation. When this event occurs before labor begins, it's assumed that the pelvic inlet is adequate. Engagement of the head proves that the head fits into the pelvic brim and indicates that the head will probably also be able to pass through the midpelvis and through the outlet. In CPD, the fetal head may be too large to fit or the overall fetal size may be prohibitively large (known as *macrosomia*, or a birthweight of more than 4,000 g [8.8 lb]).

Inlets and outlets

Inlet contraction occurs when the narrowing of the anteroposterior diameter (from the symphysis pubis to the sacral prominence) is less than 11 cm or a maximum transverse diameter (between the ischial spines) is 12 cm or less. In outlet contraction, the transverse diameter narrows at the outlet to less than 11 cm. The outlet measurement is the distance between the ischial tuberosities. Because this measurement is easy to take during the expectant mother's prenatal visits, the health care team can anticipate and prepare for outlet contraction before labor begins.

Positional faux pas

Abnormal positions of the fetus can also cause CPD. Posterior, transverse, face, brow, or breech presentations can make it difficult or impossible for the fetal presenting part to fit through the pelvis.

Fetal faux pas

Fetal anomalies such as hydrocephalus, hydrops fetalis, and tumors of the fetal head can also result in CPD.

It all adds up. To prepare for outlet contraction before labor begins, measure the distance between the ischial tuberosities during prenatal visits.

How it's detected

When engagement doesn't occur in a primigravida, a problem exists. This problem may be a fetal abnormality, such as a larger-than-usual head, or a pelvic abnormality, as in a smaller-than-usual pelvis. It's important to note that engagement doesn't usually occur in multigravidas until labor begins. In this situation, a previous delivery of a full-term neonate vaginally without problems is substantial proof that the birth canal is considered adequate.

Rule of mum

Every primigravida should have pelvic measurements taken and recorded before week 24. Based on these measurements and the assumption that the fetus will be of average size, a decision can be made about the possibility of vaginal delivery.

What to do

If the pelvic measurements are borderline or just adequate, especially the inlet measurement, and the fetal lie and position are good, the woman's practitioner or nurse-midwife may allow a trial labor to determine whether labor can progress normally. A trial labor may be allowed to continue if descent of the presenting part and dilation of the cervix are occurring. In other words, normal labor and delivery are occurring and no complications have been detected.

Giving it a try

If trial labor is anticipated, the following nursing measures are important:
• Monitor fetal heart sounds and uterine contractions continuously if possible to detect abnormalities promptly.
• Make sure that the woman's urinary bladder is kept as empty as possible, such as by urging her to void every 2 hours, to allow the fetal head to use all the space available, making delivery possible.
• After rupture of the membranes, assess fetal heart rate (FHR) carefully. If the fetal head is still high, alterations in FHR may indicate an increased danger of prolapsed cord and fetal anoxia.
• Monitor progress of labor. After 6 to 12 hours, if fetal descent and cervical dilation can't be documented or fetal distress occurs at any time, the woman should be scheduled for a cesarean birth.
• Keep in mind that a woman undertaking trial labor may feel she'll be unable to complete the process, which may lead her to feel she's being needlessly subjected to pain. Emphasize that it's best for the baby to be born vaginally, if possible.
• If the trial labor fails and cesarean birth is scheduled, explain why the procedure is necessary and why it's a better alternative for the baby at that point.
• A woman having a trial labor may feel as if she's on trial herself. She may feel she's being judged and may be self-conscious if labor doesn't go as well as hoped.
• When dilation doesn't occur, the woman may feel discouraged and inadequate, as if she's somehow at fault. A woman may not be

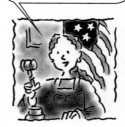

Trial labor failed! The verdict is clear: Cesarean birth is the best way to deliver a healthy baby.

aware how much she wanted the trial labor to work until she's told that it isn't working.
• Remember to support the support person. He or she may also be frightened and feel helpless when a problem occurs.
• Assure the parents that a cesarean birth isn't an inferior method of birth. Remind them that it's an alternative method. In this instance, it's the method of choice, allowing them to achieve their goal of a healthy mother and a healthy child.

Cesarean birth

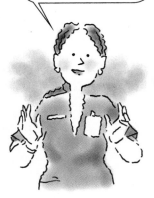

When vaginal birth isn't possible, all roads lead to cesarean birth.

Also known as *cesarean section* or *cesarean delivery*, cesarean birth is one of the oldest surgical procedures known. It may be performed as a planned surgery or an emergency procedure when vaginal birth isn't possible. (See *Cesarean factors*.)

Follow the plan

A cesarean birth is usually planned when the patient has had a previous cesarean birth and a vaginal birth after cesarean (VBAC) isn't recommended. It's considered elective because the patient and her practitioner choose the date that the cesarean birth will be performed based on her due date and the maturity of the fetus.

Still dangerous

Because it's an invasive surgical procedure, cesarean birth is considered more hazardous than vaginal birth. Thus, it's only performed when the health and safety of the mother or fetus are in jeopardy. In addition, cesarean birth is generally contraindicated

---

Cesarean factors

Cesarean birth may be a planned or an emergency procedure. Factors that lead to cesarean birth may be maternal, placental, or fetal in nature.

Maternal
• Cephalopelvic disproportion
• Active genital herpes or papilloma
• Previous cesarean birth by classic incision
• Disabling conditions, such as severe gestational hypertension and heart disease, that prevent pushing to accomplish the pelvic division of labor

Placental
• Placenta previa
• Premature separation of the placenta

Fetal
• Transverse fetal lie
• Extremely low fetal size
• Fetal distress
• Compound conditions, such as macrosomic fetus in a breech lie

when there's a documented dead fetus. In this situation, labor can be induced to avoid an unnecessary surgical procedure.

On the rise

The incidence of cesarean birth is on the rise. In the United States, between 9% and 16% of pregnancies end in cesarean birth. In perinatal centers that care for mothers with high-risk deliveries, the rate has risen to as high as 25%. Some theories have attributed this rise to recent medical and technologic advances in fetal and placental surveillance and care. However, nurse-midwifery birthing services have a lower incidence of cesarean birth than more mainstream hospital services. Some suggest that the midwifery model of continuous support during labor may be a reason for the difference.

Other possible influences on the rising rate of cesarean birth include:
- combination of the increasing safety of cesarean birth and the use of fetal monitors, which provide for early detection of fetal problems that would necessitate cesarean birth
- practitioners becoming increasingly skilled in the procedure while not acquiring comparable experience in alternative methods, such as external cephalic version and exercises to encourage a breech presentation to move into a vertex presentation
- doctors' fears of malpractice suits, which may result when a fetus is allowed to be delivered vaginally and then discovered to have suffered anoxia.

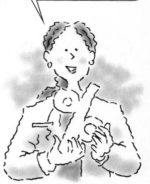

In the United States, about 15% of all pregnancies and about 25% of high-risk pregnancies end in cesarean birth.

Double trouble

Occasionally, a woman may refuse to submit to a cesarean birth. Because women have a right to decide if they'll undergo surgery, the right to refuse the procedure is respected. In some instances, however, a court order to go ahead with the procedure may be obtained when cesarean birth is seen as necessary for the life of the fetus as well as the mother. Nurses working in labor and delivery units should be aware of the opinion of their agency's ethics committee on this issue and should also be aware of the proper channels to take should this situation arise.

Body system effects

Because cesarean birth requires a surgical procedure, it can result in systemic effects, including thrombophlebitis from interference in the body's natural stress response as well as alterations in body defenses, circulatory function, organ function, self-image, and self-esteem.

Stress response

Whenever the body is subjected to stress, either physical or psychological, it responds by trying to preserve function of all major body systems. This response includes the release of epinephrine and norepinephrine from the adrenal medulla. Norepinephrine release leads to peripheral vasoconstriction, which forces blood to the central circulation and increases blood pressure. Epinephrine causes changes resulting in:
- increased heart rate
- bronchial dilation
- elevation of blood glucose levels.

These responses are considered normal and are elicited when the person is tensed. The body is then ready for action with an increased heart rate and lung function as well as glucose for energy.

Antagonize, not minimize

However, these responses may antagonize anesthetic action aimed at minimizing body activity in the mother undergoing a cesarean birth. In addition, the stress response may result in reduced blood supply to the patient's lower extremities. The pregnant patient is prone to thrombophlebitis due to the stasis of blood flow; the stress response compounds this potential, greatly increasing the risk. Combined with other effects of stress on major body systems, the stress response can significantly increase the risks associated with surgery.

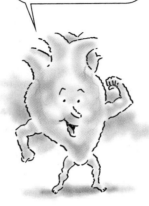

The stress response ensures that the body is ready for action with increased heart rate, lung function, and glucose for energy.

Altered body defenses

The skin is the first line of defense against bacterial invasion. When the skin is incised for a surgical procedure, as in cesarean birth, this important line of defense is automatically lost. In addition, if cesarean birth is performed after membranes have been ruptured for hours, the woman's risk of infection doubles. Of course, precautions should be taken to minimize the risk to the patient through strict adherence to sterile technique during surgery and the days following the procedure.

Altered circulatory function

During cesarean birth, blood vessels are incised, a consequence of even the simplest surgical procedure. A surgical wound results in blood loss that, if extensive, can lead to hypovolemia and decreased blood pressure. When blood pressure decreases, inadequate perfusion of body tissues results, especially if the problem isn't recognized and corrected quickly. The amount of blood lost in cesarean birth is relatively high compared with vaginal birth. Pelvic vessels are usually congested with blood needed to supply the placenta. When pressure is placed on these vessels, blood loss

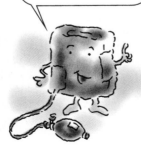

Decreased blood pressure results in inadequate perfusion—especially in cesarean birth, in which blood loss is greater than in other procedures.

occurs freely. During a vaginal birth, a woman may loose up to 500 ml of blood. This loss increases dramatically to 1,000 ml with a cesarean birth.

Altered organ function

Like any body organ, the uterus may respond to being manipulated, cut, or repaired with a temporary disruption in function. Pressure from edema or inflammation can occur as fluid moves into the injured area. This normal response can further impair function of the uterus. In addition, handling of the uterus may result in a decrease in its ability to contract, which can lead to postpartum hemorrhage. Because complications may not be evident during the procedure, close assessment of the uterus is required in the postoperative period as well as an assessment of total body function to determine the degree of disruption.

What about the others?

In addition to effects on the uterus, other organs may be directly affected. For example, to reach the uterus, the bladder must be displaced anteriorly. To perform the cesarean birth, pressure must be exerted on the intestine, possibly leading to paralytic ileus or halting of intestinal function. Because of these manipulating events, uterine, bladder, intestine, and lower circulatory function must be carefully assessed after a cesarean birth to detect complications early and avert potential problems.

Altered self-image or self-esteem

Surgical procedures almost always leave incisional scars that are noticeable to some extent afterward. In some situations, the resulting scar from a cesarean birth may be quite noticeable, such as when a horizontal incision is performed across the lower abdomen. The appearance of this scar may cause the woman to feel self-conscious later. She may also experience decreased self-esteem. This decrease may stem from a belief that she's marked as someone who can't give birth vaginally.

Incision types

Depending on the type of cesarean incision, a patient may be able to deliver vaginally after previously delivering by cesarean birth. VBAC is becoming an increasingly successful alternative to elective cesarean birth. The type of incision chosen depends on the presentation of the fetus and the speed with which the procedure can be performed. In general, there are two types of cesarean incisions: classic and low-segment.

Classic cesarean incision

In a classic cesarean incision, the incision is made vertically through the abdominal skin and the uterus. It's made high on the uterus in the case of a placenta previa to avoid cutting the placenta. The result of this incision type is a wide skin scar that runs through the active contractile portion of the uterus. This scarring pattern carries an additional risk of complication in future pregnancies. Because this type of scar could cause uterine rupture during labor, it's likely that the woman won't be able to have a subsequent vaginal birth. (See *Types of cesarean incisions*.)

Low-segment incision

Low-segment incision is the most common type of cesarean incision. Unlike the classic incision, a low-segment incision is made horizontally across the lower abdomen just over the symphysis pubis and occurs horizontally across the uterus just over the cervix. This incision type is also referred to as *Pfannenstiel's incision* or a *bikini incision* because even a low-cut bathing suit should cover it. Because it's made through the nonactive portion of the uterus, or the part of the uterus that contracts minimally, it's less likely to cause rupture in subsequent labors. Thus, the low-segment incision makes it possible for a woman to attempt VBAC. Other advantages of this incision type include:
- decreased blood loss
- ease of suturing
- minimal postpartum uterine infection risk
- decreased risk of postpartum GI complications.

The downside

The major disadvantage of this incision is that it takes longer to perform. So if the cesarean must be done in a hurry, such as in an emergency, low-segment incision becomes impractical because of time constraints.

No assumptions, please

Sometimes a skin incision is made horizontally and the uterine incision is made vertically, or vice versa. Thus, during a future pregnancy, don't assume that a small skin incision indicates a small uterine incision.

What causes it

Cesarean birth is indicated when labor or vaginal birth carries an unacceptable risk for the mother or fetus, such as in CPD and transverse lie or other malpresentations. It may also be necessary

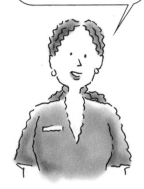

A classic cesarean incision may eliminate the option of vaginal birth in subsequent pregnancies.

Types of cesarean incisions

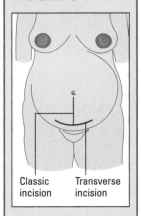

Classic incision   Transverse incision

if induction is contraindicated or difficult or if advanced labor increases the risk of morbidity and mortality.

The most common reasons for cesarean birth are:
• malpresentation of the fetus (such as shoulder or face presentation)
• evidence of fetal intolerance of labor stress
• CPD in which the pelvis is too small to accommodate the fetal head
• certain cases of toxemia or preeclampsia
• previous cesarean birth, especially with a classic incision
• inadequate progress in labor (failure of induction).

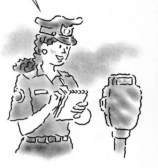

When labor or vaginal birth carries an unacceptable risk for the mother or fetus, cesarean birth is just the ticket.

Fetus in distress

Conditions causing fetal distress can also indicate a need for cesarean birth. These conditions include:
• living fetus with prolapsed cord
• fetal hypoxia
• abnormal FHR patterns
• unfavorable intrauterine environment, such as from infection
• moderate to severe rhesus factor (Rh) isoimmunization.

Mom needs help

Less commonly, maternal conditions may necessitate cesarean birth. These conditions include:
• complete placenta previa
• abruptio placentae
• placenta accreta
• malignant tumors
• chronic diseases in the mother in which delivery is indicated before term.

How it's detected

Special tests and monitoring procedures provide early indications of the need for cesarean birth:
• Magnetic resonance imaging or X-ray pelvimetry reveals CPD and malpositioning.
• Ultrasonography shows pelvic masses that interfere with vaginal birth and fetal position.
• Auscultation of FHR (by fetoscope, Doppler unit, or electronic fetal monitor) determines acute fetal intolerance of labor.

What to do

In preparation for cesarean birth, an anesthetic is administered. Patients may have general or regional anesthetic, depending on the extent of maternal or fetal distress. The woman is then positioned on the operating table. A towel may be placed under her left hip to help relocate abdominal contents so that they're up and away from the surgical field. This can also assist in lifting the uterus off the vena cava, promoting better circulation to the fetus as well as maternal blood return.

Blocking bacteria as well as the view

A metal screen or some other type of shielding may be placed at the patient's shoulder level and covered with a sterile drape. This not only serves as a courtesy to help obstruct the patient's view of the necessary surgical incision but also helps to block the flow of bacteria from the woman's respiratory tract to the incision site. Placement of the drape also blocks the support person's line of vision, preventing additional anxiety and fear that may arise from the sight of blood.

Support for the support

The support person is usually positioned at the mother's head. The incision area on the patient's abdomen is then scrubbed, and drapes are placed around the area of incision so that only a small area of skin is left exposed. In many cases, watching a cesarean birth is the first surgery the father or support person has witnessed. Thus, the person may be too overwhelmed by the whole event or too interested in the procedure to be of optimum support. He or she may become concerned about the amount of manipulation and cutting that occurs before the uterus itself is cut, assuming fetal distress isn't extreme. Remember to prepare the patient and support person for what they might see. This can help avert too much shock or surprise as well as promote open discussion about how much they would like to see or not see.

Remember to prepare the patient and support person for what they might see in the operating room.

The down side

Possible maternal complications of cesarean birth include:
• respiratory tract infection
• wound dehiscence
• thromboembolism
• paralytic ileus
• hemorrhage
• genitourinary tract infection
• bowel, bladder, or uterine injury.

Before surgery

Preoperative care measures involve both the mother and fetus. Here are some measures you should take:
• Assess maternal and fetal status frequently until delivery, as your facility's policy directs.

- If ordered, make sure that an ultrasound has been obtained. The practitioner may have ordered the test to determine fetal position.
- Explain cesarean birth to the patient and her partner, and answer any questions they may have.
- Provide reassurance and emotional support to help improve the self-esteem and self-concept of the mother and her partner. Remember that a cesarean birth is commonly performed after hours of labor, resulting in an exhausted patient and partner. Be brief but clear and stress the essential points about the procedure.
- For a scheduled cesarean birth, discuss the procedure with both parents and provide preoperative teaching.
- Observe the mother for signs of imminent delivery.
- Demonstrate use of the incentive spirometer, and have the patient practice deep breathing. Review splinting measures to decrease incisional pain with deep breathing and coughing.
- Restrict food and fluids after midnight if a general anesthetic is ordered to prevent aspiration of vomitus.
- Prepare the patient by shaving her from below the breasts to the pubic region and the upper quarter of the anterior thighs as indicated. Scrub and shave the abdomen and the symphysis pubis as ordered.
- Make sure the patient's bladder is empty, use an indwelling urinary catheter as ordered, and check for flow and patency. Tell the mother that the catheter may remain in place for 24 hours or longer.
- Administer ordered preoperative medication.
- Give the mother an antacid to help neutralize stomach acid if ordered.
- Start an I.V. infusion for fluid replacement therapy using the patient's nondominant hand if required. Use an 18G or larger catheter to allow blood administration through the I.V. if needed.
- Make sure the practitioner has ordered typing and crossmatching of the mother's blood and that two units of blood are available.

After surgery

Postoperative care measures of the mother and child include:
- As soon as possible, allow the mother to see, touch, and hold her neonate, either in the delivery room or after she recovers from the general anesthetic. Contact with the neonate promotes bonding.
- Check the perineal pad and abdominal dressing on the incision every 15 minutes for 1 hour, then every half-hour for 4 hours, every hour for 4 hours, and finally every 4 hours for 24 hours.
- Perform fundal checks at the same intervals. Gently assess the fundus.
- Check the dressing frequently for bleeding, and report it immediately. Be sure to keep the incision clean and dry.

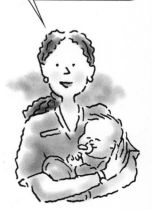

As soon as possible after delivery, allow the mother to see, touch, and hold her baby to promote bonding.

• Monitor vital signs every 5 minutes until stable. Then check vital signs when you evaluate perineal and abdominal drainage.
• The practitioner may order oxytocin mixed in with the first 1,000 to 2,000 ml of I.V. fluids infused to promote uterine contraction and decrease the risk of hemorrhage. Make sure the I.V. is patent and monitor the patient carefully for effects of the medication.
• Monitor intake and output as ordered. Expect the mother to receive I.V. fluids for 24 to 48 hours.
• Make sure the catheter is patent and urine flow is adequate. When the catheter is removed, make sure that the woman can void without difficulty and that urine color and amount are adequate.
• Maintain a patent airway for the mother and the neonate.
• Encourage the mother to cough and deep-breathe and use the incentive spirometer to promote adequate respiratory function.
• If a general anesthetic was used, remain with the patient until she's responsive.
• If regional anesthetic was used, monitor the return of sensation to the legs.
• Help the mother to turn from side to side every 1 to 2 hours.
• If ordered, show the patient how to administer patient-controlled analgesia.
• Administer pain medication as ordered, and provide comfort measures for breast engorgement as appropriate.
• If the mother wants to breast-feed, offer encouragement and help.
• Recognize afterpains in multiparas and monitor the effects of pain medication. Timing of administration of pain medication and breast-feeding may need to be coordinated so that the neonate won't receive as much of the sedating effect.
• Promote early ambulation to prevent cardiovascular and pulmonary complications. Remember to assist the mother initially and make sure she doesn't suffer from orthostatic hypotension. Warn her that lochia may flow freely when she moves from a supine to an upright position.

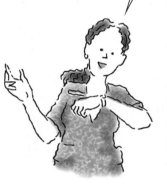

After cesarean birth, check the perineal pad and abdominal dressing every 15 minutes for 1 hour, every half-hour for 4 hours, every hour for 4 hours, and finally every 4 hours for 24 hours.

Going home

Home care instructions should also be provided to a patient who has had a cesarean birth, including:
• Instruct the patient to immediately report hemorrhage, chest or leg pain (possible thrombosis), dyspnea, or separation of the wound's edges.
• Tell her to also report signs and symptoms of infection, such as fever, difficulty urinating, and flank pain.
• Remind the patient to keep her follow-up appointment. At that time, she can talk to the practitioner about using contraception and resuming intercourse.

Fetal presentation or position

Problems can occur with the fetus's presentation or position during labor and delivery. Although most fetuses move into the proper birthing position, alternative positions and presentations can occur, making vaginal delivery difficult and, in some situations, impossible.

Problematic presentations and positions

Some presentations and positions that can be problematic include occipitoposterior position, breech presentation, face presentation, and transverse lie. A fifth type of presentation, called *brow presentation*, is rarely seen. (See *A briefing on brow presentation.*)

Occipitoposterior position

In about one-tenth of labors, the fetal position may be posterior rather than the traditional anterior position. When this occurs, the occiput, assuming the presentation is vertex, is directed diagonally and posteriorly, right occipitoposterior or left occipitoposterior. In these positions, during internal rotation, the fetal head must rotate through an arc of approximately 135 degrees, rather than the normal 90-degree arc.

This rotation through the 135-degree arc may not be possible if the fetus is above average in size or isn't in good flexion or if contractions are ineffective. Ineffective contractions may occur in:
• uterine dysfunction from maternal exhaustion
• fetal head arrested in the transverse position (transverse arrest).

1-2-3 rotate!

If rotation through the 135-degree arc doesn't occur but the fetus has reached the midportion of the pelvis, he may be rotated manually to an anterior position with forceps and then delivered. As an alternative, cesarean delivery may be preferred because the risk of a midforceps maneuver exceeds the risk of cesarean delivery. If midforceps are used for birth, the woman is at risk for reproductive tract lacerations, hemorrhage, and infection in the postpartum period.

Breech presentation

Most fetuses are in a breech presentation early in pregnancy. However, in approximately 97% of pregnancies, the fetus turns to a cephalic presentation by week 38. Although the fetal head is the widest single diameter, the fetus's buttocks (breech), plus the low-

A briefing on brow presentation

A brow presentation (the rarest of the presentations) may occur with a multipara or in an individual with relaxed abdominal muscles. Here are some key points about this type of presentation:
• It almost invariably results in obstructed labor because the head becomes jammed in the brim of the pelvis as the occipitomental diameter presents.
• Unless the presentation spontaneously corrects, cesarean birth is necessary to safely deliver the neonate.
• Because brow presentation leaves extreme ecchymotic bruising on the neonate's face and head, his parents may need additional reassurance that he's healthy.

er extremities, takes up more space. The fundus, being the largest part of the uterus, promotes fetal turning so that the buttocks and lower extremities are within it. Additionally, some evidence suggests that a breech presentation is less likely to occur if a woman assumes a knee-chest position for approximately 15 minutes three times per day during pregnancy.

Styles of breech from frank to complete

There are several types of breech presentations:
• frank breech—in which the buttocks are the presenting part and the legs are extended and rest on the fetal chest
• footling breech—which can be either one foot (single-footling) or both feet (double-footling breech) and the thighs or lower legs aren't flexed
• complete breech—in which the fetal thighs are flexed on the abdomen and both the buttocks and the tightly flexed feet are against the cervix.

Danger, danger

Breech presentation is more hazardous than a cephalic presentation because there's a greater risk of:
• anoxia from a prolapsed cord
• traumatic injury to the after-coming head, which can result in intracranial hemorrhage or anoxia
• fracture of the spine or arm
• dysfunctional labor
• early rupture of the membranes because of the poor fit of the presenting part
• meconium aspiration (the inevitable contraction of the fetal buttocks from cervical pressure commonly causes meconium to be extruded into the amniotic fluid before birth).

Same stages

In a breech birth, the same stages of flexion, descent, internal rotation expulsion, and external rotation occur as in a cephalic birth. (See *A look at breech birth*.)

Turn, turn, turn

An alternative to vaginal or cesarean birth of a fetus in breech presentation is a method called *external cephalic version*. In this method, the fetus is manually turned from a breech to a cephalic position before birth. Use of external version can decrease the number of cesarean births due to breech presentations by about 40%. To turn the fetus:

The breech and vertex of the fetus are located and grasped transabdominally by an examiner's hands on the woman's abdomen.

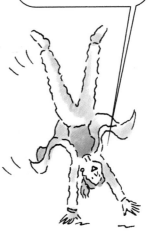

To put a different spin on things, in external cephalic version, the fetus is manually turned from a breech presentation to a cephalic position before birth.

A look at breech birth

A breech presentation follows the same stages of descent, flexion, and rotation as a cephalic presentation.

As the breech fetus enters the birth canal, descent and external rotation occur, as shown below.

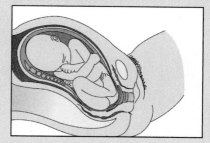

If the presenting part is the buttocks, the practitioner reaches up into the birth canal and pulls the legs down and out, as shown below. The breech delivery continues as the shoulders turn and present in the anteroposterior diameter of the mother's pelvis.

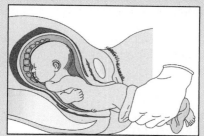

The head is then delivered by laying the neonate across the practitioner's left hand while two fingers are placed in the neonate's mouth and the other hand is placed on the back of the neck to apply gentle pressure to flex the head fully, as shown below. At the same time, gentle upward and outward traction is applied to the shoulders. An assistant may need to gently apply external abdominal wall pressure to ensure that head flexion occurs.

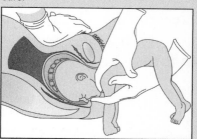

Gentle pressure is then exerted to rotate the fetus. The fetus must be moved in a forward direction to a cephalic lie. (See *A look at external cephalic version,* page 378.)

Face presentation

In a face presentation, the chin, or *mentum,* is the presenting part. Although this presentation is rare, when it does occur, birth usually can't proceed because the diameter of the presenting part is too large for the maternal pelvis. Face presentation is considered a warning sign because its cause is always some abnormality in the fetus or mother.

Transverse lie

Transverse lie occurs when the fetus lays horizontal to the uterus. Because there's no firm presenting part, a vaginal delivery isn't possible.

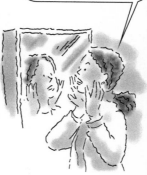

Let's face this head on. A face presentation results from some abnormality in the fetus or mother.

A look at external cephalic version

In external cephalic version, the practitioner manually rotates the fetus. The fetus is rotated by external pressure to a cephalic lie, aiding the possibility of a normal vaginal delivery.

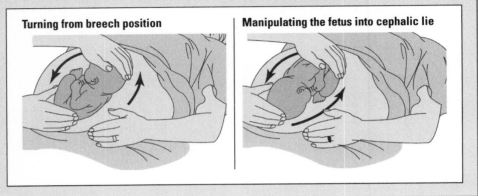

Turning from breech position

Manipulating the fetus into cephalic lie

What causes it

Contributing factors depend on the specific fetal presentation or position abnormality.

Occipitoposterior position

Posterior positions tend to occur in women with these pelvic structures:
• android pelvis
• anthropoid pelvis
• contracted pelvis.

Breech presentation

Breech presentation may occur for various reasons, including:
• gestational age younger than 40 weeks
• fetal abnormality from anencephaly, hydrocephalus, or meningocele
• hydramnios, which allows free fetal movement so the fetus doesn't have to engage for comfort
• congenital anomaly of the uterus, such as a midseptum, that traps the fetus in a breech position
• space-occupying mass in the pelvis that doesn't allow engagement, such as a fibroid tumor of the uterus and placenta previa
• pendulous abdomen in the mother that occurs when the abdominal muscles are lax, which may cause the uterus to fall so far for-

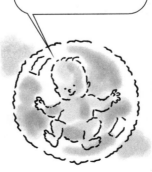

Oops! Am I early? Gestational age less than 40 weeks can contribute to breech presentation.

ward that the head comes to lie outside the pelvic brim, causing breech presentation
• multiple gestation in which the presenting fetus can't turn to a vertex position.

Face presentation

A fetus in a posterior position, instead of flexing the head as labor proceeds, may extend the head, resulting in a face presentation. The situations in which this occurs include:
• a woman with a contracted pelvis
• placenta previa
• relaxed uterus of a multipara
• prematurity
• hydramnios
• fetal malformation.

Transverse lie

Transverse lie occurs in these conditions:
• a woman with a pendulous abdomen
• a uterine mass, such as fibroid tumor, that obstructs the lower uterine segment
• contraction of the pelvic brim
• congenital uterine abnormalities
• hydramnios
• hydrocephalus or other gross abnormalities that prevent the head from engaging
• prematurity
• room for free fetal movement in the uterus
• multiple gestation (particularly in a second twin)
• short umbilical cord
• placenta previa
• fetal abnormalities.

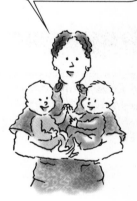

Seeing double? Multiple gestation can cause transverse lie, especially in a second twin.

How it's detected

Detection of abnormalities also depends on the specific fetal position or presentation abnormality.

Occipitoposterior position

On assessment, a posteriorly presenting head will be found to not fit the cervix as snugly as one occurring in an anterior position. Because this increases the risk of prolapse of the umbilical cord, the position of the fetus should be confirmed on vaginal examination or by sonogram.

A posterior position may also be suspected when dysfunctional labor patterns occur, such as:
- prolonged active phase
- arrested descent
- fetal heart sounds heard best at the lateral sides of the abdomen.

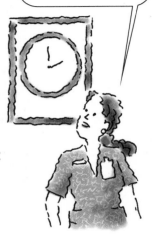

Posterior position may be suggested by a prolonged active phase.

Getting into position

Most fetuses presenting in posterior positions rotate during labor, and birth can proceed normally. This scenario is most common when the fetus is of average size and in good flexion. This rotation is also aided by forceful uterine contractions causing the fetus to rotate through the large arc. The fetus arrives at a good birth position for the pelvic outlet in these situations and can be delivered satisfactorily. The fetus may experience slightly increased molding and caput formation.

Drawing it out

One of the drawbacks to the posterior position is the duration of the labor process. Because the arc of rotation is greater, it's common for the labor to be somewhat prolonged. Labor pain is also different in this type of positioning. Because the fetal head rotates against the sacrum, the woman may experience pressure and pain in her lower back from sacral nerve compression during labor.

Breech presentation

Breech presentation is detected by these findings:
- Fetal heart sounds are commonly heard high in the abdomen.
- Leopold's maneuvers identify the fetal head in the uterine fundus.
- Vaginal examination reveals the presence of the buttocks or the foot (or both) as the presenting part, although, if the breech is complete and firmly engaged, the tightly stretched gluteal muscles may be mistaken on vaginal examination for a head and the cleft between the buttocks may be mistaken for the sagittal suture line.
- Ultrasound reveals the position of the fetus and provides information on pelvic diameter, fetal skull diameter, and the existence of placenta previa.

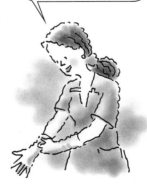

Be careful! Tightly stretched gluteal muscles can be mistaken for a head during vaginal examination for breech presentation.

Face presentation

When a face presentation is suspected, a sonogram can be performed to confirm the position of the fetus. If indicated, measurements of the pelvic diameters are made. Other signs of face presentation include:

- fetus's head that feels more prominent than normal with no engagement apparent during Leopold's maneuvers
- fetus's head and back that are both felt on the same side of the uterus with Leopold's maneuvers
- difficulty outlining the fetus's back (because it's concave)
- fetal heart tones heard on the side of the fetus where feet and arms can be palpated (in extremely concave back, which causes transmission of fetal heart tones to the forward-thrust chest)
- vaginal examination that reveals the nose, mouth, or chin as the presenting part.

Transverse lie

A transverse lie is usually obvious on inspection, when the ovoid of the uterus is found to be more horizontal than vertical. Other detection methods include:
- Leopold's maneuvers, which make it easier to palpate the fetus in a transverse lie position
- sonogram, which confirms transverse lie and provides other information (such as pelvic size).

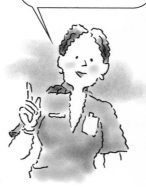

Intervention depends on the specific presentation and position.

What to do

Management of fetal position or presentation abnormalities depends on the specific type of abnormality.

Occipitoposterior position

Because labor pain may be intense when a fetus is in the occipitoposterior position, management can be a challenge. Commonly, the laboring woman asks for medication for relief of the intense pressure on and pain in her back. Consider alternative methods to help relieve back pressure, such as those mentioned here:
- Place pressure on the sacrum, such as with a back rub, or suggest a position change to relieve some of the pain.
- Apply heat or cold, depending on which is more successful in obtaining relief.
- Ask the woman to lie on the side opposite the fetal back or maintain a hands-and-knees position to help the fetus rotate.
- Encourage the woman to void approximately every 2 hours to keep the bladder empty to avoid impeding the descent of the fetus and additional discomfort.
- Because of the commonly lengthy labor, be aware of how long it has been since the patient last ate. During a long labor, she may need I.V. glucose solutions to replace glucose stores used for energy.

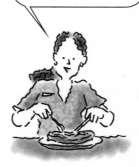

I.V. glucose may be necessary for energy in a prolonged labor when the woman hasn't eaten in a long time.

Something else to consider

Here are some other considerations for the woman delivering a baby in the occipitoposterior position:

• During labor, the woman needs a great deal of support to prevent her from becoming panicked over the length of the labor. In addition, you should provide practical, step-by-step explanations of what's happening.

• Be aware that the woman who's best prepared for labor is commonly the most frightened when deviations occur because she realizes that her labor isn't going "by the book" or as described by her birthing instructor. Provide frequent reassurance to her that, although the labor is long, her pattern of labor is still within safe, controlled limits.

Breech presentation

If the fetus in a breech presentation can be born vaginally, when full dilation is reached the woman is allowed to push and the breech, trunk, and shoulders are delivered. Here's what else you can expect:

• As the breech spontaneously emerges from the birth canal, it's steadied and supported by a sterile towel held against the neonate's inferior surface.

• The shoulders present toward the outlet, with their widest diameter anteroposterior. If the shoulders don't deliver readily, the arm of the posterior shoulder may be drawn down by passing two fingers over the neonate's shoulder and down the arm to the elbow and then sweeping the flexed arm across the neonate's face and chest and out.

• The other arm is then delivered in the same way. External rotation is allowed to occur to bring the head into the best outlet diameter.

Everything comes to a head

Birth of an aftercoming head involves a great deal of judgment and skill. Here's how it's done:

• To aid delivery of the head, the trunk of the neonate is usually straddled over the practitioner's right forearm.

• The practitioner places two fingers of his right hand in the neonate's mouth.

• The practitioner slides his left hand into the mother's vagina, palm down, along the neonate's back.

• Pressure is applied to the occiput to flex the head fully.

• Gentle traction applied to the shoulders (upward and outward) delivers the head.

Pied Piper

An aftercoming head may also be delivered using Piper forceps to control the flexion and rate of descent. (See *Using Piper forceps*.)

Head hazards

Birth of the head is the most hazardous part of a breech birth. Here are some complications to consider:
• Because the umbilicus comes before the head, a loop of cord passes down alongside the head and automatically becomes compressed. This compression is due to the pressure of the head against the pelvic brim.
• With a cephalic presentation, molding to the confines of the birth canal occurs over hours. With a breech birth, this pressure change occurs instantaneously. Tentorial tears can occur as a result of this pressure change. These tears may cause gross motor malfunction, mental problems, or lethal damage to the fetus.
• The neonate may be delivered suddenly to decrease the duration of cord compression. Doing so, however, may result in an intracranial hemorrhage.
• A neonate delivered gradually in order to reduce the possibility of intracranial injury may suffer hypoxia.

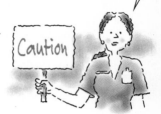

Here's a heads up. The most hazardous part of a breech birth is the birth of the head.

What happened?

Parents and health care providers usually inspect a breech neonate a little more closely than a neonate from a normal delivery for many reasons:
• The cause of the breech birth may be unknown. The parents and the person who makes the initial physical assessment of the neonate may look for the reason that made the presentation breech.

Using Piper forceps

Occasionally, the fetal head can't be easily delivered in a breech presentation. Piper forceps may be used to apply traction directly to the head, preventing damage to the fetal neck.

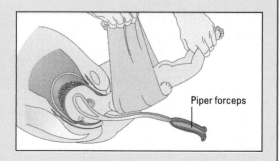

Piper forceps

• Remember that a neonate who was delivered in a frank breech position may resume his fetal position. He may keep his legs extended and at the level of the face for the first 2 to 3 days of life.
• The neonate who presented in a footling breech may keep the legs extended in a footling position for the first few days.
• Be sure to point out these possible positions to the parents to avoid undue worry or a misinterpretation of the neonate's unusual posture.

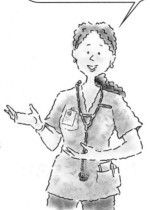

Be sure to point out these possible positions to the parents to avoid undue worry or a misrepresentation of the neonate's unusual posture.

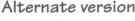
Alternate version

If external cephalic version is performed before the birth to turn the fetus to a cephalic position, remember the following considerations:
• FHR and, possibly, ultrasound should be recorded continuously.
• A tocolytic agent may be administered to help relax the uterus.
• Provide support to the woman to help her tolerate the discomfort from the pressure experienced during the procedure.
• Women who are Rh-negative should receive Rh immunoglobulin in case minimal bleeding occurs.

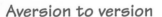
Aversion to version

Contraindications to external cephalic version include:
• multiple gestation
• severe oligohydramnios
• contraindications to vaginal birth
• a nuchal cord
• unexplained third-trimester bleeding (possibly suggesting placenta previa).

Face presentation

If the chin is anterior and the pelvic diameters are within normal limits, the fetus in face presentation may be delivered without difficulty. However, certain complications must be considered:
• There may be a long first stage of labor because the face doesn't mold well to make a snugly engaging part.
• If the chin is posterior, cesarean delivery is the optimal method of birth because a vaginal birth would require posterior-to-anterior rotation, which could take a long time. In addition, such rotation can result in uterine dysfunction or a transverse arrest.

Edema dilemma

Babies born after a face presentation have a great deal of facial edema and may be purple from ecchymotic bruising. Additional considerations include:
• Lip edema may be so severe that the neonate can't suck for 1 or 2 days.

- The neonate may need gavage feedings to obtain enough fluid until he can suck effectively.
- The neonate must be observed closely for a patent airway.
- The neonate is usually transferred to a neonatal ICU for the first 24 hours.
- Assure the parents that the edema will disappear in a few days and causes no long-term effects.

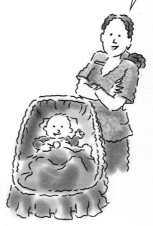

Assure parents that facial edema will disappear in a few days and causes no long-term effects.

Transverse lie

A mature fetus in a transverse lie position can't be delivered vaginally. Although the membranes usually rupture at the beginning of labor, there's no firm presenting part. Thus, the cord or arm may prolapse or the shoulder can come down and obstruct the cervix. Cesarean birth is mandatory in this instance. Thus, to manage transverse lie presentation, follow the care measures for cesarean birth.

Fetal size

The size of the fetus may be an indication of a difficult delivery. In general, a fetus who weighs more than 4,500 g (9.9 lb) may lead to a difficult delivery. An abnormally large fetal size may pose a problem at birth because it can cause fetal pelvic disproportion or uterine rupture from obstruction. The risk of perinatal mortality in larger neonates is substantially higher than in normal-sized neonates (15% versus 4%). The large neonate born vaginally also has a higher-than-normal risk of:
- cervical nerve palsy
- diaphragmatic nerve injury
- fractured clavicle because of shoulder dystocia.

Mom, too

During the postpartum period, the mother has an increased risk of hemorrhage because an overdistended uterus may not contract as readily.

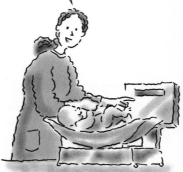

The incidence of shoulder dystocia is increasing along with the increasing average weight of neonates.

Shoulder dystocia

Shoulder dystocia is increasing in incidence along with the increasing average weight of neonates. The problem occurs at the second stage of labor when the fetal head is born but the shoulders are too broad to enter the pelvic outlet. This situation can cause vaginal or cervical tears in the mother or cord compression leading to a fractured clavicle or brachial plexus injury in the fetus.

What causes it

Large fetuses are most common in women who are diabetic. Large babies are also associated with multiparity, because each neonate born to a woman tends to be slightly heavier and larger than the one born just before. Shoulder dystocia is most apt to occur in babies of women with diabetes, multiparas, and in postdate pregnancies.

How it's detected

Although fetal size can usually be detected using palpation, it may be missed in an obese woman because the fetal contours are difficult to palpate. Also, just because she's obese doesn't mean the woman has a larger-than-usual pelvis; in fact, her pelvis may be small. Pelvimetry or sonography is the best way to compare fetal size with the woman's pelvic capacity.

Head and...shoulders?

Shoulder dystocia, however, commonly isn't identified until the head has been born. The wide anterior shoulder then seems to lock beneath the symphysis pubis. Shoulder dystocia may be suspected earlier if:
• second stage of labor is prolonged
• arrest of descent occurs
• the head, when it appears on the perineum (crowning), retracts instead of protruding with each contraction (turtle sign).

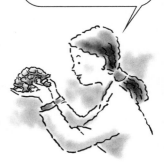

When the head of the fetus appears on the perineum and then retracts with each contraction, it's known as the turtle sign.

What to do

If the fetus is so large that the child can't be delivered vaginally, cesarean delivery becomes the method of choice. In shoulder dystocia, measures may include:
• asking the woman to flex her thighs sharply on her abdomen to widen the pelvic outlet and help the anterior shoulder deliver
• applying suprapubic pressure to help the shoulder escape from beneath the symphysis pubis.

Ineffective uterine force

Uterine contractions force the moving fetus through the birth canal. Usually, contractions are initiated at one pacemaker point in the uterus. When a contraction occurs, it sweeps down over the uterus, encircling it. Repolarization then occurs, a low resting

tone is achieved, and another pacemaker-activated contraction begins. This process is aided by:
- hormones—adenosine triphosphate, estrogen, and progesterone
- electrolytes—calcium, sodium, and potassium
- proteins—actin and myosin
- epinephrine and norepinephrine
- oxytocin
- prostaglandins.

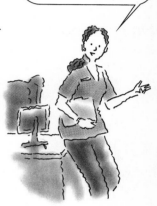

Infant mortality is higher in women who have a prolonged labor than in those who don't.

Ineffective = increased mortality

Although about 95% of labors are completed with contractions following a predictable, normal course, ineffective labor can occur. The incidence of maternal puerperal infection and hemorrhage and infant mortality is higher in women who have a prolonged labor than in those who don't. Therefore, it's vital to recognize and prevent ineffective labor.

Although effective labor can become ineffective at any time, there are two general types:

 primary (at beginning of labor)

secondary (later in labor).

Be productive

Abnormal labor can produce anxiety, fear, or discouragement in the woman as well as her partner. You should provide continuous explanations of what's happening to the woman and her support person. (See *Helping your patient reduce stress*, page 388.) In addition, there are some measures you can employ to try to promote a more productive labor. (See *Promoting productive labor*, page 389.)

When the force isn't with you

Complications due to ineffective uterine force can impede the natural course of labor. These complications include:
- hypertonic contractions
- hypotonic contractions
- uncoordinated contractions. (See *Comparing and contrasting contractions*, page 390.)

Hypertonic, hypotonic, and uncoordinated contractions are three major complications that impede the natural course of labor.

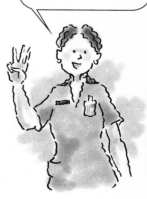

Hypertonic contractions

Hypertonic uterine contractions are marked by an increased resting tone to more than 15 mm Hg. Even so, the intensity of contractions may be no stronger than with hypotonic contractions. Hypertonic contractions tend to occur frequently. They're most commonly seen in the latent phase of labor, and may result in precipitous labor. (See *Precipitous labor*, page 391.)

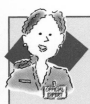

Advice from the experts

Helping your patient reduce stress

Stress results from and can lead to or increase dysfunctional labor. If a woman is tense or frightened during labor, her cervix won't dilate as rapidly, making labor prolonged.

Employ these management techniques to help your patient and her partner reduce stress:
• Ask directly if the woman has concerns.
• Offer explanations of all procedures.
• Make the support person just as welcome and comfortable as the woman herself.
• Pose questions such as, "Is labor what you thought it would be?" to both the woman and her support person to help them express concerns.
• Remember that pain is exhausting and rest promotes adequate cervical dilation. Encourage the patient to rest or sleep (if possible) in between the contractions.

• Encourage the use of nonpharmacologic comfort measures.
• Employ comfort measures, such as breathing with the woman, giving back rubs, changing sheets, and using cool washcloths. If breathing exercises are effective, the need for analgesia (which can lead to hypotonic contractions) can be reduced.
• Urge the woman to lie on her side so the uterus is lifted off the vena cava to promote comfort, increase blood supply to the uterus, and prevent hypotension.
• If a woman is more comfortable lying supine, place a hip roll under one buttock to tip her pelvis and move the uterus to the side.

Hypotonic contractions

Contractions are termed *hypotonic* when the number or frequency of contractions is low. For example, they might not increase beyond two or three in a 10-minute period. The strength of contractions doesn't rise above 25 mm Hg.

Utter exhaustion

Hypotonic contractions tend to increase the length of labor because so many of them are necessary to achieve cervical dilation. This can result in exhaustion of the mother as well as of the organs involved. This exhaustion can lead to:
• ineffective contraction of the uterus, increasing the woman's chance for postpartum hemorrhage
• risk of infection in the uterus and the fetus because of the extended period of cervical dilation.

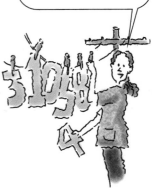

Contractions are termed hypotonic when the number or frequency of contractions is low.

Uncoordinated contractions

Uncoordinated contractions occur erratically, such as one on top of another followed by a long period without any. The lack of a regular pattern to contractions makes it difficult for the woman to rest or to use breathing exercises between contractions. Uncoordinated contractions may occur so closely together that they don't allow good filling time.

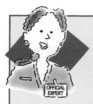

Advice from the experts

Promoting productive labor

Some measures used to promote productive labor can help avoid serious complications from ineffective labor. Consider the following measures for a patient suffering from abnormal labor.

Glucose stores
Because labor is work, it can cause a woman to deplete her glucose stores. To investigate this possibility:
• On a patient's admission to a birthing room, ask the time of her last meal to help determine if she's at risk for depleting her glucose stores. Alert the practitioner or nurse-midwife to this possibility.
• If the patient is still in early labor, she may be allowed to drink some high-carbohydrate fluid such as orange juice. I.V. fluid therapy may also be initiated to provide glucose for energy.
• Most practitioners and nurse-midwives also allow women to have lollipops or hard candy to suck on during labor to supply additional glucose.

Fluid replacement
Many women don't want to receive I.V. fluid therapy during labor. Some perceive it as losing control over their bodies or having the naturalness of labor and birth taken away.
  Take these measures to allay your patient's concerns:
• Explain the purpose of I.V. fluid therapy before arriving with the bag of fluid and tubing.
• When inserting the I.V. catheter device, try to use an insertion site in the woman's nondominant hand.
• Assure the patient that she can be out of bed and walking as well as turn freely or move about during labor as desired because none of these acts should interfere with the infusion.

What causes it

The causes of ineffective uterine force depend on the type of dysfunction.

Hypertonic contractions

Hypertonic contractions occur because the muscle fibers of the myometrium don't repolarize after a contraction, making it ready to accept a new pacemaker stimulus. They can occur when more than one pacemaker is stimulating the contractions, unlike the normal single stimulus found with normally occurring contractions. Oxytocin administration may also cause hypertonic contractions. (See *Hypertonic contractions and oxytocin*, page 392.)

Hypotonic contractions

Hypotonic contractions usually occur during the active phase of labor. They may occur when:
• analgesia has been administered too early (before cervical dilation of 3 to 4 cm)
• bowel or bladder distention is present, preventing descent or firm engagement

Hypertonic contractions can occur when more than one pacemaker stimulates contractions. It's like trying to ride two waves at once.

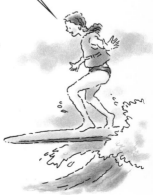

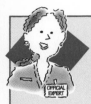

Advice from the experts

Comparing and contrasting contractions

Here are illustrations of the different uterine activity types. Depending on your assessment, you may need to intervene to promote adequate labor contractions.

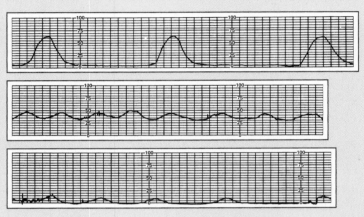

Typical contractions
Typical uterine contractions occur every 2 to 5 minutes during active labor and typically last 30 to 90 seconds.

Hypertonic contractions
Hypertonic contractions don't allow the uterus to rest between contractions, as shown by a resting pressure of 40 to 50 mm Hg.

Hypotonic contractions
Hypotonic contractions are evident by a rise in pressure of no more than 10 mm Hg during a contraction.

- the uterus is overstretched due to multiple gestation, larger-than-normal single fetus, hydramnios, or grand multiparity.

Uncoordinated contractions

With uncoordinated contractions, more than one pacemaker may initiate contractions. In addition, receptor points in the myometrium act independently of the pacemaker.

How it's detected

Ineffective uterine force is determined through physical examination and monitoring. Signs and symptoms depend on the type of dysfunction.

Hypertonic contractions

Hypertonic contractions are determined by the presence of painful uterine contractions that are either palpated or observed on an electronic monitor. On the electronic monitor, these uterine contractions show a high resting tone, and a lack of relaxation between contractions is also present. Fetal monitoring may even re-

Precipitous labor

Precipitous labor and birth occur when uterine contractions are so strong that the woman delivers with only a few rapidly occurring contractions. It's commonly defined as labor completed within less than 3 hours. Such rapid labor may occur with multiparity. It may also follow induction of labor by oxytocin or when an amniotomy is performed.

Dangerous force

In precipitous labor, contractions may be so forceful that they lead to premature separation of the placenta, placing the mother and fetus at risk for hemorrhage. The woman may also sustain injuries such as lacerations of the birth canal from the forceful delivery. Precipitous labor is also disconcerting and the woman may feel as if she has lost control.

Rapid labor poses an additional risk to the fetus as well. Subdural hemorrhage may result from the sudden release of pressure on the head.

Graphic evidence

A precipitous labor can be detected from a labor graph. This can occur during the active phase of dilation, when the rate is greater than 5 cm/hour (1 cm every 12 minutes) in a nullipara and more than 10 cm/hour (1 cm every 6 minutes) in a multipara. If this situation occurs, a tocolytic may be administered to reduce the force and frequency of contractions.

Even shorter next time

Because labors tend to be quicker with subsequent pregnancies, inform the multiparous woman by week 28 of pregnancy that her labor might be shorter than a previous one. She should plan for appropriately timed transportation to the hospital or alternative birthing center. When labor begins, alert a woman who has had a prior precipitous labor and birth that she may deliver this way again. When preparing for delivery, both grand multiparas and women with histories of precipitous labor should have the birthing room converted to birth readiness before full dilation. Then birth can be accomplished in a controlled surrounding.

veal bradycardia and fetal distress in the form of late decelerations because the absence of uterine relaxation doesn't allow the best possible uterine filling, which results in diminished oxygenation to the fetus. The woman won't be able to relax between contractions and may find it difficult to breathe with her contractions. These contractions are painful because the myometrium becomes tender as a result of inadequate relaxation.

Hypotonic contractions

Hypotonic contractions usually aren't abnormally painful because they aren't intense. However, pain is subjective; one woman's interpretation of uterine contractions may be different from another. Thus, some women may interpret these contractions as very painful.

Lack of progress

Hypotonic contractions are detected by lack of labor progression and cervical dilation. The contractions are insufficient to dilate the cervix and won't register as intense on an electronic uterine contraction monitoring strip.

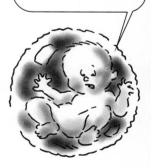

I don't want to sound like a baby, but hypertonic contractions can cause me distress.

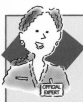

Advice from the experts

Hypertonic contractions and oxytocin

When assessing the patient receiving oxytocin, monitor for hypertonic uterine contractions. These contractions can be as high as 100 mm Hg in intensity. With these contractions, the fetus may experience late decelerations and fetal heart rate increases, as depicted here.

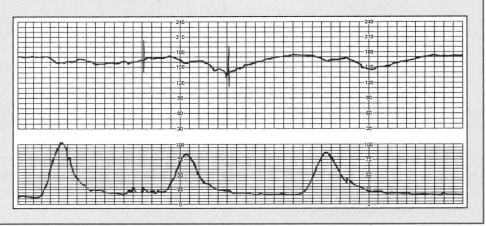

Uncoordinated contractions

Uncoordinated contraction patterns may be detected with the application of a fetal and uterine external monitor. Monitoring allows assessment of the rate, pattern, resting tone, and fetal response to contractions, revealing an abnormal pattern. Usually this pattern may be detected within 15 minutes; however, a longer time span may be necessary to show the disorganized pattern in early labor.

What to do

Management of ineffective uterine force depends on the type of dysfunction. Emotional support and other comfort measures are essential. Medication such as oxytocin may be required. (See *Oxytocin adverse effects* and *Preventing oxytocin complications*.) Cesarean delivery may be necessary if other measures are unsuccessful.

Hypertonic contractions

A woman whose pain seems out of proportion to the quality of her contractions should have both a uterine and fetal external monitor applied for at least a 15-minute interval to ensure the resting phase of the contractions is adequate and to determine that the fetal pattern isn't showing late deceleration.

Oxytocin adverse effects

When administering oxytocin, be aware of its possible adverse effects and intervene to avoid complications. Adverse effects include:
• dizziness
• headache
• nausea and vomiting
• tachycardia
• hypotension
• fetal bradycardia or tachycardia
• hypertonic contractions
• decreased urine output.

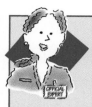

Advice from the experts

Preventing oxytocin complications

Oxytocin infusion can cause excessive uterine stimulation—leading to hypertonicity, tetany, rupture, cervical or perineal lacerations, premature placental separation, fetal hypoxia, or rapid forceful delivery—and fluid overload—leading to seizures and coma. To help prevent these complications, follow these guidelines.

Excessive uterine stimulation
• Administer oxytocin with a volumetric pump and use piggyback infusion so that the drug may be discontinued, if necessary, without interrupting the main I.V. line.
• Every 15 minutes, monitor uterine contractions, intrauterine pressure, fetal heart rate, and the character of blood loss.
• If contractions occur less than 2 minutes apart, last 90 seconds or longer, or exceed 50 mm Hg, stop the infusion, turn the patient onto her side (preferably the left), and notify the practitioner. Contractions should occur every 2½ to 3 minutes, followed by a period of relaxation.

• Keep magnesium sulfate (20% solution) available to relax the myometrium.

Fluid overload
• To identify fluid overload, monitor the patient's intake and output, especially in prolonged infusion of doses above 20 milliunits/minute.
• The risk of fluid overload also increases when oxytocin is given in hypertonic saline solution after abortion.

For good measures

Other management measures include:
• promoting rest
• providing analgesia with a drug such as morphine
• possibly inducing sedation so the woman can rest
• possibly administering morphine to relax hypertonicity
• comfort measures, such as changing the linen and the patient's gown, darkening room lights, and decreasing noise and stimulation.

If it isn't working

If decelerating FHR, an abnormally long first stage of labor, or lack of progress with pushing (second stage arrest) occurs, cesarean birth may be necessary. The woman and her support person need to understand that, although the contractions are strong, they are, in reality, ineffective and aren't achieving cervical dilation.

Hypotonic contractions

Management of hypotonic contractions includes these considerations:
• If hypotonicity is the only abnormal factor (including ruling out CPD or poor fetal presentation by sonogram), then rest and fluid intake should be encouraged.

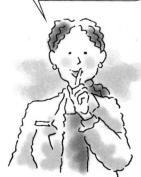

Decreasing noise and stimulation, changing the patient's linens and gown, and dimming lights are comfort measures for hypertonic contractions.

• If the membranes haven't ruptured spontaneously, rupturing them at this point may be helpful.
• Oxytocin may be administered I.V. to augment labor by causing the uterus to contract more effectively.
• If hypertension occurs, discontinue oxytocin and notify the practitioner.

Uncoordinated contractions

Management of uncoordinated contractions includes these considerations:
• Oxytocin administration may be helpful in uncoordinated labor to stimulate a more effective and consistent pattern of contractions with a better, lower resting tone.
• If hypertension occurs, discontinue oxytocin and notify the practitioner.

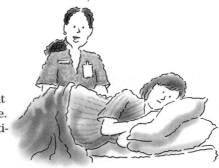

Discontinue oxytocin and notify the practitioner if hypertension occurs.

Intrauterine fetal death

Intrauterine fetal death is described as death of the fetus that occurs after a gestation of 20 weeks or longer. It can also be defined as a weight of 500 g (1.1 lb) or more.

What causes it

There are four causes of intrauterine fetal death:

 fetal

 maternal

 placental

 unknown.

Fetal fault

Fetal causes include genetic or congenital abnormalities and infection.

Maternal fault

Maternal causes include advanced maternal age, hypertension, diabetes, and pregnancy-related complications, such as preeclampsia and eclampsia, uterine rupture, Rh incompatibility, and maternal infection.

Placental fault

Placental causes include placental abruption (most common cause), prolapsed cord or a true knot in the cord, premature rupture of membranes (PROM), and twin-to-twin transfusion.

No one's fault

Sometimes, there's no clear or accountable cause for the intrauterine death.

What to look for

A pregnant woman reporting that she can no longer feel her baby move is the first sign of possible fetal death. Or, the practitioner may not be able to detect a fetal heartbeat.

What tests tell you

The only way to confirm fetal death is through an ultrasound, which can assess the cardiac movement of the fetal heart. Lack of fetal cardiac movement confirms fetal death.

How it's treated

Treatment consists of inducing labor within the next few days after it has been determined that the fetus is dead because the longer the woman carries the fetus, the greater her risk of developing DIC. If the gestation is less than 28 weeks, the woman's cervix may not be favorable for an induction; she may need to be induced with prostaglandin E_2 vaginal suppositories or oral or intravaginal misoprostol (Cytotec).

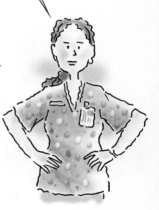

The only way to confirm fetal death is through an ultrasound.

What to do

Nursing care for a woman who has experienced an intrauterine fetal death is no different from that for a woman giving birth to a viable fetus; however, the emotional care is certainly more complex.
• Answer the woman's questions as honestly as possible.
• Encourage her to name and hold her baby, if she's able.
• Remember that each patient goes through the grieving process in different stages.
• Know that the woman and her partner may react to the death of the baby in different ways.
• Offer to call a pastor or a chaplain for the woman, her partner, and the family.

- Allow the woman, her partner, and the family time to grieve.
- Allow the woman and her partner unhurried private time with the baby to facilitate the grieving process.
- Allow the woman to assist with bathing and dressing the baby.
- Ask the woman and her partner if there's a particular religious ritual that they may wish to be performed, such as baptism or a blessing.
- According to facility policy, gather mementos such as a photograph of the baby and distribute them to the family. Some facilities take a photograph of the baby, which is kept on record for a year; if the woman refuses the photograph initially, she may later change her mind.
- Collect footprints, a lock of hair, and other reminders of the baby and give to the woman or her partner.

Multiple gestation

A woman with multiple gestation usually causes excitement in the labor room. Additional personnel are needed for the birth. Nurses are needed to attend to possible preterm neonates. Additional pediatricians or neonatal nurse practitioners are required. The woman may get lost in all this activity and may be more frightened than excited.

Multiple gestation may be delivered by cesarean birth to decrease the risk of anoxia to a subsequent fetus. This problem is more common in multiple gestation of three or more because of the increased incidence of cord entanglement and premature separation of a placenta.

Twin positions

Most twin pregnancies present with both twins in the vertex position. This is followed in frequency by vertex and breech, breech and vertex, and then breech and breech. (See *Twin presentations*.)

What causes it

Multiple gestation may occur spontaneously, especially with a history of twins or multiple births in the family. It may also occur with fertility medications, which cause multiple ova to be released simultaneously, thus increasing the chances of fertilization of more than one ovum.

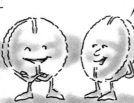

Multiple gestation may occur spontaneously or with the use of fertility drugs.

Twin presentations

There are four types of twin presentations; they are illustrated here.

Vertex	Vertex and breech	Breech	Vertex and transverse lie
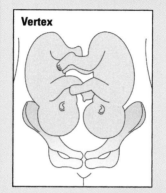	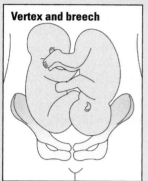	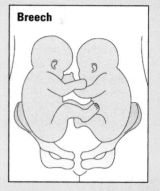	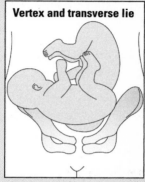

How it's detected

Multiple gestation may be suspected when several FHRs are auscultated, the mother is larger than average for gestational age of the fetus, or when palpation reveals multiple fetuses. Multiple gestation is confirmed by ultrasound.

Multiple gestation of three or more has extremely varied presentations after the birth of the first child. The lie of the second fetus is usually determined by external abdominal palpation and sonogram.

What to do

If the presentation isn't vertex, external version is attempted to make it so. If external version isn't successful, a decision for a breech delivery or cesarean delivery must be made. If a woman with multiple gestation is to deliver vaginally, she's usually instructed to come to the hospital early in labor. Here are some other considerations:

• The first stage of labor won't differ greatly from that of a single-gestation labor but coming to a hospital early may make labor seem long.

• Urge the woman to spend the early hours of labor engaged in an activity such as playing cards to make the time pass more quickly.

• Analgesia administration is given conservatively so it won't compound respiratory difficulties the neonates may have at birth because of their immaturity.

- Oxytocin infusion may be initiated to assist uterine contractions and shorten the time span between the births. It's usually begun after the first fetus is delivered.
- Nitroglycerine may be administered to relax the uterus.
- Support the use of breathing exercises to minimize the need for analgesia or anesthesia. Remember that multiple pregnancies commonly end before they're full-term, so the woman may not yet have practiced breathing exercises. The early hours of labor are an excellent opportunity to practice breathing.
- Try to monitor each FHR by a separate fetal monitor if possible.

Oxytocin may be initiated to assist uterine contractions and shorten the time span between the births.

Multiple complications

Complications such as these are common in multiple gestation:
- Because the fetuses are usually small, firm head engagement may not occur, which increases the risk of cord prolapse after rupture of the membranes.
- Uterine dysfunction from a long labor may occur.
- An overstretched uterus may result and could cause ineffective labor.
- Premature separation of the placenta after the birth of the first child is more common in multiple gestation. When separation occurs, there's sudden, profuse bleeding at the vagina, causing a risk of exsanguination for the woman.
- Because of the multiple fetuses, abnormal fetal presentation may occur.
- Anemia and gestational hypertension occur at higher-than-usual incidences in multiple gestation. Hematocrit and blood pressure should be monitored closely during labor.
- After the birth, the uterus can't contract, placing the woman at risk for hemorrhage from uterine atony.
- Separation of the first placenta may cause loosening of the additional placentas. If a common placenta is involved, the fetal heart sounds of the other fetuses immediately register distress. Careful FHR monitoring is essential. If separation occurs, the fetuses must be delivered immediately to avoid fetal death.

The risk of anemia and gestational hypertension is greater in multiple gestation.

After the event

Keep in mind the following points after the birth of multiple neonates:
- The neonates need careful assessment to determine their true gestational age and whether twin-to-twin transfusion has occurred.
- Some parents worry that the hospital will confuse their neonates through improper identification. Review with them the careful measures that are taken to ensure correct identification.
- Despite preparations for a multiple birth, the woman may have difficulty believing she has given birth to multiple neonates. She

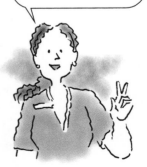

may find it helpful to discuss her feelings with you as well as view all her neonates together to become accustomed to the idea.
• The parents may be unable to inspect the neonates thoroughly immediately after the birth because of low birth weight and the danger of hypothermia. Bonding time should be promoted as soon as possible to dispel fears they may have that the babies are less than perfect.

Placental abnormalities

The normal placenta weighs in at approximately 500 g (1⅛ lb) and is 15 to 20 cm (5⅞″ to 7⅞″) in diameter and 1.5 to 3 cm (⅝″ to 1⅛″) thick. Its weight is approximately one-sixth that of the fetus. Problems can occur with the size of the placenta or the blood vessels connected to it. Other abnormalities can involve the placement of the umbilical cord or placental attachment. Types of abnormalities include:
• battledore placenta
• placenta accreta
• placenta circumvallata
• placenta succenturiata
• vasa previa
• velamentous cord insertion. (See *Abnormal placental formations*, page 400.)

What causes it

Abnormalities may be present for several reasons. For example, a placenta may be unusually enlarged in a woman with diabetes. In certain diseases, such as syphilis or erythroblastosis, the placenta may be so large that it weighs half as much as the fetus. The placenta may be wider in diameter if the uterus has scars or a septum, possibly because it was forced to spread out to find implantation space.

Well, that depends...

Other causes of placental abnormalities depend on the type of abnormality:
• Battledore placenta has no known cause.
• Placenta accreta is caused by a defect in decidua formation from implantation over uterine scars or in the lower segment of the uterus.
• Placenta circumvallata has no known cause, although formation of insufficient chorion frondosum, subchorial infarcts, and an abnormally implanted blastocyst causes part of the fetal surface to be covered by the decidua.

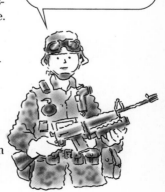

Attention! Battledore placenta has no known cause.

Abnormal placental formations

Abnormal placental formations occur for various reasons, some of which are unknown. The types of abnormal placental formations and their clinical significance are discussed here.

Battledore placenta
In battledore placenta, the umbilical cord is attached marginally, rather than centrally. It can lead to preterm labor, fetal distress, and bleeding from cord compression or vessel rupture.

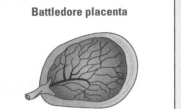

Battledore placenta

Placenta accreta
In placenta accreta, an unusually deep attachment of the placenta to the uterine myometrium doesn't allow the placenta to loosen and deliver as it should. Attempts to remove it manually may lead to extreme hemorrhage. This abnormality is associated with placenta previa, which can lead to severe maternal hemorrhage, uterine perforation, and subsequent hysterectomy.

Placenta circumvallata
In placenta circumvallata, the chorion membrane that usually begins at the edge of the placenta and spreads to envelop the fetus is missing on the fetal side of the placenta. In this condition, the umbilical cord may enter the placenta at the usual midpoint with large vessels spreading out from there. However, the vessels end abruptly at the point where the chorion folds back onto the surface. This abnormality can lead to spontaneous abortion, abruptio placentae, preterm labor, placental insufficiency, and intrapartum and postpartum hemorrhage.

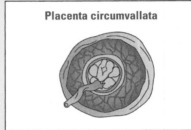

Placenta circumvallata

Placenta succenturiata
In placenta succenturiata, one or more accessory lobes are connected to the main placenta by blood vessels. Identify this abnormality through careful examination of the placenta after birth because the small lobes may be retained in the uterus, leading to severe maternal postpartum hemorrhage.

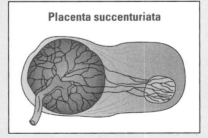

Placenta succenturiata

Vasa previa
In vasa previa, velamentous insertion of the cord is present and the unprotected and fragile umbilical vessels cross the internal os and lie in front of the presenting fetal head. This abnormal insertion may cause the cord to be delivered before the fetus, possibly causing the vessels to tear with cervical dilation, leading to hemorrhage.

Velamentous cord insertion
Velamentous cord insertion occurs when the cord separates into small vessels that reach the placenta by spreading across a fold of amnion. This form of cord insertion is found most commonly in multiple gestation and may be associated with fetal abnormalities. This condition can lead to vessel tearing and hemorrhage because the vessels are unprotected as they travel through the amnion and chorion before they form the cord.

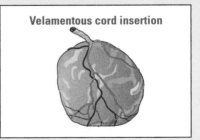

Velamentous cord insertion

- Placenta succenturiata is caused when a group of villi distant to the placenta fail to degenerate and implantation is superficial or confined to a specific site so that attachment of the trophoblast also occurs on the opposing wall. This condition can occur in the case of a bicornuate uterus.
- Vasa previa is caused by rotation of the inner cell mass and body stalk, which aligns in an eccentric insertion.
- In velamentous cord insertion, the umbilical cord inserts into the membrane, causing the vessles to run between the amnion and chorion before entering the placenta. This condition most likely occurs during implantation.

How it's detected

Placental abnormalities usually aren't detected until after the birth of the placenta. Both the umbilical cord and placenta are examined. However, if sudden painless bleeding occurs with the beginning of cervical dilation, vasa previa should be suspected. Sonogram confirms this diagnosis.

What to do

Some placental abnormalities require immediate attention, whereas others may not be significant. For example, if the patient has a placenta succenturiata, the remaining lobes must be removed from the uterus manually. This is done to prevent maternal hemorrhage from poor uterine contraction.

Look before you touch

Some abnormalities must be detected before routine care may be performed. For example, before inserting an instrument (such as an internal fetal monitor), fetal and placental structures must be identified to prevent problems. For example, accidental tearing of a vasa previa can result in sudden fetal blood loss. If vasa previa is identified, cesarean delivery of the neonate is necessary.

Abnormalities such as placenta accreta require more intense treatment. Placenta accreta requires a hysterectomy or treatment with methotrexate (Rheumatrex) to destroy the still-attached tissue.

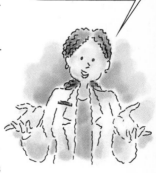

Some placental abnormalities require immediate attention, whereas others may not be significant.

Preterm labor and delivery

When labor begins earlier in gestation than normal, it's considered preterm. As with normal labor, in preterm labor rhythmic uterine contractions produce cervical change. This change may occur after fetal viability but before fetal maturity. It usually occurs between 20 and 37 weeks' gestation. Premature labor is a major cause of perinatal morbidity and mortality. Neonatal complications may include respiratory distress syndrome and intracranial bleeding. Only 5% to 10% of pregnancies end prematurely; however, about 75% of these pregnancies result in neonatal death.

Weight and length = outcome

The impact on the fetus depends on birth weight and length of gestation:
• Neonates weighing less than 737.1 g (1 lb, 10 oz) and born at fewer than 26 weeks' gestation have a survival rate of about 10%.
• Neonates weighing 737.1 g (1 lb, 10 oz) to 992.2 g (2 lb, 3 oz) and born at 27 to 28 weeks' gestation have a survival rate of more than 50%.
• Neonates weighing 992.2 g (2 lb, 3 oz) to 1,219 g (2 lb, 11 oz) and born at more than 28 weeks' gestation have a 70% to 90% survival rate.

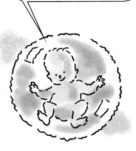

I might be a little early, but here I come!

What causes it

Causes of preterm labor include:
• PROM (30% to 50% of cases)
• hydramnios
• fetal death.

When mom is at risk

Numerous maternal risk factors also increase the incidence of preterm labor, including:
• gestational hypertension
• chronic hypertensive vascular disease
• placenta previa
• abruptio placentae
• incompetent cervix
• abdominal surgery
• trauma
• structural anomalies of the uterus
• infections (such as group B streptococci)
• genetic defect in the mother.

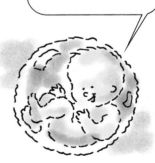

Don't blame me. It could be the genes.

Other contributors

Other factors that may cause preterm labor include:
• stimulation of the fetus via heredity. Genetically imprinted information tells the fetus that nutrition is inadequate and that a change in environment is required for well-being, thus provoking the onset of labor.

- sensitivity to the hormone oxytocin. Labor begins because the myometrium becomes hypersensitive to oxytocin, the hormone that usually induces uterine contractions.

How it's detected

As with labor at term, preterm labor produces:
- rhythmic uterine contractions
- cervical dilation and effacement
- possible rupture of the membranes
- expulsion of the cervical mucus plug
- bloody discharge.

Combination confirmation

Preterm labor is confirmed by the combined results of:
- prenatal history indicating that the patient is at 20 to 37 weeks of gestation
- ultrasonography (if available) showing the position of the fetus in relation to the mother's pelvis
- cervical examination confirming progressive cervical effacement and dilation
- continuous electronic fetal monitoring showing rhythmic uterine contractions
- possible ambulatory home monitoring with a tocodynamometer to identify preterm contractions
- differential diagnosis excluding Braxton Hicks contractions and urinary tract infection.

What to do

Treatment of premature labor aims to suppress labor when tests show:
- immature fetal pulmonary development
- cervical dilation of less than 4 cm
- absence of factors that contraindicate continuation of pregnancy.

Let's be conservative

Here are some conservative measures to suppress labor:
- A patient in preterm labor requires bed rest, close observation for signs of fetal or maternal distress, and comprehensive supportive care.
- During attempts to suppress preterm labor, make sure the patient maintains bed rest and administer medications as ordered.
- Because sedatives and analgesics may be harmful to the fetus, administer them sparingly. Minimize the need for these drugs by

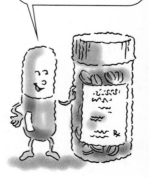

Because sedatives and analgesics may be harmful to the fetus, administer them sparingly.

providing comfort measures, such as frequent repositioning and good perineal and back care.
- Avoid preterm labor by successfully identifying patients at risk. Such patients should comply with the prescribed home treatment.
- Ensure that the woman is taking proper preventive measures, such as good prenatal care, adequate nutrition, and proper rest.
- Insertion of a purse-string suture (cerclage) can reinforce an incompetent cervix at 14 to 18 weeks' gestation to avoid preterm delivery in a patient with a history of this disorder.
- Women at risk can be treated at home and have their contractions monitored via telephone hookup.

Drug details

Pharmacologic measures to suppress labor include:
- terbutaline (Brethine) to stimulate the beta$_2$-adrenergic receptors and inhibit contractility of uterine smooth muscle. When administering this drug, monitor blood pressure, pulse rate, respirations, FHR, and uterine contraction pattern.
- magnesium sulfate to relax the myometrium and stop contractions.

Monitoring measures

Careful monitoring is essential throughout therapy. The usual monitoring of uterine contractions and fetal heart tones should be conducted. Here are some additional measures:
- If a uterine relaxant is to be given I.V., perform a baseline electrocardiogram (ECG).
- During therapy, monitor laboratory test results to detect hypokalemia, hypoglycemia, or decreased hematocrit. Report abnormal findings to the practitioner.
- Monitor the patient's cardiac status continuously and report arrhythmias.
- Check the patient's blood pressure and pulse every 10 to 15 minutes initially, then every 30 minutes or as ordered.
- Notify the practitioner if the patient's pulse rate exceeds 140 beats/minute or if her blood pressure falls 15 mm Hg or more.
- If the patient complains of palpitations or chest pain or tightness, decrease the drug dosage and notify the practitioner immediately.
- Keep emergency resuscitation equipment nearby.
- Assess pulmonary status every hour during I.V. therapy, and report crackles or increased respirations.
- Monitor intake and output and notify the practitioner if urine output drops below 50 ml/hour as pulmonary edema may result.
- If signs of pulmonary edema develop, place the patient in high-Fowler's position, administer oxygen as ordered, and notify the practitioner.

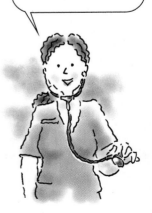

It's important to assess pulmonary status every hour during I.V. therapy, and report crackles or increased respirations.

- For 1 to 2 hours after I.V. therapy, monitor the patient's vital signs, intake and output, and fetal heart sounds.
- Perform serial ECGs as ordered.
- Immediately report tachycardia, hypotension, decreased urine output, or diminished or absent fetal heart sounds.
- Watch for maternal adverse reactions to magnesium sulfate administration, including drowsiness, slurred speech, flushing, decreased reflexes, decreased GI motility, and decreased respirations.
- Watch for fetal and neonatal adverse effects of magnesium sulfate use, including central nervous system depression, decreased respirations, and decreased sucking reflex.
- Carry out thorough patient teaching to ensure patient understanding and compliance with treatment. (See *Teaching the patient about preterm labor.*)

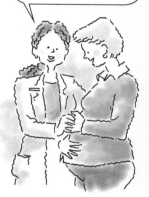

Preterm delivery may be best for mother and fetus when intrauterine infection, abruptio placentae, or severe preeclampsia is a factor.

Preterm delivery

It may be in the best interest of the fetus or the mother and fetus to allow preterm labor to progress and delivery to ensue. Maternal factors that jeopardize the mother and fetus, making preterm delivery the lesser risk, include:

- intrauterine infection
- abruptio placentae
- severe preeclampsia.

Education edge

Teaching the patient about preterm labor

Here are some guidelines for teaching a patient about preterm labor.

- Reassure her that drug effects on her neonate should be minimal.
- Tell her to notify the practitioner immediately if she experiences sweating, chest pain, or increased pulse rate.
- Teach her to check her pulse before oral drug administration. If her pulse exceeds 130 beats/minute, she shouldn't take the drug and should notify the practitioner.
- Emphasize the importance of immediately reporting contractions, lower back pain, cramping, or increased vaginal discharge.

- Instruct her to report other adverse reactions requiring a reduction in drug dosage, such as headache, nervousness, tremors, restlessness, nausea, and vomiting.
- Tell her to notify the practitioner if her urine output decreases or if she gains more than 5 lb (2.3 kg) in 1 week.
- Tell her to take her temperature every day and to report fever to the practitioner because it may be a sign of infection.
- Advise her to take oral doses of the drug with food (to avoid GI upset) and take the last dose several hours before bedtime (to avoid insomnia).
- Encourage her to remain in bed as much as possible.
- Tell her to avoid preparing her breasts for breast-feeding until about 2 weeks before her due date because this can stimulate the release of oxytocin and initiate contractions.

Factors that jeopardize the fetus can become more significant as pregnancy nears term, and so preterm delivery may be more favorable. These factors include:

- placental insufficiency
- isoimmunization
- congenital anomalies.

Ideal situation

Ideally, treatment of active preterm labor should take place in a perinatal intensive care center, where the staff is specially trained to handle this situation. The neonate can also remain close to his parents, promoting bonding. Community hospitals commonly lack the facilities for special neonatal care and transfer the neonate alone to a perinatal center.

Part of a team

Treatment and delivery require an intensive team effort focusing on:

- continuous assessment of the fetus's health through fetal monitoring
- unless contraindicated, administration of antenatal steroids to assist fetal lung development
- maintenance of adequate hydration through I.V. fluids.

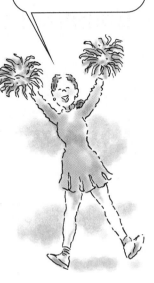

Go, team! Treatment and delivery of a preterm neonate require a team effort.

Constant concerns

Also keep in mind:

- Morphine (Duramorph) and meperidine (Demerol) may cause fetal respiratory depression. They should be administered only when necessary and in the smallest possible dose.
- Amniotomy should be avoided, if possible, to prevent cord prolapse or damage to the fetus's tender skull.
- The preterm neonate has a lower tolerance for the stress of labor and is much more likely to become hypoxic than the term neonate.
- If necessary, administer oxygen to the mother through a nasal cannula.
- Observe fetal response to labor through continuous monitoring.
- Continually reassure the mother throughout labor to help reduce her anxiety.
- Monitor fetal and maternal response to local and regional anesthetics.
- Pushing between contractions is ineffective and can damage the premature neonate's soft skull.
- Throughout labor, keep the mother informed of her progress and the condition of the fetus.
- Inform the parents of their neonate's condition. Describe his appearance and explain the purpose of supportive equipment.

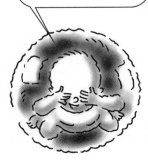

Peek-a-boo. I see you! Remember to keep tabs on my condition throughout labor.

• As necessary, before the parents leave the facility with the neonate, refer them to a community health nurse who can help them adjust to caring for a preterm neonate.

Umbilical cord anomalies

Umbilical cord anomalies include absence of an umbilical artery and an unusually long or short umbilical cord.

Absent artery

A normal umbilical cord contains one vein and two arteries. The presence of a single umbilical artery is caused by atrophy of a previously normal artery, presence of the original artery of the body stalk, or agenesis of one of the umbilical arteries. The absence of one of the umbilical arteries has been associated with congenital heart and kidney defects because the insult that caused the loss of the vessel probably led to an insult to other mesoderm germ layer structures as well.

The long...

An unusually long cord can be compromised more easily because of its greater tendency to twist or knot. When this happens, the natural pulsations of the blood through the vessels and the muscular vessel walls usually keep the blood flow adequate. A long cord that wraps around the fetus's neck is called a *nuchal cord*. If the cord is wrapped tightly enough to restrict blood flow to the fetus, it may cause stillbirth.

...and short of it

An unusually short umbilical cord can result in premature separation of the placenta or an abnormal fetal lie. It can also result in fetal asphyxia because of traction on the umbilical cord as the fetus descends.

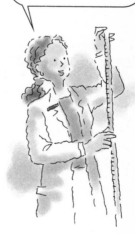

A cord that's either too long or too short can cause problems.

What causes it

The cause of differences in cord length is unknown. Some researchers suggest that reduced fetal activity, such as in the case of twinning (monoamniotic and conjoined), may be a cause and can be a genetic failure of the cord to elongate. However, the cause of unusual inversions of the cord into the placenta may be a result of rotation of the body stalk (which becomes the cord) as it implants into the placenta. The degree of rotation determines how far the umbilical cord will be from the center of the placenta.

How it's detected

Cord length abnormalities and abnormal cord insertion can be detected using ultrasound. However, detection of other umbilical cord abnormalities is only possible upon inspection of a cord at birth. Inspection should take place immediately, before the cord begins to dry because drying distorts the appearance.

What to do

Document the number of vessels present. The neonate with only two vessels needs to be observed carefully for other defects during the neonatal period.

Umbilical cord prolapse

In umbilical cord prolapse, a loop of the umbilical cord slips down in front of the presenting fetal part. This prolapse may occur at any time after the membranes rupture, especially if the presenting part isn't fitted firmly into the cervix. It happens in 1 out of 200 pregnancies. (See *Prolapse patterns*.)

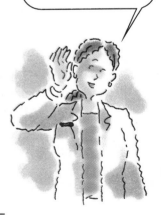

Auscultate heart sounds immediately after rupture of the membranes to rule out cord prolapse.

What causes it

Prolapse tends to occur more commonly with the following conditions:
• PROM
• fetal presentation other than cephalic
• placenta previa
• intrauterine tumors that prevent the presenting part from engaging
• small fetus
• CPD that prevents firm engagement
• hydramnios
• multiple gestation.

How it's detected

Signs of prolapse include a sudden variable deceleration FHR pattern with the cord then visible at the vulva. To rule out cord prolapse, auscultate heart sounds immediately after rupture of the membranes (occurring spontaneously or by amniotomy).

Prolapse patterns

Prolapse of the umbilical cord may occur in two ways: outwardly prolapsed or hidden. Regardless of the type of prolapse, it means that the fetal nutrient supply is compromised. Both types of prolapse can be detected by fetal monitoring.

Hidden prolapse
The cord still remains within the uterus but is prolapsed.

Outward prolapse
The cord can be seen at the vulva.

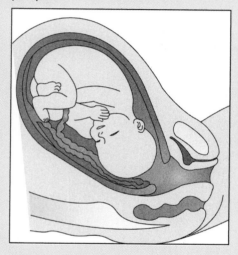 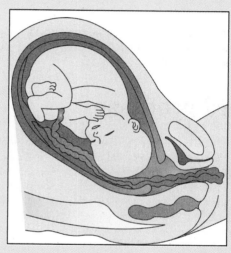

Perhaps it's prolapse

Signs of hypoxia and fetal distress suggest prolapse. In rare instances, the cord may be felt as the presenting part on vaginal examination. It can also be identified in this position on sonogram.

What to do

Cord prolapse leads to immediate cord compression because the fetal presenting part presses against the cord at the pelvic brim. Management is aimed toward relieving pressure on the cord, thereby relieving the compression and avoiding fetal anoxia.

Here are some points that you should consider if this occurs:
• If vaginal examination reveals the cord as the presenting part, cesarean birth is necessary before rupture of the membranes occurs. Otherwise, with rupture, the cord prolapses down into the vagina.

- A gloved hand may be placed in the vagina. This is done to manually elevate the fetal head off the cord.
- The woman may be placed in a knee-chest or Trendelenburg's position, which causes the fetal head to fall back from the cord.
- Administering oxygen at 10 L/minute by face mask to the mother is also helpful.
- A tocolytic agent may be used to reduce uterine activity and pressure on the fetus.
- If the cord has prolapsed so far that it's exposed to room air, drying begins, leading to atrophy of the umbilical vessels. If this happens, don't attempt to push exposed cord back into the vagina. This may add to the compression and further cause knotting or kinking. Cover the exposed portion with a sterile saline compress to prevent drying.
- If the cervix is fully dilated at the time of the prolapse, the practitioner may choose to deliver the neonate quickly, possibly with forceps, to prevent a period of anoxia.
- If dilation is incomplete, the birth method of choice is upward pressure on the presenting part by a practitioner's hand in the woman's vagina to keep pressure off the cord until a cesarean delivery can be performed.

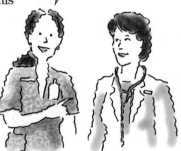

If the cervix is fully dilated at the time of prolapse, the practitioner may choose to deliver the neonate quickly to prevent a period of anoxia.

Uterine rupture

Rupture of the uterus during labor is a rare occurrence; it happens in about 1 in 1,500 births. A uterus ruptures when it undergoes more strain than it can sustain. If the situation isn't relieved, uterine rupture and death of the fetus may occur. In the placental stage, massive maternal hemorrhage may result because the placenta is loosened but then can't deliver, preventing the uterus from contracting. Uterine rupture accounts for as many as 5% of all maternal deaths. When it occurs, fetal death results 50% of the time.

The viability of the fetus depends on the extent of the rupture and the time that elapses between the rupture and abdominal extraction. The woman's prognosis depends on the extent of the rupture and blood loss. It's inadvisable for a woman to conceive again after a rupture of the uterus unless it occurred in the inactive lower segment.

What causes it

The most common cause of uterine rupture is previous cesarean birth, such as when a vertical scar from a previous incision is present. It can also be from hysterotomy repair. Contributing factors include:
- prolonged labor
- faulty presentation
- multiple gestation
- use of oxytocin
- obstructed labor
- traumatic maneuvers using forceps or traction.

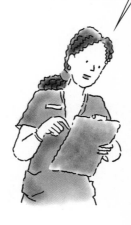

The most common cause of uterine rupture is previous cesarean birth.

How it's detected

Strong uterine contractions that occur without cervical dilation are a sign of impending rupture. A more specific sign, called a *pathologic retraction ring*, is an indentation that appears across the abdomen over the uterus just before rupture.

The things about rings

Two types of retraction rings can occur in abnormal labor:

Bandl's ring—This sign is evident at the junction of the upper and lower uterine segments. It usually appears during the second stage of labor as a horizontal indentation across the abdomen. It's formed by excessive retraction of the upper uterine segment. The uterine myometrium is much thicker above the ring than below it.

Constricting ring—This sign can occur at any point in the myometrium and at any time during labor. When it occurs in early labor, it's usually the result of uncoordinated contractions. Causes may include obstetric manipulation or administration of oxytocin. In a constricting ring, the fetus is gripped by the constricting ring and can't advance beyond that point. The undelivered placenta is also held at that point.

Retraction rings are confirmed by sonogram. This finding is extremely serious and should be reported promptly.
- Administration of I.V. morphine or the inhalation of amyl nitrite may relieve the retraction ring.
- A tocolytic may be administered to halt contractions.

Complete rupture

If the rupture is complete, here are some changes you can expect:
- The woman experiences a sudden, severe pain during a strong labor contraction and then contractions stop.

• The patient may report a tearing sensation and hemorrhaging may occur from the torn uterus into the abdominal cavity and possibly into the vagina. Rupture goes through endometrium, myometrium, and peritoneum.
• Signs of shock begin immediately, including rapid, weak pulse; falling blood pressure; cold and clammy skin; and respiratory distress.
• The woman's abdomen changes in contour. Two distinct swellings are visible: the retracted uterus and the extrauterine fetus.
• Fetal heart sounds become absent.

Incomplete rupture

If the rupture is incomplete, the signs are less dramatic:
• The woman may experience only a localized tenderness.
• She may complain of a persistent aching pain over the area of the lower segment.
• Fetal heart sounds, lack of contractions, and the woman's vital signs gradually reveal fetal and maternal distress. (See *Signs of uterine rupture*.)

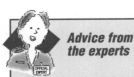

Advice from the experts

Signs of uterine rupture

Signs and symptoms of uterine rupture require prompt recognition and intervention. Intervene immediately to save the life of the mother and fetus. Signs and symptoms include:
• severe abdominal pain
• halt in contractions
• absent fetal heart rate
• possible vaginal bleeding
• falling blood pressure
• rapid weak pulse.

What to do

The uterus at the end of pregnancy is a highly vascular organ. This makes uterine rupture an immediate emergency situation. It's comparable to a splenic or hepatic rupture. Most likely, a cesarean delivery is performed to ensure safe birth of the fetus. Manual removal of the placenta under general anesthesia may be necessary in the event of placental-stage pathologic retraction rings. The following measures are also indicated:
• Administer emergency fluid replacement therapy as ordered.
• Anticipate use of I.V. oxytocin to attempt to contract the uterus and minimize bleeding.
• Prepare the woman for a possible laparotomy as an emergency measure to control bleeding and effect a repair.
• The practitioner, with consent, may perform a hysterectomy (removal of the damaged uterus) or tubal ligation at the time of the laparotomy. Explain to the patient that these procedures result in loss of childbearing ability.
• The woman may have difficulty giving her consent at this time because it isn't known whether the fetus will live.
• If blood loss is acute, the woman may be unconscious from hypotension. If this is the case, her support person must give consent, relying on the information provided by the operating surgeon to decide whether a functioning uterus can be saved.

- Be prepared to offer information and support and to inform the support person about the fetal outcome, the extent of the surgery, and the woman's safety as soon as possible.

Give time for grief

- Expect the parents to go through a grieving process for not only the loss of this child (as applicable) but also the loss of having future children through pregnancies.
- Allow them time to express these emotions without feeling threatened.

Uterine inversion

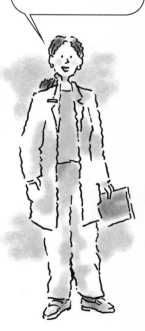

Excessive cord traction or excessive fundal pressure during the third stage of labor can cause uterine inversion.

Uterine inversion is a rare phenomenon in which the uterus turns inside out. It occurs in about 1 in 15,000 births. It may occur after the birth of the neonate, especially if traction is applied to the uterine fundus when the uterus isn't contracted. It may also occur when there's insertion of the placenta at the fundus, so that during birth, the passage of the fetus pulls the fundus down.

A matter of degrees

Uterine inversion can range from first-degree (incomplete) inversion, in which the corpus extends to the cervix but not beyond the cervical ring, to third-degree (complete) inversion. In complete inversion, the inverted uterus extends into the perineum. An additional condition, called *total uterine inversion*, involves total inversion of the uterus and the vagina.

What causes it

Causes of uterine inversion occur during the third stage of labor and include:
- excessive cord traction
- excessive fundal pressure.

How it's detected

Signs of inversion include:
- a large, sudden gush of blood from the vagina
- inability to palpate the fundus in the abdomen
- signs of blood loss (hypotension, dizziness, paleness, diaphoresis)

• signs of shock (such as increased heart rate and decreased blood pressure) if the loss of blood continues unchecked for more than a few minutes
• inability of the uterus to contract, resulting in continued bleeding (a woman could exsanguinate within a period as short as 10 minutes).

What to do

When exsanguination is imminent, follow these measures:
• Never attempt to replace the inversion because without good pelvic relaxation this may only increase bleeding.
• Never attempt to remove the placenta if it's still attached because this only creates a larger bleeding area.
• Administering an oxytocic drug only compounds the inversion.
• Start an I.V. fluid line if one isn't present. Use a large-gauge needle because blood must be replaced. Open an existing fluid line to achieve optimal fluid flow for fluid volume replacement.
• Administer oxygen by mask, and assess vital signs.
• Be prepared to perform CPR if the woman's heart fails from the sudden blood loss.
• The woman should immediately receive general anesthesia or, possibly, nitroglycerine or a tocolytic drug I.V. to relax the uterus.
• The delivering practitioner or nurse-midwife replaces the fundus manually.
• Oxytocin is administered after manual replacement, which helps the uterus to contract into place.
• Because the uterine endometrium was exposed, the woman requires antibiotic therapy postpartum to prevent infection.

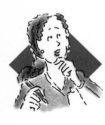

Quick quiz

1. Maternal factors indicating the need for cesarean birth include:
    A.   transverse fetal lie.
    B.   previous cesarean birth with bikini incision.
    C.   active genital herpes.
    D.   hypotension.
Answer: C. Maternal factors for cesarean birth include CPD, active genital herpes or papilloma, previous cesarean birth by classic incision, and disabling conditions, such as severe hypertension of pregnancy or heart disease, that prevent pushing to accomplish the pelvic division of labor.

2. Contraindications for cesarean birth include:
A. papilloma.
B. fetal distress.
C. transverse fetal lie.
D. dead fetus.

Answer: D. Cesarean birth is generally contraindicated when there's a documented dead fetus. In this situation, labor can be induced to avoid a surgical procedure.

3. The presence of meconium in the amniotic fluid before birth may indicate:
A. breech presentation.
B. transverse lie.
C. abruptio placentae.
D. placenta previa.

Answer: A. In breech presentation, the inevitable contraction of the fetal buttocks from cervical pressure typically causes meconium to be extruded into the amniotic fluid before birth. This, unlike meconium staining that occurs from fetal anoxia, isn't a sign of fetal distress but is expected from the buttock pressure.

4. The child born in breech presentation is at risk for:
A. hypotension.
B. hypoxia.
C. intracranial hemorrhage.
D. infection.

Answer: C. A danger of breech birth is intracranial hemorrhage. With a cephalic presentation, molding to the confines of the birth canal occurs over hours. With a breech birth, pressure changes occur instantaneously. The neonate who's delivered suddenly to reduce the amount of time of cord compression may, therefore, suffer an intracranial hemorrhage.

5. Administration of oxytocin should be discontinued when:
A. contractions are less than 2 minutes apart.
B. contractions are stronger than 50 mm Hg.
C. contractions are less than 50 seconds long.
D. contractions are irregular.

Answer: B. General guidelines for oxytocin use include that contractions should occur no more than every 2 minutes, shouldn't be stronger than 50 mm Hg, and shouldn't last longer than 70 seconds.

6. With the administration of magnesium sulfate, the woman should be observed for:
   A.   hyperactivity.
   B.   flushing.
   C.   increased reflexes.
   D.   increased respirations.

Answer: B. Magnesium sulfate relaxes the myometrium. It also produces maternal adverse effects, such as drowsiness, slurred speech, flushing, decreased reflexes, decreased GI motility, and decreased respirations.

Scoring

✰✰✰   If you answered all six questions correctly, give yourself a hand! You've got a good grip on a complicated subject.

✰✰   If you answered five questions correctly, capital! You're using your head to grasp these labor complications.

✰   If you answered fewer than five questions correctly, keep your eye on the prize. Going through the chapter again can help you see your way through.

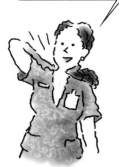

Give yourself a pat on the back for a job well done! Then let's go to the chapter on postpartum care.

Postpartum care

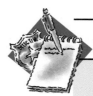

Just the facts

In this chapter, you'll learn:

♦ physiologic and psychological changes that occur during the postpartum period

♦ key components of a postpartum assessment

♦ nursing care measures required during the postpartum period

♦ physiologic events that occur during lactation

♦ two feeding methods, including their advantages and disadvantages.

A look at postpartum care

The postpartum period, or *puerperium*, refers to the 6- to 8-week period after delivery during which the mother's body returns to its prepregnant state. Some people refer to this period as the *fourth trimester of pregnancy*. Many physiologic and psychological changes occur in the mother during this time. Nursing care should focus on helping the mother and her family adjust to these changes and on easing the transition to the parenting role.

Physiologic changes

Two types of physiologic changes occur during the postpartum period: retrogressive changes and progressive changes.

Getting back to normal

Retrogressive changes involve returning the body to its prepregnancy state. Retrogressive reproductive system changes include:

- shrinkage and descent of the uterus into its prepregnancy position in the pelvis
- sloughing of the uterine lining and development of lochia
- contraction of the cervix and vagina
- recovery of vaginal and pelvic floor muscle tone.

Theory of involution

After delivery, the uterus gradually decreases in size and descends into its prepregnancy position in the pelvis—a process known as *involution*. Involution normally begins immediately after delivery, when the firmly contracted uterus lies midway between the umbilicus and symphysis pubis. Soon after, the uterus rises to the umbilicus or slightly above it. After the first postpartum day, the uterus begins its descent into the pelvis at the rate of 1 cm/day (or 1 fingerbreadth/day), or slightly less for the patient who has had a cesarean delivery. By the 10th postpartum day, the uterus lies deep in the pelvis—either at or below the symphysis pubis—and it can't be palpated.

Contraction is key

If the uterus fails to contract or remain firm during involution, uterine bleeding or hemorrhage can result. At delivery, placental separation exposes large uterine blood vessels. Uterine contraction acts as a tourniquet to close these blood vessels at the placental site. Fundal massage, the administration of synthetic oxytocics, and the release of natural oxytocics during breast-feeding help to maintain or stimulate contraction.

All systems under-go

Other body systems undergo retrogressive changes as well. These alterations include:
- reduction in pregnancy hormones, such as human chorionic gonadotropin, human placental lactogen, progestin, estrone, and estradiol
- extensive diuresis, which rids the body of excess fluid and reduces the added blood volume of pregnancy
- gradual rise in hematocrit, which occurs as excess fluid is excreted
- reactivation of digestion and absorption
- eventual fading of striae gravidarum (stretch marks), chloasma (pigmentation on face and neck), and linea nigra (pigmentation on abdomen)
- gradual return of tone to the abdominal muscles, wall, and ligaments
- return of vital signs to normal parameters
- weight loss due to rapid diuresis and lochial flow

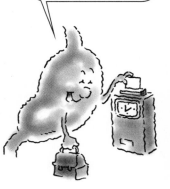

In the postpartum period, I'm working on regaining my muscle tone.

- recession of varicosities (although they may never return completely to prepregnancy appearance).

In addition, estrogen and progesterone production drops abruptly after delivery and follicle-stimulating hormone (FSH) production rises, resulting in the gradual return of ovulation and the menstrual cycle.

Making progress

Progressive changes involve the building of new tissues, primarily those that occur with lactation and the return of menstrual flow. In the postpartum period, fluid accumulates in the breast tissue in preparation for breast-feeding and breast tissue increases in size as breast milk forms. The changes associated with lactation are discussed in more detail later in this chapter.

Psychological changes

The postpartum period is a time of transition for the new mother and her family. Even if the family has other children, each family member must adjust to the neonate's arrival. The mother, in particular, undergoes many psychological changes during this time in addition to the changes that are occurring in her body.

Don't let the phases faze you

The mother goes through three distinct phases of adjustment in the postpartum period:

 taking in

 taking hold

 letting go.

In the past, each phase of the postpartum period encompassed a specific time span, with women progressing through the phases sequentially. However, with today's shorter hospitalizations for childbirth, women move through the phases more quickly and sometimes even experience more than one phase at a time. (See *Phases of the postpartum period,* page 420.)

Building relationships

The mother and her family undergo other changes as well. Ideally, these changes lead to the development of parental love for the neonate and positive relationships among all family members.

Phases of the postpartum period

This chart summarizes the three phases of the postpartum period.

Phase	Maternal behavior and tasks
Taking in (1 to 2 days after delivery)	• Contemplation of her recent birth experience • Assumption of passive role and dependence on others for care • Verbalization about labor and birth • Sense of wonderment when looking at the neonate
Taking hold (2 to 7 days after delivery)	• Increased independence in self-care • Strong interest in caring for the neonate that's often accompanied by a lack of confidence about her ability to provide care
Letting go (about 7 days after delivery)	• Adaption to parenthood and definition of new role as parent and caregiver • Abandonment of fantasized image of neonate and acceptance of real image • Recognition of neonate as a separate entity • Assumption of responsibility and care for the neonate

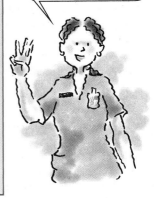

Some women move through the three phases—taking in, taking hold, and letting go—more quickly than others.

Not all change is good

In some cases, negative psychological reactions may also occur. For example, a mother may feel let down because the neonate is now the center of attention or she may feel disappointed because the neonate doesn't meet her preconceived expectations.

A mother may also feel overwhelming sadness for no discernible reason; these feelings are commonly termed *postpartum blues* or *baby blues*. A mother with postpartum blues may experience emotional lability, a let-down feeling, crying for no apparent reason, headache, insomnia, fatigue, restlessness, depression, and anger. These feelings most commonly peak around postpartum day 5 and subside by postpartum day 10. (See *Battling the baby blues*.)

First contact

Early contact and interaction between the parents, the neonate, and other siblings—including rooming in and sibling visitation—encourages bonding and helps integrate the neonate into the family.

Education edge

Battling the baby blues

For most women, having a baby is a joyous experience. However, childbirth leaves some women feeling sad, depressed, angry, anxious, and afraid. Commonly called *postpartum blues* or *baby blues,* these feelings affect about 70% to 80% of women after childbirth. In most cases, they occur within the first few days postpartum and then disappear on their own within several days.

Help is on the way
To help your patient with postpartum blues, tell her to:
• get plenty of rest
• ask for help from her family and friends
• take special care of herself
• spend time with her partner
• call her practitioner if her mood doesn't improve after a few weeks and she has trouble coping (this may be a sign of a more severe depression).

Be sure to explain to the patient that many new mothers feel sadness, fear, anger, and anxiety after having a baby. These feelings don't mean that she's a failure as a woman or as a mother. They indicate that she's adjusting to the changes that follow birth.

Blues vs. depression
Unfortunately, about 10% of women experience a more profound problem called *postpartum depression*. In these cases, maternal feelings of depression and despair last longer than a few weeks and are so intense that they interfere with the woman's daily activities. Postpartum depression can occur after any pregnancy; it isn't specifically associated with first pregnancies. It commonly requires counseling or medication to resolve.

Possible causes of postpartum depression include:
• doubt about the pregnancy
• recent stress, such as loss of a loved one, a family illness, or a recent move
• lack of a support system
• unplanned cesarean birth (may leave the woman feeling like a failure)
• breast-feeding problems, especially if a new mother can't breast-feed or decides to stop
• sharp drop in estrogen and progesterone levels after childbirth, possibly triggering depression in the same way that much smaller changes in hormone levels can trigger mood swings and tension before menstrual periods
• early birth of neonate (may cause woman to feel unprepared)
• unresolved issues of not being able to be the "perfect" mother
• feeling of failure if the mother believes that she should instinctively know how to care for her neonate
• disappointment over sex of neonate or other characteristics (neonate isn't as mother imagined).

Signs and symptoms that may indicate that postpartum blues are actually postpartum depression include:
• worsening insomnia
• changes in appetite; poor intake
• poor interaction with the neonate; views the neonate as a burden or problem
• suicidal thoughts or thoughts of harming the neonae
• feelings of isolation from social contacts and support systems
• inability to care for self or neonate due to lack or energy or desire.

Women experiencing signs of postpartum depression should seek medical help as soon as possible. (See chapter 10 for more information on postpartum depression.)

Postpartum assessment

As with any assessment, a postpartum assessment consists of a patient history and a physical examination.

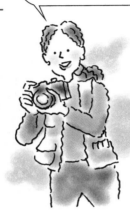

Your postpartum patient history should focus on the patient's pregnancy, labor, and birth events.

Patient history

Your postpartum patient history should focus on the patient's pregnancy, labor, and birth events. You should be able to find much of this information on the medical record. For example, the medical record should contain information about:
- problems experienced, such as gestational hypertension or gestational diabetes
- time of labor onset and admission to the birthing area
- types of analgesia and anesthesia used
- length of labor
- time of delivery
- time of placenta expulsion and appearance of the placenta
- sex, weight, and status of the neonate.

You'll need this information to plan the mother's care and promote maternal-neonate bonding.

Another reliable source

Don't rely on the medical record as your sole source of information. Always ask the mother to describe the events and fill in the details in her own words. This is also a good way to find out her emotions and feelings about pregnancy and childbirth.

Also ask the mother about her family and lifestyle, including support systems, other children, other people living in the home, her occupation, her community environment, and her socioeconomic level. This information can help you determine whether additional support, follow-up, or education about self-care and neonatal care are needed.

Always ask the mom to describe the events and fill in the details in her own words.

Physical examination

In many cases, you won't need to do a complete physical examination in the postpartum period because the mother already had a complete assessment early in the labor process. However, you should complete a review of systems, covering the following areas:
- general appearance
- skin
- energy level, including level of activity and fatigue

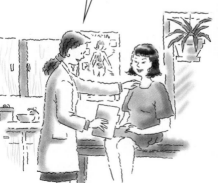

• pain, including location, severity, and aggravating factors, such as sitting and walking
• GI elimination, including bowel sounds, passage of flatus, and hemorrhoids
• fluid intake
• urinary elimination, including the time and amount of first voiding
• peripheral circulation.
  In addition, you'll need to assess these four critical areas:
• breasts
• uterus
• lochia
• perineum.

Breasts

Inspect and then palpate the breasts, noting size, shape, and color. At first, the breasts should feel soft and secrete a thin, yellow fluid called *colostrum*. However, as they fill with milk—usually around the third postpartum day—they should begin to feel firm and warm. Between feedings, the entire breast may be tender, hard, and tense on palpation. A low-grade temperature (under 101° F [38.3° C]) isn't uncommon between days 2 to 5, but it shouldn't last for more than 24 hours. (See *Engorgement or something else?* page 424.)

Land of nodule

A small, firm nodule in the breast may be caused by a temporarily blocked milk duct or milk that hasn't flowed forward into the nipple. This problem generally corrects itself when the neonate breast-feeds. Be sure to reassess the breast after the neonate feeds to determine if the problem has resolved, and report your findings—including the location of the nodule—to the practitioner

Inspect the nipples for cracks, fissures, or configuration. Cracks or breaks in the skin can provide an entry for organisms and lead to infection. Also look for other problems. Successful breast-feeding can be more challenging if the nipples are flat or inverted. A lactation consultant or a breat-feeding counselor may be helpful.

Uterus

During your examination, palpate the uterine fundus to determine uterine size, degree of firmness, and rate of descent, which is measured in fingerbreadths above or below the umbilicus. Unless the practitioner orders otherwise, perform fundal assessments every 15 minutes for the first hour after delivery, every 30 minutes for the next hour or two, every 4 hours for the rest of the first postpartum day, and then every

Memory jogger

To help you remember what to evaluate during a postpartum assessment, think of the words **BUBBLE HE.**

Breasts
Uterus
Bowel
Bladder
Lochia

Episiotomy

Homans' sign

Emotions

Keep abreast of cracks or breaks in the skin of a breast-feeding mother. They can provide an entry for organisms, leading to infection.

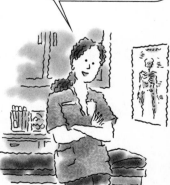

Education edge

Engorgement or something else?

Engorgement, which may result from venous and lymphatic stasis and alveolar milk accumulation, causes the entire breast to appear reddened and to feel warm, firm, and tender. The neonate will experience difficulty latching onto a severely engorged breast, which further complicates the situation. Encourage the woman to perform frequent and regular breastfeedings to help prevent this problem.

Something else

If the warmth, tenderness, and redness are localized to only one portion of the breast and the patient has a fever or flulike symptoms, suspect *mastitis*—inflammation of the glands or milk ducts.

Mastitis occurs postpartum in about 1% of mothers. It usually results from a pathogen that passes from the infant's nose or pharynx into breast tissue through a cracked nipple. Teach the mother about mastitis, and warn her to call the practitioner immediately if she has any signs or symptoms.

8 hours until the patient is discharged. Fundal assessment will need to occur more frequently if complications are noted.

Pain at the incision site makes fundal assessment especially uncomfortable for the patient who has had a cesarean birth. In such cases, provide pain medication beforehand as ordered.

Ready, set, palpate!

Before palpating the uterus, explain the procedure to the patient and provide privacy. Wash your hands and then put on gloves. Also, ask the patient to void. A full bladder makes the uterus boggier and deviates the fundus to the right of the umbilicus or +1 or +2 above the umbilicus. When the bladder is empty, the uterus should be at or close to the level of the umbilicus.

Next, lower the head of the bed until the patient is lying supine or with her head slightly elevated. Expose the abdomen for palpation and the perineum for inspection. Watch for bleeding, clots, and tissue expulsion while massaging the uterus.

Performing palpation

To palpate the uterine fundus, follow these steps:
• While supporting the lower segment of the uterus with a hand placed just above the symphysis, gently palpate the fundus with your other hand to evaluate its firmness. (See *Feeling the fundus.*)
• Note the level of the fundus above or below the umbilicus in centimeters or fingerbreadths.
• If the uterus seems soft and boggy, gently massage the fundus with a circular motion until it becomes firm. Without digging into

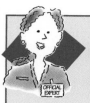

Advice from the experts

Feeling the fundus

A full-term pregnancy stretches the ligaments supporting the uterus, placing it at risk for inversion during palpation and massage. To guard against this, place one hand against the patient's abdomen at the symphysis pubis level, as shown. This steadies the fundus and prevents downward displacement. Then place the other hand at the top of the fundus, cupping it, as shown.

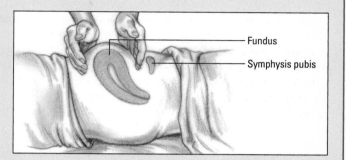

— Fundus

— Symphysis pubis

the abdomen, gently compress and release your fingers, always supporting the lower uterine segment with your other hand. Observe the vaginal drainage during massage.

• Massage long enough to produce firmness but not discomfort. You may also encourage the patient to massage her fundus for 10 to 15 seconds every 15 minutes. This is usually necessary only for a few hours.

• Notify the practitioner immediately if the uterus fails to contract and heavy bleeding occurs. If the fundus becomes firm after massage, keep one hand on the lower uterus and press gently toward the pubis to expel clots. (See *Complications of fundal palpation.*)

Remember the bladder

When assessing the uterine fundus, also assess for bladder distention. A distended bladder can impede the downward descent of the uterus by pushing it upward and, possibly, to the right side. If the bladder is distended and the patient is unable to urinate, you may need to catheterize her.

Lochia

After birth, the outermost layer of the uterus becomes necrotic and is expelled. This vaginal discharge—called *lochia*—is similar to menstrual flow and consists of blood, fragments of the decidua, white blood cells (WBCs), mucus, and some bacteria.

Education edge

Complications of fundal palpation

Because the uterus and its supporting ligaments are tender after birth, pain is the most common complication of fundal palpation and massage. Excessive massage can stimulate uterine contractions, causing undue muscle fatigue and leading to uterine atony or inversion. Lack of lochia may signal a clot blocking the cervical os. Heavy bleeding may result if a position change dislodges the clot. Take the patient's vital signs frequently to assess for hypovolemic shock.

Assessing lochia flow

Lochia is commonly assessed in conjunction with fundal assessment. (See *Three types of lochia.*)

Help the patient into the lateral Sims' position. Be sure to check under the patient's buttocks to make sure that blood isn't pooling there. Then remove the patient's perineal pad and evaluate the character, amount, color, odor, and consistency (presence of clots) of the discharge. Before removing the perineal pad, make sure that it isn't sticking to any perineal stitches. Otherwise, tearing may occur, possibly increasing the risk of bleeding.

On the lookout

Here's what to look for when assessing lochia:
- *Amount*—Although it varies, the amount of lochia is typically comparable to the amount during menstrual flow. A woman who's breast-feeding may have less lochia. Also, a woman who has had a cesarean birth may have a scant amount of lochia; however, lochia shouldn't be absent. Lochia should be present for at least 3 weeks postpartum. Lochia flow increases with activity; for example, when the patient gets out of bed the first several times (due to pooled lochia being released) or when she lifts a heavy object or walks up stairs (due to an actual increase in the amount of lochia). If your patient saturates a perineal pad in less than an hour, this is considered excessive flow, and you should notify the practitioner.
- *Color*—Lochia typically is described as lochia rubra, serosa, or alba, depending on the color of the discharge. Lochia color depends on the postpartum day. A sudden change in color—for example, from pink back to red—suggests new bleeding or retained placental fragments.
- *Odor*—Lochia should smell similar to menstrual flow. A foul or offensive odor suggests infection.
- *Consistency*—Lochia should have minimal or small clots, if any. Evidence of large or numerous clots indicates poor uterine contraction and requires further assessment.

Perineum and rectum

The pressure exerted on the perineum and rectum during birth results in edema and generalized tenderness. Some areas of the perineum may be ecchymotic, caused by the rupture of surface capillaries. Sutures for an episiotomy or laceration may also be present. Hemorrhoids are also commonly seen.

What's your position?

Assessment of the perineum and rectum mainly involves inspection and is performed at the same time that you assess the lochia. Help the patient into the lateral Sims' position. This position pro-

---

Three types of lochia

Lochia color, which typically changes throughout the postpartum period, may be categorized as:
- *lochia rubra*—red vaginal discharge that occurs from approximately day 1 to day 3 postpartum
- *lochia serosa*—pinkish or brownish discharge that occurs from approximately day 4 to day 10 postpartum
- *lochia alba*—creamy white or colorless vaginal discharge that occurs from approximately day 10 to day 14 postpartum (although it may continue for up to 6 weeks).

vides better visibility and causes less discomfort for the patient with a mediolateral episiotomy. A back-lying position can also be used for patients with midline episiotomies. Make sure you have adequate light for inspection.

Checking down under

Lift the patient's buttocks and observe for intactness of skin, positioning of the episiotomy (if one was performed), and appearance of sutures (from episiotomy or laceration repair) and the surrounding rectal area. Keep in mind that the edges of an episiotomy are usually sealed 24 hours after delivery. Note ecchymosis, hematoma, erythema, edema, drainage or bleeding from sutures, a foul odor, or signs of infection. Also observe for the presence of hemorrhoids.

Perineal care

Perineal assessment also includes perineal care. The goals of postpartum perineal care are to relieve discomfort, promote healing, and prevent infection by cleaning the perineal area. Assist and teach the patient how to perform perineal care in conjunction with a perineal assessment. Perineal care should be performed after the patient voids or has a bowel movement.

Two methods of providing perineal care are generally used: a water-jet irrigation system or a peri bottle. In either case, help the patient walk to the bathroom or place her on a bedpan; then wash your hands and put on gloves.

Water-jet system

If you're using a water-jet irrigation system, follow these steps:
• Insert the prefilled cartridge containing the antiseptic or medicated solution into the handle, and push the disposable nozzle into the handle until you hear it click into place.
• Help the patient sit on the toilet or bedpan.
• Place the nozzle parallel to the perineum and turn on the unit.
• Rinse the perineum for at least 2 minutes from front to back.
• Turn off the unit, remove the nozzle, and discard the cartridge.
• Dry the nozzle and store as appropriate for later use.

Peri bottle

If you're using a peri bottle for perineal care, follow these steps:
• Fill the bottle with cleaning solution (usually warm water).
• Help the patient sit on the toilet or bedpan.
• Tell her to pour the solution over her perineal area.
• After completion, help the patient off the toilet or remove the bedpan.
• Pat the perineal area dry, and help the patient apply a new perineal pad.

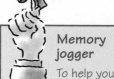

Memory jogger

To help you remember what to look for when assessing an episiotomy site or a laceration, think REEDA:

Redness

Erythema and Ecchymosis

Edema

Drainage or Discharge

Approximation (of wound edges).

Hot and cold comfort

During perineal care, note if the patient complains of pain or tenderness. If she does, you may need to apply ice or cold packs to the area for the first 24 hours after birth. This helps reduce perineal edema and prevent hematoma formation, thereby reducing pain and promoting healing.

Cold therapy isn't effective after the first 24 hours. Instead, heat is recommended because it increases circulation to the area. Forms of heat include a perineal hot pack (dry heat) or a sitz bath (moist heat).

Sitz right down

For extensive lacerations, such as third or fourth degree lacerations, the practitioner may order a sitz bath to aid perineal healing, provide comfort, and reduce edema. Because of shortened hospitalization time, you may need to teach the patient how to use a sitz bath at home. (See *Using a sitz bath.*)

> If the patient complains of pain or tenderness, you may need to apply ice or cold packs to the perineal area for the first 24 hours after birth.

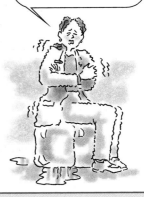

Education edge

Using a sitz bath

A sitz bath allows the postpartum patient to immerse her perineal area in warm or hot water without the bother of taking a complete bath. It relieves discomfort and promotes wound healing by cleaning the perineum and anus, increasing circulation, and reducing inflammation. It also helps relax local muscles.

How it's done

Tell the patient to follow these steps to use a sitz bath correctly:
• Assemble the equipment and wash your hands.
• Empty your bladder.
• Fill the basin to the specified line with water at the prescribed temperature (usually 100° to 105° F [37.8° to 40.6° C]). Be sure to check the water temperature frequently to ensure therapeutic effects.
• Place the basin under the commode seat, clamp the irrigation tubing to block water flow, and fill the irrigation bag with water of the same temperature as that in the basin. Attach the end of the tubing in the correct groove to secure its position in the basin.
• To create flow pressure, hang the bag above your head on a hook, towel rack, or edge of a door.

• Remove and dispose of your perineal pad and then sit on the basin.
• If your feet don't reach the floor and the weight of your legs presses against the edge of the equipment, place a small stool under your feet. Also place a folded towel or small pillow against your lower back.
• Cover your shoulders and knees with blankets or a robe to prevent chilling.
• Open the clamp on the irrigation tubing to allow a stream of water to flow continuously. Refill the bag with water of the correct temperature, as needed, and continue to regulate the flow.
• After approximately 15 to 20 minutes, clamp the tubing and rest for a few minutes before arising to prevent dizziness and light-headedness.
• Pat the perineal area dry from front to back, and apply a new perineal pad (by holding the bottom sides or ends).
• Dispose of soiled materials properly. Empty and clean the sitz bath according to the manufacturer's directions.
• Report changes in drainage amount or characteristics, light-headedness, perspiration, weakness, nausea, or irregular heart rate.

Postpartum care measures

Ongoing assessment is crucial during the postpartum period. Continue to assess the patient's vital signs, uterine fundus, lochia, breasts, and perineum as ordered. Administer medications as ordered to relieve discomfort from the episiotomy or from uterine contractions, incisional pain, or breast engorgement and assess for therapeutic effectiveness. Encourage the patient to rest after delivery and throughout the postpartum period to prevent exhaustion.

A-voiding catheterization

Assess the patient's urinary elimination. The patient should void within 6 to 8 hours after delivery. If she doesn't, help her urge to void by administering analgesics as ordered, pouring warm water over the perineum, placing the patient's hands in warm water, or running water for the patient to hear (the sound may encourage the urge to void). If all attempts fail, the patient may need to be catheterized.

Flatus foreshadows function

Finally, assess bowel function. Elimination is typically a good indicator of bowel function. The patient should have a bowel movement 1 to 2 days after delivery to avoid constipation. However, a patient who has eaten nothing by mouth for 12 to 24 hours and then has a cesarean birth may not have a bowel movement for several days. In these cases, flatus may be a better indicator of bowel function.

Encourage the patient to drink plenty of fluids and eat high-fiber foods to prevent constipation. If necessary, the practitioner may order stool softeners or laxatives. If the patient has hemorrhoids, cool witch hazel compresses may be helpful. Don't use suppositories if the patient has a third or fourth degree laceration.

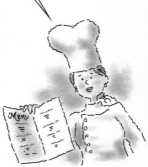

Get a move on! A postpartum patient should drink plenty of fluids and eat high-fiber foods to prevent constipation.

Patient teaching

Because of the short length of stay for most postpartum women, patient teaching is essential. Teaching should focus on maternal self-care activities and neonatal care. (See *Postpartum maternal self-care*, page 430.)

Education edge

Postpartum maternal self-care

When teaching your patient about self-care for the postpartum period, be sure to include these topic areas and instructions.

Personal hygiene

• Change perineal pads frequently, removing them from the front to the back and disposing of them in a plastic bag.
• Perform perineal care each time that you urinate or move your bowels.
• Monitor your vaginal discharge; it should change from red to pinkish brown to clear or white before stopping altogether. Notify your practitioner if the discharge returns to a previous color, becomes bright red or yellowish green, suddenly increases in amount, or develops an offensive odor.
• Follow your practitioner's instructions about using sitz baths or applying heat to your perineum.
• Shower daily.

Breasts

• Wear a firm, supportive bra.
• If nipple leakage occurs, use clean gauze pads or nursing pads inside your bra to absorb the moisture.
• Inspect your nipples for cracking, fissures, or soreness, and report areas of redness, tenderness, or swelling.
• Wash breasts daily with clear water when showering and dry with a soft towel or allow to air dry. Don't use soap on your breasts or nipples because soap is drying.
• If you're breast-feeding and your breasts become engorged, use warm compresses, stand under a warm shower, or feed your baby more frequently for relief. If the baby is unable to latch on due to engorgement, using a breast pump should help. If you aren't breast-feeding, apply cool compresses several times per day.

Activity and exercise

• Balance rest periods with activity, get as much sleep as possible at night, and take frequent rest periods or naps during the day.

• Check with your practitioner about when to begin exercising.
• If your vaginal discharge increases with activity, elevate your legs for about 30 minutes. If the discharge doesn't decrease with rest, call your practitioner.

Nutrition

• Increase your intake of protein and calories.
• Drink plenty of fluids throughout the day, including before and after breast-feeding.

Elimination

• If you have the urge to urinate or move your bowels, don't delay doing so. Urinate at least every 2 to 3 hours. This helps keep the uterus contracted and decreases the risk of excessive bleeding.
• Report difficulty urinating, burning, or pain to your practitioner.
• Drink plenty of liquids and eat high-fiber foods to prevent constipation.
• Follow your practitioner's instructions about the use of stool softeners or laxatives.

Sexual activity and contraception

• Remember that breast-feeding isn't a reliable method of contraception. Discuss birth control options with your practitioner.
• Ask your practitioner when you can resume sexual activity and contraceptive measures. Most couples can resume having sex within 3 to 4 weeks after delivery, or possibly as soon as lochia ceases.
• Use a water-based lubricant if necessary.
• Expect a decrease in intensity and rapidity of sexual response for about 3 months after delivery.
• Perform Kegel exercises to help strengthen your pelvic floor muscles. To do this, squeeze your pelvic muscles as if trying to stop urine flow, and then release them.

Lactation

Lactation refers to the production of breast milk, the preferred source of nutrition for a neonate. All patients experience the physiologic changes that occur with lactation and breast milk production regardless of whether they plan to breast-feed.

Physiology of lactation

During pregnancy, a hormone called *prolactin* prepares the woman's breasts to secrete milk. Other hormones (progesterone and estrogen) interact to suppress milk secretion while developing the breasts for lactation. Estrogen causes the breasts to grow by increasing their fat content. Progesterone causes lobule growth and develops the alveolar (acinar) cells' secretory capacity.

After birth, the mother's estrogen and progesterone levels drop abruptly. This drop in hormones triggers the release of prolactin from the anterior pituitary, which starts the cycle of synthesis and secretion of milk (See *A closer look at lactation*, page 432.)

Breast milk composition

From about the fourth month of pregnancy until the first 3 to 4 days after delivery, the acinar cells produce and secrete colostrum. Colostrum is a thick, sticky, golden-yellow fluid that contains protein, sugar, fat, water, minerals, vitamins, and maternal antibodies. It's easy for the neonate to digest because it's high in protein and low in sugar and fat. It also provides completely adequate nutrition for the neonate. The high protein level of colostrum aids in the binding of bilirubin and also has a laxative effect, which promotes early passage of the neonate's first stool, called *meconium.*

Got milk?

On about the second to fourth postpartum day, colostrum is replaced by mature breast milk. During this time, the woman produces copious amounts of breast milk. The composition of this breast milk changes with each feeding. As the neonate nurses, the bluish-white foremilk (containing part skim and part whole milk) primarily provides protein, lactose, and water-soluble vitamins to the neonate. Hindmilk, or cream, is produced within the first 10 to 20 minutes of breast-feeding and contains denser calories from fat. This transitional breast milk is replaced by true or mature breast milk by around day 10 after delivery.

A closer look at lactation

After delivery of the placenta, the drop in progesterone and estrogen levels stimulates the production of prolactin. This hormone stimulates milk production by the acinar cells in the mammary glands.

Nerve impulses caused by the neonate sucking at the breast travel from the nipple to the hypothalamus, resulting in the production of prolactin-releasing factor. This factor leads to additional production of prolactin and, subsequently, more milk production.

Go with the flow

Milk flows from the acinar cells through small tubules to the lactiferous sinuses (small reservoirs located behind the nipple). This milk, called *foremilk,* is thin, bluish, and sugary and is constantly forming. It quenches the neonate's thirst but contains little fat and protein.

When the neonate sucks at the breast, oxytocin is released, causing the sinuses to con-

tract. Contraction pushes the milk forward through the nipple to the neonate. In addition, release of oxytocin causes the smooth muscles of the uterus to contract.

That let-down feeling

Movement of the milk forward through the nipple is termed the *let-down reflex* and may be triggered by things other than the infant sucking at the breast. For example, women have reported that hearing their baby cry or thinking about him causes this reflex.

Once the let-down reflex occurs and the neonate has fed for 10 to 15 minutes, new milk—called *hindmilk*—is formed. This milk is thicker, whiter, and contains higher concentrations of fat and protein. Hindmilk contains the calories and fat necessary for the neonate to gain weight, build brain tissue, and be more content and satisfied between feedings.

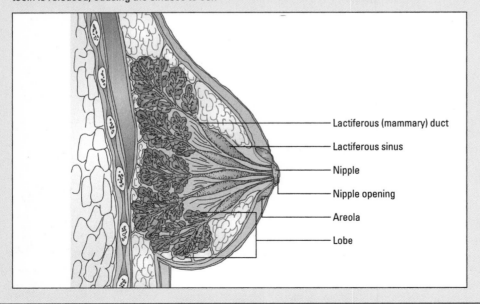

Lactiferous (mammary) duct

Lactiferous sinus

Nipple

Nipple opening

Areola

Lobe

Lactation and the menstrual cycle

After delivery of the placenta, estrogen and progesterone production ceases. As a result, the pituitary gland increases the production of FSH, which eventually leads to ovulation and resumption of the menstrual cycle.

Here we go again

Lactating women begin menstruating again at various times, anywhere from 2 to 18 months. Ovulation may occur by the end of the first month postpartum, or it may not occur for one or more menstrual cycles. Woman who aren't lactating usually resume menstruating in 6 to 10 weeks. Approximately one-half of these women ovulate with the first menstrual cycle.

Neonatal nutrition

Human milk consumed through breast-feeding is considered optimal for neonates. Despite this, not all mothers can or choose to breast-feed. Medical conditions, cultural background, anxiety, drug abuse, and various other factors can prevent a woman from breast-feeding. Furthermore, some neonates can't take in enough breast milk through breast-feeding to meet nutritional needs. Preterm or high-risk neonates may require additives or fortifiers in their breast milk to meet their unique needs while still receiving all the benefits of regular breast milk.

Breast-feeding

Breast-feeding is considered the safest, simplest, and least expensive way to provide complete infant nourishment. The American Academy of Pediatrics and the American Dietetic Association recommend breast-feeding exclusively for the first 4 to 6 months of the infant's life and then in combination with infant foods until age 1.

Contrary to popular belief

Breast-feeding is contraindicated if the mother:
• has herpes lesions on her nipples
• is receiving certain medications, such as methotrexate (Folex PFS) or lithium (Eskalith), that pass into the breast milk and may harm the neonate
• is on a restricted diet that interferes with adequate nutrient intake and subsequently affects the quality of milk produced
• has breast cancer

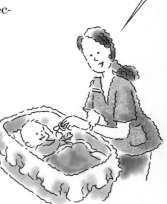

Here's food for thought. Breast-feeding is the safest, simplest, and least expensive way to provide complete infant nourishment.

• has a severe chronic condition, such as active tuberculosis, human immunodeficiency virus infection, or hepatitis.

Advantages

Breast-feeding is advantageous for the mother and the neonate. (See *Benefits of breast-feeding.*)

Maternal benefits include:

• protection against breast cancer
• assistance in uterine involution due to the release of oxytocin
• empowerment (as the woman learns to master the skill)
• less preparation time and less cost than using infant formula.

More good news about breast-feeding

Breast milk is also highly beneficial for the neonate. For example, it reduces the risk of infection because it contains:

• immunoglobulin A—an antibody that prevents foreign proteins from being absorbed by the neonate's GI tract
• lactoferrin—an iron-binding protein that interferes with bacterial growth
• lysozyme—an enzyme that actively destroys bacteria
• leukocytes—WBCs that protect against common respiratory infections
• macrophages—cells that produce interferon, which offers protection from viral invasion.

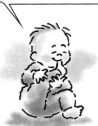

Wow! Breast-feeding is even better than sucking my toes. And it reduces my risk of infection.

Benefits of breast-feeding

Here are some of the benefits of breast-feeding.

Passive immunity
Human milk provides passive immunity. Colostrum is the first fluid secreted from the breast (occurs within the first few days after delivery) and provides immune factor and protein to the neonate. Many components of breast milk protect against infection—it contains antibodies (especially immunoglobulin A) and white blood cells that protect the baby from some forms of infection. Breast-fed babies also experience fewer allergies and intolerances.

Easily digestible
Breast milk provides essential nutrients in an easily digestible form. It contains lipase, which breaks down dietary fat, making it easily available to the baby's system.

Brain booster
The lipids in breast milk are high in linoleic acid and cholesterol, which are needed for brain development.

Low protein content
Cow's milk contains proportionally higher concentrations of electrolytes and protein than are needed by human babies. It must be cleared by the immature kidneys and thus isn't recommended until after a baby is at least 12 months old.

Convenient and inexpensive
Breast-feeding saves time and money in buying and preparing formula.

In addition, breast-feeding is advantageous to the neonate for these reasons:

• Breast milk promotes rapid brain growth because it contains large amounts of lactose, which is easily digested and can be rapidly converted to glucose.

• Breast milk's protein and nitrogen contents provide foundations for neurologic cell building.

• Breast milk contains adequate electrolyte and mineral composition for the neonate's needs without overloading the neonate's renal system.

• Breast-feeding improves the neonate's ability to regulate calcium and phosphorus levels.

• The sucking mechanism associated with breast-feeding reduces dental arch malformations.

• A breast-fed neonate's GI tract contains large amounts of *Lactobacillus bifidus*, a beneficial bacterium that prevents the growth of harmful organisms.

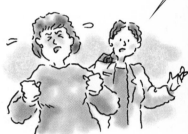

Sorry, mom, but you're wrong. Breast-feeding will NOT prevent pregnancy!

On the contrary

Breast-feeding may delay ovulation but shouldn't be considered a reliable form of contraception. In addition, evidence doesn't suggest that breast-feeding aids in weight loss after pregnancy.

Maternal nutrition and breast-feeding

Nutritional needs for a woman who's breast-feeding are only slightly different from those during her pregnancy. Folate and iron needs decrease after giving birth, and energy requirements increase.

Fueling milk production

While breast-feeding, a healthy woman should consume 2,300 to 2,700 calories/day, approximately 500 calories/day more than prepregnancy recommendations. If maternal intake is poor, which can occur when a lactating woman is dieting, the nutrient intake in her breast milk may become inadequate.

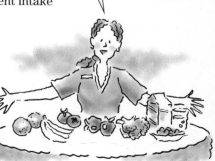

Eat up! Lactation requires more energy! Now isn't the time for mom to cut calories.

Water hydrant

Adequate hydration encourages ample milk production, so it's important for new mothers to drink plenty of fluids—2 to 3 qt (2 to 3 L)/day. The mother should also drink one 8-oz glass of fluid each time she breast-feeds to ensure she stays hydrated. Water and such beverages as fruit juices and milk are good choices to maintain adequate hydration.

Keep contaminants out!

Most substances that the mother ingests are secreted into her milk. Therefore, beverages containing alcohol and caffeine should be limited or avoided because they may be harmful to the neonate. In addition, it's important to check with a pediatrician before taking medication. Some researchers believe that components of the maternal food may contribute to colic or the neonate's fussiness.

Breast-feeding assistance

Even women who have previously breast-fed can benefit from assistance and instruction. The key is helping the patient to latch the neonate properly. Breast-feeding should occur as soon as possible after birth. However, this may not be possible, especially if the woman is overly fatigued or if a complication has developed.

Don't get comfy yet

When assisting with breast-feeding, explain the procedure and provide privacy. Encourage the mother to drink a beverage before and during or after breast-feeding to ensure adequate fluid intake, which maintains milk production. Also encourage her to use the bathroom and change the neonate's diaper before breast-feeding begins so that feeding is uninterrupted. Then wash your hands and instruct the mother to do the same.

Now, take a load off

Help the mother find a comfortable position. (See *Breast-feeding positions.*) Then follow these instructions:
• Have the mother expose one breast and rest the nape of the neonate's neck in the crook of her arm, supporting his back with her forearm.
• Inform her that uterine cramping may occur during breast-feeding until her uterus returns to its original size.
• Guiding the mother's free hand, have her place her thumb on top of the exposed breast's areola and her first two fingers beneath it, forming a C. Have her turn the neonate so that his entire body faces the breast.
• Tell the mother to stroke the neonate's cheek with her finger or the neonate's mouth with her nipple. This stimulates the rooting reflex. Emphasize that she should touch the cheek closest to the exposed breast. Touching the other cheek may cause the neonate to turn his head toward the touch and away from the breast.
• When the neonate opens his mouth and roots for the nipple, instruct the mother to move him onto the breast so that he gets as much of the areola as possible into his mouth. This helps him to exert sufficient pressure with his lips, gums, and cheek muscles on the milk sinuses below the areola.

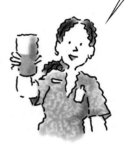

Breast-feeding moms should drink a beverage before breast-feeding as well as during or after to ensure adequate fluid intake, which maintains milk production.

Education edge

Breast-feeding positions

The position a mother uses when breast-feeding should be comfortable and efficient. Explain to the mother that changing positions periodically alters the neonate's grasp on the nipple and helps to prevent contact friction on the same area. As appropriate, suggest these three popular feeding positions.

Cradle position

The mother cradles the neonate's head in the crook of her arm. Instruct her to place a pillow on her lap for the neonate to lie on. Offer to place a pillow behind her back; this provides comfort and may also assist with correct positioning.

Side-lying position

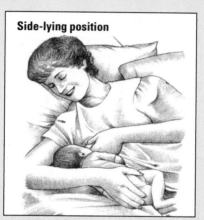

Instruct the mother to lie on her side with her stomach facing the neonate's. As the neonate's mouth opens, she should pull him toward the nipple. Inform her to place a pillow or rolled blanket behind the neonate's back to prevent him from moving or rolling away from the breast.

Football position

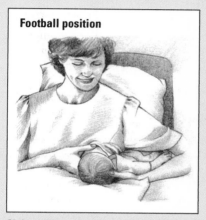

Sitting with a pillow in front of her, the mother places her hand under the neonate's head. As the neonate's mouth opens, she pulls the neonate's head near her breast. This position may be more comfortable for the woman who has had a cesarean birth.

• Show the mother how to check for occlusion of the neonate's nostrils by the breast. If this happens, she should reposition the neonate to give him room to breathe. The tip of his nose should touch the breast but not be mashed into it. The baby will breathe out of the sides of his nose.

• Suggest that the mother breast-feed for 15 minutes on each breast for the first 24 hours after birth. After that, the best advice is to never break a good latch. Remember: The neonate doesn't start receiving fat-and-protein-rich hind milk until after 15 minutes of feeding.

• To switch to the other breast, instruct the mother to slip a finger into the side of the neonate's mouth to break the seal, and then move him to the other breast.

Burping basics

Because some neonates swallow large amounts of air when feeding, encourage the mother to burp the neonate after emptying the first breast and again at the end of the feeding. Burping also helps to waken the neonate. Before burping, remind the mother to place a protective cover, such as a cloth diaper or washcloth, under the neonate's chin. The most common way to burp an neonate is to place him over one shoulder and gently pat or rub his back to help expel ingested air.

A burp is a burp is a burp

Some mothers have trouble supporting the neonate's head while patting or rubbing his back. This position may be especially awkward with small neonates because they lack the ability to control their heads. In these cases, suggest the sitting position for burping. (See *Sitting up for burping.*) A third acceptable position is placing the neonate prone across the mother's lap.

Taking a breather

When the mother finishes breast-feeding, instruct her to place the neonate in bed, lying on his back. She should let her nipples air dry for about 15 minutes after breast-feeding.

To make sure that both breasts receive equal stimulation, advise the mother to begin the next feeding using the breast on which the neonate finished this feeding. To help her remember, she can put a safety pin on her bra strap on the side last used.

Quelling concerns

Mothers commonly have questions about breast-feeding, including how often the neonate should feed, how much the neonate is getting, and what to do if the neonate is too sleepy to breast-feed. Reassure the mother that breast-feeding schedules aren't carved in stone and that developing a schedule that both she and her baby feel comfortable with takes time.

Feed me, feed me!

During the first few days of life, a neonate is usually fed as often as he's hungry, possibly every 2 hours. This helps to ensure that the neonate is satisfying his sucking needs and is receiving the necessary fluid and nutrients. Frequent feeding also helps initiate the mother's milk supply because frequent emptying stimulates more milk production.

A neonate's behavior and output helps to determine if he's getting enough breast milk. If he's content between feedings, wets approximately one diaper per day of life, and has stool once per day of age, then he's getting enough until the mother's milk comes in. For example, on the first day of life, expect one wet diaper and

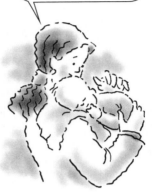

The most common way to burp a baby is to place him over one shoulder and gently pat or rub his back to expel ingested air.

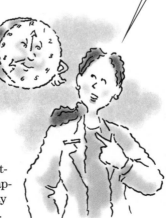

A neonate is usually fed every 2 hours, which also helps the mom, because frequent emptying stimulates more milk production.

one stool. On the second day of life, expect two wet diapers and two stools. On the third day of life, expect three wet diapers and three stools. More wet diapers or stools than expected is considered good. Once the mother's milk is evident, she can expect to see six to eight wet diapers per day and three to four stools per day. The neonate should be at or above his birthweight between 1 and 2 weeks of age.

Whetting his appetite

Sometimes neonates seem to be uninterested or fall asleep when breast-feeding. If the neonate shows little interest in breast-feeding, assist the mother in keeping him awake. If the neonate is sleepy, suggest that the mother try rubbing the baby's feet, unwrapping his blanket, changing the diaper, or changing her position or the neonate's. She may also manually express a little milk and allow the neonate to taste it. (See *Manual breast milk expression.*) If the neonate has little success or interest in breast-feeding for several feedings, refer the patient to a lactation consultant or breast-feeding specialist.

Keep up the good work!

Always encourage the mother's breast-feeding efforts. To boost these efforts, urge her to eat balanced meals, to drink at least

Sitting up for burping

If the mother indicates that placing the neonate over her shoulder for burping is awkward, suggest this alternative:
• Hold the neonate in a sitting position on your lap.
• Lean the neonate forward against one hand and support his head and neck with the index finger and thumb of that same hand, as shown below.

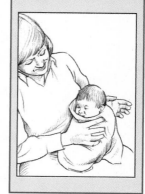

Manual breast milk expression

Manually expressing breast milk can enhance milk production and ensure an adequate supply. It's especially helpful for mothers who have problems with engorgement or those who must be away from their infants for several hours. (A mother who works outside the home or is away on a regular basis may find an electric pump quicker and more efficient.)

Express yourself

To help the mother manually express breast milk, follow these steps:
• Make sure that a clean collection container is available and that you and the patient have washed your hands.
• Explain the procedure to the patient, have her sit in a comfortable position, and provide privacy.
• Tell her to place her dominant hand on one breast with the thumb positioned on the top

and the fingers below and at the outer limit of the areola.
• Instruct her to press her thumb and fingers inward toward her chest while holding the collection container with her opposite hand directly under the nipple.
• Tell the patient to move her thumb and fingers forward, using gentle pressure in a milking type motion. Caution her not to use too much pressure because this can injure breast tissue. Milk should flow out of the nipple and into the collection container.
• Encourage the patient to move her thumb and fingers around the breast, using the same motion, to ensure complete emptying.
• Advise the patient to cover the container and place the milk in the refrigerator if it will be used within 24 hours; if not, she should freeze it.

eight 8-oz glasses of fluid daily, and to nap daily for at least the first 2 weeks after giving birth. Answer her questions about breast-feeding and provide instructional materials if available. Always provide a patient who's breast-feeding information and instructions related to possible complications. (See chapter 10, Complications of the postpartum period, for more in-depth information on complications.) Contact a lactation consultant as appropriate.

Before discharge, tell the mother about local breast-feeding and parenting support groups such as La Leche League International.

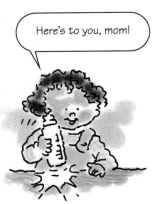

Here's to you, mom!

Daddy dearest

To involve the father, have him change the neonate's diaper before feeding or burp the neonate afterwards. Even young children can get involved by helping with burping or diaper changes.

Bottle-feeding with breast milk

In some cases, a mother may need to be away from her neonate but still desires to provide breast milk. The mother may also need to express breast milk when her breasts are engorged. Although breast-milk can be expressed by hand, pumping may be the most efficient method.

Breast pumping

Breast pumping involves the use of suction created with a manual pump or a battery-powered or electric pump to stimulate lactation. It's used when the mother and neonate are separated or while illness temporarily incapacitates one or the other.

A breast pump can also relieve engorgement, collect milk for a premature neonate with a weak sucking reflex, reduce pressure on sore or cracked nipples, or reestablish the milk supply. The mother can also use a pump to collect milk when she's unable to manually express it.

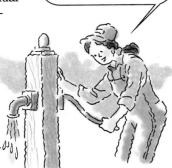

Breast pumping involves the use of suction created with a manual pump or a battery-powered or electric pump to stimulate lactation.

Preparing to pump

Before teaching the mother to use a breast pump:
• Assemble the equipment according to the manufacturer's instructions.
• Explain the procedure to the patient.
• Provide privacy.
• Wash your hands and instruct the patient to wash hers.
• Help the patient into a comfortable position and urge her to relax.

Tell the patient to drink a beverage before and after pumping. If the patient's breasts are engorged, instruct her to apply warm compresses for 5 minutes or take a warm shower before pumping.

Manual pump

To use a manual pump, instruct the patient to place the flange or shield against her breast with the nipple in the center of the device. Then have her pump each breast by operating the device according to the manufacturer's instructions. She should continue until the breast is empty and then repeat the procedure on the other breast. It's also acceptable to pump for 5 minutes on one side and then switch sides and pump for 5 minutes; then, after 5 to 10 minutes, she should switch sides again and continue pumping until milk stops flowing from each breast.

Battery-powered or electric pump

To use a battery-powered or electric pump, instruct the patient to set the suction regulator on low. Tell her to hold the collection unit upright to allow milk to flow into it. Have her place the shield against her breast with the nipple in the center. She should turn on the machine and adjust the suction regulator to a comfortable pressure.

Instruct her to start with the least amount of suction to prevent nipple damage and then gradually increase the suction. Advise her to check the operator's manual to see the pressure setting at which the pump functions most efficiently.

Keep on pumping

Instruct the patient to pump each breast for 15 to 20 minutes or until the milk stops spraying, which takes longer. She may wish to use a double pump, which allows for pumping both breasts at the same time. Using a double pump is also efficient and will save time if she uses this breast-feeding method.

When she's finished, show the patient how to remove the shield from the breast by inserting a finger between the breast and the shield to break the vacuum seal. Then return the suction regulator to the low setting and turn off the machine.

Freeze, store, or enjoy right now?

After using either type of pump, the patient should let her nipples air dry for about 15 minutes. She should also disassemble the removable parts of the pump and clean them according to the manufacturer's directions.

If she plans to store or freeze the milk, have her fill a sterile plastic bottle with milk from the collection unit. Place the milk in the refrigerator or freezer immediately. Always label the collected milk with the date, the time of collection, and the amount. Write the neonate's name on the label, if necessary. If the neonate is going to drink the milk right away, show the patient how to attach a rubber nipple to the cylinder or collection unit.

Timing is everything. Store freshly pumped breast milk in the fridge for 3 days or freeze it for up to 6 months. But after it's defrosted (in the fridge, of course), use it within 24 hours.

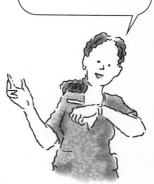

Bottle-feeding with formula

Formula-feeding is a reliable and nutritionally adequate method of feeding for neonates whose mothers are unable to breast-feed or who choose not to. Commercial formulas are designed to mimic human milk.

Types of formulas

Commercial formulas typically provide 20 calories per ounce when diluted properly and are classified as milk-based, soy-based, and elemental. Milk-based formulas are usually prescribed. Some of these formulas are lactose-free, so they can be used for neonates with galactosemia or lactose intolerance.

Health food for babies

Soy-based formulas are used for babies who could be allergic to cow's milk protein. Elemental formulas are commonly prescribed for babies who may have protein allergies or fat malnutrition. With these formulas, the amount of fat, protein, and carbohydrates is modified. However, all commercial formulas are designed to simulate the nutritional content of human milk.

Formula x four

Commercial formulas may be supplied in one of four forms:
- powdered—to be combined with water
- condensed liquid—must be diluted
- ready to feed
- disposable, individually prepared bottles.

The powdered form is the least expensive, whereas individually prepared bottles are most expensive but easiest to use. Most health care facilities use individually prepared bottles. Tell parents about the forms of formula available so they can choose what's most convenient for them.

Formula-feeding assistance

Each day, an infant requires 2.5 to 3 ounces of fluid per pound of body weight (150 to 200 ml/kg) and 50 to 55 calories per pound of body weight (100 to 120 kcal/kg). Because commercial formulas consistently provide 20 calories per ounce, only the infant's fluid needs are used to determine the amount of each feeding. Unlike breast-feeding, you can measure the amount of formula consumed.

Until about age 4 months, most infants need 6 feedings per day. After this, the number of feedings drops, but the amount at each feeding increases because the baby starts to eat cereal, fruits, and vegetables.

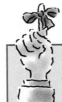

Memory jogger

To easily determine the amount of milk an infant should take in at each feeding, add 2 to 3 oz to the infant's age (in months). So, for example:

- A 1-month-old should take 3 to 4 oz at each feeding.

- A 4-month-old should take 6 to 7 oz.

- A 5-month-old should take 7 to 8 oz.

Prefeeding prep

When bottle-feeding a neonate, or helping the mother with bottle-feeding, know the type of formula that's ordered and how it's supplied. If you're using a commercially prepared formula, check the expiration date, uncap the formula bottle, and make sure that the seal isn't broken to ensure sterility and freshness. If the seal is broken, discard the formula. If the seal isn't broken, remove it.

Next, screw on the nipple and cap. Keep the protective sterile cap over the nipple until the neonate is ready to feed. If you're preparing formula, follow the manufacturer's directions or the doctor's prescription. Administer the formula at room temperature or slightly warmer.

Bottle-feeding blow by blow

Teach the mother and other family members to follow these steps when bottle-feeding the neonate:

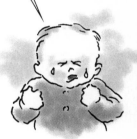

Do I need to say it again?
I WANT MILK!

- After washing your hands and preparing the formula, invert the bottle and shake some formula on your wrist to test its temperature and the patency of the nipple hole. The formula should drip freely but not stream out. If the hole is too large, the neonate may aspirate formula; if it's too small, the extra sucking effort may tire him before he can empty the bottle.
- Sit comfortably in a semireclining position and cradle the neonate in one arm to support his head and back. This position allows swallowed air to rise to the top of the stomach where it's more easily expelled. If the neonate can't be held, sit by him and elevate his head and shoulders slightly.
- Place the nipple in the neonate's mouth on top of his tongue, but not so far back that it stimulates the gag reflex. He should begin to suck, pulling in as much nipple as is comfortable. If he doesn't start to suck, stroke him under the chin or on his cheek, or touch his lips with the nipple to stimulate the sucking reflex.

Tilting does the trick

- As the neonate feeds, tilt the bottle upward to keep the nipple filled with formula and to prevent him from swallowing air. Watch for a steady stream of bubbles in the bottle. This indicates proper venting and flow of formula.
- If the neonate pushes out the nipple with his tongue, reinsert the nipple. Expelling the nipple is a normal reflex. It doesn't necessarily mean that the neonate is full.
- Always hold the bottle for a neonate. If left to feed himself, he may aspirate formula or swallow air if the bottle tilts or empties. In older infants, experts also link bottle propping with an increased incidence of otitis media and dental caries.
- Be sure to interact with the neonate during feeding.

- Burp the neonate after each ½ oz of formula because he'll usually swallow some air even when fed correctly. Use the same positions previously described for breast-feeding.
- After feeding and burping the neonate, place him on his back as recommended by the American Association of Pediatricians. This position reduces the incidence of sudden infant death syndrome.
- Don't worry if the neonate regurgitates some of the feeding. Neonates are prone to regurgitation because of an immature cardiac sphincter. Regurgitation is merely an overflow and shouldn't be confused with vomiting—a more complete emptying of the stomach accompanied by symptoms not associated with feeding.
- Discard any remaining formula and properly dispose of all equipment.

Too much or not enough

A neonate tires if he feeds too long, and his sucking needs aren't met if he doesn't feed long enough. In some cases, you or the mother may need to select a nipple of a different size or one with a larger opening to change the duration of the feeding. Additionally, be sure to note how much formula is in the bottle before and after the feeding. Use the calibrations along the side of the container to calculate the amount of formula consumed.

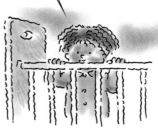

I can't decide. Did I not feed long enough to meet my need to suck, or did I feed too long and now I'm tired?

At home, go with the flow

Teach parents and other family members how to prepare and (if required) sterilize formula, bottles, and nipples. Although most health care facilities have a feeding schedule, advise the mother to switch to a more flexible demand-feeding schedule when at home.

Breast care

A mother who plans to breast-feed after the neonate's birth will need to maintain breast tissue integrity. Although postpartum care varies for breast-feeding and non-breast-feeding women, some guidelines are similar.

For breast-feeding women

Provide these instructions to a woman who's breast-feeding her neonate:
- Wash your breasts with water only to avoid washing away the natural oils and keratin.
- If your nipples are sore or irritated, apply ice compresses to them just before breast-feeding. This numbs them, making them less sensitive and easier for the neonate to grasp
- To help prevent tenderness, lubricate the nipple with a few drops of expressed breast milk before feeding.

- Place breast pads over your nipples to collect milk, and replace the pads often to reduce the risk of infection. Breasts often leak during the first few weeks you're breast-feeding.
- Be alert for a slight temperature elevation and an increase in breast size, warmth, and firmness 2 to 5 days after birth. This signals that breast milk is coming in.
- Wear a well-fitting support bra to help control engorgement.
- Apply warm compresses, massage the breasts, take a warm shower, or express some milk before feeding if your breasts are engorged and the neonate can't latch on to the nipple.

For non-breast-feeding women

Provide these instructions to a woman who isn't breast-feeding her neonate:
- Clean your breasts with water only or with soap if necessary.
- Wear a supportive bra to help minimize engorgement and decrease nipple stimulation.
- To minimize further milk production, avoid stimulating the nipples or manually expressing milk.
- Use analgesics (if ordered), ice packs, or a breast binder to minimize engorgement.

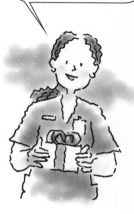

Okay, let's wrap it up. A supportive bra can help minimize engorgement.

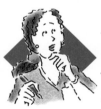

Quick quiz

1. Which option would you identify as a progressive physiologic change in the postpartum period?
    A.   Lactation
    B.   Lochia
    C.   Uterine involution
    D.   Diuresis

Answer: A. Lactation is an example of a progressive physiologic change that occurs during the postpartum period.

2. Which behavior would you expect to assess during the taking-in phase?
    A.   Strong interest in caring for the neonate
    B.   Redefinition of new role
    C.   Insecurity about ability to provide neonatal care
    D.   Passivity with dependence on others

Answer: D. During the taking-in phase, the patient assumes a passive role, relying on others for care.

3. Where would you expect to assess the uterine fundus in a patient who's 2 days postpartum?

    A.   2 cm above the level of the umbilicus

    B.   At the level of the symphysis pubis

    C.   Approximately 2 cm below the umbilicus

    D.   2 cm above the symphysis pubis

Answer: C. The uterus descends at a rate of about 1 cm/day. The fundus of a woman who's 2 days postpartum should be 2 cm below the umbilicus.

4. At the patient's 6-week follow-up appointment, you should assess:

    A.   lochia rubra.

    B.   lochia serosa.

    C.   lochia alba.

    D.   absence of lochia.

Answer: D. By 6 weeks, lochia usually has ceased. Lochia rubra typically lasts from days 1 to 3 postpartum; lochia serosa, from days 3 to 10; and lochia alba, from days 10 to 14.

5. Lactation is stimulated by:

    A.   estrogen.

    B.   prolactin.

    C.   progesterone.

    D.   FSH.

Answer: B. Prolactin is the hormone responsible for stimulating lactation.

6. Which measure would the woman who isn't breast-feeding use to minimize engorgement?

    A.   Cold compresses

    B.   Manual expression

    C.   Warm showers

    D.   Nipple stimulation

Answer: A. For the woman who isn't breast-feeding, cold compresses help to minimize engorgement.

Scoring

✩✩✩ If you answered all six questions correctly, whoa! You've certainly galloped through this chapter.

✩✩ If you answered four or five questions correctly, giddyup! Looks like you've corraled your knowledge of postpartum care.

✩ If you answered fewer than four questions correctly, stay steady. You're sure to be more stable the next time you go over this chapter.

10

Complications of the postpartum period

Just the facts

In this chapter, you'll learn:

♦ major complications that can occur during the postpartum period, including risk factors for each

♦ ways to identify complications based on key assessment findings

♦ treatments that are appropriate for each complication

♦ appropriate nursing interventions for each complication.

A look at postpartum complications

Although the postpartum period is a time of many physiologic and psychological changes and stressors, these changes are usually considered good changes—not unhealthy. During this time, the mother, the neonate, and other family members interact and grow as a family.

A cluster of complications

However, complications can develop due to a wide range of factors, such as blood loss, trauma, infection, or fatigue. Some common postpartum complications include postpartum hemorrhage, postpartum psychiatric disorders, puerperal infection, mastitis, and deep vein thrombosis (DVT). Your keen nursing skills can help to prevent problems or detect them early before they cause more stress or seriously interfere with the parent-child relationship.

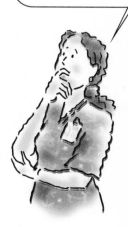

Postpartum complications can occur for a number of reasons. Some are more complicated than others.

Postpartum hemorrhage

Postpartum hemorrhage—any blood loss from the uterus that exceeds 500 ml during a 24-hour period—is the major cause of maternal mortality. The danger of postpartum hemorrhage due to uterine atony is greatest during the first hour after birth. During this time, the placenta has detached, leaving the highly vascular yet denuded uterus widely exposed. The risk continues to be high for 24 hours after birth.

After vaginal birth, blood loss of up to 500 ml is considered acceptable, although this amount may vary among health care facilities. The acceptable range for blood loss after cesarean birth is usually between 1,000 and 1,200 ml.

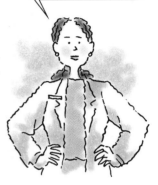

Postpartum hemorrhage is the major cause of maternal mortality.

Complicating the matter

A patient who has a birth complicated by any of these factors should be observed for the possibility of developing a postpartum hemorrhage:
- abruptio placentae
- missed abortion
- placenta previa
- uterine infection
- placenta accreta
- uterine inversion
- severe preeclampsia
- amniotic fluid embolism
- intrauterine fetal death
- precipitous labor
- macrosomia
- multiple gestation
- prolonged labor
- multiparity.

What a difference a day makes

Postpartum hemorrhage is classified as early or late, depending on when it occurs. *Early postpartum hemorrhage* refers to blood loss in excess of 500 ml that occurs during the first 24 hours postpartum. *Late postpartum hemorrhage* refers to uterine blood loss in excess of 500 ml that occurs during the remaining 6-week postpartum period but after the first 24 hours.

What causes it

Uterine atony, lacerations, retained placenta or placental fragments, and disseminated intravascular coagulation (DIC) are the leading causes of postpartum hemorrhage.

Relax—don't do it!

The primary cause of postpartum hemorrhage, especially early postpartum hemorrhage, is uterine atony (uterine relaxation). When the uterus doesn't contract properly, vessels at the placental site remain open, allowing blood loss. Any condition that interferes with the ability of the uterus to contract can lead to uterine atony and, subsequently, postpartum hemorrhage. (See *Relaxation is risky*.)

> You're kidding. Relaxation is bad? When the uterus relaxes, blood loss can occur, causing postpartum hemorrhage.

Blame it on lacerations

Lacerations of the cervix, birth canal, or perineum can also lead to postpartum hemorrhage. Cervical lacerations may result in profuse bleeding if the uterine artery is torn. This type of hemorrhage usually occurs immediately after delivery of the placenta, while the patient is still in the delivery area. Suspect lacerations when bleeding persists but the uterus is firm.

Stuck on you

Entrapment of a partially or completely separated placenta by an hourglass-shaped uterine constriction ring (a condition that prevents the entire placenta from expelling) can cause placental fragments to be retained in the uterus. Poor separation of the placenta is common in preterm births of 20 to 24 weeks' gestation.

The reason for abnormal adherence is unknown but it may result from the implantation of the zygote in an area of defective endometrium. This abnormal implantation leaves a zone of separation between the placenta and the decidua. If the fragment is large, bleeding may be apparent in the early postpartum period. If the fragment is small, however, bleeding may go unnoticed for several days, after which time the woman suddenly has a large amount of bloody vaginal discharge.

To clot or not to clot

DIC is a fourth cause of postpartum hemorrhage. Any woman is at risk for DIC after childbirth. However, it's more common in women with abruptio placentae, missed abortion, placenta previa, uterine infection, placenta accreta, uterine inversion, severe preeclampsia, amniotic fluid embolism, or intrauterine fetal death.

Relaxation is risky

Risk factors for uterine atony include:
- polyhydramnios
- delivery of a macrosomic neonate, usually more than 4.1 kg (9 lb)
- use of magnesium sulfate during labor
- multiple gestation
- delivery that was rapid or required operative techniques, such as forceps or vacuum suction
- injury to the cervix or birth canal, such as from trauma, lacerations, or hematoma development
- use of oxytocin to initiate or augment labor or prolonged use of tocolytic agents
- dystocia (dysfunctional labor)
- previous history of postpartum hemorrhage
- use of deep analgesia or anesthesia
- infection, such as chorioamnionitis or endometritis.

What to look for

Bleeding is the key assessment finding for postpartum hemorrhage. It can occur suddenly in large amounts or over time, as seeping or oozing of blood. Expect a patient with postpartum hemorrhage to saturate perineal pads more quickly than usual.

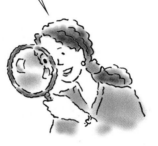

Uh oh. Is that blood I see? Bleeding is the key assessment finding for postpartum hemorrhage.

Soft and boggy

When uterine atony is the cause, the uterus feels soft and relaxed. The bladder may be distended, displacing the uterus to the right or left side of midline and preventing it from contracting properly. The fundus may also be pushed upward.

A cut above

When a laceration is the cause of postpartum hemorrhage, you may notice bright-red blood with clots oozing continuously from the site and a uterus that remains firm.

Left behind

Bleeding caused by a retained placenta or placental fragments usually starts as a slow trickle, oozing, or frank hemorrhage. In the case of retained placental fragments, also expect to find the uterus soft and noncontracting.

The fourth culprit: DIC

When the patient's bleeding is continuous and uterine atony, lacerations, and retained placenta or fragments have been ruled out, coagulation problems may be the cause of the bleeding.

The shocking truth

If blood loss is sufficient, the patient exhibits signs and symptoms of hypovolemic shock, such as increasing restlessness, light-headedness, and dizziness as cerebral tissue perfusion decreases. Inspection may also reveal pale skin, decreased sensorium, increased pulse rate, and rapid, shallow respirations. Urine output usually falls below 25 ml/hour. Palpation may disclose rapid, thready peripheral pulses and cool skin that becomes cold and clammy.

Auscultation of blood pressure usually detects a mean arterial pressure below 60 mm Hg and a narrowing pulse pressure. Capillary refill at the nail beds is delayed 3 to 5 seconds.

What tests tell you

Diagnostic testing reveals a decrease in hemoglobin level and hematocrit. The patient's hemoglobin level typically decreases 1 to 1.5 g/dl and hematocrit drops 2% to 4% from baseline. If the patient has retained placental fragments, you may also find that serum human chorionic gonadotropin levels are elevated.

Coagulating the matter

When DIC is the cause of postpartum hemorrhage, platelet and fibrinogen levels are decreased and clotting times (prothrombin time [PT] and partial thromboplastin time [PTT]) are prolonged. Blood tests also reveal decreased fibrinogen levels and fragmented red blood cells (RBCs). Fibrinolysis increases and then decreases. Coagulation factors are decreased, with decreased antithrombin III, an increased D-dimer test, and a normal or prolonged euglobulin lysis time.

> Treating postpartum hemorrhage involves correcting the underlying cause, controlling blood loss, and minimizing hypovolemic shock.

How it's treated

Treatment of postpartum hemorrhage focuses on correcting the underlying cause and instituting measures to control blood loss and to minimize the extent of hypovolemic shock.

Pump up the tone

For the patient with uterine atony, initiate uterine massage. The goal is to increase uterine tone and contractility to minimize blood loss. If clots are present, they should be expressed. If the patient's bladder is distended, she should try to empty her bladder because a distended bladder prevents the uterus from fully contracting. If these efforts are ineffective or fail to maintain the uterus in a contracted state, oxytocin (Pitocin) or methylergonovine (Methergine) may be given I.M. or I.V. to produce sustained uterine contractions. Prostaglandins (Carboprost Tromethamine) can also be given I.M. to promote strong, sustained uterine contractions.

Source search

If the uterus is firm and contracted and the bladder isn't distended, the source of the bleeding must still be identified. Perform visual or manual inspection of the perineum, vagina, uterus, cervix, and rectum. A laceration requires sutures. If a hematoma is found, treatment may involve observation, cold therapy, ligation of the bleeding vessel, or evacuation of the hematoma. Depending on the extent of fluid loss, replacement therapy may be indicated.

Remove the stragglers

Retained placental fragments typically are removed manually or, if manual extraction is unsuccessful, via dilatation and curettage (D&C). If the placenta is adhered to the uterine wall or has implanted into the myometrium, a hysterectomy may need to be performed to stop uterine bleeding.

Supportive to specific

Successful management of DIC requires prompt recognition and adequate treatment of the underlying disorder. Treatment may be supportive (for example, when the underlying disorder is self-limiting) or highly specific. If the patient isn't actively bleeding, supportive care alone may reverse DIC. Active bleeding may require administration of blood, fresh-frozen plasma, platelets, or packed RBCs to support hemostasis.

Heparin (Hep-loc) therapy for DIC is controversial. It may be used early in the disease to prevent microclotting but may be considered a last resort in the patient who's actively bleeding. If thrombosis occurs, heparin therapy is usually mandatory. In most cases, it's administered in combination with transfusion therapy.

Making up for lost fluids

Emergency treatment relies on prompt and adequate blood and fluid replacement to restore intravascular volume and to raise blood pressure and maintain it above 60 mm Hg. Rapid infusion of lactated Ringer's solution and, possibly, albumin or other plasma expanders may be needed to expand volume adequately until whole blood can be matched.

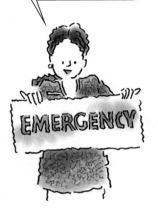

Emergency treatment of DIC relies on prompt and adequate blood and fluid replacement.

What to do

Close, frequent assessment in the hour following delivery is crucial to prevent complications or allow early identification and prompt intervention should hemorrhage occur.

Here are other steps you should take in case of postpartum hemorrhage:

• Assess the patient's fundus and lochia every 15 minutes for 1 hours after birth to detect changes. Notify the practitioner if the fundus doesn't remain contracted or if lochia increases.

• Perform fundal massage, as indicated, to assist with uterine involution. Stay with the patient, frequently reassessing the fundus to ensure that it remains firm and contracted. Keep in mind that the uterus may relax quickly when massage is completed, placing the patient at risk for continued hemorrhage.

• If you suspect postpartum hemorrhage, weigh perineal pads to estimate blood loss.

• Turn the patient onto her side and inspect under the buttocks for pooling of blood.

• Inspect the perineal area closely for oozing from possible lacerations.

• Monitor vital signs frequently for changes, noting trends such as a continuously rising pulse rate and a drop in blood pressure. Report changes immediately. (See *Managing low blood pressure*.)

• Assess intake and output, and report urine output less than 30 ml/hour. Encourage the patient to void frequently to prevent bladder distention from interfering with uterine involution. If she can't void, you may need to insert an indwelling urinary catheter.

A shocking development

Here are the steps you should take if the patient develops signs and symptoms of hypovolemic shock:
• Begin an I.V. infusion with lactated Ringer's solution delivered through a large-bore (14G to 18G) catheter.
• Administer colloids (albumin) and blood products as ordered.
• Monitor the patient for fluid overload.
• Monitor for signs and symptoms of infection, such as increased temperature, foul-smelling lochia, or redness and swelling of the incision.
• Record blood pressure, pulse and respiratory rates, and peripheral pulse rates every 15 minutes until stable.
• Monitor cardiac rhythm continuously.
• During therapy, assess skin color and temperature and note changes. Cold, clammy skin may signal continuing peripheral vascular constriction and progressive shock.
• Monitor capillary refill and skin turgor.
• Watch for signs of impending coagulopathy, such as petechiae, bruising, and bleeding or oozing from gums or venipuncture sites.
• Anticipate the need for fluid replacement and blood component therapy, as ordered.
• Obtain arterial blood samples to measure arterial blood gas (ABG) levels. Administer oxygen by nasal cannula, face mask, or airway to ensure adequate tissue oxygenation. Adjust the oxygen flow rate as ABG measurements indicate.
• Obtain venous blood specimens as ordered for a complete blood count, electrolyte measurements, typing and crossmatching, and coagulation studies.
• If the patient has received I.V. oxytocin for treatment of uterine atony, continue to assess the fundus closely. The action of oxytocin, although immediate, is short in duration, so atony may recur. Monitor for nausea and vomiting.
• Monitor the patient for hypertension if methylergonovine is administered. This medication shouldn't be administered if the patient's baseline blood pressure is 140/90 mm Hg or greater.
• If the practitioner orders I.M. administration of prostaglandin, be alert for possible adverse effects, such as nausea, diarrhea, tachycardia, headache, fever, and hypertension.
• Provide emotional support to the patient, and explain all procedures to help alleviate fear and anxiety.
• Monitor the patient's level of consciousness (LOC) for signs of hypoxia (decreased LOC).

Advice from the experts

Managing low blood pressure

If the patient's systolic blood pressure drops below 80 mm Hg, increase the oxygen flow rate and notify the practitioner immediately. Systolic blood pressure below 80 mm Hg usually results in inadequate coronary artery blood flow, cardiac ischemia, arrhythmias, and further complications of low cardiac output.

Another ominous sign
Notify the practitioner and increase the infusion rate if the patient has a progressive drop in blood pressure (30 mm Hg or less from baseline) accompanied by a thready pulse. This usually signals inadequate cardiac output from reduced intravascular volume. Assess the patient's level of consciousness. As cerebral hypoxia increases, the patient becomes more restless and confused.

- Prepare the patient for possible treatments, such as bimanual massage, surgical repair of lacerations, or D&C.

Postpartum psychiatric disorders

Three distinct psychiatric disorders have been recognized during the postpartum period; postpartum blues (or baby blues), postpartum depression, and postpartum psychosis.

Blue, blue, my world is blue

Baby blues are the most common of the postpartum psychiatric disorders and the least severe. Approximately 50% of all postpartum women experience some form of baby blues. Baby blues usually occur within 3 to 5 days after birth. They are a normal, hormonally generated postpartum occurrence that is thought to foster maternal-neonatal attachment. Mothers who have delivered prematurely, and those who have an infant in the newborn intensive care unit, are at particularly high risk.

From blue to black

Postpartum depression and postpartum psychosis are mood disorders recognized by the American Psychiatric Association's *Diagnostic and Statistical Manual of Mental Disorders*, Fourth Edition, Text Revision. Approximately 400,000 women a year (10% to 20% of postpartum women) develop postpartum depression or postpartum psychosis.

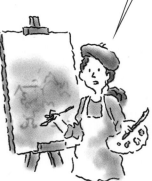

I think I'm definitely in my blue period. About 50% of all postpartum women experience some form of baby blues.

Postpartum depression

Postpartum depression affects as many as 15% of new mothers. This number may be higher because many cases probably aren't reported due to the stigma of a psychiatric illness. Not only does postpartum depression interfere with the mother-infant relationship; it is thought to also interfere with child development and the relationship the child has with other children, family, and friends.

What causes it

The exact cause is unknown, but some prenatal risk factors may contribute to the development of postpartum depression.

A major key

A major risk factor for developing postpartum depression is a previous history of depression or a psychiatric illness before or during the pregnancy. Anxiety during the pregnancy, a teenage pregnancy, multiple births, lack of social support, stressful life situations other than the pregnancy, and conflict with a spouse or significant other during the pregnancy can also be major risk factors.

A minor key

Some minor risk factors include the socioeconomic status of the mother and obstetric complications.

The result

Untreated depression during pregnancy can lead to poor self-care; noncompliance with prenatal care; a negative effect on maternal-infant bonding; a higher risk of obstetric complications; drug, tobacco, or alcohol abuse; termination of the pregnancy; and suicide.

What to look for

Some distinct signs and symptoms help distinguish postpartum depression from postpartum baby blues, including:
- feeling sad or down
- decreased interest in normal activities
- appetite problems and weight changes
- anxiety and agitation
- difficulty sleeping
- fatigue and reduced energy
- feeling guilty or worthless
- feelings of suicide or thoughts of harming the infant.

What tests tell you

There are no specific diagnostic tests for postpartum depression, but women can be screened during the prenatal period. One such screening method is the Postpartum Depression Predictors Inventory. (See *Postpartum depression predictors inventory (PDPI)-revised*, page 456.)

How it's treated

Treatment can usually be accomplished on an outpatient basis. Selective serotonin reuptake inhibitors, such as paroxetine (Paxil), fluoxetine (Prozac), and sertraline (Zoloft), are prescribed. These agents are thought to be safe for breast-feeding women.

What to do

- Teach the postpartum patient about the warning signs of postpartum depression and provide resource material.
- Include teaching about postpartum depression as part of the patient's discharge teaching plan.

Postpartum depression predictors inventory (PDPI)-revised

The PDPI-Revised identifies risk factors for which nursing interventions can be planned to address each mother's problems. The first 10 predictors can be assessed during pregnancy and the postpartum period. The last three risk factors are assessed after a mother has delivered.

During pregnancy — Check one

Marital status
1. Single ☐
2. Married/cohabitating ☐
3. Separated ☐
4. Divorced ☐
5. Widowed ☐
6. Partnered ☐

Socioeconomic status
1. Low ☐
2. Middle ☐
3. High ☐

Self-esteem — Yes / No
1. Do you feel good about yourself as a person? ☐ ☐
2. Do you feel worthwhile? ☐ ☐
3. Do you feel you have a number of good qualities as a person? ☐ ☐

Prenatal depression
1. Have you ever felt depressed during your pregnancy? ☐ ☐
   If yes, when and how long have you been feeling this way? _____
   If yes, how mild or severe would you consider your depression? _____

Prenatal anxiety
1. Have you ever felt anxious during your pregnancy? _____
   If yes, how long have you been feeling this way? _____

Unplanned/unwanted pregnancy
1. Was the pregnancy planned? ☐ ☐
2. Is the pregnancy wanted? ☐ ☐

History of previous depression — Yes / No
1. Before this pregnancy, have you ever been depressed? ☐ ☐
   If yes, when did you experience this depression? _____
   If yes, have you been under a physician's care for this past depression? _____
   If yes, did the physician prescribe any medication for your depression? _____

Social support
1. Do you feel you have received adequate support from your partner? ☐ ☐
2. Do you feel you have received adequate instrumental support from your partner (e.g., help with household chores or babysitting)? ☐ ☐
3. Do you feel you can rely on your partner when you need help? ☐ ☐
4. Do you feel you can confide in your partner? ☐ ☐
(Repeat the same questions for family and again for friends.)

Marital satisfaction
1. Are you satisfied with your marriage (or living arrangement)? ☐ ☐
2. Are you currently experiencing any marital problems? ☐ ☐
3. Are things going well between you and your partner? ☐ ☐

Life stress — Yes / No
1. Are you currently experiencing any stressful events in your life such as:
   Financial problems ☐ ☐
   Marital problems ☐ ☐
   Death in the family ☐ ☐
   Serious illness in the family ☐ ☐
   Moving ☐ ☐
   Unemployment ☐ ☐
   Job changes ☐ ☐

After delivery, add the following items:

Child Care Stress
1. Is your infant experiencing any health problems? ☐ ☐
2. Are you having problems with your baby feeding? ☐ ☐
3. Are you having problems with your baby sleeping? ☐ ☐

Infant temperament
1. Would you consider your baby irritable or fussy? ☐ ☐
2. Does your baby cry a lot? ☐ ☐
3. Is your baby difficult to console or soothe? ☐ ☐

Maternity blues
1. Did you experience a brief period of tearfulness and mood swings during the first week after delivery? ☐ ☐

Comments: _____

Reprinted with permission from Beck, C.T., et al. "Postpartum Depression Predictors Inventory—revised (PDPI)," *Journal of Obstetric Gynecological Neonatal Nursing* 35(6):735, November/December 2006.

• Encourage the woman to verbalize her feelings about the pregnancy.
• Help the woman understand that it's normal to feel sadness or a lack of enthusiasm about motherhood.
• Instruct the woman and her family that postpartum depression can occur at any time after delivery.
• Advise the family of the warning signs of postpartum depression. Inform them that it's important not to ignore even the subtlest of signs. Urge them to immediately report these signs to the practitioner.
• Assist the woman in contacting a support group that can help to alleviate her feelings of isolation.

Postpartum psychosis

Postpartum psychosis usually appears within the first 2 to 3 weeks after birth but can occur as early as the first or second day. This condition affects about 1 to 2 women in every 1,000 births and is an emergency situation that requires immediate intervention.

What causes it

The exact cause is unknown but some predisposing factors may contribute to the development of postpartum psychosis. These include changing hormone levels, lack of support systems, low sense of self-esteem, financial difficulties, and major life changes.

What to look for

Signs and symptoms of postpartum psychosis may be similar to those of any psychosis. For example, the woman may experience symptoms associated with schizophrenia, bipolar disorder, or major depression. As a postpartum patient, she may also experience:
• feelings that her baby is dead or defective
• hallucinations that may include voices telling her to harm the baby or herself
• severe agitation, irritability, or restlessness
• poor judgment and confusion
• feelings of worthlessness, guilt, isolation, or overconcern with the baby's health
• sleep disturbances
• euphoria, hyperactivity, or little concern for self or infant.

What tests tell you

There are no specific diagnostic tests for postpartum psychosis, but women can be screened during the prenatal period. One such screening method is the Postpartum Depression Predictors Inventory.

How it's treated

Postpartum psychosis is a medical emergency and requires immediate hospitalization. Medications such as antipsychotics and antidepressants are used. It may also be necessary to institute suicide precautions. The family should also be involved in the patient's treatment plan.

What to do

• Teach the postpartum patient about the warning signs of postpartum depression and psychosis. Provide resource material.
• Include teaching about postpartum depression and psychosis as part of the patient's discharge teaching plan.
• Instruct the woman and her family that postpartum depression and psychosis can occur at any time after delivery.
• Advise the family of the warning signs of postpartum depression and psychosis. Inform them that it's important not to ignore even the subtlest of signs. Urge them to immediately report these signs to the practitioner.

Postpartum psychosis is a medical emergency and requires immediate hospitalization.

Puerperal infection

Infection during the puerperal period (immediately following childbirth) is a common cause of childbirth-related death. Puerperal infection affects the uterus and structures above it with a characteristic fever pattern. It can result in endometritis, parametritis, pelvic and femoral thrombophlebitis, and peritonitis.

In the United States, puerperal infection develops in about 6% of maternity patients. The prognosis is good in these cases with treatment. There are also certain precautions you can take to prevent puerperal infection. (See *Preventing puerperal infection.*)

What causes it

Microorganisms that commonly cause puerperal infection include group A, B, or G hemolytic streptococcus, *Gardnerella vaginalis*, *Chlamydia trachomatis*, and coagulase-negative staphylococci. Less common causative agents are *Clostridium perfringens*, *Bacteroides fragilis*, Klebsiella, *Proteus mirabilis*, Pseudomonas, *Staphylococcus aureus*, and *Escherichia coli*.

Normal unless predisposed

Most of these organisms are considered normal vaginal flora. However, they can cause puerperal infection in the presence of the following predisposing factors:

- prolonged (more than 24 hours) or premature rupture of the membranes
- prolonged (more than 24 hours) or difficult labor, allowing bacteria to enter while the fetus is still in utero
- frequent or unsterile vaginal examinations or unsterile delivery
- delivery requiring the use of instruments, which may traumatize the tissue, providing an entry portal for microorganisms
- internal fetal monitoring, which may introduce organisms when electrodes are placed
- retained products of conception (such as placental fragments), which cause tissue necrosis and provide an excellent medium for bacterial growth
- hemorrhage, which weakens the patient's overall defenses
- maternal conditions, such as anemia, diabetes mellitus, immunosuppression, or debilitation from malnutrition, that lower the woman's ability to defend against microorganism invasion
- cesarean birth (places patient at a 30% to 50% increased risk for puerperal infection)
- existence of localized vaginal infection or other type of infection at delivery, which allows direct transmission of infection
- bladder catheterization
- episiotomy or lacerations
- history of urinary tract infection
- pneumonia
- venous thrombosis.

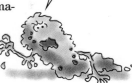

Normal? Who you callin' "normal"?

What to look for

A characteristic sign of puerperal infection is fever (a temperature of at least 100.4° F [38° C]) that occurs during the first 10 days postpartum (except during the first 24 hours) and lasts for 2 consecutive days. The fever can spike as high as 105° F (40.6° C) and is commonly accompanied by chills, headache, malaise, restlessness, and anxiety.

Care to accompany me?

Accompanying signs and symptoms depend on the extent and site of infection and may include:

- localized perineal infection—pain, elevated temperature, edema, redness, firmness, and tenderness at the wound site; sensa-

tion of heat; burning on urination; discharge from the wound; or
separation of the wound
• endometritis—heavy, sometimes foul-smelling lochia; tender,
enlarged uterus; backache; severe uterine contractions persisting
after childbirth; temperature greater than 100.4° F; chills; and increased pulse rate
• parametritis (pelvic cellulitis)—vaginal tenderness and abdominal pain and tenderness (pain may become more intense as infection spreads).

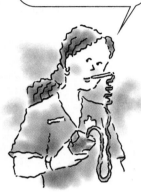

A characteristic
sign of puerperal
infection is a
temperature of at
least 100.4° F that
lasts for 48 hours.

Spreading far and wide

The inflammation may remain localized, may lead to abscess formation, or may spread through the blood or lymphatic system.
Widespread inflammation may cause these conditions, signs, and
symptoms:
• septic pelvic thrombophlebitis—severe, repeated chills and dramatic swings in body temperature; lower abdominal or flank pain;
and, possibly, a palpable tender mass over the affected area,
which usually develops near the second postpartum week
• peritonitis—rigid, boardlike abdomen with guarding (usually
the first sign); elevated body temperature; tachycardia (greater
than 140 beats/minute); weak pulse; hiccups; nausea; vomiting; diarrhea; and constant, possibly excruciating, abdominal pain.

What tests tell you

Development of the typical clinical features—especially fever for
48 hours or more after the first postpartum day—suggests a diagnosis of puerperal infection. Uterine tenderness is also highly suggestive. Typical clinical features usually suffice for a diagnosis of
endometritis and peritonitis. In parametritis, pelvic examination
shows induration without purulent discharge.

You're so cultured

A culture of lochia, incisional exudate (from cesarean incision or
episiotomy), uterine tissue, or material collected from the vaginal
cuff that reveals the causative organism may help confirm the diagnosis. However, such cultures are generally contaminated with
vaginal flora and aren't considered helpful. A sensitivity test is
also done to determine if the proper antibiotic has been administered. Blood cultures are performed for a temperature above
101° F (38.3° C).

White cell uprising

Normal white blood cell (WBC) count during pregnancy is 5,000 to
15,000 µl. WBCs can increase to 30,000 µl during labor due to the

stress response and decreases after recovery. A sudden increase of 30% above the baseline WBC count over a 6-hour period or the presence of bands in the differential WBC count is a sign of infection after birth. Erythrocyte sedimentation rate may also be elevated.

How it's treated

Treatment of puerperal infection usually begins with I.V. infusion of a broad-spectrum antibiotic. This controls the infection and prevents its spread while you await culture results. After identifying the infecting organism, the doctor may prescribe a more specific antibiotic. (An oral antibiotic may be prescribed after discharge.)

Ancillary measures include analgesics for pain, antiseptics for local lesions, and antiemetics for nausea and vomiting from peritonitis.

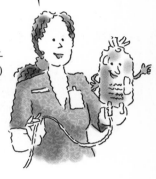

Treatment of puerperal infection usually begins with I.V. infusion of a broad-spectrum antibiotic.

Stick to the standards

A mother with a contagious disease is usually placed in a private room and should be isolated, but not from her neonate. The neonate should be isolated from other neonates and should remain in the room with the mother.

If the mother isn't contagious, she doesn't need to be isolated but you should follow standard precautions. Follow the guidelines of the Centers for Disease Control and Prevention and your facility to determine whether isolation precautions are necessary.

A break from breast-feeding?

Whether the mother can continue breast-feeding, if applicable, depends on the type of antibiotic she's receiving and her physical ability to breast-feed. A mother can't breast-feed if she's receiving metronidazole (Flagyl) or acyclovir (Zovirax). If she plans to breast-feed after her course of antibiotics, help her to pump her breasts and discard the breast milk produced while she's on the medication.

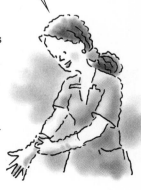

Standard precautions are a must, even if your patient isn't contagious.

Support, surgery, and drugs

Supportive care includes bed rest, adequate fluid intake, I.V. fluids when necessary, and measures to reduce fever. Surgery may also be necessary to remove remaining products of conception or retained placental fragments or to drain local lesions such as an abscess in parametritis.

If the patient develops septic pelvic thrombophlebitis, treatment consists of heparin anticoagulation for about 10 days in conjunction with broad-spectrum antibiotic therapy.

What to do

If your postpartum patient develops an infection, perform these interventions:
• Monitor vital signs every 4 hours (or more frequently depending on the patient's condition).
• Assess capillary refill and skin turgor as well as mucous membranes.
• Assess intake and output closely.
• Enforce strict bed rest.
• Provide a high-calorie, high-protein diet to promote wound healing.
• Provide fluids (3,000 to 4,000 ml), unless otherwise contraindicated.
• Encourage the patient to void frequently, which empties the bladder and helps to prevent infection.
• Inspect the perineum often. Assess the fundus and palpate for tenderness (subinvolution may indicate endometritis). Note the amount, color, and odor of vaginal drainage and document your observations.
• Encourage the patient to change perineal pads frequently, removing them from front to back. Help her change pads, if necessary. Be sure to wear gloves when helping the patient change a perineal pad.
• Administer antibiotics and analgesics, as ordered. Assess and document the type, degree, and location of pain as well as the patient's response to analgesics. Give the patient an antiemetic to relieve nausea and vomiting, as needed.
• Provide sitz baths or warm or cool compresses for local lesions, as ordered.
• Change bed linens, perineal pads, and underpads frequently.
• Provide warm blankets and keep the patient warm.
• Thoroughly explain all procedures to the patient and her family. Offer reassurance and emotional support.
• If the mother is separated from her neonate, reassure her often about his progress. Encourage the father to reassure the mother about the neonate's condition as well.

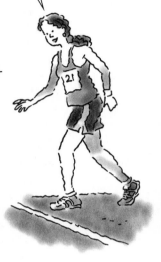

Prevention is best, but prompt treatment runs a close second.

Mastitis

Mastitis is a parenchymatous inflammation of the mammary glands that disrupts normal lactation. It occurs postpartum in about 1% of women, mainly in primiparas who are breast-feeding. It occurs only occasionally in nonlactating females. The prognosis for a woman with mastitis is good.

What causes it

Mastitis develops when trauma due to incorrect latching or removal from the breast allows introduction of organisms from the neonate's nose or pharynx into the maternal breast. The pathogen that most commonly causes mastitis is *Staphylococcus aureus;* less frequently, *Staphylococcus epidermidis* and beta-hemolytic streptococci are the culprits. Rarely, mastitis may result from disseminated tuberculosis or the mumps virus.

Predisposing factors include a fissure or abrasion on the nipple, blocked milk ducts, and an incomplete let-down reflex, usually due to emotional trauma. Blocked milk ducts can result from wearing a tight-fitting bra or waiting prolonged intervals between breast-feedings.

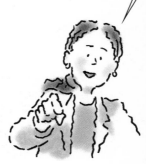

Master the treatment of mastitis adequately and promptly, so it can't progress to breast abscess.

What to look for

Mastitis may develop anytime during lactation, but it usually begins 1 to 4 weeks postpartum with fever (101° F [38.3° C], or higher in acute mastitis), chills, malaise, and flulike symptoms. Mastitis is generally unilateral and localized but, in some cases, both breasts or the entire breast is affected.

Inspection and palpation may uncover redness, swelling, warmth, hardness, tenderness, nipple cracks or fissures, and enlarged axillary lymph nodes. Unless mastitis is treated adequately, it may progress to breast abscess.

Which kind is it?

Mastitis must be differentiated from normal breast engorgement, which generally starts with the onset of lactation (day 2 to day 5 postpartum). During this time, the breasts undergo changes similar to those in mastitis and body temperature may also be elevated.

Engorgement may be mild, causing only slight discomfort, or severe, causing considerable pain. A severely engorged breast can prevent a neonate from feeding properly because he can't latch on to the nipple of the swollen, rigid breast.

What tests tell you

Cultures of expressed breast milk are used to confirm generalized mastitis; cultures of breast skin are used to confirm localized mastitis. These cultures are also used to determine antibiotic therapy. Differential diagnosis should exclude breast engorgement, breast abscess, viral syndrome, and a clogged duct.

How it's treated

Antibiotic therapy, the primary treatment for mastitis, generally consists of oral cephalosporins or either cloxacillin (Cloxapen) or dicloxacillin (Dynapen) to combat staphylococcus. Azithromycin (Zithromax) or vancomycin (Vancocin) may be used for patients who are allergic to penicillin. Although symptoms usually subside after 24 to 48 hours of antibiotic therapy, antibiotic therapy should continue for 10 days.

Other appropriate measures include analgesics for pain and, on the rare occasions when antibiotics fail to control the infection and mastitis progresses to breast abscess, incision and drainage of the abscess.

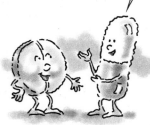

Whadda ya say we treat our friend mastitis here to our own kind of therapy, eh?

What to do

Here's what you should do to treat a patient with mastitis:
• Explain mastitis to the patient and why infection control measures are necessary.
• Establish infection control measures for the mother and neonate to prevent the spread of infection to other nursing mothers.
• Obtain a complete patient history, including a drug history, especially allergy to penicillin.
• Administer antibiotic therapy, as ordered.
• Assess and record the cause and amount of discomfort. Give analgesics, as needed.
• Reassure the mother that breast-feeding during mastitis won't harm her neonate because he's the source of the infection.
• Tell the mother to offer the neonate the affected breast first to promote complete emptying and prevent clogged ducts. However, if an open abscess develops, she must stop breast-feeding with this breast and use a breast pump until the abscess heals. She should continue to breast-feed on the unaffected side.
• Suggest applying a warm, wet towel to the affected breast or taking a warm shower to relax and improve her ability to breast-feed. Cold compresses may also be used to relieve discomfort.
• Advise the patient to wear a supportive bra.
• Provide good skin care.
• Show the patient how to position the neonate properly to prevent cracked or sore nipples.
• Tell the patient to empty her breasts as completely as possible with each feeding.
• Tell the patient to get plenty of rest and drink sufficient fluids to help combat fever.
• Encourage the patient to wear a supportive bra.

Education edge

Preventing mastitis

With today's shortened hospital stays for childbirth, postpartum teaching is more important than ever. If your patient is breast-feeding, be sure to include these instructions about breast care and preventing mastitis in your teaching plan.

• Wash your hands after using the bathroom, before touching your breasts, and before and after every breast-feeding.

• If necessary, apply a warm compress or take a warm shower to help facilitate milk flow.

• Position the neonate properly at the breast, and make sure that he grasps the nipple and entire areola area when feeding.

• Empty your breasts as completely as possible at each feeding.

• Alternate feeding positions and rotate pressure areas.

• Release the neonate's grasp on the nipple before removing him from the breast.

• Expose your nipples to the air for part of each day.

• Drink plenty of fluids, eat a balanced diet, and get sufficient rest to enhance the breast-feeding experience.

• Don't wait too long between feedings or wean the infant abruptly.

An ounce of prevention

Before your breast-feeding patient leaves the hospital, teach her about breast care and how to prevent mastitis. (See *Preventing mastitis*.)

Deep vein thrombosis

DVT, also called *deep vein thrombophlebitis*, is an inflammation of the lining of a blood vessel that occurs in conjunction with clot formation. It typically occurs at the valve cusps because venous stasis encourages the accumulation and adherence of platelets and fibrin.

Thrombophlebitis usually begins with localized inflammation (phlebitis), but this rapidly provokes thrombus formation. Rarely, venous thrombosis develops without associated inflammation of the vein (phlebothrombosis).

Any vein will do

DVT can affect small veins, such as the lesser saphenous vein, or large veins, such as the iliac, femoral, pelvic, and popliteal veins and the vena cava. It's more serious than superficial vein thrombophlebitis because it affects the veins deep in the leg musculature that carry 90% of the venous outflow from the leg.

What causes it

DVT may be idiopathic, but it's more likely to occur along with certain diseases, treatments, injuries, or other factors. In the postpartum woman, DVT most commonly results from an extension of endometritis.

Risky business

Risk factors for developing DVT in the postpartum period include:
- history of varicose veins
- obesity
- previous DVT
- multiple gestations
- increased age (older than age 30)
- family history of DVT
- smoking
- cesarean birth
- multiparity.

> You're old enough to hear this. Being over 30 increases your risk of developing DVT during the postpartum period.

Compounding the risk

These risk factors are compounded by specific occurrences during labor and delivery. For example, blood clotting increases postpartally as a result of elevated fibrinogen levels. Also, pressure from the fetal head during pregnancy and delivery causes veins in the lower extremities to dilate, leading to venous stasis. Finally, lying in the lithotomy position for a long time with the lower extremities in stirrups promotes venous pooling and stasis.

Bad news x 2

During the postpartum period, two major types of DVT may occur: femoral or pelvic. Pelvic DVT runs a long course, usually 6 to 8 weeks. (See *Comparing femoral and pelvic DVT.*)

What to look for

The signs and symptoms for femoral and pelvic DVT differ, but both types require careful assessment.

Femoral DVT

With femoral thrombophlebitis, the patient's temperature increases around the 10th day postpartum. Other signs and symptoms include malaise, chills, and pain, stiffness, or swelling in a leg or in the groin.

Comparing femoral and pelvic DVT

This table outlines the major differences between femoral and pelvic deep vein thrombosis (DVT), including the vessels affected, time of onset, assessment findings, and treatment.

Characteristic	Femoral DVT	Pelvic DVT
Vessels affected	• Femoral • Saphenous • Popliteal	• Ovarian • Uterine • Hypogastric
Onset	Approximately postpartum day 10	Approximately postpartum day 14 to 15
Assessment findings	• Associated arterial spasm, making leg appear milky-white or drained • Edema • Fever • Malaise • Diminished peripheral pulses • Positive Homans' sign • Chills • Pain • Redness and stiffness of affected leg • Shiny white skin on extremity	• Extremely high fever • Tachycardia • Chills • General malaise • Possible pelvic abscess • Abdominal and flank pain
Treatment	• Bed rest • Elevation of affected extremity • Never massaging affected area • Anticoagulants • Moist heat applications • Analgesics	• Complete bed rest • Anticoagulants • Antibiotics • Incision and drainage if abscess develops

With leg swelling, the affected extremity appears reddened or inflamed, edematous below the level of the obstruction, and possibly shiny and white. This white appearance may be related to an accompanying arterial spasm, which results in a decrease in arterial circulation to the area. When measured, the thigh and calf of the affected leg are typically larger than the unaffected extremity.

Man, Homan oh man!

Pain may occur in the calf of the affected leg when the foot is dorsiflexed. This finding—a positive Homans' sign—suggests DVT but isn't a reliable indicator. Even if the patient is negative for Homans' sign, the possibility of an obstruction can't be ruled out. Always elicit Homans' sign passively; active dorsiflexion could lead to embolization of a clot.

What's your sign?

A positive Rielander's sign (palpable veins inside the thigh and calf) or Payr's sign (calf pain when pressure is applied on the inside of the foot) also suggests femoral DVT.

Pelvic DVT

The patient with pelvic DVT appears acutely ill with a sudden onset of a high fever, severe repeated chills, and general malaise. In most cases, body temperature fluctuates widely. The patient may complain of lower abdominal or flank pain, and you may be able to palpate a tender mass over the affected area

What tests tell you

Diagnosis of DVT is based on these characteristic test findings:
• Doppler ultrasonography identifies reduced blood flow to a specific area and obstruction to venous flow, particularly in iliofemoral DVT
• More sensitive than ultrasonography in detecting DVT, plethysmography shows decreased circulation distal to the affected area.
• Venography usually confirms the diagnosis and shows filling defects and diverted blood flow.

How it's treated

Treatment for DVT includes bed rest, with elevation of the affected arm or leg; application of warm, moist compresses; and administration of analgesics, antibiotics, and anticoagulants. After the acute episode subsides, the patient may begin to ambulate while wearing antiembolism stockings (applied before she gets out of bed).

Bring on the meds

Drug therapy typically includes anticoagulants to prolong clotting time, starting with heparin for 5 to 7 days and then changing to another anticoagulant, such as warfarin (Coumadin), for 3 months.

> Drug therapy for DVT typically includes anticoagulants, starting with heparin and then changing to another anticoagulant such as warfarin.

For lysis of acute, extensive DVT, treatment should include streptokinase if the risk of bleeding doesn't outweigh the potential benefits of thrombolytic treatment.

Kicking the treatment up a notch

Rarely, DVT may cause complete venous occlusion, which requires venous interruption through simple ligation, vein plication, or clipping. Embolectomy may be done if clots are being shed to the pulmonary and systemic vasculature and other treatments are unsuccessful.

Caval interruption with transvenous placement of an umbrella filter can trap emboli, preventing them from traveling to the pulmonary vasculature. If the patient develops a pulmonary embolism, heparin may be initiated until the embolism resolves; then subcutaneous heparin or an oral anticoagulant may be continued for 6 months.

Pelvic DVT in particular

In addition, treatment for pelvic DVT focuses on complete bed rest and administration of antibiotics along with anticoagulants. If the patient develops a pelvic abscess, a laparotomy for incision and drainage may be done. Because this procedure may cause tubal scarring and may interfere with fertility, the patient may need additional surgery later to remove the vessel before becoming pregnant again.

What to do

Prevention of DVT is key. Assess the patient for risk factors, and teach her ways to reduce her risk. (See *Preventing DVT*.)

Education edge

Preventing DVT

Incorporate these instructions in your teaching plan to reduce a woman's risk of developing deep vein thrombosis (DVT).
• Check with your practitioner about using a side-lying or back-lying (supine recumbent) position for birth instead of the lithotomy position (on your back with your legs in stirrups). These alternative positions reduce the risk of blood pooling in the lower extremities.
• If you must use the lithotomy position for birth, ask the practitioner to pad the stirrups well so that you put less pressure on your calves.
• Change positions frequently if on bed rest.
• Avoid deeply flexing your legs at the groin or sharply flexing your knees.

• Don't stand in one place for too long or sit with your knees bent or legs crossed. Elevate your legs slightly to improve venous return.
• Don't wear garters or constrictive clothing.
• Wiggle your toes and perform leg lifts while in bed to minimize venous pooling and help increase venous return.
• Use a sequential compression device or wear thigh-high stockings during and after cesarean birth until you're ambulating.
• Walk as soon as possible after birth.
• Wear antiembolism or support stockings as ordered. Put them on before getting out of bed in the morning.

In addition, because postpartal DVT commonly results from an endometrial infection:
• be alert to signs and symptoms of endometritis
• notify the practitioner if signs and symptoms of endometritis occur
• institute treatment promptly, as ordered.

Fighting back

To combat DVT, take the following measures:
• Enforce bed rest as ordered, and elevate the patient's affected arm or leg. If you use pillows for elevation of a leg, place the pillows so that they support its entire length to avoid compressing the popliteal space.
• Apply warm compresses or a covered aquathermia pad to increase circulation to the affected area and to relieve pain and inflammation.
• Give analgesics to relieve pain as ordered.
• Assess uterine involution and note changes in fundal consistency such as the inability to remain firm or contracted.
• Monitor vital signs closely, at least every 4 hours or more frequently if indicated. Report changes in pulse rate or blood pressure as well as temperature elevations.
• Administer I.V. anticoagulants as ordered, using an infusion monitor or pump to control the flow rate, if necessary. Have an anticoagulant antidote, such as protamine sulfate (for heparin therapy), readily available.
• Because neither heparin nor warfarin is excreted in significant amounts in breast milk, breast-feeding is allowed.
• If the mother is hospitalized, have her pump her breast milk for the neonate.
• Administer antibiotic and antipyretic therapy for the patient with pelvic DVT.
• Mark, measure, and record the circumference of the affected extremity at least once daily, and compare it to the other extremity. To ensure accuracy and consistency of serial measurements, mark the skin over the area and measure at the same spot daily.
• Obtain coagulation studies, such as International Normalized Ratio (INR), PTT, and PT, as ordered. Keep in mind that therapeutic anticoagulation values usually are considered to be 1½ to 2 times the control value; INR should be between 2 and 3.5.

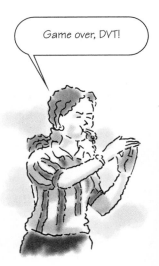

Game over, DVT!

On the lookout for lochia

• Monitor the patient for increased amounts of lochia. Encourage her to change perineal pads frequently, and weigh the pads to estimate the amount of blood loss.
• Watch for signs and symptoms of bleeding, such as tarry stools, coffee-ground vomitus, and ecchymoses. Note oozing of blood at

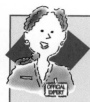

Advice from the experts

Dealing with pulmonary embolism

A woman with deep vein thrombosis is at high risk for developing a pulmonary embolism. Be alert for the classic signs and symptoms of pulmonary embolism, such as:
• chest pain
• dyspnea
• tachypnea
• tachycardia
• hemoptysis
• sudden changes in mental status
• hypotension.

Also, be vigilant in monitoring for these problems, which may occur along with the classic signs and symptoms:
• chills
• fever
• abdominal pain
• signs and symptoms of respiratory distress, including tachypnea, tachycardia, restlessness, cold and clammy skin, cyanosis, and retractions.

Nip it in the bud

A pulmonary embolism is a life-threatening event that can lead to cardiovascular collapse and death. You should intervene at once if pulmonary embolism is suspected. Follow these steps:
• Elevate the head of the bed to improve the work of breathing.
• Administer oxygen via face mask at 8 to 10 L per minute, as ordered.
• Begin I.V. fluid administration, as ordered.
• Monitor oxygen saturation rates continuously via pulse oximetry.
• Obtain arterial blood gas samples for analysis as ordered to evaluate gas exchange.

• Assess vital signs frequently, as often as every 15 minutes.
• Anticipate the need for continuous cardiac monitoring to evaluate for arrhythmias secondary to hypoxemia and for insertion of a pulmonary artery catheter to evaluate hemodynamic status and gas exchange.
• Administer emergency drugs, such as dopamine (Intropin) for pressure support and morphine (Duramorph) for analgesia, as ordered.
• Expect the patient to be transferred to the critical care unit.
• Administer analgesics without aspirin for pain relief.
• Administer anticoagulants or thrombolytics, as ordered.

I.V. sites, and assess gums for excessive bleeding. Report positive findings to the practitioner immediately.
• Assess the patient for signs and symptoms of pulmonary emboli, such as crackles, dyspnea, hemoptysis, sudden changes in mental status, restlessness, and hypotension. (See *Dealing with pulmonary embolism*.)
• Provide emotional support to the woman and her family, and explain all procedures and treatments.
• Prepare the patient for surgery, if indicated.
• Emphasize the importance of follow-up blood studies to monitor anticoagulant therapy.
• If the patient is discharged on heparin therapy, teach her or a family member how to give subcutaneous injections. If additional assistance is required, arrange for a home health care referral and follow-up.

- Teach the patient how to properly apply and use antiembolism stockings. Tell her to report complications, such as toes that are cold or blue.
- To prevent bleeding, encourage the patient to avoid medications that contain aspirin and to check with the practitioner before using over-the-counter medications. Teach the patient the signs and symptoms of bleeding, such as easy bruising or blood in the urine or stool.
- Tell her to use a soft toothbrush and an electric razor to prevent tissue damage and bleeding.
- Advise her to use contraception because oral anticoagulants are teratogenic.
- Tell the patient not to increase her vitamin K intake while taking oral anticoagulants because vitamin K counteracts the anticoagulant effects.
- Stress that the patient should report her history of DVT to the practitioner if she becomes pregnant again so that preventative measures can be started early.

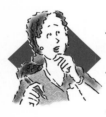

Quick quiz

1. What's considered the major cause of early postpartum hemorrhage?

    A.   Uterine atony
    B.   Perineal laceration
    C.   Retained placental fragments
    D.   DIC

Answer: A. Although all of the above complications are possible causes of postpartum hemorrhage, uterine atony (relaxation of the uterus) is considered the primary and most common cause of early postpartum hemorrhage.

2. Which finding would lead you to suspect that a woman has developed hypovolemic shock secondary to postpartum hemorrhage?

    A.   Respiratory rate of 22 breaths/minute
    B.   Pale-pink, moist skin
    C.   Urine output below 25 ml/hour
    D.   Bounding peripheral pulses

Answer: C. A urine output below 25 ml/hour suggests hypovolemic shock secondary to decreased renal perfusion. Other findings include rapid and shallow respirations; pale, cold, clammy skin; rapid, thready peripheral pulses; mean arterial pressure below 60 mm Hg; and narrowed pulse pressure.

3. Which factor predisposes a patient to a puerperal infection?
   A. External fetal monitoring during labor
   B. Rupture of membranes 15 hours ago
   C. Labor lasting 20 hours
   D. Cesarean birth

Answer: D. A cesarean birth increases a woman's risk for puerperal infection by as much as 20 times. The use of internal fetal monitoring, prolonged (more than 24 hours) or premature rupture of membranes, and prolonged (more than 24 hours) or difficult labor also increase the risk for puerperal infection.

4. A patient reports foul-smelling lochia with strong uterine contractions persisting after birth. Her temperature has been elevated, ranging from 102.2° (39° C) to 104° F (40° C), for the past 2 days. Her uterus is firm but tender, and her abdomen is soft with no guarding noted. You would suspect:
   A. localized perineal infection.
   B. peritonitis.
   C. endometritis.
   D. parametritis.

Answer: C. Endometritis may cause heavy, foul-smelling lochia; a tender, enlarged uterus; backache; severe uterine contractions that persist after childbirth; and elevated temperature for 2 or more days after the first 24 hours.

5. Which microorganism most commonly causes mastitis?
   A. *Staphylococcus aureus*
   B. *Staphylococcus epidermis*
   C. Beta hemolytic streptococcus
   D. Mumps virus

Answer: A. Although all are possible causative organisms, *Staphylococcus aureus* is the most common. Mastitis caused by the mumps virus is rare.

6. If your patient has DVT, for which complication should you watch?
   A. Endometritis
   B. Pulmonary embolism
   C. Hematoma
   D. Mastitis

Answer: B. A possible life-threatening complication of DVT, pulmonary embolism occurs when the clot breaks off and travels to the pulmonary vascular bed, interfering with gas exchange.

Scoring

☆☆☆ If you answered all seven questions correctly, great going! You've summed it up totally.

☆☆ If you answered five or six questions correctly, fantastic! You've added immeasurably to your knowledge of the subject.

☆ If you answered fewer than five questions correctly, no problem. Count on doing better when you read through the chapter once more.

11

Neonatal assessment and care

Just the facts

In this chapter, you'll learn:

♦ changes that occur in the neonate after birth

♦ the proper way to perform a neonatal assessment

♦ nursing interventions critical to neonatal care.

Adapting to extrauterine life

After birth, a neonate must quickly adapt to extrauterine life, even though many of the neonate's body systems are still developing. During this time of adaptation, the nurse must be aware of normal neonatal physiologic characteristics and assessment findings in order to detect possible problems and initiate appropriate interventions. (See *Physiology of the neonate*, page 476.)

Respiratory system

The major adaptation for the neonate is that he must breathe on his own rather than depend on fetal circulation. At birth, air is substituted for the fluid that filled the neonate's respiratory tract in the alveoli during gestation. In a normal vaginal delivery, some of this fluid is squeezed out during birth. After delivery, the fluid is absorbed across the alveolar membrane into the capillaries.

At first breath

The onset of the neonate's breathing is stimulated by several factors:
• low blood oxygen levels
• increased blood carbon dioxide (CO_2) levels
• low blood pH
• temperature change from the warm uterine environment to the cooler extrauterine environment.

Physiology of the neonate

This chart provides a summary of the physiologic characteristics of a neonate after birth, including adaptations the neonate must make to cope with extrauterine life.

Body system	Physiology after birth
Respiratory	• Onset of breathing occurs as air replaces the fluid that filled the lungs before birth.
Cardiovascular	• Functional closure of fetal shunts occurs. • Transition from fetal to postnatal circulation occurs.
Renal	• System doesn't mature fully until after the first year of life; fluid imbalances may occur.
Gastrointestinal	• System continues to develop. • Uncoordinated peristalsis of the esophagus occurs. • The neonate has a limited ability to digest fats.
Thermogenic	• The neonate is susceptible to rapid heat loss due to acute change in environment and thin layer of subcutaneous fat. • Nonshivering thermogenesis occurs. • The presence of brown fat (more in mature neonate; less in preterm neonate) warms the neonate by increasing heat production.
Immune	• The inflammatory response of the tissues to localized infection is immature.
Hematopoietic	• Coagulation time is prolonged.
Neurologic	• Presence of primitive reflexes and time in which they appear and disappear indicate the maturity of the developing nervous system.
Hepatic	• The neonate may demonstrate jaundice.
Integumentary	• The epidermis and dermis are thin and bound loosely to each other. • Sebaceous glands are active.
Musculoskeletal	• More cartilage is present than ossified bone.
Reproductive	• Females may have a mucoid vaginal discharge and pseudomenstruation due to maternal estrogen levels. • In males, testes descend into the scrotum. • Small, white, firm cysts called *epithelial pearls* may be visible at the tip of the prepuce. • Scrotum may be edematous if the neonate presented in breech position.

Noise, light, and other sensations related to the birth process
may also influence the neonate's initial breathing.

Delicate and developing

Although the neonate can breathe on his own, his respiratory system isn't as developed as an adult's is. The neonate is an obligatory nose breather. In addition, the neonate has a relatively large tongue whereas the trachea and glottis are small.

Other significant differences between a neonate's respiratory system and an adult's system include:
• airway lumens that are narrower and collapse more easily
• respiratory tract secretions that are more abundant
• mucous membranes that are more delicate and susceptible to trauma
• alveoli that are more sensitive to pressure changes
• a capillary network that's less developed
• rib cage and respiratory musculature that are less developed.

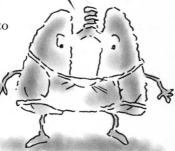

Careful! A neonate's mucous membranes are more susceptible to trauma than an adult's.

Cardiovascular system

The neonate's first breath triggers the start of several cardiopulmonary changes that help him transition from fetal circulation to postnatal circulation. During this transition, the foramen ovale, ductus arteriosis, and ductus venosus close. These closures allow blood to start flowing to the lungs.

Ovale to no avail

When the neonate takes his first breath, the lungs inflate. When the lungs are inflated, pulmonary vascular resistance to blood flow is reduced and pulmonary artery pressure drops. Pressure in the right atrium decreases, and the increased blood flow to the left side of the heart increases the pressure in the left atrium. This change in pressure causes the foramen ovale (the fetal shunt between the left and right atria) to close. Increased blood oxygen levels then influence other fetal shunts to close.

From ducts to ligaments

The ductus arteriosus, located between the aorta and pulmonary artery, eventually closes and becomes a ligament. The ductus venosus, between the left umbilical vein and the inferior vena cava, closes because of vasoconstriction and lack of blood flow; then it also becomes a ligament. The umbilical arteries and vein and the hepatic arteries also constrict and become ligaments.

Renal system

After birth, the renal system is called into action because the neonate can no longer depend on the placenta to excrete waste products. However, renal system function doesn't fully mature until after the first year, which means that the neonate is at risk for chemical imbalances. The neonate's limited ability to excrete drugs because of renal immaturity, coupled with excessive neonatal fluid loss, can rapidly lead to acidosis and fluid imbalances.

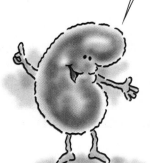

Hey, I'm new to the job. Give me a chance to mature or I might easily develop acidosis and fluid imbalances.

Gastrointestinal system

At birth, the neonate's GI system isn't fully developed because normal bacteria aren't present in the digestive tract. The lower intestine contains meconium, which usually starts to pass within 24 hours. It appears greenish black and viscous.

Ongoing developments

As the GI system starts to develop, these characteristics appear:
• audible bowel sounds 1 hour after birth
• uncoordinated peristaltic activity in the esophagus for the first few days of life
• limited ability to digest fats because amylase and lipase are absent at birth
• frequent regurgitation because of an immature cardiac sphincter.

Thermogenic system

Among the many adaptations that occur after birth, the neonate must regulate his body temperature by producing and conserving heat. This can be difficult for the neonate because he has a thin layer of subcutaneous fat and his blood vessels are closer to the surface of the skin. In addition, the neonate's vasomotor control is less developed, his body surface area to weight ratio is high, and his sweat glands have minimal thermogenic function until he's age 4 weeks or older.

Where's the heat?

The neonate's body also has to work against four routes of heat loss:

 convection—the flow of heat from the body to cooler air

radiation—the loss of body heat to cooler, solid surfaces near (but not in direct contact with) the neonate

evaporation—heat loss that occurs when liquid is converted to a vapor

conduction—the loss of body heat to cooler substances in direct contact with the neonate.

Warming things up

To maintain body temperature, the neonate must produce heat through a process called *nonshivering thermogenesis*. This involves an increase in the neonate's metabolism and oxygen consumption. Thermogenesis mainly occurs in the heart, liver, and brain. Brown fat (brown adipose tissue) is another source of thermogenesis that's unique to the neonate.

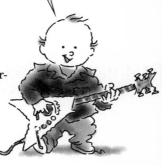

I'd like to heat things up a little. This next number is something I like to call thermogenesis.

Immune system

The neonatal immune system depends largely on three immunoglobulins: immunoglobulin (Ig) G, IgA, and IgM.

Fighting infection with shear numbers

IgG (which can be detected in the fetus at 3 months' gestation) consists of bacterial and viral antibodies. It's the most abundant immunoglobulin and is found in all body fluids. In utero, IgG crosses from the placenta to the fetus. After birth, the neonate produces his own IgG during the first 3 months while the leftover maternal antibodies in the neonate break down.

The enforcer of bacterial growth

IgA, an immunoglobulin that limits bacterial growth in the GI tract, is produced gradually. Maximum levels of IgA are reached during childhood. The neonate obtains IgA from maternal colostrum and breast milk.

First responder

IgM, found in blood and lymph fluid, is the first immunoglobulin to respond to infection. It's produced at birth, and by age 9 months the IgM level in the neonate reaches the level found in adults.

Still in training

Even though these immunoglobulins are present in the neonate, the inflammatory response of the tissues to localized infection is still immature. All neonates, especially preterm neonates, are at high risk for infection during the first several months of life.

Hematopoietic system

In the neonatal hematopoietic system, blood volume accounts for 80 to 85 ml/kg of body weight. Immediately after birth, the neonatal blood volume averages 300 ml; however, it can drop to as low as 100 ml depending on how long the neonate remains attached to the placenta via the umbilical cord. In addition, neonatal blood has a prolonged coagulation time because of decreased levels of vitamin K.

Neurologic system

The neurologic system at birth isn't completely integrated, but it's developed enough to sustain extrauterine life. Most functions of this system are primitive reflexes. The full-term neonate's neurologic system should produce equal strength and symmetry in responses and reflexes. Diminished or absent reflexes may indicate a serious neurologic problem, and asymmetrical responses may indicate that trauma, such as nerve damage, paralysis, or fracture, occurred during birth.

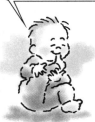

My reflexes are primitive—neurologically speaking, that is.

Hepatic system

Jaundice (yellowing of the skin) is a major concern in the neonatal hepatic system. It's caused by hyperbilirubinemia, a condition that occurs when serum levels of unconjugated bilirubin increase because of increased red blood cell lysis, altered bilirubin conjugation, or increased bilirubin reabsorption from the GI tract.

A mellow yellow

Jaundice resulting from physiologic hyperbilirubinemia occurs in 50% of full-term neonates and 80% of preterm neonates. It's a mild form of jaundice that appears after the first 24 hours of extrauterine life and usually disappears in 7 days (9 or 10 days in preterm neonates). However, if bilirubin levels rise, pathologic conditions such as bilirubin encephalopathy may develop.

Shades of an underlying condition

Jaundice resulting from pathologic hyperbilirubinemia is evident at birth or within the first 24 hours of extrauterine life. It may be caused by hemolytic disease, liver disease, or severe infection. Prognosis varies depending on the cause.

Education edge

Protecting neonates from the sun

Neonates are more susceptible to the harmful effects of the sun because the amount of melanin (pigment) in the skin is low at birth. Teach parents the importance of avoiding sun exposure by giving them these tips.
• Keep a hat with a visor on the neonate when outside.
• Make sure that the hood of the stroller covers the neonate.
• Use a blanket to shade the neonate from the sun when necessary.
• Be especially careful in the car. Sun roofs and windows may expose the neonate to too much sun. Use commercially available window shades and visors.

Integumentary system

At birth, all of the structures of the integumentary system are present, but many of their functions are immature. The epidermis and dermis are bound loosely to each other and are very thin. In addition, the sebaceous glands are very active in early infancy because of maternal hormones. (See *Protecting neonates from the sun.*)

Musculoskeletal system

At birth, the skeletal system contains more cartilage than ossified bone. The process of ossification occurs very rapidly during the first year of life. The muscular system is almost completely formed at birth.

Reproductive system

The ovaries of the female neonate contain thousands of primitive germ cells. These germ cells represent the full potential for ova. The number of ova decreases from birth to maturity by about 90%. After birth, the uterus undergoes involution and decreases in size and weight because, in utero, the fetal uterus enlarges from the effects of maternal hormones.

For 97% of male neonates, the testes descend into the scrotum before birth. However, spermatogenesis doesn't occur until puberty.

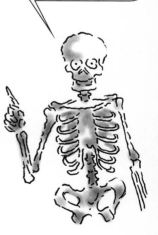

Here's an interesting fact: At birth, the skeletal system contains more cartilage than ossified bone.

Neonatal assessment

Neonatal assessment includes initial and ongoing assessments, a head-to-toe physical examination, and neurologic and behavioral assessments.

Initial assessment

The initial neonatal assessment involves draining secretions, assessing abnormalities, and keeping accurate records. To complete an initial assessment, follow these steps:

• For infection control purposes, all caregivers should wash their hands and wear gloves when assessing or caring for a neonate until after his initial bath.

• Ensure a proper airway by suctioning, and administer oxygen as needed.

• Dry the neonate under the warmer while keeping his head lower than his trunk (to promote the drainage of secretions)

• Apply a cord clamp and monitor the neonate for abnormal bleeding from the cord; check the number of cord vessels.

• Observe the neonate for voiding and meconium; document the first void and stools.

• Assess the neonate for gross abnormalities and clinical manifestations of suspected abnormalities.

• Continue to assess the neonate by using the Apgar score criteria even after the 5-minute score is received.

• Obtain clear footprints and fingerprints. (In some facilities, the neonate's footprints are kept on a record that also includes the mother's fingerprints.)

• Apply identification bands with matching numbers to the mother (one band) and the neonate (two bands) before they leave the delivery room. Some facilities also give the father or significant other an identification band.

• Promote bonding between the mother and the neonate by putting the neonate to the mother's breast or having the mother and neonate engage in skin-to-skin contact.

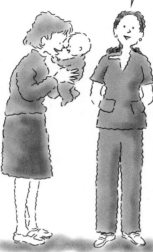

Mother and neonate bonding can be helped by skin-to-skin contact.

Apgar scoring

During the initial examination of a neonate, expect to calculate an Apgar score and make general observations about the neonate's appearance and behavior. Developed by anesthesiologist Dr. Virginia Apgar in 1952, Apgar scoring evaluates neonatal heart rate, respiratory effort, muscle tone, reflex irritability, and color. Evaluation of each category is performed 1 minute after birth and again at 5 minutes after birth. Each item has a maximum score of 2 and

Recording the Apgar score

Use this chart to determine the neonatal Apgar score at 1-minute and 5-minute intervals after birth. For each category listed, assign a score of 0 to 2, as shown. A total score of 7 to 10 indicates that the neonate is in good condition; 4 to 6, fair condition (the neonate may have moderate central nervous system depression, muscle flaccidity, cyanosis, and poor respirations); 0 to 3, danger (the neonate needs immediate resuscitation, as ordered). Each component should be assessed at 1, 5, 10, 15, and 20 minutes after delivery, as necessary. Resuscitation efforts such as oxygen, endotracheal intubation, chest compressions, positive pressure ventilation or nasal continuous positive airway pressure, and epinephrine administration should also be documented.

Sign	Apgar score		
	0	1	2
Heart rate	Absent	Less than 100 beats/minute	More than 100 beats/minute
Respiration	Absent	Weak cry, hypoventilation	Good crying
Muscle tone	Flaccid	Some flexion	Active motion
Reflex irritability	No response	Grimace or weak cry	Cry or active withdrawal
Color	Pallor, cyanosis	Pink body, blue extremities	Completely pink

a minimum score of 0. The final Apgar score is the sum total of the five items; a maximum score is 10.

Evaluation at 1 minute quickly indicates the neonate's initial adaptation to extrauterine life and whether resuscitation is necessary. The 5-minute score gives a more accurate picture of his overall status. (See *Recording the Apgar score*.)

First and foremost

Assess heart rate first. If the umbilical cord still pulsates, you can palpate the neonate's heart rate by placing your fingertips at the junction of the umbilical cord and the skin. The neonate's cord stump continues to pulsate for several hours and is a good, easy place (next to the abdomen) to check heart rate. You can also place two fingers or a stethoscope over the neonate's chest at the fifth intercostal space to obtain an apical pulse. For accuracy, the heart rate should be counted for 1 full minute.

Second to one

Next, check the neonate's respiratory effort, the second most important Apgar sign. Assess the neonate's cry, noting its volume and vigor. Then auscultate his lungs using a stethoscope. Assess his respirations for depth and regularity. If the neonate exhibits ab-

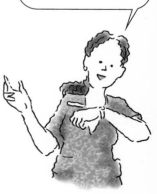

Got a minute? An easy place to check heart rate is the neonate's cord stump. Be sure to count for a full minute.

normal respiratory responses, begin neonatal resuscitation according to the guidelines of the American Heart Association and the American Academy of Pediatrics. Then use the Apgar score to judge the progress and success of resuscitation efforts. (See *Monitoring for effects of medication.*)

Move along to the muscles

Determine muscle tone by evaluating the degree of flexion in the neonate's arms and legs and their resistance to straightening. This can be done by extending the limbs and observing their rapid return to flexion—the neonate's normal state.

Assess reflex irritability by evaluating the neonate's cry for presence, vigor, and pitch. Initially he may not cry, but you should be able to elicit a cry by flicking his soles. The usual response is a loud, angry cry. A high-pitched or shrill cry is abnormal.

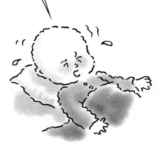

Stop trying to straighten my arms and legs or I'll tell my mommy!

Now add a little color

Finally, observe skin color for cyanosis. A neonate usually has a pink body with blue extremities. This condition, called *acrocyanosis*, appears in about 85% of normal neonates 1 minute after birth. Acrocyanosis results from decreased peripheral oxygenation caused by the transition from fetal to independent circulation. When assessing a non-White neonate, observe for color changes in the mucous membranes of the mouth, conjunctivae, lips, palms, and soles.

Gestational age and birth weight

Perinatal mortality and morbidity are related to gestational age and birth weight. Classifying a neonate by both weight and gestational age provides a more accurate method for assessing mortality risk and offers guidelines for treatment. The neonate's age and weight classifications should also be considered during future assessments.

How old are you now?

The clinical assessment of gestational age classifies a neonate as *preterm* (fewer than 37 weeks' gestation), *term* (37 to 42 weeks' gestation), or *postterm* (42 weeks' gestation or longer). The Ballard scoring system uses physical and neurologic findings to estimate a neonate's gestational age within 1 week, even in extremely preterm neonates. This evaluation can be done at any time between birth and 42 hours after birth, but the greatest reliability is between 30 and 42 hours after birth. (See *Ballard gestational-age assessment tool.*)

Advice from the experts

Monitoring for effects of medication

Closely observe a neonate whose mother has received heavy sedation just before delivery or magnesium sulfate during labor. Even if he has a high Apgar score at birth, he may exhibit secondary effects of sedation later. Be alert for respiratory depression or unresponsiveness. Monitor the neonate whose mother received magnesium sulfate during labor for hypotonia.

Too small, too big, just right

Normal birth weight is 2,500 g (5 lb, 8 oz) or greater. A neonate is considered to have a low birth weight if he weighs between 1,500 g (3 lb, 5 oz) and 2,499 g. A neonate of very low birth weight ranges between 1,000 g (2 lb, 3 oz) and 1,499 g. A neonate weighing less than 1,000 g has an extremely low birth weight.

Postnatal growth charts are used to assess the neonate based on head circumference, weight, length, and gestational age.

(Text continues on page 488.)

Ballard gestational-age assessment tool

To use this tool, evaluate and score the neuromuscular and physical maturity criteria, total the score, and then plot the sum in the maturity rating box to determine the neonate's corresponding gestational age.

Posture
With the neonate supine and quiet, score as follows:
- Arms and legs extended = 0
- Slight or moderate flexion of hips and knees = 1
- Moderate to strong flexion of hips and knees = 2
- Legs flexed and abducted, arms slightly flexed = 3
- Full flexion of arms and legs = 4

Square window
Flex the hand at the wrist. Measure the angle between the base of the thumb and the forearm. Score as follows:
- > 90 degrees = −1
- 90 degrees = 0
- 60 degrees = 1
- 45 degrees = 2
- 30 degrees = 3
- 0 degrees = 4

Arm recoil
With the neonate supine, fully flex the forearm for 5 seconds, then fully extend by pulling the hands and releasing. Observe and score the reaction according to this criteria:
- Remains extended 180 degrees or displays random movements = 0
- Minimal flexion (140 to 180 degrees) = 1
- Small amount of flexion (110 to 140 degrees) = 2
- Moderate flexion (90 to 110 degrees) = 3
- Brisk return to full flexion (< 90 degrees) = 4

Popliteal angle
With the neonate supine and the pelvis flat on the examining surface, use one hand to flex the leg and then the thigh. Then use the other hand to extend the leg. Score the angle attained:
- 180 degrees = −1
- 160 degrees = 0
- 140 degrees = 1
- 120 degrees = 2
- 100 degrees = 3
- 90 degrees = 4
- < 90 degrees = 5

Scarf sign
With the neonate supine, take his hand and draw it across the neck and as far across the opposite shoulder as possible. You may assist the elbow by lifting it across the body. Score according to the location of the elbow:
- Elbow reaches or nears level of opposite shoulder = −1
- Elbow crosses opposite anterior axillary line = 0
- Elbow reaches opposite anterior axillary line = 1
- Elbow at midline = 2
- Elbow doesn't reach midline = 3
- Elbow doesn't cross proximate axillary line = 4

Heel to ear
With the neonate supine, hold his foot with one hand and move it as near to the head as possible without forcing it. Keep the pelvis flat on the examining surface. Score as shown in the chart.

(continued)

Ballard gestational-age assessment tool (continued)

NEUROMUSCULAR MATURITY

Neuromuscular maturity sign	Score							Record score here
	−1	0	1	2	3	4	5	
Posture	—						—	
Square window (wrist)	>90°	90°	60°	45°	30°	0°	—	
Arm recoil	—	180°	140° to 180°	110° to 140°	90° to 110°	< 90°	—	
Popliteal angle	180°	160°	140°	120°	100°	90°	<90°	
Scarf sign							—	
Heel to ear							—	

Total neuromuscular maturity score

Ballard gestational-age assessment tool (continued)

PHYSICAL MATURITY

Physical maturity sign	Score							Record score here
	−1	0	1	2	3	4	5	
Skin	Sticky, friable, transparent	Gelatinous, red, translucent	Smooth, pink; visible vessels	Superficial peeling or rash; few visible vessels	Cracking; pale areas; rare visible vessels	Parchment-like; deep cracking; no visible vessels	Leathery, cracked, wrinkled	
Lanugo	None	Sparse	Abundant	Thinning	Bald areas	Mostly bald	—	
Plantar surface	Heel-to-toe 40 to 50 mm: −1; < 40 mm: −2	> 50 mm; no crease	Faint red marks	Anterior transverse crease only	Creases over anterior two-thirds	Creases over entire sole	—	
Breast	Impercep-tible	Barely perceptible	Flat areola; no bud	Stippled areola; 1- to 2-mm bud	Raised areola; 3- to 4-mm bud	Full areola; 5- to 10-mm bud	—	
Eye and ear	Lids fused, loosely: −1; tightly: −2	Lids open; pinna flat, stays folded	Slightly curved pinna; soft, slow, recoil	Well-curved pinna; soft but ready recoil	Formed and firm; instant recoil	Thick cartilage; ear stiff	—	
Genitalia (male)	Scrotum flat, smooth	Scrotum empty; faint rugae	Testes in upper canal; rare rugae	Testes descending; few rugae	Testes down; good rugae	Testes pendulous; deep rugae	—	
Genitalia (female)	Clitoris prominent; labia flat	Prominent clitoris; small labia minora	Prominent clitoris; enlarging minora	Majora and minora equally prominent	Majora large; minora small	Majora cover clitoris and minora	—	

Total physical maturity score

(continued)

Ballard gestational-age assessment tool *(continued)*

SCORE

Neuromuscular: _____

Physical: _____

Total maturity score: _____

GESTATIONAL AGE (Weeks)

By dates: _____

By ultrasound: _____

By score: _____

Total maturity score	−10	−5	0	5	10	15	20	25	30	35	40	45	50
Gestational age (weeks)	20	22	24	26	28	30	32	34	36	38	40	42	44

Adapted with permission from Ballard, J.L., et al. "New Ballad Score, expanded to include extremely premature infants," *Journal of Pediatrics* 119(3):417-23, 1991. Used with permission from Mosby–Year Book, Inc.

Neonates who are small for gestational age have a birth weight less than the 10th percentile on postnatal growth charts; weight appropriate for gestational age signifies a birth weight within the 10th and 90th percentiles; and weight large for gestational age means a birth weight greater than the 90th percentile. (See *Caring for a preterm neonate*.)

Ongoing assessment

Ongoing neonatal physical assessment includes observing and recording vital signs and administering prescribed medications. To perform ongoing assessment, follow these steps:
- Assess the neonate's vital signs.
- Measure and record the neonate's vital statistics.
- Administer prescribed medications such as vitamin K (AquaMEPHYTON), which is a prophylactic to the transient deficiency of coagulation factors II, VII, IX, and X.
- Administer erythromycin ointment (Ilotycin), the drug of choice for neonatal eye prophylaxis, to prevent damage and blindness from conjunctivitis caused by *Neisseria gonorrhoeae* and *Chlamydia*; treatment is required by law.
- Perform laboratory tests.
- Monitor glucose levels and hematocrit (test results aid in assessing for hypoglycemia and anemia).

Vital signs

Measuring vital signs establishes the baseline of any neonatal assessment. Vital signs include the respiratory rate, heart rate (taken

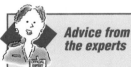

Advice from the experts

Caring for a preterm neonate

When caring for a preterm neonate, be alert for problems—even if the neonate is of average size. A preterm neonate who's an appropriate weight for his gestational age is more prone to respiratory distress syndrome, apnea, patent ductus arteriosus with left-to-right shunt, and infection. A preterm neonate who's small for his gestational age is more likely to experience asphyxia, hypoglycemia, and hypocalcemia.

Reviewing normal neonatal vital signs

This list includes the normal ranges for neonatal vital signs.

Respiration
• 30 to 50 breaths/minute

Heart rate (apical)
• 110 to 160 beats/minute

Temperature
• Rectal: 96° to 99.5° F (35.6° to 37.5° C)
• Axillary: 97.5° to 99° F (36.4° to 37.2° C)

Blood pressure
• Systolic: 60 to 80 mm Hg
• Diastolic: 40 to 50 mm Hg

Counting neonatal respirations

When counting a neonate's respiratory rate, observe abdominal excursions rather than chest excursions. Auscultation of the chest or placing the stethoscope in front of the mouth and nares are other ways to count respirations.

apically), and the first neonatal temperature (this is taken rectally to verify rectal patency). Subsequent temperature readings are axillary to avoid injuring the rectal mucosa. Blood pressure readings may be assessed by sphygmomanometer or by palpation or auscultation. An electronic vital signs monitor may be used. (See *Reviewing normal neonatal vital signs.*)

Determining respiratory rate

Observe respirations first, before the neonate becomes active or agitated. Watch and count respiratory movements for 1 minute and record the result. A normal respiratory rate is usually between 30 and 50 breaths/minute. Also, note any signs of respiratory distress, such as cyanosis, tachypnea, sternal retractions, grunting, nasal flaring, or periods of apnea. Short periods of apnea (less than 15 seconds) are characteristic of the neonate. (See *Counting neonatal respirations.*)

Assessing heart rate

Use a pediatric stethoscope to determine the neonate's apical heart rate. Place the stethoscope over the apical impulse on the fourth or fifth intercostal space at the left midclavicular line over the cardiac apex. To ensure an accurate measurement, count the beats for 1 minute. A normal heart rate ranges from 110 to 160 beats/minute. Variations during sleeping and waking states are normal.

Taking a rectal temperature

The technique for taking a rectal temperature in a neonate is relatively simple. With the neonate lying in a supine position, place a diaper over the penis (if applicable) and firmly grasp his ankles with your index finger between them. Then insert a lubricated thermometer into the rectum, no more than ½″ (1.3 cm). Place your palm on his buttocks, and hold the thermometer between your index and middle fingers. If resistance is met while inserting the thermometer, withdraw the thermometer and notify the practitioner.

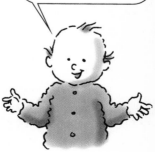

You're not really going to put the thermometer there, are you?

Hold it

Hold a mercury thermometer in place for 3 minutes and an electronic thermometer in place until the temperature registers. Remove the thermometer and record the result.

Body temperature in neonates is less constant than in adults and can fluctuate during the course of a day, without reason. The normal range for a rectal temperature is 96° to 99.5° F (35.6° to 37.5° C).

Taking an axillary temperature

To take an axillary temperature, make sure that the axillary skin is dry. Place the thermometer in the axilla and hold it along the lateral aspect of the neonate's chest between the axillary line and the arm. Hold the thermometer in place until the temperature registers. Normal axillary temperature is 97.5° to 99° F (36.4° to 37.2° C).

Reassess axillary temperature in 15 to 30 minutes if the first measurement registers outside the normal range. If the temperature remains abnormal, notify the doctor.

The low-down on low temperatures

Decreased temperatures by either the rectal or axillary route could suggest:
• prematurity
• infection
• low environmental temperature
• inadequate clothing
• dehydration.

Why it may be high

Possible reasons for increased temperatures include:
• infection
• high environmental temperature
• excessive clothing
• proximity to heating unit or direct sunlight
• drug addiction
• diarrhea and dehydration.

Determining blood pressure

If possible, measure a neonate's blood pressure when he's in a quiet or relaxed state. Make sure that the blood pressure cuff is small enough for the neonate (cuff width should be about one-half the circumference of the neonate's arm). Then wrap the cuff one or two fingerbreadths above the antecubital or popliteal area. With the stethoscope held directly over the chosen artery, hold the cuffed extremity firmly to keep it extended and inflate the cuff no faster than 5 mm Hg/second.

Normal systolic readings are 60 to 80 mm Hg and normal diastolic readings are 40 to 50 mm Hg. A drop in systolic blood pressure (about 15 mm Hg) during the first hour after birth is common. Crying and movement result in blood pressure changes.

From top to bottom

Compare blood pressures in the upper and lower extremities at least once to detect abnormalities. Remember that blood pressure readings from the thigh will be approximately 10 mm Hg higher than the arm. If the blood pressure reading in the thigh is the same or lower than the arm, notify the practitioner. This could indicate coarctation of the aorta, a congenital heart defect, and should be investigated further.

Size and weight

Size and weight measurements establish the baseline for monitoring growth. Size and weight measurements can also be used to detect such disorders as failure to thrive and hydrocephalus. (See *Average neonatal size and weight.*)

Average neonatal size and weight

In addition to weight, anthropometric measurements include head and chest circumferences and head-to-heel length. Together, these measurements serve as a baseline and show whether neonatal size is within normal ranges or whether there may be a significant problem or anomaly—especially if values stray far from the mean.

Average initial anthropometric ranges are:
- head circumference—13" to 14" (33 to 35.5 cm)
- chest circumference—12" to 13" (30.5 to 33 cm)
- head to heel—18" to 21" (46 to 53 cm)
- weight—2,500 to 4,000 g (5 lb, 8 oz to 8 lb, 13 oz).

Head circumference

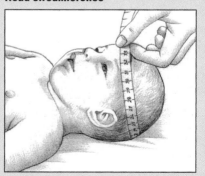

Chest circumference

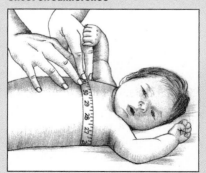

Head-to-heel length

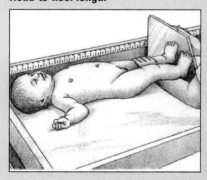

Measuring head circumference

Head circumference reflects the rate of growth of the head and its contents. To measure head circumference, slide the tape measure under the neonate's head at the occiput and draw the tape around snugly, just above the eyebrows. Normal neonatal head circumference is 13″ to 14″ (33 to 35.5 cm). Cranial molding or caput succedaneum from a vaginal delivery may affect this measurement.

Measuring chest circumference

Measure chest circumference by placing the tape under the back, wrapping it snugly around the chest at the nipple line, and keeping the back and front of the tape level. Take the measurement after the neonate inspires and before he begins to exhale. Normal neonatal chest circumference is 12″ to 13″ (30.5 to 33 cm).

Measuring head-to-heel length

Fully extend the neonate's legs with the toes pointing up. Measure the distance from the heel to the top of the head. A length board may be used if available. Normal length is 18″ to 21″ (46 to 53 cm).

Weighing the neonate

A neonate should be weighed before a feeding and the scale should be balanced. Remove the diaper and place the neonate in the middle of the scale tray. Keep one hand poised over the neonate at all times; never leave the neonate unattended on the scale. Average weight is 2,500 to 4,000 g (5 lb, 8 oz to 8 lb, 13 oz).

Return the neonate to the bassinet or examination table. Be sure to document if the neonate had any clothing or equipment on him (such as an I.V.). Take the neonate's weight at the same time each day, and on the same scale, if possible. Be careful to prevent heat loss.

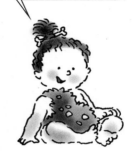

Sometimes it's good to have a big head. Head circumference should be about 1″ (2.5 cm) larger than chest circumference.

Head-to-toe assessment

The neonate should receive a thorough physical examination of each body part. However, before each body part is examined, assess the general appearance and posture of the neonate. Neonates usually lie in a symmetrical, flexed position—the characteristic "fetal position"—as a result of their position while in utero.

Skin

The term neonate has beefy red skin for a few hours after birth. Then the skin turns to its normal color. It commonly appears mottled or blotchy, especially on the extremities.

Findings can be skin deep

Common findings in a neonatal assessment may include:
• acrocyanosis (caused by vasomotor instability, capillary stasis, and high hemoglobin level) for the first 24 hours after birth
• milia (clogged sebaceous glands) on the nose or chin
• lanugo (fine, downy hair) appearing after 20 weeks of gestation on the entire body, except the palms and soles
• vernix caseosa (a white, cheesy protective coating composed of desquamated epithelial cells and sebum)
• erythema toxicum neonatorum (a transient, maculopapular rash)
• telangiectasia (flat, reddened vascular areas) appearing on the neck, upper eyelid, or upper lip
• sudamina or miliaria (distended sweat glands), which cause minute vesicles on the skin surface, especially on the face
• Mongolian spots (bluish black areas of pigmentation more commonly noted on the back and buttocks of dark-skinned neonates [regardless of race]).

Make general observations about the appearance of the neonate's skin in relationship to his activity, position, and temperature. Usually, the neonate is redder when crying or hot. He may also have transient episodes of cyanosis with crying. Cutis marmorata is transient mottling when the neonate is exposed to cooler temperatures.

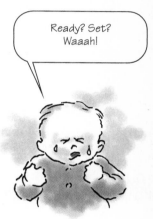

Ready? Set? Waaah!

Roll with it, baby

Palpate the skin to assess skin turgor. To do this, roll a fold of skin on the neonate's abdomen between your thumb and forefinger. Assess consistency, amount of subcutaneous tissue, and degree of hydration. A well-hydrated infant's skin returns to normal immediately upon release.

Head

The neonate's head is about one-fourth of its body size. Six bones make up the cranium:
• the frontal bone
• the occipital bone
• two parietal bones
• two temporal bones.

Bands of connective tissue, called *sutures*, lie between the junctures of these bones. At the junction of the sutures are wider spaces of membranous tissues, called *fontanels*.

Fontanel facts

The neonatal skull has two fontanels. The anterior fontanel is diamond-shaped and located at the juncture of the frontal and parietal bones. It measures 1⅛" to 1⅝" (3 to 4 cm) long and ¾" (2 cm) to 1⅛" wide. The anterior fontanel closes in about 18 months. The posterior fontanel is triangle-shaped. It's located at the juncture of the occipital and parietal bones and measures about ¾" across. The posterior fontanel closes in 8 to 12 weeks.

The fontanels should feel soft to touch but shouldn't be depressed. A depressed fontanel indicates dehydration. In addition, fontanels shouldn't bulge. Bulging fontanels require immediate attention because they may indicate increased intracranial pressure (ICP). Pulsations in the fontanels reflect the peripheral pulse.

Molding under the pressure

Molding refers to asymmetry of the cranial sutures due to difficulties during vaginal delivery; it isn't seen in neonates born by cesarean delivery. There are two types of cranial abnormalities:

Cephalhematoma occurs when blood collects between a skull bone and the periosteum. It's caused by pressure during delivery and tends to spontaneously resolve in 3 to 6 weeks. A cephalhematoma doesn't cross cranial suture lines.

Caput succedaneum is a localized edematous area of the presenting part of the scalp. It's also caused by pressure during delivery, but disappears spontaneously in 3 to 4 days and can cross cranial suture lines.

Heads up!

The degree of head control the neonate has should also be evaluated during this part of the examination. If neonates are placed down on a firm surface, they'll turn their heads to the side to maintain an open airway. They also attempt to keep their heads in line with their body when raised by their arms. Although head lag is normal in the neonate, marked head lag is seen in neonates with Down syndrome or brain damage and in hypoxic infants.

Eyes

Neonates tend to keep their eyes tightly shut. Observe the lids for edema, which is normally present for the first few days of life. The eyes should also be assessed for symmetry in size and shape. Here are some common findings of neonatal eye examination:
• The neonate's eyes are usually blue or gray because of scleral thinness. Permanent eye color is established within 3 to 12 months.
• Lacrimal glands are immature at birth, resulting in tearless crying for up to 2 months.
• The neonate may demonstrate transient strabismus.

• The doll's eye reflex (when the head is rotated laterally, the eyes deviate in the opposite direction) may persist for up to 10 days.
• Subconjunctival hemorrhages may appear from vascular tension changes during birth.
• The corneal reflex is present but generally isn't elicited unless a problem is suspected.
• The pupillary reflex and the red reflex are present.

Nose

Observe the neonate's nose for:
• shape
• symmetry
• placement
• patency
• bridge configuration.
　　Because neonates are obligatory nose breathers for the first few months of life, nasal passages must be kept clear to ensure adequate respiration. Neonates instinctively sneeze to remove obstruction. Test the patency of the nasal passages by occluding each naris alternately while holding the neonate's mouth closed. (See *Monitoring for respiratory distress*.)

Mouth and pharynx

The neonate's mouth usually has scant saliva and pink lips. Inspect the mouth for its existing structures. The palate is usually narrow and highly arched. Inspect the hard and soft palates for clefts.

Pearls of wisdom on pearls

Epstein's pearls (pinhead-size, white or yellow, rounded elevations) may be found on the gums or hard palate. These are caused by retained secretions and disappear within a few weeks or months. The frenulum of the upper lip may be quite thick. Precocious teeth may also be apparent. The pharynx can be best assessed when the neonate is crying. Tonsillar tissue generally isn't visible.

Ears

Assess the neonate's ears for:
• symmetry
• placement on head
• amount of cartilage
• open auditory canal
• hearing.
　　The neonate's ears are characterized by incurving of the pinna and cartilage deposition. The pinna is usually flattened against the

Advice from the experts

Monitoring for respiratory distress

Nasal flaring is a serious sign of air hunger from respiratory distress. If you assess nasal flaring or seesaw respirations; pale, gray skin; periods of apnea; or bradycardia, alert the practitioner. These may be signs of respiratory distress syndrome.

side of the head from pressure in utero. The top of the ear should be above or parallel to an imaginary line from the inner to the outer canthus of the eye. Low-set ears are associated with several syndromes, including chromosomal abnormalities.

Before you go

Procedures to screen for hearing in neonates have become common practice before a neonate leaves the hospital or birthing facility. Testing can detect permanent bilateral or unilateral sensory or conductive hearing loss. (See *Universal neonatal hearing screening.*)

Now hear this!

Auditory assessment is performed by noninvasive, objective, physiologic measures that include otoacoustic emissions or auditory brainstem response. Both testing methods are painless and can be performed while the neonate rests. If the neonate doesn't pass the screening test, the test is usually repeated at age 3 months.

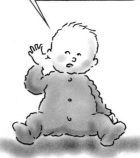

Say what? Auditory assessment can include otoacoustic emissions or auditory brainstem response.

Neck

The neonate's neck is typically short and weak with deep folds of skin. Observe for:
• range of motion

Weighing the evidence

Universal neonatal hearing screening

Considerable data has been collected to support the early screening of neonates to detect early loss and to provide for early intervention in those infants determined to have hearing loss.

In view of this supporting evidence, the Joint Commission on Infant Hearing (JCIH) Year 2000 Position Statement recommends the early detection of and intervention for infants with hearing loss.

According to JCIH recommendations:
• All infants should have hearing screening using a physiologic measure.

• Neonates who receive routine care should have access to hearing screening during their hospital birth admission.
• Neonates born in alternative care centers such as home birth settings should have access to and are referred to the hearing screening before 1 month of age.
• All neonates who require neonatal intensive care should receive hearing screening before discharge.
• All infants who don't pass the birth admission screen and any subsequent rescreening will begin appropriate audiologic and medical evaluations to confirm the presence of hearing loss before 3 months of age.

Material reprinted courtesy of the American Academy of Audiology

- shape
- abnormal masses.

Also, palpate each clavicle and sternocleidomastoid muscle. Note the position of the trachea. The thyroid gland generally isn't palpable.

Chest

Inspect and palpate the chest, noting:
- shape
- clavicles
- ribs
- nipples
- breast tissue
- respiratory movements
- amount of cartilage in rib cage.

The neonatal chest is characterized by a cylindrical thorax (because the anteroposterior and lateral diameters are equal) and flexible ribs. Slight intercostal retractions are usually seen on inspiration. The sternum is raised and slightly rounded, and the xiphoid process is usually visible as a small protrusion at the end of the sternum.

Breast engorgement from maternal hormones may be apparent, and the secretion of "witch's milk" may occur. Supernumerary nipples may be located below and medial to the true nipples.

Lungs

Normal respirations of the neonate are abdominal with a rate between 30 and 50 breaths/minute. After the first breaths to initiate respiration, subsequent breaths should be easy and fairly regular. Occasional irregularities may occur with crying, sleeping, and feeding.

Hush little baby, don't say a word

It's easiest to auscultate the lung fields when the neonate is quiet. Bilateral bronchial breath sounds should be heard. Crackles soon after birth represent the transition of the lungs to extrauterine life.

Heart

The neonate's heart rate is normally between 110 and 160 beats/minute. Because neonates have a fast heart rate, it's difficult to auscultate the specific components of the cardiac cycle. Heart sounds during the neonatal period are generally of higher pitch, shorter duration, and greater intensity than in later life. The first sound is usually louder and duller than the second, which is sharp in quality. Murmurs are commonly heard, especially over the base

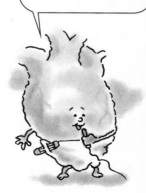

I'm so excited to be here, my heart's beating fast—between 110 and 160 beats/minute.

of the heart or at the third or fourth intercostal space at the left sternal border, due to incomplete functional closure of the fetal shunts.

The apical impulse (point of maximal impulse) is at the fourth intercostal space and to the left of the midclavicular line.

Abdomen

Neonatal abdominal assessment should include:
- inspection and palpation of the umbilical cord
- evaluation of the size and contour of the abdomen
- auscultation of bowel sounds
- assessment of skin color
- observation of movement with respirations
- palpation of internal organs.

Stop, look, listen...

The neonatal abdomen is usually cylindrical with some protrusion. Bowel sounds are heard a few hours after birth. A scaphoid appearance indicates a diaphragmatic hernia. The umbilical cord is white and gelatinous with two arteries and one vein and begins to dry within 1 to 2 hours after delivery.

...and feel

The liver is normally palpable 1″ (2.5 cm) below the right costal margin. Sometimes the tip of the spleen can be felt, but a spleen that's palpable more than ⅓″ (1 cm) below the left costal margin warrants further investigation. Both kidneys should be palpable; this is easiest done soon after delivery, when muscle tone is lowest. The suprapubic area should be palpated for a distended bladder. The neonate should void within the first 24 hours of birth.

Femoral pulses should also be palpated at this point in the examination. Inability to palpate femoral pulses could signify coarctation of the aorta.

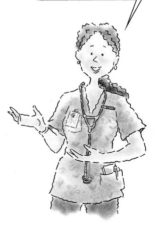

Palpate femoral pulses while examining the neonate. Inability to do so could indicate coarctation of the aorta, a congenital heart defect.

Genitalia

Characteristics of a male neonate's genitalia include rugae on the scrotum and testes descended into the scrotum. Scrotal edema may be present for several days after birth due to the effects of maternal hormones. The urinary meatus is located in one of three places:

at the penile tip (normal)

on the dorsal surface (epispadias)

on the ventral surface (hypospadias).

In the female neonate, the labia majora cover the labia minora and clitoris. These structures may be prominent due to maternal hormones. Vaginal discharge may also occur and the hymenal tag is present.

Extremities

The extremities should be assessed for range of motion, symmetry, and signs of trauma. All neonates are bowlegged and have flat feet. The hips should be assessed for dislocation, suggestive of developmental dysplasia of the hip. Hyperflexibility of joints is characteristic of Down syndrome. Some neonates may have abnormal extremities. They may be polydactyl (more than five digits on an extremity) or syndactyl (two or more digits fused together).

Note the nails

The nail beds should be pink, although they may appear slightly blue due to acrocyanosis. Persistent cyanosis indicates hypoxia or vasoconstriction.

Reading palms

The palms should have the usual creases. A bilateral transverse palmar crease, called a *simian crease*, suggests Down syndrome.

Expect resistance

Assess muscle tone. Extension of any extremity is usually met with resistance and, upon release, returns to its previously flexed position.

Spine

The neonatal spine should be straight and flat, and the anus should be patent without any fissure. Dimpling at the base of the spine is commonly associated with spina bifida. The shoulders, scapulae, and iliac crests should line up in the same plane.

Neurologic assessment

An examination of the reflexes provides useful information about the neonate's nervous system and his state of neurologic maturation. Some reflexive behaviors in the neonate are necessary for survival whereas other reflexive behaviors act as safety mechanisms.

Reflex revelations

Normal neonates display several types of reflexes. Abnormalities are indicated by absence, asymmetry, persistence, or weakness in these reflexes:

- sucking—begins when a nipple is placed in the neonate's mouth
- Moro reflex—when the neonate is lifted above the bassinet and suddenly lowered; the arms and legs symmetrically extend and then abduct while the thumb and forefinger spread to form a "C"
- rooting—when the neonate's cheek is stroked, the neonate turns his head in the direction of the stroke
- tonic neck (fencing position)—when the neonate's head is turned while he's lying in a supine position, the extremities on the same side straighten and those on the opposite side flex
- Babinski's reflex—when the sole on the side of the neonate's small toe is stroked and the toes fan upward
- grasping—when a finger is placed in each of the neonate's hands, the neonate's fingers grasp tightly enough to be pulled to a sitting position
- stepping—when the neonate is held upright with the feet touching a flat surface, he responds with dancing or stepping movements
- startle—a loud noise such as a hand clap elicits neonatal arm abduction and elbow flexion and the neonate's hands stay clenched
- trunk incurvature—when a finger is run laterally down the neonate's spine, the trunk flexes and the pelvis swings toward the stimulated side
- blinking—the neonate's eyelids close in response to bright light
- acoustic blinking—both eyes of the neonate blink in response to a loud noise
- Perez reflex—when the neonate is suspended prone in one of the practitioner's hands and the thumb of the other hand is moved firmly up the neonate's spine from the sacrum, the neonate's head and spine extend, the knees flex, the neonate cries, and he may empty his bladder.

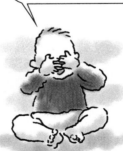

Geez! That's a lot of reflexes to display!

Behavioral assessment

Behavioral characteristics are an important part of neonatal development. To assess whether a neonate is exhibiting normal behavior, be aware of the neonate's principal behaviors of sleep, wakefulness, and activity (such as crying) as well as his social capabilities and ability to adapt to certain stimuli.

Factors that affect behavioral responses include:
- gestational age
- time of day
- stimuli
- medication.

Why cry?

The neonate should begin life with a strong cry. Variations in this initial cry can indicate abnormalities. For example, a weak, groaning cry or grunt during expiration usually signifies respiratory disturbances. Absent, weak, or constant crying suggests brain damage. A high-pitched shrill cry may be a sign of increased ICP.

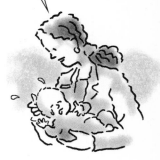

Absent, weak, or constant crying indicates neonatal brain damage.

Are you sleeping, are you sleeping?

Another aspect of behavioral assessment is observing the neonate's sleep-wake cycles (the variations in the neonate's consciousness). The nurse should assess how the neonate handles transitions from one state in the cycle to the next. Six specific sleep-activity states have been defined:

deep sleep—regular breathing, eyes closed, no spontaneous activity

light sleep—eyes closed, rapid eye movements (REM), random movements and startles, irregular breathing, sucking movements

drowsy—eyes open, dull, heavy eyelids, variable activity, delayed response to stimuli

alert—bright, seems focused, minimal motor activity

active—eyes open, considerable motor activity, thrusting movements, briefly fussy

crying—high motor activity.
Sleep-wake cycles are highly influenced by the environment.

Social senses

Neonates possess sensory capabilities that indicate their readiness for social interaction. An absence of these behavioral responses is cause for concern:
• sensitivity to light—a neonate opens his eyes when the lights are dim and his responses to movement are noticeable
• selective listening—a neonate tends to exhibit selective listening to his mother's voice
• response to touch—a neonate responds to touch, such as calming when touched softly, suggesting that he's ready to receive tactile messages
• taste preferences—a series of studies have demonstrated that neonates prefer sweet fluids to those that are sour or bitter
• sense of smell—studies have shown that neonates prefer pleasant smells and that they have the ability to learn and remember odors.

Filtering stimuli

Each neonate has a unique temperament and varies in his ability to handle stimuli from the external world. Through habituation, the neonate can control the type and amount of stimuli processed, which decreases his response to constant or repeated stimuli. A neonate presented with new stimuli becomes wide-eyed and alert but eventually shows decreased interest. Habituation enables the neonate to respond to select stimuli, such as human voices, that encourage continued learning about the social world.

The ability to habituate depends on the neonate's:

- state of consciousness
- hunger
- fatigue
- temperament.

Factor this in

These factors also affect behaviors:

- consolability—the ability of the neonate to console himself or be consoled
- cuddliness—the neonate's response to being held
- irritability—how easily a neonate is upset
- crying—the ability of the neonate to communicate different needs with his cry.

Neonatal care

Physical care for the neonate includes:

- protecting from infection and injury
- maintaining a patent airway
- maintaining a stable body temperature.

Neonatal eye prophylaxis

Neonatal eye prophylaxis involves instilling 0.5% erythromycin ointment into the neonate's eyes. Its purpose is to prevent ophthalmia neonatorum and *Neisseria gonorrhoeae* or *Chlamydia trachomatis* infections, which the neonate may have acquired from the mother as he passed through the birth canal. Erythromycin provides the antimicrobial effects of a broad-spectrum antibiotic.

It's the law

Neonatal eye prophylaxis is required by law in all 50 states. Before this treatment, gonorrheal conjunctivitis was a common cause of permanent eye damage and blindness.

Break for bonding

To perform neonatal eye prophylaxis, you'll need ophthalmic antibiotic ointment as ordered and gloves. Although the drug may be administered in the birthing room, treatment can be delayed for up to 1 hour to allow initial parent-child bonding. Antibiotic prophylaxis may not be effective if the infection was acquired in utero from premature rupture of the membranes.

> Neonatal eye prophylaxis can be delayed for up to 1 hour to allow initial parent-child bonding.

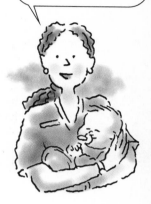

Step by step

To perform neonatal eye prophylaxis follow these steps:
• Wash your hands, and put on gloves.
• To ensure comfort and effectiveness, shield the neonate's eyes from direct light and tilt his head slightly to the side that will receive the treatment.
• Using your nondominant hand, gently raise the neonate's upper eyelid with your index finger and pull the lower eyelid down with your thumb.
• Using your dominant hand, instill the ointment into the lower conjunctival sac.
• Close and manipulate the eyelids to spread the medication over the eye.
• Repeat the procedure for the other eye.
• A single-dose ointment tube should be used to prevent contamination and the spread of infection.
• If the neonate's parents are present, explain that the procedure is required by state law. Tell them that it may temporarily irritate the neonate's eyes and make him cry but that the effects are transient. (See *Complications of neonatal eye prophylaxis*.)

Write it down!

Be sure to document neonatal eye prophylaxis appropriately. If it's done in the delivery room, record the treatment on the delivery room form. If you perform it in the nursery, document it in your notes.

Skin care

Skin care is an important aspect of neonatal care. The first bath should be performed as soon as the neonate's body temperature has been established and maintained for at least 4 hours.

Glove up

Wear gloves when touching the neonate before the first bath. Don't use soap on the eyes but soap may be used on the neonate's body, especially on the hair to remove vernix and blood. Be careful to remove all of the blood to minimize transmission of blood-

Complications of neonatal eye prophylaxis

Complications of neonatal eye prophylaxis include chemical conjunctivitis (which may cause redness, swelling, and drainage) or discoloration of the skin around the neonate's eyes. If such complications occur, reassure the parents that these temporary effects will subside within a few days.

borne pathogens to the neonate or health care providers. Running a comb gently through the hair will help remove blood. You may not be able to remove all of the vernix but that's okay because it serves as a lubricant and a natural protection against infection.

Hot or cold?

When the bath is finished, check the neonate's temperature again. If the temperature is below 97.5° F (36.4° C), return the neonate to the radiant warmer until he can maintain his temperature.

Bundle up

When the neonate's temperature is within normal limits, dress him in a shirt, diaper, and cap, swaddle him in blankets before placing him in an open bassinet.

Thermoregulation

Because the neonate has a relatively large surface-to-weight ratio, reduced metabolism per unit area, and small amounts of insulating fat, he's susceptible to hypothermia. The neonate keeps warm by metabolizing brown fat, which has a greater concentration of energy-producing mitochondria in its cells, enhancing its capacity for heat production. This kind of fat is unique to neonates. Brown fat metabolism is effective, but only within a very narrow temperature range.

Without careful external thermoregulation, the neonate may become chilled, which can result in:

- hypoxia
- acidosis
- hypoglycemia
- pulmonary vasoconstriction
- death.

Keep it neutral

The object of thermoregulation is to provide a neutral thermal environment that helps the neonate maintain a normal core temperature with minimal oxygen consumption and caloric expenditure. The core temperature varies with the neonate but is about 97.7° F (36.5° C). Cold stress and its complications can be prevented with proper interventions. (See *Understanding thermoregulators*, page 505.)

To perform thermoregulation, you'll need:

- radiant warmer or incubator (if necessary)
- blankets
- washcloths or towels
- skin probe

See? It says right there: Core temperature for neonates is about 97.7° F.

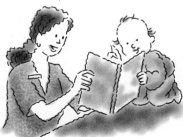

Understanding thermoregulators

Thermoregulators preserve neonatal body warmth in various ways. A radiant warmer maintains the neonate's temperature by radiation. An incubator maintains the neonate's temperature by conduction and convection.

Temperature settings
Radiant warmers and incubators have two operating modes: nonservo and servo. The nurse manually sets temperature on nonservo equipment; a probe on the neonate's skin controls temperature settings on servo models.

Other features
Most thermoregulators come with alarms. Incubators have the added advantage of providing a stable, enclosed environment, which protects the neonate from evaporative heat loss.

Radiant warmer

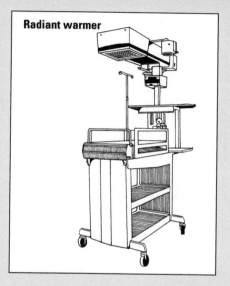

Incubator

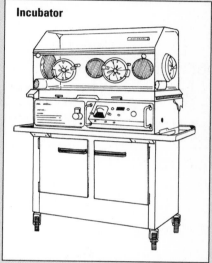

- adhesive pad
- water-soluble lubricant
- thermometer
- clothing, including a cap.

While you wait

While preparing for the neonate's birth, turn on the radiant warmer in the delivery room and set it to the desired temperature. Warm the blankets, washcloths, or towels under a heat source.

After the arrival

In the birthing room:
• Place the neonate under the radiant warmer, dry him with warm washcloths or towels, then cover his head with a cap to prevent heat loss.
• Perform required procedures quickly and wrap him in the warmed blankets. If his condition permits, give him to his parents to promote bonding. Initiate breast-feeding if appropriate.
  If the neonate is stable, dry him quickly, place a cap on his head, and then place the neonate skin-to-skin with the mother or

father. Cover them both with a blanket. This is called *kangaroo care*. Transport the neonate to the nursery in the warmed blankets; use a transport incubator as necessary.

In the nursery:
- Remove the blankets and cap and place the neonate under the radiant warmer.
- Use the adhesive pad to attach the temperature control probe to his skin in the upper-right abdominal quadrant. If the neonate will lie prone, put the skin probe on his back. Don't cover the device with anything because this could interfere with the servo control.
- Take the neonate's rectal temperature on admission, then take axillary temperatures thereafter every 15 to 30 minutes until the temperature stabilizes, then every 4 hours to ensure stability. (See *Preventing heat loss.*)

Sponge bathe the neonate under the warmer only after his temperature stabilizes and his glucose level is normal. Leave him under the warmer until his temperature remains stable. If the temperature doesn't stabilize, place the neonate under a plastic heat shield or in a warmed incubator, as per facility policy. Check for signs of infection, which can cause hypothermia.

Incubator involvement

Apply a skin probe to a neonate in an incubator as you would for a neonate in a radiant warmer. Move the incubator away from cold walls or objects. Perform all required procedures quickly and close portholes in the hood after completion. If procedures must be performed outside the incubator, do them under a radiant warmer.

To leave the facility or to move to a bassinet, a neonate must be weaned from the incubator by slowly reducing the temperature to that of the nursery. Check periodically for hypothermia. When the neonate's temperature stabilizes, dress him, put him in a bassinet, and cover him with a blanket. Also, be sure to instruct the parents on the importance of maintaining body temperature. (See *Maintaining the neonate's body temperature.*)

Noteworthy items

In your nursing notes, be sure to document:
- the name and temperature of the heat source used
- the neonate's temperature
- complications resulting from use of thermoregulatory equipment.

Advice from the experts

Preventing heat loss

Follow these steps to prevent heat loss in the neonate.

Conduction
- Preheat the radiant warmer bed and linen.
- Warm stethoscopes and other instruments before use.
- Before weighing the neonate, pad the scale with a paper towel or a preweighed, warmed sheet.

Convection
- Place the neonate's bed out of a direct line with an open window, fan, or air-conditioning vent.

Evaporation
- Dry the neonate immediately after delivery.
- When bathing the neonate, expose only one body part at a time; wash each part thoroughly, and then dry it immediately.

Radiation
- Keep the neonate and examination tables away from outside windows and air conditioners.

Education edge

Maintaining the neonate's body temperature

To help parents understand the importance of maintaining the neonate's temperature, instruct them to:
• keep the neonate wrapped in a blanket and out of drafts when he isn't in the bassinet
• avoid placing the bassinet next to a window, a fan, an air conditioner, or an air conditioner vent

• keep the stockinette cap on his head because a neonate loses considerable heat through his head
• remove any wet linens from on or around the neonate as soon as possible
• avoid placing the neonate on a cold surface such as a counter without placing a towel or blanket down first.

Oxygen administration

Oxygen relieves neonatal respiratory distress, which can be caused by cyanosis, pallor, tachypnea, nasal flaring, bradycardia, hypothermia, retractions (intercostal, subcostal marginal, suprasternal), hypotonia, hyporeflexia, or expiratory grunting.

Too much of a good thing

No matter how it's administered, oxygen therapy can be hazardous to the neonate. When given in high concentrations and for prolonged periods, it can cause retinopathy of prematurity, which may result in blindness in preterm neonates, and can contribute to bronchopulmonary dysplasia. Because of the neonate's size and special respiratory requirements, oxygen administration commonly requires special techniques and equipment.

Hands-on in an emergency

In emergency situations, give oxygen through a manual resuscitation bag and mask of appropriate size until more permanent measures can be initiated.

A method for every occasion

When the neonate merely requires additional oxygen above the ambient concentration, it can be delivered using an oxygen hood. When the neonate requires continuous positive airway pressure (CPAP) to prevent alveolar collapse at the end of an expiration, as in respiratory distress syndrome (hyaline membrane disease), administer oxygen through nasal prongs or an endotracheal (ET) tube connected to a manometer. If the neonate can't breathe on his own, deliver oxygen through a ventilator. Oxygen must be warmed and humidified to prevent hypothermia and dehydration, to which the neonate is especially susceptible.

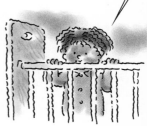

Oh, and one more thing: I like my oxygen warmed and humidified to prevent hypothermia and dehydration.

The right tools for the job

To begin oxygen therapy, you'll need:
- an oxygen source (wall, cylinder, or liquid unit)
- a compressed air source
- flowmeters
- large and small bore sterile oxygen tubing
- a blood gas analyzer
- a stethoscope
- a nasogastric (NG) tube.

For handheld resuscitation bag and mask delivery, you'll also need:
- a specially sized mask with handheld resuscitation bag and pressure release valve
- a manometer with connectors.

For delivery via an oxygen hood, you'll need:
- an appropriate-sized oxygen hood
- an oxygen analyzer.

For delivery through nasal prongs, other equipment includes:
- nasal prongs
- water-soluble lubricant.

For CPAP delivery, you'll also need:
- a manometer with connectors
- a nasopharyngeal or ET tube, or nasal CPAP prongs
- water-soluble lubricant
- hypoallergenic tape
- an exhaled CO_2 monitor.

For delivery with a ventilator, you'll need:
- a ventilator unit with manometer and in-line thermometer
- specimen tubes for arterial blood gas (ABG) analysis
- an ET tube
- an exhaled CO_2 monitor
- a pulse oximeter or transcutaneous oxygen monitor.

Be prepared

To prepare for oxygen administration, wash your hands and gather and assemble the necessary equipment. To calibrate the oxygen analyzer, turn the analyzer on and read the results. Room air should be about 21% oxygen. Expose the analyzer probe to 100% oxygen, adjust the sensitivity, and recheck the amount of oxygen in room air.

By hand

To use a handheld resuscitation bag and mask:
- Place the assembled resuscitation bag and mask in the bassinet.
- Turn on the oxygen and compressed air flowmeters and place the mask on the neonate's nose and mouth.

• Check pressure settings and mask size.
• Have another staff member notify the practitioner immediately.
• Provide 40 to 60 breaths/minute, using enough pressure to cause a visible rise and fall of the chest. Provide enough oxygen to maintain pink nail beds and mucous membranes.
• Continuously watch the neonate's chest movements and listen to breath sounds, avoiding overventilation. If the neonate's heart rate falls below 100 beats/minute, continue to use the handheld resuscitation bag until the heart rate rises to 100 beats/minute or greater.
• Insert an NG tube to vent air from the neonate's stomach.

By hood

To use an oxygen hood:
• Attach the oxygen hood to the connecting tubing and place an in-line thermometer close to the neonate.
• Activate oxygen and compressed air source, if needed, at ordered flow rates.
• Place the oxygen hood over the neonate's head.
• Measure the amount of oxygen the neonate is receiving with the oxygen analyzer. Be sure to place the analyzer probe close to the neonate's nose.
• Adjust the oxygen to the prescribed amount.

By prongs

When using nasal prongs:
• Match the prong size to the neonate's nose.
• Apply a small amount of water-soluble lubricant to the outside of the prongs.
• Turn on the oxygen and compressed air, if necessary.
• Connect the prongs to the oxygen source.
• Insert the prongs into the nose and secure them.
• Be sure to keep the prongs clean to ensure patency.

By CPAP

Here are some pointers if the neonate needs CPAP.

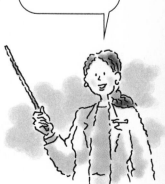

If the neonate needs CPAP to prevent alveolar collapse at the end of each breath (as in respiratory distress syndrome), he may receive this through an ET or nasopharyngeal tube or nasal CPAP prongs. To use CPAP:
• Position the neonate on his back with a rolled towel under his neck to keep the airway open; avoid hyperextending the neck.
• Assist with intubation if necessary.
• Turn on the oxygen and compressed air source and attach the delivery system to the ET tube or nasal CPAP prongs.
• If an ET tube is in place, confirm placement by using an exhaled CO_2 monitor and tape the tube in place.

- Insert an NG or orogastric tube to keep the stomach decompressed, if ordered. Leave the tube open to air unless the neonate is receiving gavage feedings.
    To use a ventilator:
- Turn on the ventilator and set the controls as ordered.
- Help with ET tube insertion and attach it to the ventilator.
- Confirm placement of the ET tube with the exhaled CO_2 monitor and tape it securely.
- Watch the manometer to maintain pressure at the prescribed level and monitor the in-line thermometer for correct temperature.

Knowing the know-how

Know how to perform neonatal chest auscultation correctly to pick up subtle respiratory changes. Also, be able to identify signs of respiratory distress and perform emergency procedures. If required, perform chest physiotherapy and percussion as ordered and follow with suctioning to remove secretions.

Monitor ABG levels every 15 to 20 minutes (or at another reasonable interval) after any changes in oxygen concentration or pressure. If ordered, monitor oxygen perfusion via either pulse oximetry or mixed venous oxygen saturation monitoring. Keep the practitioner aware of ABG levels so he can order appropriate changes in oxygen concentration.

As ordered, discontinue oxygen administration when the neonate's fraction of inspired oxygen (FIO_2) is at room air level (20% to 21%) and his arterial oxygen is stable at 60 to 90 mm Hg. Repeat ABG measurements 20 to 30 minutes after discontinuing oxygen and thereafter as ordered by the practitioner or by facility policy.

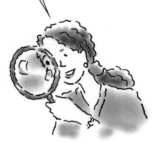

Keep a sharp eye on the neonate for complications of oxygen administration.

On the watch

Assess the neonate for complications of oxygen administration, including:
- signs and symptoms of infection
- hypothermia
- metabolic and respiratory acidosis
- pressure ulcers on the neonate's head, face, and nose
- signs of a pulmonary air leak, including pneumothorax, pneumomediastinum, pneumopericardium, and interstitial emphysema.

Safety first

When administering oxygen, always take safety precautions to avoid fire or explosion. Take measures to keep the neonate warm because hypothermia impedes respiration. (See *Hazards of oxygen therapy.)*

Hazards of oxygen therapy

No matter which system delivers the oxygen, oxygen therapy is potentially hazardous to a neonate. The gas must be warmed and humidified to prevent hypothermia and dehydration. Given in high concentrations over prolonged periods, oxygen can cause retinopathy of prematurity, leading to blindness. With low oxygen concentration, hypoxia and central nervous system damage may occur. Also, depending on how it's delivered, oxygen can contribute to bronchopulmonary dysplasia.

Other worries

Here are some other possible complications of oxygen therapy in neonates:

• Infection or "drowning" can result from overhumidification. Overhumidification, in turn, allows water to collect in tubing, providing a growth medium for bacteria or suffocating the neonate.

• Hypothermia can increase oxygen consumption and can result from administering cool oxygen.

• Metabolic and respiratory acidosis may follow inadequate ventilation.

• Pressure ulcers may develop on the neonate's head, face, and around the nose during prolonged oxygen therapy.

• A pulmonary air leak (pneumothorax, pneumomediastinum, pneumopericardium, interstitial emphysema) may arise spontaneously with respiratory distress or result from forced ventilation.

• Decreased cardiac output may result from excessive continuous positive airway pressure.

For the record

When documenting oxygen administration, be sure to include:

• type of respiratory distress requiring oxygen administration
• oxygen concentration given
• oxygen delivery method used
• each change in oxygen concentration
• routine checks of oxygen concentration
• neonate's F_{IO_2} (as measured by the oxygen analyzer)
• ABG values, noting the time each sample was obtained
• each time suctioning is performed
• amount and consistency of mucus
• type of continuous oxygen monitoring, if any
• complications
• neonate's condition during oxygen therapy, including respiratory rate, breath sounds, and signs of additional respiratory distress.

Circumcision

Circumcision is the removal of the penile foreskin. It's thought to promote a clean glans, minimize the risk of phimosis (foreskin tightening) later in life, and reduce the risk of penile cancer and cervical cancer in sexual partners. However, after 40 years of research on the risks and benefits of circumcision, the American Academy of Pediatrics has concluded that it can't recommend a policy of routine neonate circumcision. (See *Circumcision and religion*.)

Bells and clamps (but no whistles)

One method of circumcision involves removing the foreskin by using a Gomco clamp to stabilize the penis. With this device, a cone fits over the glans, providing a cutting surface and protecting the glans penis. Another technique uses a plastic circumcision bell (Plastibell) over the glans and a suture that's tied tightly around the base of the foreskin. This method prevents bleeding, and the resultant ischemia causes the foreskin to slough off in 5 to 8 days. It's thought to be painless because it stretches the foreskin, which inhibits sensory conduction.

When it's a no-go

Contraindications to circumcision include:
• illness
• bleeding disorders
• ambiguous genitalia
• congenital penile anomalies, such as hypospadias or epispadias (because the foreskin may be needed for later reconstructive surgery).

Prep the parents

The neonate experiences pain during the circumcision. Explain the procedure to the parents or caregivers, and tell them that a local anesthetic will be administered and that the neonate will be given sucrose on a pacifier to reduce crying. The neonate needs to be restricted from feeding for 1 hour before the procedure to reduce the possibility of emesis, aspiration, or both. Tell the parents that it's necessary to restrain the neonate for the procedure. Make sure that the parent has signed a consent form for the procedure (many facilities require this before the circumcision is performed).

Gather what's needed

The following equipment is necessary:
• circumcision tray (contents vary, but usually include circumcision clamps, various-sized cones, scalpel, probe, scissors, forceps, sterile basin, sterile towel, and sterile drapes)
• povidone-iodine solution
• restraining board with arm and leg restraints
• sterile gloves
• petroleum gauze
• sterile 4″ × 4″ gauze pads

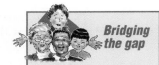

Bridging the gap

Circumcision and religion

For those of Jewish faith, circumcision takes place in a religious ritual called a *Bris Milah*. It's performed by a mohel 8 days after birth, when the neonate is officially given his name. Because most neonates are sent home before this time, the Bris is rarely done in the hospital.

- anesthetic agent
- pacifier with sucrose (for pain relief).

Optional equipment includes: sutures, a plastic circumcision bell, antimicrobial ointment, topical anesthetic, and an overhead warmer.

Be prepared

To prepare for the procedure:
- Assemble the sterile tray and other equipment in the procedure area.
- Open the sterile tray and pour povidone-iodine solution into the sterile basin.
- Using aseptic technique, place sterile 4″ × 4″ gauze pads and petroleum gauze on the sterile tray.
- Arrange the restraining board and direct adequate light on the area.

If a plastic circumcision bell is being used, you won't need a circumcision tray; however, assemble sterile gloves, sutures, restraining board, petroleum gauze and, if ordered, antibiotic ointment.

Set up for the assist

- Place the neonate on the restraining board, and restrain his arms and legs. Don't leave him unattended.
- Assist the doctor as necessary throughout the procedure, and comfort the neonate as needed.
- After putting on sterile gloves, the doctor will clean the penis and scrotum with povidone-iodine, drape the neonate, and administer a local anesthetic.

Clamp champ

When using a Gomco clamp, the doctor:
- applies the Gomco clamp to the penis, loosens the foreskin, and inserts the cone under it to provide a cutting surface for the removal of the foreskin and to protect the penis
- covers the wound with sterile petroleum gauze to prevent infection and control bleeding.

Over and done

When the procedure is complete, remove the neonate from the restraining board and check for bleeding. His diaper should be changed as soon as he voids. At each diaper change, apply antimicrobial ointment, petroleum jelly, or petroleum gauze until the wound appears healed. (See *Caring for the circumcised neonate*.)

Advice from the experts

Caring for the circumcised neonate

Here are some points to consider when caring for a neonate who has been circumcised:
- Avoid leaving a circumcised neonate under the radiant warmer after placing petroleum gauze on the penis because the area may burn.
- Apply diapers loosely to prevent irritation.
- If the dressing falls off, clean the wound with warm water to minimize pain on the circumcised area from the urine.
- Don't remove the original dressing until it falls off.
- Check for bleeding every 15 minutes for the first hour and then every hour for the next 24 hours. If bleeding occurs, apply pressure with sterile gauze pads. Notify the practitioner if bleeding continues.

Education edge

Teaching proper care of a circumcision

Always be sure to show parents the circumcision before discharge so that they can ask questions. Teach them these tips for proper care of a circumcision:
• Reapply fresh antimicrobial ointment, peroleum jelly, or petrolatum gauze after each diaper change, if applicable.
• Don't use premoistened towelettes to clean the penis because they contain alcohol, which can delay healing and cause discomfort.
• Don't attempt to remove exudate that forms around the penis. Removing exudate can cause bleeding.
• Change the neonate's diaper at least every 4 hours to prevent it from sticking to the penis.

• Check to make sure that the neonate urinates after being circumcised. He should have 6 to 10 wet diapers in a 24-hour period. If he doesn't, notify the practitioner.
• Wash the penis with warm water to remove urine or feces until the circumcision is healed. Soap can be used after the circumcision has healed.
• Notify the practitioner if redness, swelling, or discharge is present on the penis. These signs may indicate infection. Note that the penis is dark red after circumcision and then becomes covered with a yellow exudate in 24 hours.

A bell below the belt

When using a plastic circumcision bell, the doctor:
• slides the plastic bell device between the foreskin and the glans penis
• ties a suture tightly around the foreskin at the coronal edge of the glans.

The foreskin distal to the suture becomes ischemic and then atrophic. After 5 to 8 days, the foreskin drops off with the plastic bell attached, leaving a clean, well-healed excision. No special care is required but the parents should watch for swelling, which may indicate infection or interfere with urination (See *Teaching proper care of a circumcision.*)

After the fact

Stay alert for these complications of circumcision:
• urethral fistulae and edema
• infection or bleeding (if a Gomco clamp was used)
• delayed healing or infection, indicated by pus or bloody discharge
• scarring or fibrous bands, from adherence of penile shaft skin to the glans

• incomplete foreskin amputation from use of a plastic circumcision bell.

In your notes, be sure to document:

• circumcision date and time
• parent teaching provided
• excessive bleeding
• time that the neonate urinates before discharge.

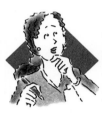

Quick quiz

1. Which factor doesn't stimulate the onset of breathing?
  A. Decreased CO_2 levels
  B. Increased CO_2 levels
  C. Decreased blood pH
  D. Decreased blood oxygen levels

Answer: A. Decreased CO_2 levels don't stimulate breathing.

2. Which option correctly describes the normal anatomy of the umbilical cord?
  A. One artery and one vein
  B. One artery and one ligament
  C. Two arteries and one vein
  D. One artery and two veins

Answer: C. The umbilical cord should consist of two arteries and one vein.

3. Apgar scoring evaluates:
  A. heart rate, respiratory rate, color, blood pressure, and temperature.
  B. heart rate, respiratory effort, muscle tone, reflex irritability, and color.
  C. respiratory rate, blood pressure, reflex irritability, muscle tone, and temperature.
  D. temperature, heart rate, color, muscle tone, and blood pressure.

Answer: B. Apgar scoring involves evaluating the neonate's heart rate, respiratory effort, muscle tone, reflex irritability, and color.

4. A sign of respiratory distress in a neonate is:
  A. acrocyanosis.
  B. nasal flaring.
  C. abdominal movements.
  D. short periods of apnea (less than 15 seconds).

Answer: B. Nasal flaring is a sign of respiratory distress in the neonate. Acrocyanosis, abdominal movements, and short periods of apnea are all normal findings.

5.   Which finding is normal for a neonate's fontanels?
   A.   They're soft to touch.
   B.   They're depressed.
   C.   They're bulging.
   D.   They're closed.

Answer: A. The fontanels should feel soft to the touch.

6.   Where's the apical impulse best assessed on the neonate?
   A.   Second intercostal space, right sternal border
   B.   Fifth intercostal space, left midclavicular line
   C.   Fifth intercostal space, left sternal border
   D.   Apex of the heart

Answer: B. The apical impulse is best assessed at the fifth intercostal space, left midclavicular line.

7.   During which sleep-wake cycle does the neonate experience REM?
   A.   Deep sleep
   B.   Light sleep
   C.   Drowsy
   D.   Crying

Answer: B. During light sleep the eyes are closed and the neonate experiences REM, random movements and startles, irregular breathing, and sucking movements.

Scoring

☆☆☆   If you answered all seven questions correctly, give yourself a high five! Then toddle on over to the next chapter!

☆☆   If you answered five or six questions correctly, stand tall! There's no holding you back!

☆   If you answered fewer than five questions correctly, roll with the punches! Get a leg up by revisiting this chapter!

12

High-risk neonatal conditions

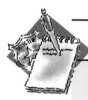

Just the facts

In this chapter, you'll learn:

♦ characteristics of selected neonatal disorders

♦ tests used to diagnose certain high-risk neonatal conditions

♦ medical treatments and therapies for high-risk neonatal conditions

♦ nursing interventions for high-risk neonatal conditions.

A look at the high-risk neonate

A neonate is considered to be high-risk if he has an increased chance of dying during or shortly after birth or has a congenital or perinatal problem that requires prompt intervention. As medicine continues to develop more treatments for perinatal problems, high-risk neonates are more likely to survive. Many of these neonates have few or no residual effects from the crisis that marked their first hours after birth.

A shaky start

Parents of high-risk neonates may experience grief and difficulty coping as they adjust to their neonate's condition. They may also feel a sense of loss and have difficulty bonding because their neonate isn't the perfect, healthy baby they anticipated. The family of a neonate with a chronic illness or congenital anomaly must find ways to cope with long-term grief and develop strategies to provide the special care the condition will require (and perhaps to balance these care needs with those of other children). If the neonate is stillborn or dies within a few hours or days after birth, family members must complete their bonding with the neonate, then detach themselves gradually so they can focus again on the family's life and needs.

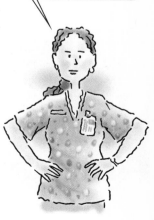

Because they feel a sense of loss, parents may have difficulty bonding with a high-risk neonate.

Although the neonate's condition dictates the specifics of nursing care, the main nursing goals for all high-risk neonates are to:
- ensure oxygenation, ventilation, thermoregulation, nutrition, and fluid and electrolyte balance
- prevent and control infection
- encourage parent-neonate bonding
- provide developmental care.

Drug addiction

Neonatal drug addiction and its associated signs and symptoms of withdrawal result from addictive drug use by the neonate's mother during pregnancy. As in all aspects of health care, care for the drug-addicted neonate should be provided in a nonjudgmental manner, especially because the neonate is an innocent victim of substance abuse by another person.

Lowdown on drug effects

Pregnant women who use addictive drugs are at higher risk for:
- abruptio placentae
- spontaneous abortion
- preterm labor
- precipitous labor
- psychotic responses.
    Complications seen in the neonate may include:
- urogenital malformations
- cerebrovascular complications
- low birth weight
- decreased head circumference
- respiratory problems
- death.

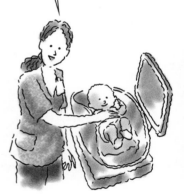

Low birth weight and respiratory problems are some of the complications seen in drug-addicted neonates.

What causes it

Neonatal drug addiction can occur if the mother uses addictive drugs while pregnant. These drugs have teratogenic effects, causing abnormalities in embryonic or fetal development.

What to look for

Intrauterine drug exposure may cause obvious physical anomalies, neurobehavioral changes, or withdrawal. Signs and symptoms of a neonate's drug dependence vary and may include physical and behavioral changes. These changes depend on:
- specific drug or combination of drugs used

Opiate withdrawal syndrome

Be alert for these signs and symptoms of opiate withdrawal syndrome in the neonate.

Central nervous system
- Seizures
- Tremors
- Irritability
- Increased wakefulness
- High-pitched cry
- Increased muscle tone
- Increased deep tendon reflexes
- Increased Moro reflex
- Increased yawning
- Increased sneezing
- Rapid changes in mood
- Hypersensitivity to noise and external stimuli
- Sleep distrubances
- Sweating

GI system
- Poor feeding
- Uncoordinated and constant sucking
- Vomiting
- Diarrhea
- Dehydration
- Poor weight gain

Autonomic nervous system
- Increased sweating
- Nasal stuffiness
- Fever
- Mottling
- Temperature instability
- Increased respiratory rate
- Increased heart rate

- dosage
- route of administration
- metabolism and excretion by the mother and fetus
- timing of drug exposure
- length of drug exposure.

Benzodiazepines

Diazepam (Valium), a benzodiazepine, is one of the most commonly prescribed drugs in the world. It easily crosses the placental barrier to the fetus and is eliminated slowly by the fetus. Withdrawal signs and symptoms may appear hours to weeks afer birth and may persist for months. Common signs and symptoms of withdrawal include:
- hypothermia
- hyperbilirubinemia
- central nervous system (CNS) depression.

Opiates

Clinical presentation of opiate withdrawal in the neonate can last 2 to 3 weeks. Withdrawal signs and symptoms generally include dysfunction of the CNS and GI system. (See *Opiate withdrawal syndrome*.)

Heroin

Neonates who have been exposed to heroin generally have low birth weights and are small for gestational age. They may also exhibit these signs and symptoms:

- jitters and hyperactivity
- shrill and persistent cry
- frequent yawning or sneezing
- increased deep tendon reflexes
- decreased Moro reflex
- poor feeding and sucking
- increased respiratory rate
- vomiting
- diarrhea
- hypothermia or hyperthermia
- increased sweating
- abnormal sleep cycle.

Methadone

Withdrawal from methadone resembles that from heroin but tends to be more severe and prolonged. It includes:

- increased incidence of seizures
- disturbed sleep patterns
- higher birth weight in neonates who are appropriate size for gestational age
- higher risk of sudden infant death syndrome.

Marijuana

Neonates born to mothers who used marijuana while pregnant tend to be born at earlier gestations. An increased incidence of precipitous labor and meconium staining also occurs in this population of neonates. Neonates may exhibit tremors, jitteriness, and impaired sleep. When the mother abuses marijuana and alcohol during pregnancy, there's a fivefold increase in the risk of fetal alcohol syndrome (FAS).

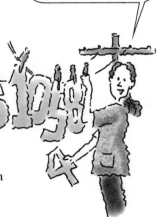

The risk of FAS increases fivefold if a mother abuses marijuana and alcohol during pregnancy.

Amphetamines

Women who use amphetamines while pregnant may have preterm neonates or neonates of low birth weight. Other characteristics these neonates may have include:

- drowsiness
- jitters
- respiratory distress soon after birth
- frequent infections
- poor weight gain
- emotional disturbances

- delays in gross motor and fine motor development in early childhood
- heart murmurs
- transient bradycardia and tachycardia.

What tests tell you

The signs and symptoms of addiction and withdrawal may be mistaken for other common neonatal problems, especially if the mother's drug use is unknown. You'll need to differentiate between neonatal drug withdrawal and CNS irritability caused by infectious or metabolic disorders, such as hypoglycemia, hypomagnesemia, or hypocalcemia. You'll also need to rule out hyperthyroidism, CNS hemorrhage, and anoxia.

Assessing the systems

The Neonatal Abstinence Scoring System is a scoring tool that can be used for term neonates. It assesses and scores areas of response in neonates with CNS, metabolic, vasomotor, respiratory, and GI disturbances. The higher the overall score, the more likely the need for medication administration for withdrawal. The test is repeated at specific intervals based on previous scores.

When it's withdrawal

If the clinical signs and symptoms are consistent with drug withdrawal, obtain specimens of urine and meconium for drug testing. Meconium testing can detect drug use over a 20-week period. Be aware that urine screening may have a high false-negative rate because only neonates with recent exposure test positive. Also keep in mind that although meconium drug testing isn't conclusive if results are negative, this method is more reliable than urine testing.

How it's treated

Initial treatment of the neonate who's experiencing withdrawal should be supportive. This includes:
- swaddling
- holding the neonate
- pacifiers
- reducing environmental stimuli (lights, noise)
- frequent, small feedings of hypercaloric (24 calories/ounce) formula
- observing sleep habits
- observing for temperature instability, weight gain or loss, or changes in clinical status that might suggest another disease process

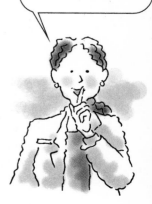

Reducing environmental stimuli and swaddling are some of the initial treatments for supporting neonates experiencing withdrawal.

Weighing the evidence

Narcan and drug withdrawal

Over the years, it has become common practice to administer naloxone (Narcan) in the birthing room to a neonate who's exhibiting central nervous system depression and whose mother recently received an opioid.

The American Academy of Pediatrics has determined that using naloxone is contraindicated in a neonate whose mother is a known or suspected opioid abuser because of the potential for neonatal seizures, which can develop as a result of the abrupt withdrawal of the drug.

Source: American Academy of Pediatrics. "Neonatal Drug Withdrawal," *Pediatrics* 101(6):1079-1088, June 1998.

Drugs for withdrawal

Drugs used to treat withdrawal include:
• chlorpromazine (Thorazine)
• clonidine (Duraclon)
• diazepam (Valium)
• methadone (Dolophine)
• morphine
• paregoric
• phenobarbital
• tincture of opium.

• fluid and electrolyte replacement
• infection control
• respiratory care.

Treating drugs with drugs

Indications for pharmacologic therapy include:
• seizures
• poor feeding
• diarrhea
• vomiting leading to weight loss and dehydration
• inability to sleep
• fever unrelated to infection.

If pharmacologic therapy is needed, specific therapy from the same drug class is preferred. (See *Drugs for withdrawal* and *Narcan and drug withdrawal*.)

What to do

Nursing interventions for neonatal drug addiction include:
• initiating preventive measures
• identifying neonates at risk
• assessing the neonate
• providing supportive care.

Stop addiction before it starts

Preventing maternal drug use is the ideal approach to eradicating the problem of neonatal drug addiction. Patient teaching and sup-

port are essential. To identify a woman and neonate at risk for drug addiction:
- Obtain a detailed maternal prescription and nonprescription drug history.
- Assess the social habits of the parents.

Screen those on the scene

To screen for drug exposure, perform maternal and neonatal assessments. Maternal findings that may indicate a need for neonatal drug testing include:
- lack of prenatal care
- previous unexplained fetal demise
- precipitous labor
- altered nutrition
- abruptio placentae
- hypertensive episodes
- severe mood swings
- stroke
- myocardial infarction (MI)
- recurrent spontaneous abortions.

Neonatal characteristics that may be associated with maternal drug use include:
- preterm labor
- cardiac defects
- unexplained intrauterine growth retardation
- neurobehavioral abnormalities
- urogenital anomalies
- atypical vascular incidents (stroke, MI, or necrotizing enterocolitis in an otherwise healthy term neonate).

Ongoing neonatal assessment should include monitoring for changes in:
- respiratory system
- reflexes (including suck, swallow, and gag)
- CNS
- feeding and growth
- vital signs.

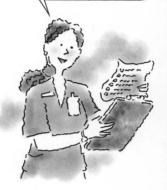

Obtaining a detailed drug history is the first step in identifying those at risk for drug addiction.

Aiding the addicted

Supportive care of the neonate with a drug addiction includes:
- maintaining the neonate's airway
- assessing breath sounds frequently
- supporting and monitoring ventilation
- providing supplemental oxygen
- managing mechanical ventilation
- making sure that resuscitative equipment is available
- monitoring pulse oximetry (and arterial blood gas [ABG] studies if pulse oximetry is abnormally low)

- decreasing CNS excitability by keeping the neonate tightly wrapped (swaddling)
- offering a pacifier for nonnutritive sucking
- using an undershirt with hand mittens to decrease facial scratching
- aspirating nasal mucus as needed
- organizing care to decrease stress due to handling
- decreasing stimuli by reducing light in the room
- monitoring the neonate with seizures
- preventing trauma
- administering medications as ordered
- promoting rest
- promoting nutritional intake
- feeding in small, frequent amounts with the head elevated and the nipple positioned correctly so that sucking is effective
- maintaining fluid and electrolyte balance
- monitoring intake and output
- giving supplemental fluids as ordered
- evaluating serum electrolytes as ordered
- maintaining skin integrity and providing skin care
- changing the neonate's position
- reporting signs of distress.

Fetal alcohol syndrome

A cluster of birth defects that are caused by in utero exposure to alcohol is referred to as *fetal alcohol syndrome (FAS)*. It can result in abnormalities in the CNS, growth retardation, and facial malformations.

What causes it

FAS is caused by the exposure of a fetus to alcohol in utero. Although prenatal alcohol exposure doesn't always result in FAS, the safe level of alcohol consumption during pregnancy isn't known. Alcohol crosses through the placenta and enters the fetal blood supply, and it can interfere with the healthy development of the fetus. In fact, birth defects associated with prenatal alcohol exposure can occur in the first 3 to 8 weeks of pregnancy, before a woman even knows she's pregnant. Variables that affect the extent of damage caused to the fetus by alcohol include the amount of alcohol consumed, the timing of consumption, and the pattern of alcohol use.

What to look for

Affected neonates may display these signs within the first 24 hours of life:
- difficulty establishing respirations
- irritability
- lethargy
- seizure activity
- tremulousness
- opisthotonos
- poor sucking reflex
- abdominal distention.

Overalls

Overall signs of FAS include CNS dysfunction, abnormal development of the midline structures of the brain, growth deficiency, and a characteristic set of minor facial abnormalities that tend to normalize as the child grows. (See *Common facial characteristics of FAS*.)

Typical CNS problems for neonates with FAS may include:
- mental retardation
- microcephaly
- poor coordination
- decreased muscle tone

Common facial characteristics of FAS

This illustration shows the distinct craniofacial features associated with fetal alcohol syndrome (FAS).

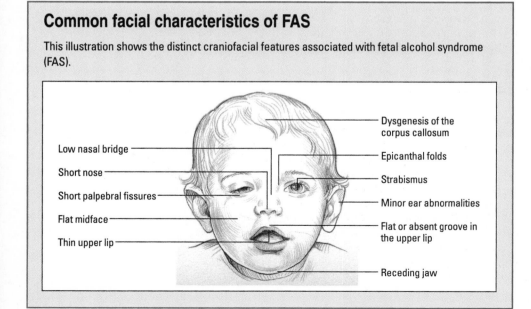

Low nasal bridge

Short nose

Short palpebral fissures

Flat midface

Thin upper lip

Dysgenesis of the corpus callosum

Epicanthal folds

Strabismus

Minor ear abnormalities

Flat or absent groove in the upper lip

Receding jaw

- small brain
- behavioral abnormalities
- irritability
- tremors
- poor feeding.

   Growth deficiencies may manifest in a failure to thrive or a disproportionate decrease in adipose tissue. Length and weight in neonates with FAS typically measures 3% less than the average neonate.

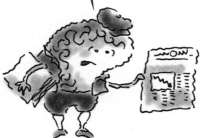

Not so great news. FAS can cause mental retardation and behavioral abnormalities.

Hits to the other systems

Abnormalities may also be seen in the cardiac system, skeletal system, urogenital system, and skin. Potential complications include:

- cardiac murmurs
- limited joint movement
- finger and toe deformities
- aberrant palmar creases
- kidney defects
- labial hypoplasia
- hemangiomas.

   As children and adults, individuals with FAS also commonly display:

- defects in intellectual functioning
- difficulties with memory, attention, and problem solving
- learning disabilities
- problems with mental health
- difficulties with social interaction.

What tests tell you

Identifying clinical problems and assessment findings characteristic of FAS leads to diagnosis. Respiratory distress and neurologic dysfunction may be present. Feeding difficulties may also be noted. Radiographic studies may be used to reveal renal or cardiac defects.

How it's treated

Treatment of FAS is supportive and depends on the individual neonate. The initial difficulties may be managed by preventing stimulation that may precipitate seizures, administering sedative or anticonvulsant medications, and providing supportive measures. Because the effects of alcohol in utero vary, care must be individualized to focus on the neonate's specific abnormalities and deficits.

What to do

A fundamental nursing intervention for FAS is helping to prevent it. This can be achieved by:
• increasing public awareness
• increasing women's access to prenatal care
• providing educational programs
• screening women of reproductive age for alcohol problems
• using appropriate resources and strategies for decreasing alcohol use.

FASe out respiratory problems

Caring for neonates with FAS involves preventing or treating respiratory distress.
• Place the neonate on a cardiac monitor and set the alarms.
• Assess breath sounds frequently and be alert for signs of distress.
• Suction as needed.
• Place the neonate in a position in which he displays the least distress.

EmFASize nutrition

Special emphasis should be placed on following weight gain, assessing feeding behaviors, and devising strategies to increase nutritional intake.
• Encourage feeding to promote bonding with the parents.
• Elevate the neonate's head during and after feeding.
• Evaluate different nipples.
• Burp the neonate well during and after feedings.
• Monitor the neonate's weight.
• Measure intake and output.

FAScillitate bonding

To promote mother-neonate attachment:
• Encourage visits.
• Encourage physical contact.
• Educate parents about the neonate's complications.
• Provide emotional support.

Gestational size variations

Whether they're preterm, term, or postterm, neonates are classified by weight in three ways:

Large for gestational age (LGA) neonates are above the 90th percentile for weight.

Appropriate for gestational age (AGA) neonates are between the 10th and 90th percentile for weight.

Small for gestational age (SGA) neonates are below the 10th percentile for weight.

What causes it

Variations in gestational size are caused by different factors.

SGA neonates

Factors that can contribute to a neonate being SGA include:
- congenital malformations
- chromosomal anomalies
- maternal infections
- gestational hypertension
- advanced maternal diabetes due to decreased blood flow to the placenta
- intrauterine malnutrition due to poor placental function or maternal malnutrition
- maternal smoking
- maternal drug or alcohol use
- multiple gestation.

LGA neonates

Neonates may become LGA because of genetic factors. For example, neonates tend to be larger if they're male, if their parents are larger, or if the mother is a multipara. Neonates of mothers with diabetes also tend to be LGA because high maternal glucose levels stimulate continued insulin production by the fetus. This constant state of hyperglycemia leads to excessive growth and fat deposition.

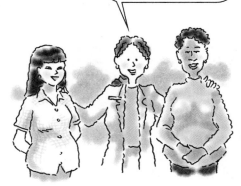

Congenital abnormalities or maternal infections can result in LGA neonates.

What to look for

Assessment findings depend on whether the neonate is SGA or LGA.

SGA neonates

SGA neonates are more likely to experience respiratory distress and hypoxia. They may also appear wide-eyed and alert at birth because of prolonged prenatal hypoxia. In addition, SGA neonates are prone to meconium aspiration because fetal hypoxia allows meconium to pass through a relaxed anal sphincter, thus causing the neonate to experience reflexive gasping. Hypoglycemia can occur in SGA neonates and can be noted from birth to day 4 of life. Decreased subcutaneous fat and a large ratio of body surface area to weight put the SGA neonate at risk for problems with thermoregulation.

LGA neonates

LGA neonates generally weigh more than 4,000 g (8 lb, 13 oz) and appear plump and full-faced. The LGA neonate may experience hypoxia during labor and be exposed to excessive trauma, such as fractures and intracranial hemorrhage, during vaginal delivery. Hypoglycemia may be noted at birth and during the transition period.

What tests tell you

Neonates of mothers with diabetes should have laboratory work to determine their hematocrit and glucose, calcium, and bilirubin levels. They should also be monitored for hypoglycemia, hyperbilirubinemia, and respiratory distress syndrome.

How it's treated

Treatment of gestational age size abnormalities varies depending on whether the neonate is SGA or LGA.

SGA neonates

Treatment of the SGA neonate should be supportive and individualized with nutrition being the primary focus. SGA neonates have higher caloric needs and benefit from frequent feedings. Care of the SGA neonate also includes glucose monitoring and careful respiratory assessments.

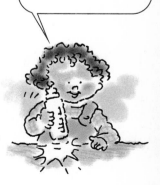

Time to eat yet? SGA neonates have higher caloric needs and benefit from frequent feedings.

LGA neonates

During delivery of an LGA neonate, the mother may need additional help, such as an episiotomy, change in position, or the use of forceps or a vacuum. After birth, glucose monitoring and evaluation of jaundice is essential in LGA neonates. Any birth traumas also need to be managed.

What to do

Nursing interventions for SGA and LGA neonates include:
- supporting respiratory efforts
- providing a neutral thermal environment
- protecting the neonate from infection
- providing appropriate nutrition
- maintaining adequate hydration
- conserving the neonate's energy
- assessing glucose level
- preventing skin breakdown
- facilitating growth and development
- keeping parents informed
- providing support to the entire family.

Human immunodeficiency virus infection

Today, pregnant women have the opportunity to be tested for human immunodeficiency virus (HIV). Such testing has led to an increase in the number of neonates known to be exposed to HIV, which in turn has allowed for early diagnosis and treatment.

What causes it

HIV can be transmitted to the neonate in one of three ways:

 transplacentally during pregnancy

 during labor and delivery

 through breast milk.

Risk factors for perinatal transmission can be either maternal or neonatal. (See *Risk factors for perinatal transmission of HIV.*)

Risk factors for perinatal transmission of HIV

Neonatal and maternal factors can contribute to perinatal transmission of the human immunodeficiency virus (HIV).

Neonatal factors
- Bacterial infection
- Being the first-born twin
- Breast-feeding
- Prematurity

Maternal factors
- Chorioamnionitis
- Low CD4+ count
- High CD8+ count
- High viral load
- New onset of disease
- Ongoing drug abuse
- Prolonged or complicated labor

What to look for

Most neonates exposed to HIV are born at term and are of AGA size. Normal physical findings are usually present. Physical findings, such as adenopathy or hepatosplenomegaly, are absent at birth because HIV infection is believed to occur at delivery. These findings may develop later and suggest HIV infection.

> Physical findings of HIV infection aren't usually present at birth, but they may develop later.

What tests tell you

The Centers for Disease Control and Prevention recommends testing for HIV within 48 hours of birth, at age 1 to 2 months, and again at age 3 to 6 months. Two positive tests at different ages are required to make a positive diagnosis. Diagnostic tests used to detect HIV include HIV deoxyribonucleic acid (DNA) polymerase chain reactions (PCR), HIV p24 antigen assay, HIV antibody, HIV culture, and immunologic testing.

PCR preferred

The HIV DNA PCR test is the preferred method for diagnosing HIV in neonates. It's highly sensitive and specific. Positive results can be detected in 93% of infected neonates by day 14 of life. This test should be performed at birth and between ages 1 and 2 months. The test should be repeated at age 4 months if the infant remains asymptomatic and the previous test results were negative.

Assay you, assay me

HIV p24 antigen assay may be used to assess HIV infection in infants older than 1 month, but the sensitivity is less than PCR testing. The absence of the p24 antigen, however, doesn't rule out HIV infection.

Antibody home?

The HIV antibody test uses enzyme-linked immunosorbent assay and Western blot analysis to determine whether HIV antibodies are present as a result of exposure to the virus. However, this test doesn't differentiate between maternal and neonatal infection. In addition, diagnosis can be complicated by the presence of the maternal, anti-HIV immunoglobulin (Ig) G antibody in the neonate. Because of this complication, cord blood should never be used for HIV testing.

A positive HIV antibody test obtained at age 18 months (after the maternal IgG in the neonate has broken down) indicates infection. For infants exposed to HIV whose previous testing was negative, a final HIV antibody test at age 24 months is recommended.

An uncommon culture

An HIV culture is a test that isn't readily available. It's also expensive to perform, requires a large blood sample, and the results may not be available for 2 to 4 weeks. If performed, an HIV culture should be taken at birth and again between ages 1 and 2 months. If the initial result is positive, the test should be repeated immediately to confirm. If an infant remains asymptomatic after testing negative, repeat the HIV culture at age 4 months.

More monitoring

Immunologic testing, including lymphocyte subsets (CD4+, CD8+, CD4+–CD8+ ratio) and quantitative immunoglobulins (IgG, IgM, IgA) should be performed on all neonates born to HIV-positive mothers. Children born to HIV-infected mothers should also undergo hematologic monitoring. This includes assessing complete blood count (CBC), differential leukocyte count, and platelet count during the first 6 months of life. Monitoring should continue in infected children and in those whose infection status is undetermined at age 6 months.

To be free from HIV

A neonate is considered uninfected with HIV when:
• no physical findings consistent with HIV are present
• immunologic test results are negative
• virologic tests are negative
• after 12 months, two or more HIV antibody tests are negative.

How it's treated

To help prevent perinatal transmission of HIV, zidovudine (Retrovir) is given to HIV-positive women during the second and third trimesters of pregnancy as well as during labor and delivery. The drug is also given to neonates born to HIV-positive mothers during the first 6 weeks of life. Such treatment has been shown to dramatically decrease perinatal transmission of HIV. Zidovudine therapy is discontinued at age 6 weeks. (See *Complications of zidovudine therapy in the neonate.*)

But wait, there's more

After zidovudine therapy is completed, prophylaxis for *Pneumocystis carinii* pneumonia (PCP) should start. PCP prophylaxis is recommended for all neonates born to HIV-infected women—regardless of the infant's initial test results—because PCP infection commonly occurs between ages 3 and 6 months, when many HIV-exposed infants haven't yet been identified as being infected. PCP prophylaxis should be initiated at age 6 months (after completion of a zidovudine regimen). It should then continue until at least age

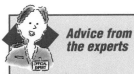

Advice from the experts

Complications of zidovudine therapy in the neonate

Zidovudine may cause transient anemia. To monitor for this adverse effect, a complete blood count and differential leukocyte count should be performed at birth as a baseline and again at ages 4 and 6 weeks.

Education edge

Caring for a neonate exposed to HIV

When teaching a woman and her family about caring for a neonate exposed to human immunodeficiency virus (HIV), emphasize the need for:
- frequent follow-up
- testing to determine infection status
- zidovudine (Retrovir) administration to decrease the risk of infection
- prophylaxis for *Pneumocystis carinii* pneumonia
- taking precautions to prevent the spread of HIV infection.

Patient teaching should also include signs of possible HIV infection in the neonate, including:
- recurrent infections
- unusual infections
- failure to thrive
- hematologic manifestations
- renal disease
- neurologic manifestations.

12 months—even if the infant's infection status hasn't been determined.

Co-trimoxazole (Bactrim) is the recommended chemoprophylaxis regimen for PCP in infants. When initiating therapy, first obtain a baseline CBC, differential leukocyte count, and platelet count. These measurements should be checked monthly while the infant receives prophylaxis treatment. If this regimen isn't tolerated, dapsone may be used.

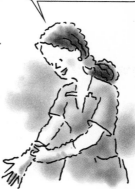

If a pregnant woman is infected with HIV, follow standard precautions during delivery.

What to do

Whether the HIV-infected woman is delivering vaginally or by cesarean birth, follow standard precautions. Be sure to wear gloves, a gown, and protective eyewear. Prompt and careful removal of blood and amniotic fluid from the neonate's skin is important. Isolation, however, isn't required. Inform the mother that breast-feeding isn't recommended, and instruct her and her family on caring for the neonate exposed to HIV. (See *Caring for a neonate exposed to HIV.*)

Hydrocephalus

Hydrocephalus is an excessive accumulation of cerebrospinal fluid (CSF) within the ventricular spaces of the brain. This accumulation of fluid forces the ventricles to dilate, which can put harmful pressure on brain tissue. Such pressure on brain tissue and cerebral blood vessels may lead to ischemia and, eventually, cell death.

Are we communicating?

Hydrocephalus may be communicating or noncommunicating. Communicating hydrocephalus occurs because CSF isn't absorbed properly. Noncommunicating hydrocephalus occurs because normal CSF flow is obstructed. Congenital hydrocephalus is present at birth. Acquired hydrocephalus develops at the time of birth or later in life.

What causes it

The cause of hydrocephalus isn't exactly known. Possible causes include:
- genetic inheritance
- neural tube defects, such as spina bifida and encephalocele
- complications of premature birth such as intraventricular hemorrhage
- meningitis
- tumors
- traumatic head injury
- subarachnoid hemorrhage
- prenatal maternal infections.

What to look for

Assessment findings vary. Be aware that a neonate's ability to tolerate the accumulation of CSF differs from an adult's—the neonate's skull can expand because the sutures haven't yet closed.

On the lookout

Findings in neonates that may suggest hydrocephalus include:
- rapid increase in head circumference or an unusually large head size disproportionate to neonate's growth
- distended scalp veins
- bulging fontanels
- thin, shiny, fragile-looking scalp skin
- downward deviation of the eyes ("sunsetting" eyes)
- sluggish pupils with unequal response to light
- seizures
- high-pitched, shrill cry
- irritability
- projectile vomiting
- feeding problems (because the head is 1⅛″ [3 cm] larger than the chest).

In addition, the neonate may cry when picked up or rocked and be quiet when still.

What tests tell you

Hydrocephalus is diagnosed by clinical assessment and imaging techniques, such as:
- ultrasound
- computed tomography
- magnetic resonance imaging
- pressure monitoring techniques.

The appropriate diagnostic tool should be chosen based on age, clinical presentation, and presence of known or suspected abnormalities of the brain or spinal cord.

How it's treated

Hydrocephalus is commonly treated with the surgical insertion of a shunt. The shunt, consisting of a catheter and a valve, leads from a ventricle in the brain to the peritoneum or an atrial chamber of the heart, thus allowing CSF to drain to an area where it can be absorbed into the circulation. The valve maintains one-way flow and regulates the rate at which CSF is drained.

Aw shunts

Potential complications of shunt systems include:
- mechanical failure
- infection
- obstruction
- need to lengthen or replace catheter.

Patients with surgically implanted shunt systems require regular medical follow-up.

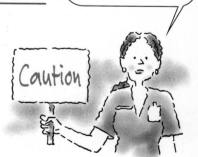

If hydrocephalus is suspected, watch closely for signs of increasing ICP.

What to do

The neonate with diagnosed or suspected hydrocephalus must be observed carefully for signs of increasing intracranial pressure (ICP). The nurse must be alert for:
- irritability
- lethargy
- seizure activity
- altered vital signs
- altered feeding behavior.

Flexible and frequent feedings

Another aspect of nursing care for the neonate with hydrocephalus is maintaining adequate nutrition. Keep feeding schedules flexible to help accommodate for various procedures. Offer small, frequent feedings, and allow extra time for feeding in case the neonate has difficulty.

Support after surgery

Postoperative care involves:
- positioning the neonate on the side opposite the shunt
- observing for signs of increased ICP
- monitoring intake and output carefully
- preventing infection
- providing skin care.

On the home front

Hydrocephalus poses risks to the neonate's cognitive and physical development. The prospect of dealing with chronic disabilities or delayed development can be overwhelming to parents. Providing support to the family is crucial to helping them cope. Allow them to express their concerns, and refer them to appropriate resources and rehabilitation services, as needed.

Hyperbilirubinemia

Hyperbilirubinemia is an excess of bilirubin in the blood that results in serum bilirubin levels above 5 mg/dl. The elevated levels are due to unconjugated bilirubin depositing in the mucous membranes and on the skin, resulting in jaundice—which can be physiologic or pathologic. (See *Ethnic groups susceptible to severe hyperbilirubinemia.*)

Physiologic jaundice is hyperbilirubinemia that results from abnormal bilirubin metabolism. It usually resolves in 7 to 10 days.

In pathologic jaundice, total bilirubin levels and total serum bilirubin levels increase.

If left untreated, hyperbilirubinemia may result in bilirubin encephalopathy, a neurologic syndrome caused by unconjugated bilirubin depositing in the brain cells. Survivors may develop cerebral palsy, epilepsy, or mental retardation, or they may have only minor aftereffects, such as perceptual-motor disabilities and learning disorders.

What causes it

As erythrocytes break down at the end of their neonatal life cycle, hemoglobin separates into globin (protein) and heme (iron) fragments. Heme fragments form unconjugated bilirubin. Unconjugated bilirubin then binds with albumin and is transported to liver cells to conjugate with glucuronide and form direct bilirubin. During this process, unconjugated bilirubin may escape to extravascular tissue, causing hyperbilirubinemia.

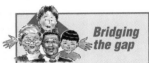

Bridging the gap

Ethnic groups susceptible to severe hyperbilirubinemia

Severe hyperbilirubinemia tends to be more common in individuals of East Asian or Native American descent. Individuals from these ethnic groups have a mean peak of unconjugated bilirubin that's about twice the average level.

Conversely, Blacks tend to have a decreased risk of developing severe hyperbilirubinemia.

Developing news

Several factors may affect whether a neonate develops hyperbilirubinemia:

• Certain drugs (such as aspirin, tranquilizers, and sulfonamides) or conditions (such as hypothermia, anoxia, hypoglycemia, and hypoalbuminemia) can disrupt conjugation and usurp albumin-binding sites.

• Decreased hepatic function can result in reduced bilirubin conjugation.

• Increased erythrocyte production or breakdown or Rh or ABO incompatibility can accompany hemolytic disorders.

• Maternal enzymes present in breast milk can inhibit the neonate's glucuronosyltransferase conjugating activity.

• If the neonate has glucose-6-phosphate dehydrogenase deficiency, he has an increased risk of developing jaundice.

What to look for

The predominant sign of hyperbilirubinemia is jaundice, which doesn't become clinically apparent until serum bilirubin levels reach about 7 mg/dl.

Physiologic jaundice

Physiologic jaundice typically develops within 3 to 4 days after birth in 60% of term neonates and in 80% of preterm neonates. It generally disappears by day 7 in term neonates and by day 9 or 10 in preterm neonates. Throughout physiologic jaundice, the serum unconjugated bilirubin level doesn't exceed 12 mg/dl and then declines rapidly over the first week after birth. Most neonates have been discharged by the time the jaundice peaks (72 hours).

Pathologic jaundice

Pathologic jaundice appears within the first 24 hours of life when the total serum bilirubin level increases by more than 5 mg/dl/day and the total bilirubin level is higher than 17 mg/dl in a full-term neonate.

What tests tell you

Jaundice and elevated levels of serum bilirubin confirm hyperbilirubinemia. Inspection of the neonate in a well-lit room (without yellow or gold lighting) reveals yellowish skin coloration, particularly in the sclerae. To verify jaundice, press the skin on the cheek or abdomen lightly with one finger, then release pressure and observe skin color immediately. Signs of jaundice necessitate measuring and charting serum bilirubin levels every 4 hours. Testing may include direct and indirect bilirubin levels, particularly for pathologic jaundice. Bilirubin levels that are excessively elevated or vary daily suggest a pathologic process.

Connecting the cause

Identifying the underlying cause of hyperbilirubinemia requires:
• a detailed patient history (including prenatal history)
• a detailed family history (paternal Rh factor, inherited red blood cell defects)
• present status of the neonate (immaturity, infection)
• blood testing of the neonate and mother (blood group incompatibilities, hemoglobin level, serum bilirubin or transcutaneous bilirubin level, hematocrit).

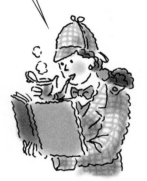

Suspect pathologic jaundice if bilirubin levels are excessively high or vary daily,

How it's treated

Depending on the underlying cause, treatment may include:
• exchange transfusions
• high-intensity phototherapy
• albumin infusion
• I.V. globulin (in isoimmune hemolytic disease).

Uneven exchange

An exchange transfusion replaces the neonate's blood with fresh blood (blood that's less than 48 hours old), thus removing some of the unconjugated bilirubin in serum.

Photo albumin

Phototherapy uses fluorescent light to decompose bilirubin in the skin by oxidation. Implemented after the initial exchange transfusion, phototherapy is usually discontinued after bilirubin levels fall below 10 mg/dl and continue to decrease for 24 hours. (See *Performing phototherapy.*)

Other therapy for excessive bilirubin levels may include albumin administration (1 g/kg of 25% salt-poor albumin), which provides additional albumin for binding unconjugated bilirubin. This may be done 1 to 2 hours before an exchange transfusion or as a substitute for a portion of the plasma in the transfused blood.

What to do

Nursing interventions for the neonate with hyperbilirubinemia include:
• Administer $Rh_o(D)$ immune globulin (human), as ordered, to an Rh-negative mother after amniocentesis or to an Rh-negative

Performing phototherapy

To perform phototherapy, follow these steps:
• Set up the phototherapy unit above the neonate's bassinet according to manufacturer's recommendations and verify placement of the light-bulb shield. If the neonate is in an incubator, place the phototherapy unit above the incubator according to the manufacturer's recommendations and turn on the lights. Place a photometer probe in the middle of the bassinet to measure the energy emitted by the lights.
• If the bilirubin level is extremely high and needs to be reduced rapidly, it may be necessary to line the sides of the bassinet with aluminum foil or white pads and to place a phototherapy unit below the neonate.
• Explain the procedure to the parents.
• Record the neonate's initial bilirubin level and his axillary temperature.
• Place the opaque eye mask over the neonate's closed eyes and fasten securely.
• Undress the neonate and place a diaper under him. Cover male genitalia with a surgical mask or small diaper to catch urine and prevent possible testicular damage from the heat and light waves.

• Take the neonate's axillary temperature every 2 hours and provide additional warmth by adjusting the warming unit's thermostat.
• Monitor elimination and weigh the neonate twice daily. Watch for signs of dehydration (dry skin, poor turgor, depressed fontanels) and check urine specific gravity with a urinometer to gauge hydration status.
• Take the neonate out of the bassinet, turn off the phototherapy lights, and unmask his eyes at least every 3 to 4 hours with feedings. Assess his eyes for inflammation or injury.
• Reposition the neonate every 2 hours to expose all body surfaces to the light and to prevent head molding and skin breakdown from pressure.
• Check the bilirubin level at least once every 24 hours—more often if levels rise significantly. Turn off the phototherapy unit before drawing venous blood for testing because the lights may degrade bilirubin in the blood. Notify the doctor if the bilirubin level nears 20 mg/dl in full-term neonates or 15 mg/dl in premature neonates.

mother during the third trimester to prevent hemolytic disease after the neonate is born.
• Assess and record the neonate's jaundice and note the time it began. Report the jaundice and serum bilirubin levels immediately.
• Maintain oral intake. Don't skip feedings because fasting stimulates the conversion of heme to bilirubin.
• Offer extra water to promote bilirubin excretion.
• Reassure parents that most neonates experience some degree of jaundice.
• Explain hyperbilirubinemia, its causes, diagnostic tests, and treatment.
• Explain to the parents that the neonate's stools contain some bile and may be greenish.
• Advise the parents that they'll need to make a follow-up appointment with the pediatrician within 48 hours after discharge. Discharge may need to be delayed if the neonate is at risk for severe bilirubinemia and a follow-up appointment can't be made.

Meconium aspiration syndrome

Meconium is a thick, sticky, greenish black substance that constitutes the neonate's first feces. It's present in the bowel of the fetus as early as 10 weeks' gestation. Meconium aspiration syndrome results when the neonate inhales meconium that's mixed with amniotic fluid. It typically occurs while the neonate is in utero or with the neonate's first breath. The meconium partially or completely blocks the neonate's airways so that air becomes trapped during exhalation. Also, the meconium irritates the neonate's airways, making breathing difficult.

In the thick of it

The severity of meconium aspiration syndrome depends on the amount of meconium aspirated and the consistency of the meconium. Thicker meconium generally causes more damage.

Increased effort

Neonates with meconium aspiration syndrome increase their respiratory efforts to create greater negative intrathoracic pressures and improve air flow to the lungs. Hyperinflation, hypoxemia, and acidemia cause increased peripheral vascular resistance. Right-to-left shunting commonly follows.

What causes it

Meconium aspiration syndrome is commonly related to fetal distress during labor. Meconium is released in utero because the anal sphincter relaxes secondary to a hypoxic episode. Occasionally, healthy neonates pass meconium before birth. In either case, if the neonate gasps or inhales the meconium, meconium aspiration syndrome can develop. The resulting lack of oxygen may lead to brain damage.

Risk factors for meconium aspiration syndrome include:
- maternal diabetes
- maternal hypertension
- difficult delivery
- fetal distress
- intrauterine hypoxia
- advanced gestational age (greater than 40 weeks)
- poor intrauterine growth.

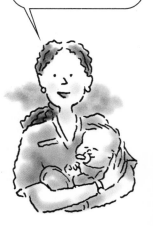

Maternal diabetes and maternal hypertension are some of the risk factors for meconium aspiration syndrome.

What to look for

Signs and symptoms of meconium aspiration syndrome include:
• dark greenish staining or streaking of the amniotic fluid
• obvious presence of meconium in the amniotic fluid
• skin with a greenish stain (if the meconium was passed long before delivery)
• limp appearance at birth
• cyanosis
• rapid breathing
• labored breathing
• apnea
• signs of postmaturity such as peeling skin and long nails
• low heart rate before birth
• low Apgar score
• hypothermia
• hypoglycemia
• hypocalcemia
• nasal flaring
• grunting
• tachypnea
• irregular gasping respirations.

What tests tell you

The most accurate way to diagnose meconium aspiration syndrome is to observe the vocal cords for meconium staining. Assess breath sounds for coarse, crackly sounds, which are common in neonates with meconium aspiration syndrome. ABG analysis helps assess for acidosis (low blood pH and hypoxemia). A chest X-ray can show patches or streaks of meconium in the lungs and reveal if hyperexpansion and air trapping have occurred.

How it's treated

If meconium aspiration is present or suspected, the neonate's nose and mouth should be suctioned as soon as the head is delivered. Tracheal suctioning may be necessary to remove all of the meconium before the first breath is taken; saline solution may be instilled to remove particularly thick meconium. Close monitoring of the infant is necessary after delivery.
    Additional treatments may include:
• chest physiotherapy
• antibiotics
• use of a radiant warmer

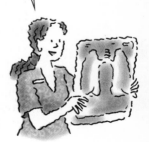

Every picture tells a story. A chest X-ray may reveal patches or streaks of meconium in the lungs.

- supplemental oxygen
- mechanical ventilation.

    If complications arise, further treatments may be necessary. (See *Complications of meconium aspiration syndrome.*)

What to do

Assess risk factors before delivery if possible. Other nursing responsibilities include:
- amniotic fluid assessment
- fetal monitoring
- immediate intervention in delivery room
- performing chest physiotherapy
- maintaining thermoregulation
- pulmonary assessment
- administering respiratory support, such as oxygen and mechanical ventilation
- being alert for potential complications
- supporting family members by providing education and reassurance and promoting parent-neonate attachment.

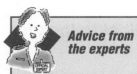

Advice from the experts

Complications of meconium aspiration syndrome

Meconium aspiration syndrome may cause:
- aspiration pneumonia
- bronchopulmonary dysplasia
- cerebral palsy
- mental retardation
- pneumothorax
- seizures.

Phenylketonuria

Phenylketonuria (PKU) is a rare hereditary condition. It's characterized by the inability of the body to metabolize phenylalanine, an essential amino acid that's found in protein-containing foods. Excess phenylalanine can affect normal development of the brain and CNS as well as levels of tyrosine, an amino acid that plays a role in the production of melanin, epinephrine, and thyroxine.

What causes it

PKU is inherited as an autosomal recessive trait. Both parents must pass the gene on for the child to be affected. In PKU, there's almost no activity of phenylalanine hydroxylase, an enzyme that helps convert phenylalanine to tyrosine. Phenylalanine accumulates in the blood and urine, resulting in low tyrosine levels. (See *Incidence of PKU.*)

PKU is an autosomal recessive trait. Both parents must have the gene and pass it on for the child to be affected.

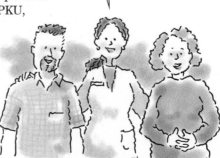

What to look for

Clinical manifestations of PKU in a neonate include:
- seizures
- microcephaly
- hyperactivity
- irritability
- purposeless, repetitive motions
- musty odor from skin and urine excretion of phenylacetic acid
- tremors
- jerking movements of arms and legs
- unusual hand posturing.

PKU phenotypes

Because PKU tends to decrease melanin production, children affected with it have similar phenotypes, including blond hair, blue eyes, and fair skin.

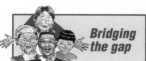

Bridging the gap

Incidence of PKU

Phenylketonuria (PKU) has a high incidence among people of Irish and Scottish descent. Incidence is lower among Blacks and Ashkenazic Jews.

What tests tell you

Diagnostic tests for PKU include:
- enzyme assay to detect whether the parents are carriers of the trait
- chorionic villus sampling and amniocentesis during pregnancy to diagnose the fetus prenatally
- PKU screening (mandatory in most states).

It's in the blood

The Guthrie blood test uses a heelstick blood sample from the neonate to screen for PKU. The test detects serum phenylalanine levels of greater than 4 mg/dl (normal level is 2 mg/dl).

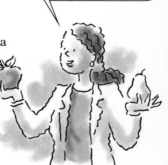

Here's a fruitful idea. A diet that includes foods low in phenylalanine, such as fruits and vegetables, can control PKU.

How it's treated

Treatment involves maintaining a diet that's extremely low in phenylalanine. Adult women with PKU should strictly adhere to a low phenylalanine diet before and during pregnancy because a strong correlation between maternal phenylalanine levels and improved fetal outcome exists. Increased phenylalanine levels in mothers with PKU can affect embryologic development, causing low birth weight, congenital malformations, microcephaly, and mental retardation.

Eating towards healthy levels

Advise the parents of neonates with PKU to consult with a registered dietitian. A proper diet should meet the neonate's nutritional needs for optimum growth while maintaining a safe phenylalanine level (2 to 8 mg/dl). Phenylalanine levels greater than 10 to 15 mg/dl can lead to brain damage; levels less than 2 mg/dl can lead to protein catabolism and growth retardation.

Foods that can't miss

Special formulas such as Lofenalac are made for infants with PKU. They can be initiated before the neonate is 3 weeks old and are used throughout life as a protein source for individuals with PKU. Foods with low levels of phenylalanine include:
- vegetables
- fruits
- juices
- some cereals, breads, and starches.

Foods to take off the list

To avoid toxicity to the brain and CNS, foods high in phenylalanine should be avoided, including:
- dairy products
- eggs
- meat
- foods or drinks containing aspartame (NutraSweet).

What to do

The principal nursing intervention for PKU is teaching the family about dietary restrictions. (See *Teaching parents about PKU*.) Parents also have the burden of knowing that they passed this disorder on to their children. They must make serious decisions regarding future children. Refer these families to genetic counseling and to a dietitian.

Preterm neonates

A neonate is considered preterm if he's born before 37 weeks' gestation. The preterm neonate is at risk for complications because the organ systems are immature. The degree of complications depends on gestational age. The closer the neonate is to 40 weeks' gestation, the easier the transition to extrauterine life will be.

What causes it

It may be necessary to deliver a neonate before term if evidence of a maternal complication exists. For example, preeclampsia is a

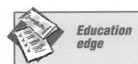

Education edge

Teaching parents about PKU

Parents of neonates with phenylketonuria (PKU) need to have a basic understanding of the disorder. They also need practical suggestions for meal planning because preparing meals can be stressful for parents who have to worry about calculating phenylalanine levels. Be sure to instruct the family on how to:
- eliminate or restrict foods high in phenylalanine
- measure to see if foods are low in phenylalanine
- avoid using artificial sweeteners with aspartame (such as NutraSweet).

condition that can develop in the second or third trimester of pregnancy. Signs of preeclampsia include elevated blood pressure, fluid retention, and protein in the urine. The only treatment for preeclampsia is to deliver the neonate. If left untreated, the mother can suffer severe organ damage and seizures. Kidney disease, heart disease, diabetes, or infection in the mother may also require preterm delivery of the neonate.

Additional risk factors for a preterm neonate include:
- multiple pregnancy
- adolescent pregnancy
- lack of prenatal care
- substance abuse
- smoking
- previous preterm delivery
- high, unexplained alpha fetoprotein level in second trimester
- abnormalities of the uterus
- cervical incompetence
- premature rupture of membranes
- placenta previa
- gestational hypertension.

What to look for

Preterm neonates have characteristics that are distinctive at various stages of development. These characteristics can give clues to the neonate's gestational age and physiologic capabilities.

First findings

Initial assessment findings typical of preterm neonates include:
- low birth weight
- minimal subcutaneous fat deposits
- proportionally large head in relation to body
- prominent sucking pads in the cheeks
- wrinkled features
- thin, smooth, shiny skin that's almost translucent
- veins that are clearly visible under the thin, transparent epidermis
- lanugo (soft, downy hair) over the body
- sparse, fine, fuzzy hair on the head
- soft, pliable ear cartilage
- minimal creases in the soles and palms
- skull and rib bones that feel soft
- closed eyes
- few scrotal rugae (males)
- undescended testes (males)
- prominent labia and clitoris (females).

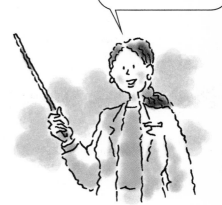

Low birth weight and wrinkled features are typical findings in a preterm neonate.

Physical findings

Physical examination findings include:
- inability to maintain body temperature
- limited ability to excrete solutes in the urine
- increased susceptibility to infection
- periodic breathing, hypoventilation, and periods of apnea
- increased susceptibility to hyperbilirubinemia
- increased susceptibility to hypoglycemia
- ability to bring the neonate's elbow across the chest when eliciting the scarf sign
- ability to easily bring the neonate's heel to his ear.

System signs

The neonate's neurologic status is assessed by observing:
- active movements
- response to stimulation
- response to passive movements.
    CNS evaluation may reveal:
- inactivity (although neonate may be unusually active immediately after birth)
- extension of extremities
- absence of suck reflex
- weak swallow, gag, and cough reflexes
- weak grasp reflex.

What tests tell you

These tests may indicate the extent of physiologic maturity and may assist caregivers in the management of the neonate:
- chest X-ray
- ABG analysis
- head ultrasounds
- echocardiography
- eye examination by a retinal specialist
- serum glucose
- serum calcium
- serum bilirubin
- euglobulin lysis time
- CBC.

How it's treated

Preterm neonates are cared for by a specially trained staff in the neonatal intensive care unit (NICU). The top priority in treating a preterm neonate is supporting the cardiac and respiratory systems as needed. If the neonate isn't breathing or respiratory efforts are poor, an endotracheal tube may be inserted and mechanical ventilation started. Supplemental oxygen may also be given. Medications to increase the heart rate or maintain blood pressure may be administered as part of the resuscitative effort. Other essential interventions include providing thermoregulation and starting I.V. or gavage nutrition.

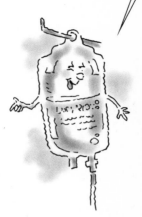

Help is on the way! I.V. nutrition is an essential intervention for preterm neonates.

Three goals

Meticulous care and observation in the NICU is necessary until the neonate:
- receives oral feedings
- maintains body temperature
- weighs about 5 pounds.

Preemie problems

Certain complications may occur:
- **Respiratory distress syndrome (RDS)** is a leading cause of morbidity and mortality among preterm neonates. The lungs lack surfactant, which prevents alveolar collapse at the end of respiration. Treatment involves administration of surfactant, oxygen administration, and mechanical ventilation.
- **Intraventricular hemorrhage (IVH)** is bleeding in or around the ventricles of the brain. It's most common in neonates born before 32 weeks' gestation. Damage to brain function and long-term effects vary.
- **Retinopathy of prematurity (ROP)** is a disease caused by abnormal growth of retinal blood vessels. Prematurity may cause abnormal vessels to grow. Supplemental oxygen is also thought to contribute to this growth. ROP can cause mild to severe eye and vision problems. Treatment may involve laser surgery or cryotherapy.
- **Patent ductus arteriosus** occurs when the ductus arteriosus reopens after birth due to lowered oxygen tension associated with respiratory impairment. Treatment involves fluid regulation, respiratory support, administration of indomethacin (Indocin), and surgical ligation (if the neonate doesn't respond to other therapies).
- **Necrotizing enterocolitis (NEC)** is an inflammatory disease of the GI mucosa. (See *A close look at necrotizing enterocolitis*, page 548.)
- **Bronchopulmonary dysplasia (BPD)** is also called *chronic lung disease*. The lungs may be less compliant because of the damage caused by being a preterm neonate, infection, or mechanical ventilation. Treatment involves supplying oxygen, maintaining good nutrition, and preventing respiratory illness.
- **Apnea of prematurity** is a common phenomenon in the preterm neonate. It occurs because neurologic and chemical respiratory control mechanisms are immature. The number of apneic spells

A close look at necrotizing enterocolitis

Necrotizing enterocolitis is an inflammatory disease of the GI mucosa. Here are its causes, pathophysiolgy, and signs as well as tests used to diagnose it and ways in which it's treated.

Causes
• Uncertain; appears to occur in neonates whose GI tract has suffered vascular compromise

Pathophysiology
• Blood flow to gastric mucosa is decreased due to shunting of blood to vital organs.
• Mucosal cells lining the bowel wall die.
• Protective, lubricating mucus isn't secreted.
• Bowel wall is attacked by proteolytic enzymes.
• Bowel wall swells and breaks down.

Signs
• Distended abdomen
• Gastric retention
• Blood in stools or gastric contents
• Lethargy
• Poor feeding
• Hypotension
• Apnea
• Vomiting

Diagnostic tests
• Radiographic studies show intestinal dilation and free air in the abdomen (indicating perforation).

• Laboratory studies show anemia, leukopenia, leukocytosis, electrolyte imbalance.

Treatment
• Prevention
• Discontinuation of enteral feedings
• Nasogastric suction
• Administration of I.V. antibiotics
• Administration of parenteral fluids
• Surgery

tends to increase the younger the gestational age of the neonate. The condition can be treated with such medications as theophylline and caffeine.

Additional complications that may occur include:
• infection
• jaundice
• anemia
• hypoglycemia
• delayed growth and development.

What to do

Nursing interventions for the preterm neonate should focus on maintaining an environment that's similar to the intrauterine environment. Care should be based on knowledge of the preterm neonate's physiologic problems and the need to conserve energy for growth and repair.

Specific nursing responsibilities include:
• rapid initial evaluation
• resuscitative measures if needed
• thermoregulation
• administration of respiratory support measures
• electronic monitoring
• parenteral fluids as ordered
• medications as ordered
• blood sample analysis as ordered.

Education edge

Teaching parents of preterm neonates

To help the parents of a preterm neonate cope with this difficult situation, follow these guidelines:

• Orient them to the neonatal intensive care unit environment and introduce them to all caregivers.

• Orient them to the machinery and monitors that may be attached to their neonate. Reassure them that the staff is alert to alarms as well as the cues of their child.

• Tell them what to expect.

• Teach them the characteristics of a preterm neonate.

• Teach them how to handle their neonate.

• Instruct them on feeding, whether it's through gavage, breast, or bottle.

• Inform them of potential complications.

• Offer discharge planning.

• Make appropriate referrals.

The right touch

Stimulation needs to be individualized to the development and tolerance of each neonate. Touch should be smooth and sure. Stroking and rubbing are discouraged. The head should be supported and the extremities held close to the body during position changes. This type of touch decreases motor disorganization and stress.

Hard to swallow

Preterm neonates born before 34 weeks' gestation aren't coordinated enough to maintain the suck, swallow, and breathe regimen necessary for oral feeding. These neonates need to be fed I.V. or by gavage. Be alert for potential complications, such as NEC. Nonnutritive sucking, such as using a pacifier while being fed by gavage, may help to ease the transition to oral feeding that occurs later.

Keep up the communication

Nursing care also involves keeping the parents informed and educated about what's involved in the care of their preterm neonate. (See *Teaching parents of preterm neonates*.)

Respiratory distress syndrome

RDS occurs when the lungs are immature. It's seen almost exclusively in preterm neonates and carries a high risk of long-term respiratory and neurologic complications.

What causes it

RDS is characterized by poor gas exchange and ventilatory failure. It's caused by a lack of pulmonary surfactant, a phospholipid secreted by the alveolar epithelium that normally appears in mature lungs. Surfactant coats the alveoli, keeping them open so that gas exchange can occur. In preterm neonates, the lungs may not be fully developed and, therefore, may not have a sufficient amount of surfactant. This leads to:

- atelectasis
- increased work of breathing
- respiratory acidosis
- hypoxemia.

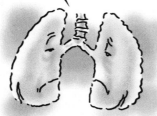

Low surfactant. Poor gas exchange. Looks like we're in trouble!

Changing the flow of things

As atelectasis worsens, pulmonary vascular resistance increases, which decreases blood flow to the lungs. Blood then shunts from right to left, perpetuating fetal circulation by keeping the foramen ovale and ductus arteriosus patent.

One membrane too many

The alveoli may become necrotic, and the capillaries may become damaged. Ischemia allows fluid to leak into the interstitial and alveolar spaces, causing a hyaline membrane to form. This membrane hinders respiratory function by decreasing the compliance of the lungs.

Risk factors for RDS include:

- preterm birth
- maternal diabetes
- stress during delivery that produces acidosis in the neonate.

What to look for

RDS can produce respiratory distress acutely after birth or over a period of a few hours. Initial assessment may reveal:

- increased respiratory rate
- retractions
- satisfactory color
- good air movement on auscultation.

Obvious observations

As respiratory distress becomes more obvious, the nurse may note:

- further increase in respiratory rate
- labored breathing
- more pronounced substernal retractions

- fine crackles on auscultation
- expiratory grunting
- nasal flaring
- cyanosis.

It gets worse

If treatment isn't started or if the neonate isn't responding to treatment, the nurse may observe:
- worsening cyanosis
- flaccidity
- unresponsiveness
- apneic episodes
- decreased breath sounds.

What tests tell you

Results of laboratory data, such as hypoxemia, hypercapnia, and acidosis, are nonspecific to RDS. Specific tests must be carried out to evaluate the neonate for complicating factors. These include:
- blood, urine, and CSF cultures
- blood glucose analysis
- serum calcium
- ABG measurements.
   Radiographic evaluation reveals:
- alveolar atelectasis (a diffuse, granular pattern that resembles ground glass) over lung fields
- dilated bronchioles (appear as dark streaks within the granular pattern).

Phospholipid lingo

Prenatal tests can evaluate lung maturity while the fetus is in utero. This is done by evaluating the lecithin and sphingomyelin ratio of the amniotic fluid. Lecithin and sphingomyelin are two surfactant phospholipids. Evaluation of fetal lung maturity gives insight into how the fetus will fare after birth and may precipitate treatment of the mother to delay labor or to mature the neonate's lungs before delivery.

How it's treated

Because RDS is a disease related to gestational age and lung maturity, one management technique is to prevent preterm delivery. If that isn't possible, surfactant production can be stimulated before

Since prevention of preterm delivery decreases my chance of suffering from RDS, I think I'll hang out here a while longer.

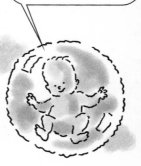

the neonate is born by administering corticosteroids to the mother before birth.

Supportive steps

RDS treatment after birth is mainly supportive and includes general measures used to treat preterm neonates, including:
- thermoregulation
- oxygen administration
- mechanical ventilation if needed
- prevention of hypotension
- prevention of hypovolemia
- correcting respiratory acidosis by ventilatory support
- correcting metabolic acidosis with the administration of sodium bicarbonate
- parenteral feedings.

Gavage feedings and oral feedings aren't recommended during the acute stage of RDS because such situations that increase respiratory rate or oxygen consumption should be avoided.

Respiratory remedies

Respiratory support can be given by:
- oxygen administration via nasal cannula
- continuous positive airway pressure (CPAP)
- mechanical ventilation.

Sometimes the use of a high-frequency oscillator is needed. Positive end-expiratory pressure (PEEP) may be used via mechanical ventilation. PEEP prevents alveolar collapse during expiration, thereby allowing more time for gas exchange to occur.

The goals of oxygen therapy are to:
- maintain adequate oxygenation to the tissues
- prevent lactic acidosis
- avoid toxic effects of oxygen.

Complications of oxygen therapy and mechanical ventilation may occur despite efforts to prevent them. They include:
- pneumothorax
- pneumomediastinum
- ROP
- BPD
- infection
- IVH.

Myriad of meds

Management of RDS also includes the administration of surfactant. Surfactant can prevent atelectasis and contribute to fluid clearance from the alveoli. Other medications that are commonly used to treat neonates with RDS include antibiotics, sedatives, paralytics, and diuretics.

What to do

Continuous monitoring of the neonate with RDS is essential because of the constant threat of hypoxemia. Nursing responsibilities include:
- collecting blood samples
- monitoring pulse oximetry
- suctioning
- implementing thermoregulation
- monitoring nutrition
- administering medication
- providing mouth and skin care.

Do not disturb

To help decrease oxygen consumption, make efforts to limit how often the neonate with RDS is disturbed. Feeding is generally given parenterally during the acute phase of the disease. Keep the neonate in a dark, quiet, thermal neutral environment as much as possible.

In addition to the general patient teaching for parents of preterm neonates, parents of neonates with RDS need to be educated about the syndrome, especially during the acute stage. Refer the parents to social services, a chaplain, and other sources of support as needed.

Transient tachypnea of the neonate

Transient tachypnea of the neonate (TTN) is a mild respiratory problem in neonates. It begins after birth and generally lasts about 3 days. TTN is also known as *wet lungs* or *type II RDS*.

What causes it

TTN results from the delayed absorption of fetal lung fluid after birth. Before birth, the fetus doesn't use his lungs to breathe. Instead, the fetal lungs are filled with fluid. All of the fetus' nutrients and oxygen come from the mother through the placenta. During the birth process, some of the neonate's lung fluid is squeezed out as he passes through the birth canal. After birth, the remaining fluid is pushed out of the lungs as the lungs fill with air. Fluid that remains is later coughed out or absorbed into the blood stream.

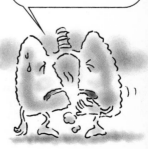

TTN results when fluid remains in the lungs, forcing the neonate to breathe harder and faster to get adequate oxygen.

TTN results when fluid remains in the lungs, forcing the neonate to breathe harder and faster to get adequate oxygen.

Risk factory

TTN is commonly observed in neonates delivered by cesarean birth. These neonates don't receive the thoracic compression that helps to expel fluid during vaginal delivery. Other risk factors for TTN include:

- preterm delivery of the neonate
- maternal smoking during pregnancy
- maternal diabetes
- size that's SGA
- macrosomia
- maternal asthma
- maternal drug abuse
- birth asphyxia
- maternal fluid overload (especially with oxytocin [Pitocin] administration)
- prolonged labor
- delayed clamping of the cord
- excessive maternal sedation.

Neonates who are small or preterm, or who were born rapidly by vaginal delivery, may not have received effective squeezing of the thorax to remove fetal lung fluid.

What to look for

Common signs of TTN include:

- tachypnea (rate greater than 60 breaths/minute)
- labored breathing
- expiratory grunting
- nasal flaring
- retractions
- cyanosis
- tachycardia.

These signs and symptoms typically occur immediately after birth. However, these could also be indicative of a more serious condition; observe the neonate closely.

What tests tell you

Laboratory tests and imaging studies are used to diagnose TTN. For example:

- ABG results may indicate hypoxemia and decreased carbon dioxide levels.

- Increased carbon dioxide levels may be a sign of fatigue and impending respiratory failure.
- Pulse oximetry is used to noninvasively monitor tissue oxygenation and allow titration of supplemental oxygen.
- A CBC with differential may be done to evaluate for signs of infection.
- Chest X-ray, the diagnostic standard for TTN, will reveal streaking that correlates with lymphatic engorgement of retained fetal lung fluid, hyperexpansion of the lungs, a mild to moderately enlarged heart, and flattening of the diaphragm.

Abnormal findings

Abnormalities in diagnostic test results resolve with resolution of the condition, usually within 72 hours.

How it's treated

Specific treatment for TTN depends on:
- the neonate's gestational age, overall health, and medical history
- the extent of respiratory distress
- tolerance of medical therapies
- expectations for the course of the disease.

Be supportive

Care is mainly supportive as the retained lung fluid is reabsorbed. Treatment may involve:
- monitoring heart rate, respiratory rate, and oxygen levels
- providing supplemental oxygen
- maintaining CPAP
- monitorng intake and output
- using mechanical ventilation
- providing proper nutrition.

Generally, a neonate with TTN is supported with I.V. fluids or gavage feedings. The increased respiratory rate and increased work of breathing makes oral feeding difficult because the neonate must coordinate the mechanisms of sucking, swallowing, and breathing. The rapid respiratory rate puts the neonate at high risk for aspiration.

Minimal meds

Medication use in TTN is minimal. Antibiotic therapy may be administered until sepsis is ruled out. The regimen usually consists of penicillin (usually ampicillin) and an aminoglycoside (usually gentamicin [Garamycin]) or a cephalosporin (usually cefotaxime [Claforan]).

What to do

A neonate with TTN may be cared for in an NICU. Nursing interventions include:
- monitoring heart and respiratory rates and oxygenation
- providing respiratory support
- maintaining a neutral thermal environment
- minimizing stimulation by decreasing lights and noise levels
- administering medication as ordered
- providing proper nutrition
- providing parental education and emotional support.

Symptoms typically resolve within 72 hours. The neonate usually recovers completely and has no increased risk of further respiratory problems.

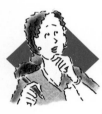

Quick quiz

1. Testing a neonate for drug exposure while in utero involves collecting and analyzing:

 A. urine and meconium.
 B. blood and urine.
 C. CSF and meconium.
 D. CSF and blood.

Answer: A. Urine and meconium specimens are collected when testing a neonate for drug exposure while in utero.

2. Neonates classified as SGA have a birth weight that's:

 A. below the 5th percentile.
 B. below the 10th percentile.
 C. below the 15th percentile.
 D. below the 20th percentile.

Answer: B. Neonates classified as SGA have a birth weight below the 10th percentile.

3. Which option is a neonatal risk factor for HIV transmission?

 A. Being born preterm
 B. Being a second-born twin
 C. Being bottle-fed
 D. Being born postterm

Answer: A. Preterm birth is neonatal risk factor for HIV infection.

4. Downward deviation of the eyes ("sunsetting eyes") is a classic assessment finding of:

    A.   FAS.

    B.   hydrocephalus.

    C.   preterm birth.

    D.   HIV infection.

Answer: B. Downward deviation of the eyes is a characteristic finding in neonates with hydrocephalus.

5. Which is the most accurate diagnostic tool for meconium aspiration syndrome?

    A.   Chest X-ray

    B.   ABG analysis

    C.   Evaluation of the vocal cords using a laryngoscope

    D.   Amniotic fluid testing for meconium

Answer: C. The most accurate way to diagnose meconium aspiration syndrome is to evaluate the vocal cords for meconium staining using a laryngoscope.

6. What's the role of surfactant in the lungs?

    A.   It coats the alveoli to help keep them open so that gas exchange can occur.

    B.   It increases pulmonary capillary blood flow.

    C.   It increases respiratory rate to correct acidemia.

    D.   It prevents bronchospasm.

Answer: A. Surfactant is a phospholipid secreted by the alveolar epithelium that coats the alveoli, keeping them open so that gas exchange can occur.

7. Which maternal disorder increases the chances that the mother will have a neonate who develops TTN?

    A.   Sickle cell anemia

    B.   Hyperemesis gravidarum

    C.   Macrosomia

    D.   Asthma

Answer: D. Maternal disorders that increase the risk of having a neonate who develops TTN include a history of asthma, drug abuse, diabetes, excessive sedation, prolonged labor, and fluid overload.

Scoring

☆☆☆ If you answered all seven questions correctly, ooh la la! You have a definite flair for neonatal care!

☆☆ If you answered five or six questions correctly, magnifique! You've outfitted yourself with a fine knowledge of high-risk neonates!

☆ If you answered fewer than five questions correctly, très bien! You can go back and look this over in your own fashion to get a better view of this chapter!

Appendices and index

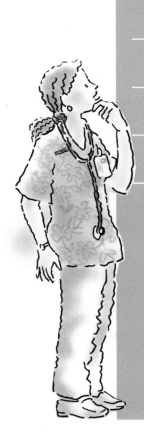

Laboratory values for pregnant
and nonpregnant patients   561

Selected maternal
daily dietary allowances   563

Normal neonatal laboratory values   565

NANDA-I taxonomy II   569

Glossary   573

Selected references   579

Index   581

Laboratory values for pregnant and nonpregnant patients

	Pregnant	Nonpregnant
Hemoglobin	11.5 to 14 g/dl	12 to 16 g/dl
Hematocrit	32% to 42%	37% to 47%
White blood cells	5,000 to 15,000/µl	4,500 to 10,000/µl
Neutrophils	60% ±10%	60%
Lymphocytes	15% to 40%	38% to 46%
Platelets	150,000 to 350,000/µl	150,000 to 350,000/µl
Serum calcium	7.8 to 9.3 mg/dl	8.4 to 10.2 mg/dl
Serum sodium	Increased retention	136 to 146 mmol/L
Serum chloride	Slight elevation	98 to 106 mmol/L
Serum iron	65 to 120 mcg/dl	75 to 150 mcg/dl
Fibrinogen	400 mg/dl	250 mg/dl
Red blood cells	1,500 to 1,900/µl	1,600/µl
Fasting blood glucose	65 mg/dl	70 to 80 mg/dl
2-hour postprandial blood glucose	<140 mg/dl (after a 100 g carbohydrate meal)	60 to 110 mg/dl
Blood urea nitrogen	Decreased	20 to 25 mg/dl
Serum creatinine	Decreased	0.5 mg/dl to 1.1 mg/dl
Renal plasma flow	Increased by 25%	490 to 700 ml/minute
Glomerular filtration rate	Increased by 50% to 160 to 198 ml/minute	105 to 132 ml/minute
Serum uric acid	Decreased	2 to 6.6 mg/dl
Erythrocyte sedimentation rate	30 to 90 mm/hour	20 mm/hour
Prothrombin time	Decreased slightly	60 to 70 seconds
Partial thromboplastin time	Decreased slightly during pregnancy and again during second and third stages of labor (indicating clotting at placental site)	12 to 14 seconds

Selected maternal daily dietary allowances

This chart shows selected daily dietary allowances for pregnant and breast-feeding women.

Nutrient	Pregnant women	Breast-feeding women
Calories	2,500	2,700
Calcium	1,000 mg	1,000 mg
Folate	600 mcg	500 mcg
Iodine	220 mcg	290 mcg
Iron	27 mg	9 mg
Magnesium	350 mg	310 mg
Niacin (B$_3$)	18 mg	17 mg
Phosphorus	700 mg	700 mg
Protein	80 g	80 g
Riboflavin (B$_2$)	1.4 mg	1.6 mg
Thiamine (B$_1$)	1.5 mg	1.5 mg
Vitamin A	770 mcg	1,300 mcg
Vitamin B$_6$	1.9 mg	2 mg
Vitamin B$_{12}$	2.6 mcg	2.8 mcg
Vitamin C	85 mg	120 mg
Vitamin D	5 mcg	5 mcg
Vitamin E	15 mg	19 mg
Zinc	11 mg	12 mg

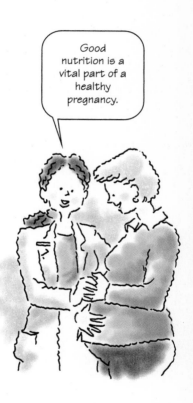

Good nutrition is a vital part of a healthy pregnancy.

Normal neonatal laboratory values

This chart shows laboratory tests that may be ordered for neonates, including the normal ranges for full-term infants. Note that ranges may vary among institutions. Because test results for preterm neonates usually reflect weight and gestational age, ranges for preterm neonates vary.

Test	Normal range
Blood	
Albumin	3.6 to 5.4 g/dl
Alkaline phosphatase	150 to 400 units/L (1 week) (SI, 150 to 400 units/L)
Alpha-fetoprotein	up to 10 mg/L, with none detected after 21 days
Ammonia	13 to 48 mcg/dl (SI, 9 to 34 µmol/L)
Amylase	5 to 65 units/L (SI, 5 to 65 units/L)
Bicarbonate	20 to 25 mEq/L (SI, 20 to 25 mmol/L)
Bilirubin, conjugated	0 to 0.2 mg/dl (SI, 0 to 3.4 µmol/L)
Bilirubin, total	less than 2 mg/dl (cord blood) (SI, less than 34 µmol/L)
• 0 to 1 day	less than 6 mg/dl (SI, less than 103 µmol/L) (peripheral blood)
• 1 to 2 days	less than 8 mg/dl (SI, less than 137 µmol/L) (peripheral blood)
• 3 to 5 days	less than 12 mg/dl (SI, less than 205 µmol/L) (peripheral blood)
Bleeding time	2 minutes
Arterial blood gases • ph • $Paco_2$ • Pao_2	 7.35 to 7.45 35 to 45 mm Hg 50 to 90 mm Hg
Venous blood gases • pH • Pco_2 • Po_2	 7.35 to 7.45 41 to 51 mm Hg 20 to 49 mm Hg

Test	Normal range
Blood (continued)	
Calcium, ionized	4.48 to 4.92 mg/dl (SI, 1.12 to 1.23 mmol/L)
Calcium, total	7 to 12 mg/dl (SI, 1.75 to 3 mmol/L)
Chloride	95 to 110 mEq/L (SI, 1.75 to 3 mmol/L)
Clotting time (2 tube)	5 to 8 minutes
Creatine kinase	76 to 600 units/L (SI, 76 to 600 units/L)
Creatinine	0.3 to 1 mg/dl (SI, 27 to 88 µmol/L)
Digoxin level	greater than 2 ng/ml possible; greater than 30 ng/ml probable
Fibrinogen	200 to 400 mg/dl (SI, 2 to 4 g/L)
Glucose	20 to 100 mg/dl (SI, 1.1 to 6.1 mmol/L)
Gamma glutamyltransferase	0 to 130 units/L (SI, 0 to 130 units/L)
Hematocrit	56% 51% (cord blood)
Hemoglobin	18.5 g/dl 16.5 g/dl (cord blood)
Immunoglobulins • IgG • IgM • IgA	 6.4 to 16 g/L 0.06 to 0.24 g/L 0 to 0.5 g/L
Iron	110 to 270 mcg/dl (SI, 20 to 48 µmol/L)
Iron-binding capacity	59 to 175 mcg/dl (SI, 10.6 to 31.3 µmol/L)
Lactate dehydrogenase	160 to 1,500 international units/L (SI, 160 to 1,500 international units/L)
Magnesium	1.5 to 2 mEq/L (SI, 0.75 to 1 mmol/L)
Osmolality	285 to 295 mOsm/kg (SI, 285 to 295 mmol/kg)
Partial thromboplastin time	40 to 80 seconds
Phenobarbital level	15 to 40 mcg/dl

Test	Normal range
Blood *(continued)*	
Phosphorus	4.2 to 9 mg/dl (SI, 1.36 to 2.91 mmol/L)
Platelets	100,000 to 300,000/µl
Potassium	3.5 to 6 mEq/L (SI, 3.5 to 6 mmol/L)
Protein, total	5 to 7.1 g/dl (SI, 50 to 71 g/L)
Prothrombin time	12 to 21 seconds
Red blood cell count	5.1 to 5.8 (1,000,000/µl)
Reticulocytes	3% to 7% (cord blood)
Sodium	135 to 145 mEq/L (SI, 135 to 145 mmol/L)
Theophylline level	5 to 10 mcg/ml
Thyroid-stimulating hormone	0 to 17.4 microinternational units/ml (SI, 0 to 17.4 microunits/L) (cord blood)
Thyroxine, (T_4) (total)	7.4 to 13 mcg/dl (SI, 95 to 168 mmol/L) (cord blood)
Urea nitrogen	5 to 20 mg/dl (SI, 2 to 7 µmol/L)
White blood cell (WBC) count • eosinophils-basophils • immature WBCs • lymphocytes • monocytes • neutrophils	18,000/µl 3% 10% 30% 5% 45%
Urine	
Casts, WBC	present first 2 to 4 days
Osmolality	50 to 1,200 mOsm/kg
pH	5 to 7
Protein	present first 2 to 4 days
Specific gravity	1.006 to 1.008

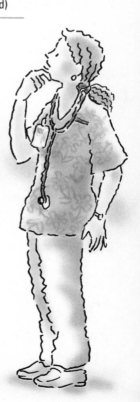

NANDA-I taxonomy II

The following is a list of the 2007-2008 current nursing diagnosis classifications according to their domains.

DOMAIN: HEALTH PROMOTION
- Effective therapeutic regimen management
- Health-seeking behaviors (specify)
- Impaired home maintenance
- Ineffective community therapeutic regimen management
- Ineffective family therapeutic regimen management
- Ineffective health maintenance
- Ineffective therapeutic regimen management
- Readiness for enhanced immunization status
- Readiness for enhanced nutrition
- Readiness for enhanced therapeutic regimen management

DOMAIN: NUTRITION
- Deficient fluid volume
- Excess fluid volume
- Imbalanced nutrition: Less than body requirements
- Imbalanced nutrition: More than body requirements
- Impaired swallowing
- Ineffective infant feeding pattern
- Readiness for enhanced fluid balance
- Risk for deficient fluid volume
- Risk for imbalanced fluid volume
- Risk for imbalanced nutrition: More than body requirements
- Risk for impaired liver function
- Risk for unstable blood glucose level

DOMAIN: ELIMINATION/EXCHANGE
- Bowel incontinence
- Constipation
- Diarrhea
- Functional urinary incontinence
- Impaired gas exchange
- Impaired urinary elimination
- Overflow urinary incontinence
- Perceived constipation
- Readiness for enhanced urinary elimination
- Reflex urinary incontinence
- Risk for constipation
- Risk for urge urinary incontinence
- Stress urinary incontinence
- Total urinary incontinence
- Urge urinary incontinence
- Urinary retention

DOMAIN: ACTIVITY/REST
- Activity intolerance
- Bathing/hygiene self-care deficit
- Decreased cardiac output
- Deficient diversional activity
- Delayed surgical recovery
- Dressing/grooming self-care deficit
- Dysfunctional ventilatory weaning response
- Energy field disturbance
- Fatigue
- Feeding self-care deficit
- Impaired bed mobility
- Impaired physical mobility
- Impaired spontaneous ventilation
- Impaired transfer ability
- Impaired walking
- Impaired wheelchair mobility
- Ineffective breathing pattern
- Ineffective tissue perfusion (specify type: renal, cerebral, cardiopulmonary, gastrointestinal, peripheral)
- Insomnia
- Readiness for enhance self-care
- Readiness for enhanced sleep
- Risk for activity intolerance
- Risk for disuse syndrome
- Sedentary lifestyle
- Sleep deprivation
- Toileting self-care deficit

DOMAIN: PERCEPTION/COGNITION

- Acute confusion
- Chronic confusion
- Deficient knowledge (specify)
- Disturbed sensory perception (specify: visual, auditory, kinesthetic, gustatory, tactile)
- Disturbed thought processes
- Impaired environmental interpretation syndrome
- Impaired memory
- Impaired verbal communication
- Readiness for enhanced communication
- Readiness for enhanced decision making
- Readiness for enhanced knowledge (specify)
- Risk for acute confusion
- Unilateral neglect
- Wandering

DOMAIN: SELF-PERCEPTION

- Chronic low self-esteem
- Disturbed body image
- Disturbed personal identity
- Hopelessness
- Powerlessness
- Readiness for enhanced power
- Risk for compromised human dignity
- Readiness for enhanced hope
- Readiness for enhanced self-concept
- Risk for loneliness
- Risk for powerlessness
- Risk for situational low self-esteem
- Situational low self-esteem

DOMAIN: ROLE RELATIONSHIPS

- Caregiver role strain
- Dysfunctional family processes: Alcoholism
- Effective breast-feeding
- Impaired parenting
- Impaired social interaction
- Ineffective breast-feeding
- Ineffective role performance
- Interrupted breast-feeding
- Interrupted family processes
- Parental role conflict

- Readiness for enhanced family processes
- Readiness for enhanced parenting
- Risk for caregiver role strain
- Risk for impaired parent/infant/child attachment
- Risk for impaired parenting

DOMAIN: SEXUALITY

- Ineffective sexuality pattern
- Sexual dysfunction

DOMAIN: COPING/STRESS TOLERANCE

- Anxiety
- Autonomic dysreflexia
- Chronic sorrow
- Complicated grieving
- Compromised family coping
- Death anxiety
- Decreased intracranial adaptive capacity
- Defensive coping
- Disabled family coping
- Disorganized infant behavior
- Fear
- Grieving
- Ineffective community coping
- Ineffective coping
- Ineffective denial
- Post-trauma syndrome
- Rape-trauma syndrome
- Rape-trauma syndrome: Compound reaction
- Rape-trauma syndrome: Silent reaction
- Readiness for enhanced community coping
- Readiness for enhanced coping (individual)
- Readiness for enhanced family coping
- Readiness for enhanced organized infant behavior
- Relocation stress syndrome
- Risk for autonomic dysreflexia
- Risk for complicated grieving
- Risk for disorganized infant behavior
- Risk for post-trauma syndrome
- Risk for relocation stress syndrome
- Risk-prone health behavior
- Stress overload

DOMAIN: LIFE PRINCIPLES
- Decisional conflict (specify)
- Impaired religiosity
- Moral distress
- Noncompliance (specify)
- Readiness for enhanced decision making
- Readiness for enhanced religiosity
- Readiness for enhanced spiritual well-being
- Readiness for enhanced hope
- Risk for impaired religiosity
- Risk for spiritual distress
- Spiritual distress

DOMAIN: SAFETY/PROTECTION
- Contamination
- Hyperthermia
- Hypothermia
- Impaired dentition
- Impaired oral mucous membrane
- Impaired skin integrity
- Impaired tissue integrity
- Ineffective airway clearance
- Ineffective protection
- Ineffective thermoregulation
- Latex allergy response
- Readiness for enhanced immunization status
- Risk for aspiration
- Risk for contamination
- Risk for falls
- Risk for imbalanced body temperature
- Risk for impaired skin integrity
- Risk for infection
- Risk for injury
- Risk for latex allergy response
- Risk for other-directed violence
- Risk for perioperative positioning injury
- Risk for peripheral neurovascular dysfunction
- Risk for poisoning
- Risk for self-directed violence
- Risk for self-mutilation
- Risk for sudden infant death syndrome
- Risk for suffocation
- Risk for suicide
- Risk for trauma
- Self-mutilation

DOMAIN: COMFORT
- Acute pain
- Chronic pain
- Nausea
- Readiness for enhanced comfort
- Social isolation

DOMAIN: GROWTH/DEVELOPMENT
- Adult failure to thrive
- Delayed growth and development
- Risk for delayed development
- Risk for disproportionate growth

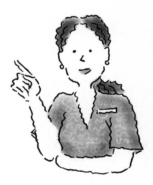

Glossary

aberration:
a deviation from what's typical or normal

acme:
the peak of a contraction

adnexal area:
accessory parts of the uterus, ovaries, and fallopian tubes

agenesis:
failure of an organ to develop

amnion:
the inner of the two fetal membranes that forms the amniotic sac and houses the fetus and the fluid that surrounds it in utero

amniotic:
relating to or pertaining to the amnion

amniotic fluid:
fluid surrounding the fetus, derived primarily from maternal serum and fetal urine

amniotic sac:
membrane that contains the fetus and fluid during gestation

analgesic:
pharmacologic agent that relieves pain without causing unconsciousness

anesthesia:
use of pharmacologic agents to produce partial or total loss of sensation, with or without loss of consciousness

anomaly:
an organ or a structure that's malformed or in some way abnormal due to structure, form, or position

artificial insemination:
mechanical deposition of a partner's or donor's spermatozoa at the cervical os

autosomes:
any of the paired chromosomes other than the X and Y (sex) chromosomes

basal body temperature:
temperature when body metabolism is at its lowest, usually below 98° F (36.7° C) before ovulation and above 98° F after ovulation

Bishop score:
method of assessing cervical dilation, effacement, station, consistency, and position to determine readiness for induction of labor

c-peptide:
an enzyme predictor of early hyperinsulinemia

cephalocaudal development:
principle of maturation that development proceeds from the head to the tail (rump)

chorion:
the fetal membrane closest to the uterine wall; gives rise to the placenta and is the outer membrane surrounding the amnion

conduction:
loss of body heat to a solid, cooler object through direct contact

congenital disorder:
disorder present at birth that may be caused by genetic or environmental factors

convection:
loss of body heat to cooler ambient air

corpus luteum:
yellow structure formed from a ruptured graafian follicle that secretes progesterone during the second half of the menstrual cycle; if pregnancy occurs, the corpus luteum continues to produce progesterone until the placenta assumes that function

cotyledon:
one of the rounded segments on the maternal side of the placenta, consisting of villi, fetal vessels, and an intervillous space

cryptorchidism:
undescended testes

cul-de-sac:
pouch formed by a fold of the peritoneum between the anterior wall of the rectum and the posterior wall of the uterus; also known as *Douglas' cul-de-sac*

decidua:
mucous membrane lining of the uterus during pregnancy that's shed after birth

dilation:
widening of the external cervical os

dizygotic:
pertaining to or derived from two fertilized ova, or zygotes (as in dizygotic twins)

doll's eye sign:
movement of a neonate's eyes in a direction opposite to which the head is turned; this reflex typically disappears after 10 days of extrauterine life

Down syndrome:
abnormality involving the occurrence of a third chromosome, instead of the normal pair (trisomy 21), that characteristically results in mental retardation and altered physical appearance

dystocia:
difficult labor

effleurage:
gentle massage to the abdomen during labor for the purpose of relaxation and distraction

effacement:
thinning and shortening of the cervix

embryo:
conceptus from the time of implantation to 8 weeks

endometrium:
inner mucosal lining of the uterus

engagement:
descent of the fetal presenting part to at least the level of the ischial spines

Epstein's pearls:
small, white, firm epithelial cysts on the neonate's hard palate

evaporation:
loss of body heat that occurs as fluid on the body surface changes to a vapor

fetus:
conceptus from 8 weeks until term

follicle-stimulating hormone:
hormone produced by the anterior pituitary gland that stimulates the development of the graafian follicle

fontanel:
space at the junction of the sutures connecting fetal skull bones

gamete intrafallopian tube transfer:
placement of an ovum and spermatozoa into the end of the fallopian tube via laparoscope; also called in vivo fertilization

gene:
factor on a chromosome responsible for the hereditary characteristics of the offspring

general anesthesia:
use of pharmacologic agents to produce loss of consciousness, progressive central nervous system depression, and complete loss of sensation

hematoma:
collection of blood in the soft tissue

hereditary disorder:
disorder passed from one generation to another

heterozygous:
presence of two dissimilar genes at the same site on paired chromosomes

Homans' sign:
calf pain on leg extension and foot dorsiflexion that's an early sign of thrombophlebitis

homozygous:
presence of two similar genes at the same site on paired chromosomes

human chorionic gonadotropin:
hormone produced by the chorionic villi that serves as the biologic marker in pregnancy tests

hyperinsulinemia:
prediabetic state marked by insulin resistance

hypoxia:
reduced oxygen availability to tissues or fetus

increment:
period of increasing strength of a uterine contraction

induction of labor:
artificial initiation of labor

informed consent:
written consent obtained by the doctor after the patient has been fully informed of the planned treatment, potential adverse effects, and alternative management choices

intensity:
the strength of a uterine contraction (if measured with an intrauterine pressure device, measured and recorded in millimeters of mercury [mm Hg]; if measured externally, a relative measurement may be used)

interval:
period between the end of one uterine contraction and the beginning of the next uterine contraction

intervillous space:
irregularly-shaped areas in the maternal portion of the placenta that are filled with blood and serve as the site for maternal-fetal gas, nutrient, and waste exchange

in vitro fertilization:
fertilization of an ovum outside the body, followed by reimplantation of the blastocyte into the woman

involution:
reduction of uterine size after delivery; may take up to 6 weeks

karyotype:
schematic display of the chromosomes within a cell arranged to demonstrate their numbers and morphology

lanugo:
downy, fine hair that covers the fetus between 20 weeks' gestation and birth

lecithin:
a phospholipid surfactant that reduces surface tension and increases pulmonary tissue elasticity; presence in amniotic fluid is used to determine fetal lung maturity

lecithin-sphingomyelin ratio:
measurement of the relation of lecithin (which rises sharply around 35 weeks' gestation) and sphingomyelin (which remains stable) that's used as an indicator of fetal lung maturity; also known as *L/S ratio*

leukorrhea:
white or yellow vaginal discharge

lie:
relationship of the long axis of the fetus to the long axis of the pregnant patient

linear terminalis:
imaginary line that separates the true pelvis from the false pelvis

local anesthesia:
blockage of sensory nerve pathways at the organ level, producing loss of sensation only in that organ

lochia:
discharge after delivery from sloughing of the uterine decidua

luteinizing hormone:
hormone produced by the anterior pituitary gland that stimulates ovulation and the development of the corpus luteum

meiosis:
process by which germ cells divide and decrease their chromosomal number by one-half

mifepristone:
a progesterone antagonist that prevents implantation of fertilized egg; also called *RU-486*

mitosis:
process of somatic cell division in which a single cell divides but both of the new cells have the same number of chromosomes as the first

molding:
shaping of the fetal head caused by shifting of sutures in response to pressure exerted by the maternal pelvis and birth canal during labor and delivery

myometrium:
middle muscular layer of the uterus that's made up of three layers of smooth, involuntary muscles

neonate:
an infant between birth and the 28th day

nidation:
implantation of the fertilized ovum in the uterine endometrium

Nitrazine paper:
a treated paper used to detect pH used in determining if amniotic fluid is present

NuvaRing:
vaginal contraceptive ring that contains estrogen and progesterone

oligohydramnios:
severely reduced and highly concentrated amniotic fluid

oocyte:
incompletely developed ovum

oogenesis:
formation and development of the ovum

ovum:
conceptus from time of conception until primary villi appear (approximately 4 weeks after the last menstrual period)

perimetrium:
outer serosal layer of the uterus

polyhydramnios:
abnormally large amount (more than 2,000 ml) of amniotic fluid in the uterus

premonitory:
serving as a warning

primordial:
existing in the most primitive form

puerperium:
interval between delivery and 6 weeks after delivery

radiation:
loss of body heat to a solid cold object without direct contact

regional anesthesia:
blockage of large sensory nerve pathways in an organ and its surrounding tissue, producing loss of sensation in that organ and in the surrounding region

ripening:
softening and thinning of the cervix in preparation for active labor

Ritgen maneuver:
manual pressure applied through the perineum to the occiput of the head as the fetus is extending and emerging during birth

rugae:
folds in the vaginal mucosa and scrotum

semen:
white, viscous secretion of the male reproductive organs that consists of spermatozoa and nutrient fluids ejaculated through the penile urethra

smegma:
whitish secretions around the labia minora and under the foreskin of the penis

sperm:
male sex cell

spermatogenesis:
formation and development of spermatozoa

sphingomyelin:
a general membrane phospholipid that isn't directly related to lung maturity but is compared with lecithin to determine fetal lung maturity; levels remain constant during pregnancy

station:
relationship of the presenting part to the ischial spines

strabismus:
condition characterized by imprecise muscular control of ocular movement

subinvolution:
failure of the uterus to return to normal size after delivery

surrogate mothering:
conceiving and carrying a pregnancy to term with the expectation of turning the infant over to contracting, adoptive parents

sutures:
narrow areas of flexible tissue on the fetal scalp that allow for slight adjustment during descent through the birth canal

teratogen:
any drug, virus, irradiation or other nongenetic factor that can cause fetal malformation

tocolytic agent:
medication that stops premature contractions

tocotransducer:
an external mechanical device that translates one physical quantity to another, most often seen in capturing fetal heart rates and transmitting and recording the value onto a fetal monitor

trisomy:
condition where a chromosome exists in triplicate instead of in the normal duplicate pattern

Wharton's jelly:
whitish, gelatinous material that surrounds the umbilical vessels within the cord

X chromosome:
sex chromosome in humans which exist in duplicate in the normal female and singly in the normal male

Y chromosome:
sex chromosome in the human male that's necessary for development of the male sex glands, or gonads

zygote intrafallopian tube transfer:
fertilization of the ovum outside the mother's body, followed by reimplantation of the zygote into the fallopian tube via laparoscope

Selected references

Côté-Arsenault, D., et al. "Watching & Worrying: Early Pregnancy After Loss Experiences," *Maternal Child Nursing* 31(6):356-63, November-December 2006.

Heaman, M. "Breastfeeding Support and Early Cessation," *MCN American Journal of Maternal Child Nursing* 31(5):336, September-October 2006.

Kyle, T. *Essentials of Pediatric Nursing.* Philadelphia: Lippincott Williams & Wilkins, 2007.

Leifer, G. *Introduction to Maternity and Pediatric Nursing.* Philadelphia: W.B. Saunders Co., 2006.

Logsdon, M.C., and Hutti, M.H. "Readability: An Important Issue Impacting Healthcare for Women with Postpartum Depression," *Maternal Child Nursing* 31(6):350-55, November-December 2006.

Lowdermilk, D., and Perry, S. *Maternity & Women's Healthcare*, 9th ed. St. Louis: Mosby, 2006.

Maternal-Neonatal Nursing Made Incredibly Quick, 2nd ed. Philadelphia: Lippincott Williams & Wilkins, 2008.

Pillitteri, A. *Maternal and Child Health Nursing Care of the Childbearing and Childrearing Family*, 5th ed. Philadelphia: Lippincott Williams & Wilkins, 2006.

Scott-Ricci, S. *Essentials of Maternity, Newborn, and Women's Health Nursing.* Philadelphia: Lippincott Williams & Wilkins, 2006.

Shorten, A., et al. "Making Choices for Childbirth: A Randomized Controlled Trial of a Decision-Aid for Informed Birth After Cesarean," *Birth* 32(4):252-61, December 2005.

Symon, A. *Risk and Choice in Maternity Care.* London: Churchill Livingstone, 2007.

Zwelling, E., et al. "How to Implement Complementary Therapies for Laboring Women," *Maternal Child Nursing* 31(6):364-70, November-December 2006.

Index

A

Abdomen, neonatal assessment of, 498
Abdominal contents, crowding of, during pregnancy, 128-129, 129i
Abdominal discomfort, minimizing, 197t, 206
Abortion
  as ethical dilemma, 20
  medically induced, 90-91
  surgically induced, 91
  spontaneous, 284-288
Abruptio placentae, 213-217
  complications of, 214
  degrees of separation in, 214-215, 215i
  nursing care in, 216-217
  pathophysiology of, 214
  predisposing factors for, 213
  signs and symptoms of, 214-215
  testing for, 215
  treatment of, 216
Abstinence, 62
Acceptance of pregnancy
  influences that affect, 135-136
  phases of, 135
  promoting, 137-138
Acoustic blinking reflex, 500
Acrocyanosis, 493
Activity changes, adaptation to, 143
Activity level, labor onset and, 312
Acupressure for pain relief, 350
Acupuncture for pain relief, 350
Adoptive family, 8
Adrenal gland, effect of pregnancy on, 118-119
Age of family members, response to pregnancy and, 19-20
Albumin therapy for neonate, 538
Alcohol during pregnancy, 190. See also Fetal alcohol syndrome.
Alpha-fetoprotein testing, prenatal, 184-185
Ambivalence, trimester of, 138-139

Amenorrhea, 104, 105t
American Nurses Association's Child Health Nursing Practice, 2
Amniocentesis, 175-176
Amniotic fluid, 52, 54
  analysis of, 177t, 258
Amniotic fluid embolism, 362-363
Amniotic sac, 52, 53i
Amniotomy, 306-307
  complications of, 307
Amphetamine use, neonatal characteristics associated with, 520-521
Androgens, 32
Ankle edema, minimizing, 197t, 202
Antepartum period of pregnancy, 2
Antibody screening tests, prenatal, 182-184, 257
Aorta, fetal, **C8**
Apnea of prematurity, 547-548
Appetite during pregnancy, 130-131
Arrhythmias during pregnancy, 121
Artificial sweeteners during pregnancy, 190
Assessment
  neonatal, 482-502
  as nursing process step, 11-12
  postpartum, 422-428
  prenatal, 148-167
Association of Women's Health, Obstetric, and Neonatal Nurses, 2
Atria, fetal, **C8**
Axillary temperature, neonatal, 489, 490

B

Babinski's reflex, 500
Baby blues, 420, 421, 454
Back, prenatal assessment of, 162
Backache, minimizing, 197t, 203-204
Ballard gestational-age assessment tool, 485-488i
Ballottement, 106t, 110
Bandl's ring, 411
Barrier methods, 79-81, 82i, 83-85, 83i, 86i

Bartholin's glands, 35, 36i
Basal body temperature as contraceptive method, 64-65
  patient teaching for, 66-67i
Battledore placenta, 400i
Behavioral assessment, neonatal, 500-502
Benzodiazepine withdrawal in neonate, 519
Billings method, 65-68
Biophysical profile, 180, 181t
Birthing environments, 3
Birthing partner or coach, 346
Birth plans, development of, 144-145
Birth weight, assessing, 485, 488, 491, 492
Bishop's score, 304, 305t
Bladder, **C1, C4, C5**
  effect of pregnancy on, 125, 127, 129i
Blastocyst, 48i
Blastomeres, 48i
Blended family, 8
Blinking reflex, 500
Blood glucose monitoring, 226
Blood loss
  after cesarean birth, 448
  in postpartum hemorrhage, 448
  after vaginal birth, 448
Blood pressure
  neonatal, 489, 490-491
  during pregnancy, 122, 123i
Blood studies, prenatal, 181-185
Blood typing, prenatal, 181
Blood volume
  in neonate, 480
  during pregnancy, 123-124
Bloody show, 314
Body image changes, acceptance of, 144
Body temperature, neonatal, maintaining, 479, 504-507, 505i

i refers to an illustration; t refers to a table; **boldface** refers to color pages.

Bottle-feeding
  with breast milk, 440-441
  with formula, 442-444
Bowel function, postpartum, 429, 430
Braxton Hicks contractions, 106t, 110
  labor onset and, 312-313
  minimizing, 206
Breast changes, pregnancy and,
  104, 105t
Breast engorgement, 424, 463
Breast-feeding, 433-440. *See also* Lactation.
  adequacy of, 438-439
  advantages of, 434-435
  assistance with, 436-440
  breast care and, 444-445
  burping and, 438, 439i
  contraindications for, 433-434
  frequency of, 438
  maternal nutrition and, 435-436,
    439-440
  positions for, 436, 437i
  puerperal infection and, 461
  risk of human immunodeficiency virus
    transmission and, 248
  sleepy neonate and, 439
Breast milk
  bottle-feeding with, 440-441
  composition of, 431
  manual expression of, 439
Breast pumping, 440-441
Breasts, 40, 40i
  effect of pregnancy on, 115-116, 116i
  postpartum assessment of, 423, 424
  postpartum care of, 430
    for breast-feeding women, 444-445
    for non-breast-feeding women, 445
  prenatal assessment of, 161-162
Breast stimulation for labor stimulation, 306
Breast tenderness, minimizing, 197t, 200
Breathing techniques, 346-349

Breech presentation, 299i, 300-301,
  375-377, 377i
  causes of, 378-379
  detection of, 380
  management of, 382-384, 383i
Bromocriptine, 97
Bronchopulmonary dysplasia, prematurity and, 547
Brow cephalic presentation, 297,
  298i, 375
Bulbourethral glands, 31, **C4**

C

Caffeine use during pregnancy, 190
Calcium requirements, 193-194
Calendar method, 63-64, 64i
Caloric requirements, 190-191
  for pregnant woman with diabetes, 226
Candida infection during pregnancy, 115
Caput succedaneum, 494
Carbohydrate metabolism, effect of
  pregnancy on, 131
Cardiac disease, 217-222
  causes of, 217-218
  classification of, 218t
  high-risk pregnancy and, 211
  nursing care in, 221-222
  signs and symptoms of, 218-219
  testing for, 220
  treatment of, 220-221
Cardiac output during pregnancy, 122
Cardiovascular system
  during active labor, 318t
  effect of pregnancy on, 121-125
  neonatal, 476t, 477
Care plan, guidelines for developing, 13
Carpal tunnel syndrome, 132
Cephalhematoma, 494
Cephalic presentation, 297, 298i, 299-300
Cephalopelvic disproportion, 363-366, **C6**
Cervical cap, 83-84, 83i
Cervical effacement and dilation, 339i
Cervical examination, 338-340
Cervical lacerations
  as postpartum hemorrhage cause, 449
  signs of, 450

Cervical mucus method, 65-68
Cervix, 37i, 38, **C1, C5**
  effect of pregnancy on, 114-115
  ripening of, 313
Cesarean birth, 366-374
  altered body defenses and, 368
  altered circulatory function and,
    368-369
  altered organ function and, 369
  altered self-esteem and, 369
  altered self-image and, 369
  factors leading to, 366
  home care instructions after, 374
  incision types for, 369-370, 370i
  indications for, 370-371, **C6-C7**
  maternal complications of, 372
  postoperative care for, 373-374
  preoperative care for, 372-373
  preparing patient for, 371-372
  rising incidence of, 367
  stress response and, 368
  testing in, 371
  woman's refusal to submit to, 367
Cesarean delivery. *See* Cesarean birth.
Cesarean section. *See* Cesarean birth.
Chadwick's sign, 106t, 110
Chest, neonatal assessment of, 497
Chest circumference, measuring,
  491i, 492
Childbearing practices, cultural beliefs
  and, 17-18
Chin cephalic presentation, 298i, 300
Chlamydia, pregnancy and, 277t
Chloasma, 106t, 108
Cholesterol during pregnancy, 190
Chorion, 52, 53i
Chorionic villi, 53i
Chorionic villi sampling, 176-179, 178i
Chronic lung disease, prematurity
  and, 547
Circulation
  fetoplacental, 55, **C8**
  during pregnancy, 123
  uteroplacental, 54

i refers to an illustration; t refers to a table; **boldface** refers to color pages.

Circumcision, 511-515
  aftercare for, 513
  complications of, 514-515
  contraindications for, 512
  documenting, 515
  methods of, 512
  parent teaching for, 514
  preparing parents for, 512
  religion and, 512
Climacteric years, 41
Clinical nurse specialist, functions of, 5
Clitoris, 35, 36i, **C1**
Clomiphene, 96-97
Coagulation, effect of pregnancy on, 123
Coagulation factor I during pregnancy,
      125
Cohabitation family, 7
Coitus interruptus, 69
Cold application for pain relief, 349
Colostrum, 423, 431
Communal family, 8
Complete abortion, 285
Complete blood count, prenatal, 181-182
Complete breech presentation, 299i,
      301, 376
Complete extension in fetal attitude,
      293-294
Complete flexion in fetal attitude, 292
Compound presentation, 298i, 302
Conception, 27-56
Conception issues, 22-23
Condyloma acuminata, pregnancy
      and, 277t
Constipation, minimizing, 197t, 203
Constricting ring, 411
Continuous external electronic monitor-
      ing, 328-331
  applying devices for, 330i
  tips for, 362
Contraception, 60-86
  choosing method of, 60-61
  implementing, 61
  methods of, 62-69, 64i, 66-67i, 70i,
      71-81, 78i, 82i, 83-85, 83i, 86i
  in postpartum period, 430
  teaching tips on, 61

Contraceptives. *See also* Contraception.
  choosing, 60
  implementing, 61
  oral, 71-73
Contraction stress test, 187-188
Corona, 28, 29i, **C4**
Corpus, 37i, 39
Corpus cavernosum, 28, 29i, **C4**
Corpus luteum, 42
  changes in, during pregnancy, 51, 55
Corpus spongiosum, 28, 29i, **C4**
Counterpressure for pain relief, 349
Couvade syndrome, 141
Crowning, 320
Crying in neonate, 501
Cultural background
  assessment considerations and, 151
  childbearing practices and, 17-18
  family's response to pregnancy and,
      15-16
  high-risk pregnancy and, 212
  pain management and, 342, 343
  pregnancy acceptance and, 136
  views of pregnancy and, 151

D
Danazol, effect of, on fertility, 95
Decidua, development of, 52, 53i, 113
Deep vein thrombophlebitis. *See* Deep
      vein thrombosis.
Deep vein thrombosis, 465-472
  causes of, 466
  femoral versus pelvic, 466, 467t
  nursing care in, 469-472
  preventing, 469
  pulmonary embolism as complication
      of, 471
  risk factors for, 466
  signs and symptoms of, 466-468, 467t
  testing for, 468
  treatment of, 468-469
Delivery date, calculating, 47
Depo-Provera, 76-77
Descent, 320, 321i, 322

Diabetes mellitus, 222-228
  causes of, 223-224
  classifications of, 222
  complications of, 223
  dietary recommendations for, 226
  glucose control and, 223
  high-risk pregnancy and, 211
  nursing care in, 227-228
  signs and symptoms of, 224
  teaching topics for pregnant patients
      with, 228
  testing for, 224-225, 225t
  treatment of, 225-227
Diagonal conjugate, 166, 166i
Diaphragm, 80-81
  inserting, 82i
Diastasis, pregnancy and, 132
Dietary recommendations for pregnant
      woman with diabetes, 226
Dilatation and vacuum extraction, 91
Dilation, labor pain and, 341
Direct monitoring. *See* Internal electron-
      ic monitoring.
Disseminated intravascular coagulation
  as postpartum hemorrhage cause, 449
  signs of, 450
  testing for, 451
  treatment of, 452
Distention, labor pain and, 341
Division of labor within family, 9
Doll's eye reflex, 495
Doppler ultrasound stethoscope,
      167, 170i
Drug addiction, neonatal, 518-524
  causes of, 518
  nursing interventions for, 522-524
  signs and symptoms of, 518-521
  testing for, 521
  treatment of, 521-522
Ductus arteriosus, fetal, **C8**
Ductus deferens, **C4**
Ductus venosus, fetal, **C8**
Dyspnea, 120

E

Ears
  neonatal assessment of, 495-496
  prenatal assessment of, 161
Eclampsia, 235, 237. *See also* Gestational hypertension.
Economic resources, family's response to pregnancy and, 19
Ectoderm, 49i
Ectopic pregnancy, 228-232
  complications of, 228-229
  conditions that cause, 229-230
  nursing care for, 231-232
  signs and symptoms of, 230
  sites of, 229i
  testing for, 230
  treatment of, 231
Effleurage, 347, 348i
Ejaculatory duct, 29i, 30-31, **C4**
Elective termination of pregnancy, 90-91
Elimination, changes in, during pregnancy, 127
Embryo, 47, 49i
  development of, to fetus, 50i
Embryo donation, 100
Embryonic development, 47, 49i
Emergency contraception, 73-74
Endocrine system
  during active labor, 318t
  effect of pregnancy on, 117-119
Endoderm, 49i
Endometritis, puerperal infection and, 460
Endometrium, 37i, 39, 48i
  effect of pregnancy on, 113
Engagement, 302-303, 303i
Entrapment neuropathies, 134
Epididymis, 29i, 30, 32, **C4**
Epidural block, 352-355, 353i
Epstein's pearls, 495
Epulides, 133
Erythema toxicum neonatorum, 493

Estrogen levels
  during pregnancy, 55, 117
  serum assays of, 173
Ethical and legal issues, 20-25
Eugenics as ethical issue, 23-24
Exchange transfusion, 538
Exercise
  postpartum, 430
  preventing hypoglycemia during, 227
Expulsion as cardinal movement of labor, 321i, 323
Extended family, 7
Extension as cardinal movement of labor, 321i, 322-323
External rotation as cardinal movement of labor, 321i, 323
Extremities
  neonatal assessment of, 499
  prenatal assessment of, 162
Eye prophylaxis, neonatal, 502-503
  complications of, 503
Eyes
  neonatal assessment of, 494-495
  prenatal assessment of, 161

F

Face cephalic presentation, 297, 299-300, 377
  causes of, 379
  detection of, 380-381
  management of, 384-385
Fallopian tubes, 37i, 39, **C1**
False labor, signs and symptoms of, 311t
Family-centered care, 6-11
  family structures and, 6-8
  family tasks and, 9-11
Family dynamics, response to pregnancy and, 18-19
Family history
  high-risk pregnancy and, 212-213
  prenatal assessment and, 153-154
Family nurse practitioner, functions of, 4
Family planning, 59
  contraception and, 60-86
  natural methods of, 62-69, 64i, 66-67i, 70i
  surgical methods of, 86-91

Fatherhood, preparation for, 140-141
Father image, development of, 142
Fatigue, 105t, 107
  minimizing, 197t, 200
Fat requirements, 192
Female condom, 85
  inserting, 86i
Female reproductive system, 34-35, 36-37i, 38-41, 40i, 42-43i, 44
  neonatal assessment of, 499
Femoral deep vein thrombosis, 466-468, 467t. *See also* Deep vein thrombosis.
Fertilization, 44, 45i, 46, **C3**
Fetal activity determination, 172
Fetal alcohol syndrome, 524-527
  cause of, 524
  nursing interventions for, 527
  signs of, 525-526, 515i
  testing for, 526
  treatment of, 526-527
Fetal attitude, 292-294
Fetal development, 27-56
  stages of, 47, 51
Fetal distress, monitoring for, 172
Fetal heart monitor, 330i
Fetal heart rate
  audible, as sign of pregnancy, 107t, 111
  baseline irregularities in, 335-337i
  external monitoring of, 167-169, 170i, 329-331, 330i
  intermittent monitoring of, 337-338
  internal monitoring of, 332i, 333-334
  reading monitor strip for, 333i
  variability in, 334t
Fetal lie, 294
Fetal membranes, development of, 53i
Fetal monitoring in woman with diabetes, 227
Fetal movement as sign of pregnancy, 107t, 111
Fetal position, 295
  abbreviations for, 295t
  determining, 296i

i refers to an illustration; t refers to a table; **boldface** refers to color pages.

Fetal presentation, 291-303
  abnormalities of, 375-385, 377i, 378i, 383i, **C6**
  engagement and, 302-303, 303i
  factors that determine, 292-295, 295t, 296i
  types of, 297, 298-299i, 299-302
Fetal size, abnormally large, 385-386
Fetal station, 303, 303i
Fetal tissue research as ethical issue, 23
Fetoplacental circulation, 55
Fetoscopy, 167, 170i, 180
Fetus
  development of, 47, 51
  embryonic development to, 50i
Fibrinogen levels during pregnancy, 125
First stage of labor, 315, 316-319
  active phase of, 317-318
    systemic changes in, 318t
  latent phase of, 316-317
  transition phase of, 319
First trimester, psychosocial changes in, 138-141
Flexion as cardinal movement of labor, 322
Fluid requirements, 196
Fluid retention during pregnancy, 126
Fluoride, pregnancy and, 195
Focusing for pain relief, 344, 345
Folic acid, foods high in, 234
Folic acid deficiency, 193
Folic acid deficiency anemia, 232-234
  causes of, 232-233
  nursing care in, 233-234
  prenatal vitamins to prevent, 234
  as risk factor, 232
  signs and symptoms of, 233
  testing for, 233
  treatment of, 233
Follicle-stimulating hormone, 33
Fontanels, 493-494
Food additives during pregnancy, 190
Food consumption during pregnancy, 130-131
Food guide pyramid, 189, 189i

Footling breech presentation, 299i, 301, 376
Foramen, ovale, fetal, **C8**
Foremilk, 431, 432i
Formula
  bottle-feeding with, 442-444
  feeding assistance with, 442-444
  types of, 442
Foster family, 8
Fourth stage of labor, 315, 326-327
Frank breech presentation, 299i, 301, 376
Fundal height
  measuring, 164i
  throughout pregnancy, 113, 114i
Fundus, 37i, 39
  postpartum assessment of, 424-425, 425i
    complications of, 425

G

Gallbladder, effect of pregnancy on, 130
Gamete intrafallopian transfer, 100
Gastrointestinal system
  during active labor, 318t
  effect of pregnancy on, 128-131, 129i
  neonatal, 476t, 478
Gay family, 8
Gene manipulation as ethical issue, 23-24
Genital herpes, pregnancy and, 278t
Germ layers, 49i
Gestation, 46
Gestational age, assessing, 484, 485-488i
Gestational diabetes, 222, 224. *See also* Diabetes mellitus.
Gestational hypertension, 234-240
  causes of, 235
  changes associated with, 236i
  classifying, 235
  complications of, 235
  emergency interventions for, 238
  nursing care in, 238-240
  signs and symptoms of, 235-237
  testing for, 237
  treatment of, 237-238
Gestational size variations, 528-530

Gestational trophoblastic disease, 240-243
  classifying, 240
  complications of, 240
  conditions associated with, 241
  incidence of, 241
  nursing care in, 243
  signs and symptoms of, 241
  testing for, 241-242
  treatment of, 242
Gingival granuloma gravidarum, 133
Glans penis, 28, 28i, **C4**
Glomerular filtration rate during pregnancy, 126, 127
Glucose in urine, 127, 128
Glucose tolerance testing, prenatal, 185
Glycosuria, 127, 128
Gonadotropins, 33
Gonorrhea, pregnancy and, 278t
Goodell's sign, 106t, 110
Grasping reflex, 500
Group B streptococci infection, pregnancy and, 278-279t
GTPAL classification system, 158
GTPALM classification system, 158
Guthrie screening test, 543
Gynecologic history
  high-risk pregnancy and, 210-211
  prenatal assessment and, 154-155

H

Habitual abortion, 285, 287
Habituation in neonate, 502
Head
  neonatal assessment of, 493-494
  prenatal assessment of, 159
Head circumference, measuring, 491i, 492
Head-to-heel length, measuring, 491i, 492
Health history
  postpartum, 422
  prenatal, 148-158
    formidable findings in, 150
    tips for, 149
Health status of family members, response to pregnancy and, 19

Heartburn, minimizing, 201-202
Heart
  effect of pregnancy on, 121
  neonatal assessment of, 497-498
  prenatal assessment of, 162
Heart failure, 219
Heart rate
  neonatal, 489
  during pregnancy, 121-122
Heart sounds during pregnancy, 121
Heat application for pain relief, 349
Heat loss in neonate
  complications of, 504
  preventing, 506
  sources of, 478-479
  thermoregulation and, 504-507, 505i
Hegar's sign, 106t, 110
HELLP syndrome, 244-245
  causative factors in, 244
  nursing care in, 245
  signs and symptoms of, 244
  testing for, 244
  treatment of, 245
Hematocrit during pregnancy, 124
Hematologic changes during pregnancy,
    124-125
Hematopoietic system, neonatal,
    476t, 480
Hemodynamic changes during pregnan-
    cy, 121-124
Hemoglobin level during pregnancy, 124
Hemorrhoids, minimizing, 197t, 203
Hepatic system, neonatal, 476t, 480
Hepatitis B, prenatal testing for, 183
Heroin withdrawal in neonate, 520
High-risk pregnancy, 209-288
  factors that contribute to, 209-213
High-risk neonate, 517-556
  ethical issues and, 24
Hindmilk, 431, 432i
Homans' sign, 467
Home pregnancy tests, 109
Hormones
  female sexual development and, 41,
    42-43i, 44
  male sexual development and, 32-34

Human chorionic gonadotropin, 109, 117
  monitoring levels of, 243
  serum assay of, 174-175
Human chorionic somatomammotropin.
    See Human placental lactogen.
Human immunodeficiency virus antibody
    test, 531
Human immunodeficiency virus
    culture, 532
Human immunodeficiency virus deoxyri-
    bonucleic acid polymerase chain
    reactions test, 531
Human immunodeficiency virus infec-
    tion, 245-249
  cause of, 246
  incidence and prevalence of, 245-246
  neonatal, 530-533
  nursing care in, 248-249
  opportunistic infections associated
    with, 247
  risk of, to neonate, 246
  signs and symptoms of, 247
  testing for, 247-248
  transmission of, 246
    perinatal risk factors for, 530
  treatment of, 248
Human immunodeficiency virus p24 anti-
    gen assay, 531
Human immunodeficiency virus testing,
    prenatal, 183-184
Human placental lactogen, 56, 117
  serum assay of, 173-174
Hydatidiform mole. See Gestational
    trophoblastic disease.
Hydrocephalus, 533-536
  assessment findings in, 534
  nursing care in, 535-536
  possible causes of, 534
  testing for, 535
  treatment of, 535
Hyperbilirubinemia, 536-539
  causes of, 536-537
  complications of, 536
  ethnic groups susceptible to, 536
  nursing interventions for, 538-539
  signs and symptoms of, 537
  testing for, 537-538

Hyperbilirubinemia (continued)
  treatment of, 538, 539
Hyperemesis gravidarum, 249-252
  complications of, 249-250
  nursing care in, 252
  possible causes of, 250
  signs and symptoms of, 250
  testing for, 250-251
  treatment of, 251
Hypergonadotrophic anovulation, 95
  treatment of, 97
Hyperprolactinemic anovulation, 94
  treatment of, 97
Hypertonic contractions, 387
  causes of, 389
  detection of, 390-391
  management of, 392-393
  oxytocin and, 392i
Hypnosis for pain relief, 350
Hypoglycemia, preventing, during exer-
    cise, 227
Hypogonadotrophic anovulation, 94-95
  treatment of, 97
Hypotonic contractions, 388
  causes of, 389-390
  detection of, 391
  management of, 393-394
Hypovolemic shock
  management of, 453
  signs and symptoms of, 450
Hysteroscopy, 101
Hysterotomy, 91

I

Imagery for pain relief, 344-345
Immune system
  effect of pregnancy on, 134
  neonatal, 476t, 479
Immunoglobulins, neonate and, 479
Immunologic testing, 532
Implantation, **C3**
Implementation as nursing process
    step, 14
Incomplete abortion, 285
Incomplete breech presentation, 299i,
    301, 376
Incubator, 505i

Indigestion, minimizing, 201-202
Indirect Coombs' test, 182
Individual temperament, pregnancy
    acceptance and, 136
Inevitable abortion, 285
Infant mortality rates, decline in, 1-2
Inferior vena cava, fetal, **C8**
Infertility, 92-101
    conditions for conception and, 93
    rising rates of, 92
    sex-specific causes of, 93-95
    teaching topics for, 93
    treatment options for, 95-101, 99i
Insomnia, minimizing, 205
Insulin therapy, pregnancy and, 226
Integumentary system
    effect of pregnancy on, 132-133
    neonatal, 476t, 481
Intermittent fetal heart rate monitoring,
    337-338
Internal electronic monitoring, 331-334
    applying devices for, 332i
Internal rotation as cardinal movement
    of labor, 321i, 322
Interstitial cell-stimulating hormone. *See*
    Luteinizing hormone.
Intestines, effect of pregnancy on,
    128-129
Intrapartum period of pregnancy, 2
Intrauterine device, 77-79
    inserting, 78i
Intrauterine fetal death, 394-396
    causes of, 394
    nursing care for, 395-396
    signs of, 395
    testing for, 395
    treatment of, 395
Intravaginal contraceptive method,
    74-75
Intraventricular hemorrhage, prematuri-
    ty and, 547
In vitro fertilization as ethical issue, 22
In vitro fertilization–embryo transfer,
    97-98, 99i
Involution, 326, 418

Iodine requirements during preg-
    nancy, 194
Iron deficiency anemia, 252-256
    causes of, 252-253
    complications of, 252
    nursing care in, 254-256, 255i
    signs and symptoms of, 253
    testing for, 253-254
    treatment of, 254
Iron requirements during pregnancy,
    124, 194-195
Iron supplements, 124
    teaching topics on, 256
Ischial tuberosity, 167
Isoimmunization, 256-260
    causes of, 257
    complications of, 256-257
    nursing care in, 259-260
    pathogenesis of, 258i
    signs and symptoms of, 257
    testing for, 257-258
    treatment of, 259

JK

Jaundice, 480. *See also* Hyperbilirubine-
    mia.
    pathologic, 536, 537
    physiologic, 536, 537

L

Labia majora, 34, 36i
Labia minora, 34-35, 36i
Labor and birth, 291-358
    cardinal movements of, 320, 321i,
        322-323
    comfort and support during, 340-358,
        348i, 353i, 356i
    complications of, 361-414
    false, 311t
    fetal presentation and, 291-295, 295t,
        296i, 297, 298-299i, 299-303, 303i
    nursing procedures performed during,
        327-334, 330i, 332i, 333i, 334t,
        335-337t, 337-340, 339i
    onset of, 310-315, 311t
    precipitous, 391

Labor and birth *(continued)*
    preliminary signs and symptoms of,
        311-313, 311t
    premature, 268-272
    preparation for, 144
    productive, promoting, 389
    stages of, 315-320, 318t, 321i, 322-327
    stimulation of, 304, 305t, 306-310
    true, 311t, 313-315
Laboratory tests for pregnancy, 106t, 109
Labor stimulation, 304-310
    Bishop's score and, 304, 305t
    conditions for, 304, 306
    methods of, 306-310
Lactation, 431-433. *See also* Breast-
    feeding.
    menstrual cycle and, 433
    physiology of, 431, 432i
    preparation for, 431
Lactiferous ducts, 40, 40i, **C5**
Lamaze method, 346-347
Lanugo, 493
Laparoscopy, 100-101
Large for gestational age, 528
    assessment findings in, 529
    causes of, 528
    nursing interventions for, 530
    treatment of, 530
Lecithin/sphingomyelin ratio, 551
Leg cramps, minimizing, 197t, 204
Leopold's maneuvers, performing, 168,
    168-169i
Lesbian family, 8
Let-down reflex, 432i
Letting go as postpartum phase, 420t
Levator ani muscle, **C1**
Leydig's cells, 33
Lightening, 311-312
Light-headedness, minimizing, 204-205
Linea nigra, 106t, 107-108, 108i
Lipid metabolism, effect of pregnancy
    on, 131
Liver, effect of pregnancy on, 129i, 130
Local anesthesia during labor,
    355-356, 356i
Local infiltration for pain relief, 356, 356i

i refers to an illustration; t refers to a table; **boldface** refers to color pages.

Lochia, 425
  assessing, 426
  types of, 426
Longitudinal fetal lie, 294
Lumbar epidural anesthesia,
    352-355, 353i
Lungs
  fetal, **C8**
  neonatal assessment of, 497
  prenatal assessment of, 162
Luteinizing hormone, 33

M

Macrosomia, 364
Magnesium sulfate
  for premature labor, 270
  safe administration of, 239
Maintenance of order as family task, 10
Male condom, 84-85
Male reproductive system, 28-34, 29i, **C4**
  neonatal assessment of, 498
Mammary glands, 40, 40i
Marijuana withdrawal in neonate, 520
Mask of pregnancy, 106t, 108
Mastitis, 424, 462-465
  causes of, 463
  nursing care in, 464
  predisposing factors for, 463
  preventing, 465
  signs and symptoms of, 463
  testing for, 463
  treatment of, 464
Maternal age
  family's response to pregnancy and, 15
  high-risk pregnancy and, 210
Maternal illness, family's response to
    pregnancy and, 20
Maternal lifestyle, high-risk pregnancy
    and, 211
Maternal mortality rates, decline in, 1-2
Maternal-neonatal nursing
  ethical and legal issues and, 20-25
  family-centered care and, 6-11
  family response to pregnancy and,
    14-20, 136
  goals of, 2

Maternal-neonatal nursing *(continued)*
  nursing process and, 11-14
  practice settings for, 3
  roles and functions of, 3-5
Maternal parity, high-risk pregnancy
    and, 210
Maternal self-care, postpartum 430
Maternal serum alpha-fetoprotein test,
    184-185
Maternal serum assays, 173-175
Meconium, 431
Meconium aspiration syndrome, 540-542
  causes of, 540
  complications of, 540, 542
  nursing interventions for, 542
  risk factors for, 540
  signs and symptoms of, 541
  testing for, 541
  treatment of, 541-542
Medical history
  high-risk pregnancy and, 211
  prenatal assessment and, 150, 152-153
Medroxyprogesterone injections, 76-77
Melasma, 106t, 108
Menarche, 34
Menopause, 41, 44
Menstrual cycle, 41, 42-43i
  lactation and, 433
  ovarian and uterine changes
    during, **C2**
Mentum cephalic presentation, 298i, 300
Mesoderm, 49i
Methadone withdrawal in neonate, 520
Mifepristone, 90-91
Milia, 493
Miliaria, 493
Mineral requirements, 193-195
Missed abortion, 285
Mitochondrial sheath, **C3**
Moderate flexion in fetal attitude, 293
Molar pregnancy. *See* Gestational
    trophoblastic disease.
Molding, 494
Mongolian spots, 493
Mons pubis, 34, 36i

Morning-after pill, 73-74
Morning sickness, 130
Moro reflex, 500
Morula, 48i
Mother image, development of, 141-142
Mouth
  effect of pregnancy on, 128
  neonatal assessment of, 495
  prenatal assessment of, 161, 162
Multigenerational family, 7
Multiple gestation. *See* Multiple
    pregnancy.
Multiple pregnancy, 260-264,
    396-399, 397i
  causes of, 262, 396
  complications of, 260, 261-262, 398
  detection of, 397
  management of, 397-399
  nursing care in, 263-264
  signs and symptoms of, 262
  testing for, 263
  treatment of, 263
  types of, 261, 261i
Muscles, effect of pregnancy on, 132
Musculoskeletal system
  during active labor, 318t
  effect of pregnancy on, 131-132
  neonatal, 476t, 481
Music therapy for pain relief, 345-346
Myometrium, 37i, 39

N

Nägele's rule, 47, 155
Nasal stuffiness, minimizing, 197t, 199
Natural family planning methods, 62-69,
    64i, 66-67i, 70i
Nausea and vomiting, 104, 105t, 130-131
  minimizing, 198, 199
Neck
  neonatal assessment of, 496-497
  prenatal assessment of, 161
Necrotizing enterocolitis, 548
Neonatal Abstinence Scoring
    System, 521

Neonatal assessment, 482-502
  Apgar scoring in, 482-484, 483t
  behavioral, 500-502
  of birth weight, 485, 488
  of gestational age, 484, 485-488i
  head-to-toe, 492-499
  initial, 482-485, 483t, 485-488i, 488
  monitoring for medication effects
      in, 484
  neurologic, 499-500
  ongoing, 488-492, 491i
Neonatal hearing screening, 496
Neonatal nurse practitioner, functions
    of, 5
Neonate. *See also* Neonatal assess-
    ment.
  adaptation of, to extrauterine life,
      475-481
  body temperature in, maintaining, 507
  circumcision of, 511-515
  eye prophylaxis for, 502-503
    complications of, 503
  habituation in, 502
  heat loss in, preventing, 506
  high-risk, 517-556
  human immunodeficiency virus infec-
      tion and, 530-533
  oxygen therapy for, 507-511
    hazards of, 511
  physiology of, 476t
  preterm, 544-549
    caring for, 488
  sensory capabilities of, 501
  skin care for, 503-504
  size of, 491-492, 491i
    variations in, 528-530
  sun protection and, 481
  thermoregulation for, 504-506, 505i
  sleep-wake cycle in, 501
Nerves, effect of pregnancy on, 132
Neurologic system
  during active labor, 318t
  effect of pregnancy on, 134
  neonatal, 476t, 480, 499-500
Nipple stimulation contraction stress
    test, 188

Nonstress testing, 186-187
Normogonadotrophic anovulation, 94
  treatment of, 96-97
Nose
  neonatal assessment of, 495
  prenatal assessment of, 161
Nuclear family, 6-7
Nucleolus, **C3**
Nucleus, **C3**
Nurse-midwife, certified, functions of, 4
Nurse practitioners, functions of, 4-5
Nursing diagnosis as nursing process
    step, 12-13
Nursing process, 11-14
  assessment and, 11-12
  implementation and, 14
  nursing diagnosis and, 12-13
  outcome evaluation and, 14
  planning and, 13
Nutritional care during pregnancy,
    188-196, 189i
Nutritional status
  high-risk pregnancy and, 212
  postpartum, 430
  prenatal assessment and, 152
Nutritional therapy for pregnant woman
    with diabetes, 226
NuvaRing, 74-75

O

Oblique fetal lie, 294
Obstetric history
  high-risk pregnancy and, 210-211
  prenatal assessment and, 150, 155-158
Occipitoposterior position, 375
  causes of, 378
  detection of, 379-380
  management of, 381-382
Oocytes, 54
Ooplasm, **C3**
Opiate withdrawal syndrome in neonate,
    519
Opioids during labor, 351-352
Oral contraceptives, 71-73
  teaching tips on, 72

Oral glucose challenge test,
    224-225, 225t
Outcome evaluation as nursing
    process step, 14
Ova donation, 98-99
Ovaries, 37i, 39, **C1**
  changes in, during pregnancy, 51, 112
Ovulation awareness as contraceptive
    method, 69
  home test for, 70i
Ovum, **C3**
Oxygen therapy for neonate, 507-511
  complications of, 510
  documenting, 511
  hazards of, 511
  monitoring, 510
  using continuous positive airway pres-
      sure, 509-510
  using handheld resuscitation bag and
      mask, 508-509
  using nasal prongs, 509
  using oxygen hood, 509
Oxytocin
  administration of, 307-310
    complications of, 309
  adverse effects of, 392
  hypertonic contractions and, 392
  preventing complications of, 393

P

Pain, labor
  cultural influences on, 342, 343
  nonpharmacologic relief of,
      343-350, 348i
  nursing interventions for, 357-358
  perception of, 341-342
  pharmacologic relief of, 350-356,
      353i, 356i
  sources of, 340-341
Palmar erythema, 133
Pancreas, effect of pregnancy on, 119
Parametritis, puerperal infection
    and, 460
Parathyroid gland, effect of pregnancy
    on, 118
Parenting, preparation for, 144

Partial extension in fetal attitude, 293

Partner support, 144

Patent ductus arteriosus, 547

Payr's sign, 468

Pediatric nurse practitioner, 5

Pelvic cellulitis, puerperal infection and, 460

Pelvic deep vein thrombosis, 460, 467t, 468, 469. *See also* Deep vein thrombosis.

Pelvic examination, prenatal, 163-164

Pelvic inflammatory disease, signs of, 79

Pelvic size, estimation of, 164-167, 165i, 166i

Pelvic structures
female, **C1**
male, **C4**

Penis, 28, 29i, **C4**

Percutaneous umbilical blood sampling, 179-180

Perez reflex, 500

Pergolide, 97

Peri bottle for postpartum perineal care, 427

Perimenopause, 41

Perineal care, postpartum, 427-428

Perineal infection, localized, puerperal infection and, 459-460

Perineum, 35, 36i
postpartum assessment of, 426-427

Peritoneum, **C4**

Peritonitis, 460

Pharynx, neonatal assessment of, 495

Phenylketonuria, 542-544
cause of, 542
incidence of, 543
parent teaching for, 544
signs and symptoms of, 543
testing for, 543
treatment of, 543-544

Phosphorus requirements during pregnancy, 193-194

Phototherapy, 538, 539

Physical assessment
postpartum, 422-428
prenatal care and, 158-167, 164i, 165i, 166i

Physical maintenance as family task, 10

Pigmentation, changes in, during pregnancy, 133

Piper forceps, 383, 383i

Pituitary gland, effect of pregnancy on, 118

Placement of family members into society, 10-11

Placenta, 54-56, 55i, 117, **C5**

Placenta accreta, 400i

Placenta circumvallata, 400i

Placental abnormalities, 399-401
causes of, 399, 401
detection of, 401
management of, 401
types of, 400i

Placental abruption. *See* Abruptio placentae.

Placental entrapment
as postpartum hemorrhage cause, 449
signs of, 450
testing for, 450-451
treatment of, 451

Placental expulsion, 325

Placental separation, 324-325

Placenta previa, 264-268, **C7**
causative factors in, 265
nursing care in, 267-268
signs and symptoms of, 265-266
testing for, 266
treatment of, 266-267
types of, 264-265, 265i

Placenta succenturiata, 400i

Planned versus unplanned pregnancy, family's response to, 16

Planning as nursing process step, 13

Pneumocystis carinii, prophylaxis for, in neonate, 532-533

Portal vein, fetal, **C8**

Positioning for pain relief, 344

Postmenopause, 44

Postpartum blues, 420, 421, 454

Postpartum care, 417-445
assessment and, 422-428, 425i
lactation and, 431, 432i, 433
maternal self-care in, 429, 430
neonatal nutrition and, 433-445, 437i, 439i
nursing care in, 429
physiologic changes and, 417-419
psychological changes and, 419-421

Postpartum depression, 421, 454-457
nursing care in, 455, 457
predictors inventory for, 456i
risk factors for, 454-455
signs and symptoms of, 455
treatment of, 455

Postpartum hemorrhage, 448-454
blood loss in, 448
causes of, 449
classifying, 448
monitoring blood pressure in, 453
nursing care in, 452-454
predisposing conditions for, 448
signs and symptoms of, 450
testing for, 450-451
treatment of, 451-452

Postpartum period, 2
complications of, 447-472
phases of, 419, 420t

Postpartum psychosis, 457-458
nursing care in, 458
predisposing factors for, 457
prenatal screening for, 457-458
signs and symptoms of, 457
treatment of, 458

Practice settings, 3

Preeclampsia, 235, 236-238. *See also* Gestational hypertension.

Pre-embryonic development, 47, 48i

Pregnancy
anatomic changes during, **C5**
assessing, by trimester, 160
classification system for, 156-158
drug addiction and, 518
ectopic, 228-232
effect of, on reproductive system, 111-116, 114i, 116i

Pregnancy *(continued)*
elective termination of, 90-91
family response to, 14-16, 18-20
foods to avoid during, 190
high-risk, 209-288
influences that affect acceptance of, 135-136
minimizing discomforts of, 196, 197t, 198-206
molar, 240-243
multiple, 260-264
periods of, 2
phases of acceptance of, 135
physiology of, 46-47, 48i, 49i, 50i, 51-52, 53i, 54-56, 55i
positive signs of, 107t, 110-111
presumptive signs of, 104, 105-106t, 107-108, 108i
probable signs of, 106t, 109-110
promoting acceptance of, 137-138
psychosocial changes in, 135-145
sexually transmitted diseases and, 276-280
Pregnancy-induced hypertension. *See* Gestational hypertension.
Premature labor, 268-272, 401-405
causes of, 268-269, 402
detection of, 403
fetal survival rate in, 268
nursing care in, 270-272
patient teaching for, 405
risk factors for, 402-403
signs and symptoms of, 269
testing for, 269, 403
treatment of, 269-270, 403-405
Premature rupture of membranes, 272-275
complications of, 273
nursing care in, 275
patient teaching for, 275
predisposing factors for, 273
signs and symptoms of, 274
testing for, 274
treatment of, 274-275
Prenatal bonding, 142-143

Prenatal care, 147-206
assessment and, 148-167, 164i, 165i, 166i
nutritional needs and, 188-196, 189i
prenatal testing and, 167-188, 168-169i, 170i, 177t, 178i, 181t
pre-pregnancy, 147
Prenatal screening, ethical issues and, 21
Pressure on adjacent organs, labor pain and, 341
Preterm delivery, 405-407
Preterm labor. *See* Premature labor.
Preterm neonate, 544-549
assessment findings in, 545-546
causes of, 544-545
complications of, 547-548
ethical issues and, 24
nursing interventions for, 548-549
parent teaching for, 549
risk factors for, 545
testing of, 546
treatment of, 546-547
Progesterone levels during pregnancy, 55, 56, 117
Progressive changes, postpartum, 419
Prolactin, 52, 431, 432i
Prostaglandins, 52, 117
Prostate gland, 29i, 31, **C4**
Protein metabolism, effect of pregnancy on, 131
Protein requirements during pregnancy, 191-192
Proteinuria, 128
Psychosocial changes
in first trimester, 138-141
in second trimester, 141-143
in third trimester, 143-145
Puberty, male, 33-34
Puerperal infection, 458-462
causes of, 458-459
complications of, 460
nursing care in, 462
predisposing factors for, 459
preventing, 459
signs and symptoms of, 459-460

Puerperal infection *(continued)*
testing for, 460-461
treatment of, 461
Puerperium. *See* Postpartum period.
Pulmonary embolism as deep vein thrombosis complication, 471

Q
Quickening, 105t, 107

R
Radiant warmer, 505i
Recruitment of family members, 10
Rectal temperature, neonatal, 489-490
Rectum, **C1**
postpartum assessment of, 426-427
prenatal assessment of, 162
Regional anesthesia during labor, 352-355, 353i
Registered nurse, functions of, 3-4
Relaxation techniques for pain relief, 343-346
Relaxin, 52, 117, 128-129
Release of family members, 10
Renal function during pregnancy, 126-127
Renal plasma flow during pregnancy, 126
Renal system. *See also* Urinary system, effect of pregnancy on.
during active labor, 318t
neonatal, 476t, 478
Renal tubular resorption during pregnancy, 127
Reproduction of family members, 10
Reproductive system
effect of pregnancy on, 111-116, 114i, 116i
neonatal, 476t, 481
Resources, distribution of, within family, 9
Respiratory distress, monitoring for, 495
Respiratory distress syndrome, 549-553
assessment findings in, 550-551
causes of, 550
nursing care in, 553
prematurity and, 547

Respiratory distress syndrome *(continued)*
   risk factors for, 550
   testing for, 551
   treatment of, 551-553
Respiratory rate, neonatal, 489
Respiratory system
   during active labor, 318t
   effect of pregnancy on, 119-120
   neonatal, 475-477, 476t
Retinopathy of prematurity, 547
Retraction rings, 411
Retrogressive changes, postpartum, 417-419
Rh incompatibility. *See* Isoimmunization.
RhoGAM, 259
   administering, 260
Rhythm method, 63-64, 64i
Rielander's sign, 468
Ripening agent application, 310
Rooting reflex, 500
Rubella titer, 182

S
Safeguarding motivation and morale as family tasks, 11
SalEst test, 173
Saline induction, 91
Scrotum, 29-30, 29i
Second stage of labor, 315, 319-323
   cardinal movements in, 320, 321i, 322-323
Second trimester, psychosocial changes in, 141-143
Semen, 31
Seminal vesicles, 29i, 31, **C4**
Sensory capabilities in neonate, 501
Septic abortion, 285
Serologic testing, prenatal, 184
Sexual activity in postpartum period, 430
Sexuality changes, acceptance of, 144
Sexually transmitted diseases, 276-280. *See also specific disease.*
   causes of, 276
   nursing care in, 276, 280
   signs and symptoms of, 276
   treatment of, 276

Shortness of breath, minimizing, 205
Shoulder dystocia, 385-386
Shoulder presentation, 298i, 301-302
Sickle cell anemia, 280-284
   cause of, 281
   complications of, 280, 281
   nursing care in, 283-284
   race and, 281
   signs and symptoms of, 281
   testing for, 281-282
   treatment of, 283
Sickle cell crisis, 281, 282i
Sickle cell trait, 281
Sinciput cephalic presentation, 298i
Single-parent family, 7
Sitz bath, 428
Skeleton, effect of pregnancy on, 131
Skene's glands, 35, 36i
Skin
   neonatal assessment of, 492-493
   prenatal assessment of, 162
Skin changes, 106t, 107-108, 108i, 132-133
Sleep-wake cycle in neonate, 501
Small for gestational age, 528
   assessment findings in, 529
   factors that contribute to, 528
   nursing interventions for, 530
   treatment of, 529
Socialization of family members, 9
Social resources, family's response to pregnancy and, 19
Sodium requirements, 195
Spermatocytes, 32, 54
Spermatogenesis, 32
Spermatogonia, 32
Spermatozoa, 32, 46
Spermatozoon, 44, 45i, 46, **C3**
Spermicidal products, 79-80
Spinal anesthesia, 355
Spine, neonatal assessment of, 499
Spontaneous abortion, 284-288
   causative factors in, 284-286
   nursing care in, 287
   patient teaching for, 288
   signs and symptoms of, 286
   testing for, 286

Spontaneous abortion *(continued)*
   treatment of, 286-287
   types of, 285
Spontaneous rupture of membranes, 314-315
Startle reflex, 500
Stepping reflex, 500
Stomach, effect of pregnancy on, 128, 129i
Stress, reducing, 388
Stretch marks, 106t, 108, 108i, 132-133
Striae gravidarum, 106t, 108, 108i, 132-133
Substance abuse, high-risk pregnancy and, 212
Sucking reflex, 500
Sudamina, 493
Superior vena cava, fetal, **C8**
Supine hypotension, 122, 123i
Surrogate embryo transfer, 100
Surrogate motherhood as ethical and legal issue, 22-23
Symphysis pubis, 29i, 37i, **C1, C5**
Symptothermal method, 68-69
Syphilis, pregnancy and, 279t

T
Taking hold as postpartum phase, 420t
Taking in as postpartum phase, 420t
Teeth, prenatal assessment of, 162
Telangiectasia, 493
Tension, labor pain and, 341
Terbutaline for premature labor, 270
   administering, 271
Testes, 29i, 30
Testosterone, 32, 33
Therapeutic touch and massage for pain relief, 345
Thermogenic system, neonatal, 476t, 478-479
Thermoregulation, 504-507, 505i
Third stage of labor, 315, 324-325
   placental expulsion in, 325
   placental separation in, 324-325
Third trimester, psychosocial changes in, 143-145

i refers to an illustration; t refers to a table; **boldface** refers to color pages.

Threatened abortion, 285
Thyroid gland, effect of pregnancy on, 118
Tocotransducer, 330i
Tonic neck reflex, 500
TPAL classification system, 156-157
Transcutaneous electrical nerve stimulation for pain relief, 350
Transdermal contraceptive patch, 75-76
Transient tachypnea of the neonate, 553-556
  causes of, 553-554
  nursing interventions for, 556
  risk factors for, 554
  signs and symptoms of, 554
  testing for, 554-555
  treatment of, 555
Transverse fetal lie, 294, 377
  causes of, 379
  detection of, 381
  management of, 385
Trichomoniasis, pregnancy and, 280t
Triple screening, 185
Trophoblast, 48i
True conjugate, 166-167
True labor, 310-311
  signs and symptoms of, 311t, 313-315
Trunk curvature reflex, 500
Tubal sterilization, 88-90, 89i
Twins
  presentation of, 263, 397i
  risk for complications in, 262
  types of, 261, 261i
Type II respiratory distress syndrome.
    See Transient tachypnea of the neonate.

U
Ultrasonography
  pregnancy and, 106t, 107t, 110, 111
  prenatal testing and, 170-171
Umbilical arteries, 54, 55i, C8
Umbilical cord, 54, 55i, C5
  anomalies of, 407-408

Umbilical cord prolapse, 307, 408-410, C7
  causes of, 408
  detection of, 408-409
  management of, 409-410
  patterns of, 409i
Umbilical vein, 54, 55i, C8
Umbilicus, maternal, 132, C5
Uncoordinated contractions, 388
  causes of, 390
  detection of, 392
  management of, 394
Ureters, C1, C4
  effect of pregnancy on, 125, 127
Urethra, 29i, 31
Urethral meatus, 35, 36i
Urinalysis, maternal, 172
Urinary elimination, postpartum, 429, 430
Urinary frequency, 104, 105t
  minimizing, 197t, 199
Urinary system, effect of pregnancy on, 125-128. See also Renal system.
Urine output during pregnancy, 126
Urine specific gravity during pregnancy, 126
Uterine atony
  as postpartum hemorrhage cause, 449
  risk factors for, 449
  signs of, 450
  treatment of, 451
Uterine bleeding during pregnancy, 114
Uterine contraction palpation, 327-328
Uterine contractions
  comparing and contrasting, 390i
  external monitoring of, 329-331, 330i
  hypertonic, 387, 389, 390-391, 392-393, 392i
  hypotonic, 388, 389-390, 391, 393-394
  internal monitoring of, 331-332, 332i
  pain and, 341
  true labor and, 313-314
  uncoordinated, 388, 390, 392, 394
  without relaxation, 329
Uterine enlargement, 105t, 107
Uterine force, ineffective, 386-394
  causes of, 389-390
  complications of, 387

Uterine force, ineffective (continued)
  detecting, 390-392
  management of, 392-394
Uterine inversion, 413-414
Uterine rupture, 410-413
  causes of, 411
  detection of, 411-412
  management of, 412-413
  signs of, 412
Uteroplacental circulation, 54
Uterus, 37i, 39, C1, C5
  changes in
    during menstrual cycle, C2
    during pregnancy, 52, 53i, 54-56, 112-113, 114i
  postpartum assessment of, 423-425, 425i

V
Vagina, 37i, 38, C1, C5
  effect of pregnancy on, 115
Vaginal discharge, minimizing, 197t, 200-201
Vaginal orifice, 35, 36i
Varicocelectomy, 100
Varicosities, minimizing, 197t, 202-203
Vasa previa, 400i
Vascular growth during pregnancy, 114
Vascular spiders, 133
Vas deferens, 29i, 30-31, 32, C4
Vasectomy, 87-88, 87i
Velamentous cord insertion, 400i
Vernix caseosa, 493
Vertex cephalic presentation, 297, 298i
Viral load testing, 247-248
Vital signs
  neonatal, 488-491
  prenatal, 158, 159
Vitamin requirements during pregnancy, 192-193

WX
Water-jet irrigation system for postpartum perineal care, 427
Wet lungs. See Transient tachypnea of the neonate.

White blood cell count during pregnancy, 124
Women's health nurse practitioner, functions of, 4

Y

Yoga for pain relief, 350
Yolk sac, 54

Z

Zidovudine therapy in neonate, complications of, 532
Zinc requirements during pregnancy, 195
Zona pellucida, 48i, **C3**
Z-track injection for iron, 255, 255i
Zygote, 27, 46, 47, 48i

Notes

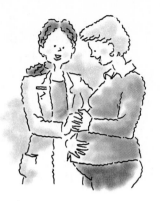

Notes

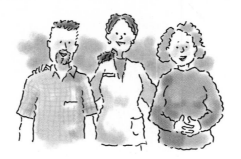

Notes

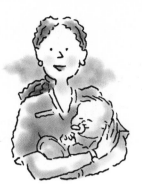

Notes

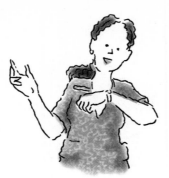

Notes

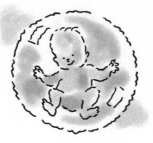

Notes

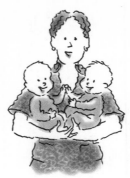

Notes

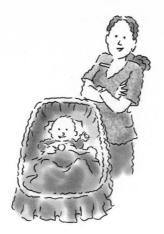

Maternal-neonatal nursing is made even easier with the bonus features on your *Incredibly Easy* CD-ROM!

The *Maternal-Neonatal Nursing Made Incredibly Easy, 2nd Edition* CD-ROM contains more than 250 NCLEX®-style practice questions, a list of nursing diagnoses by medical disorder, and concept maps for commonly encountered medical problems. The program is easy to use and install; just slip the disc into your PC and you're ready to go!

Technical stuff

To operate the *Maternal-Neonatal Nursing Made Incredibly Easy, 2nd Edition* CD-ROM, we recommend that you have the following minimum system requirements:
- Windows XP Home Edition
- Acrobat Reader
- Pentium 4
- 512 MB RAM
- 40 MB of free hard-disk space
- SVGA monitor with high color (16-bit); display area set to 800 × 600
- CD-ROM drive.

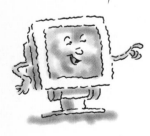

For technical support, call toll-free 1-800-638-3030, Monday through Friday, 8:30 a.m. to 5 p.m. Eastern Time. Or, e-mail us at wkhealth-support@wolterskluwer.com.

Getting started

- Start Windows.
- Place the CD in your CD-ROM drive. After a few moments, the install process will automatically begin. *Note:* If the install process doesn't automatically begin, click the Start menu and select Run. Type *D:\setup.exe* (where *D:* is the letter of your CD-ROM drive) and then click OK.
- Follow the on-screen instructions for the installation type you want.

It's that easy!